Professional Issues in Speech-Language Pathology and Audiology

4th edition

Professional Issues in Speech-Language Pathology and Audiology

Rosemary Lubinski, Ed.D.
Professor of Communicative Disorders and Sciences University at Buffalo, State University of New York

Melanie W. Hudson, M.A.
National Director
EBS Healthcare

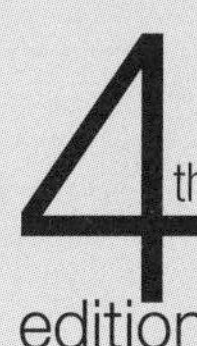

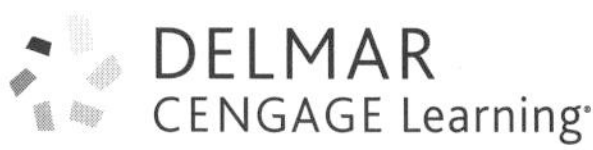

Australia • Brazil • Japan • Korea • Mexico • Singapore • Spain • United Kingdom • United States

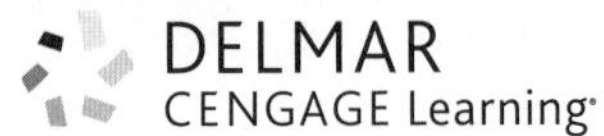

Professional Issues in Speech-Language Pathology and Audiology, 4th Edition
Rosemary Lubinski, Ed.D.
and Melanie W. Hudson, M.A.

Vice President, Careers & Computing: Dave Garza

Associate Acquisitions Editor: Tom Stover

Director, Development—Careers & Computing: Marah Bellegarde

Senior Product Manager: Laura J. Wood

Editorial Assistants: Anthony Souza, Cassie Cloutier

Brand Manager: Wendy E. Mapstone

Marketing Development Manager: Jonathan Sheehan

Senior Director, Education Production: Wendy A. Troeger

Production Manager: Andrew Crouth

Senior Content Project Manager: Kara A. DiCaterino

Senior Art Directors: David Arsenault, Benj Gleeksman

Media Editor: William Overocker

Cover Images:
© R-studio/www.Shutterstock.com
© Barauskaite/www.Shutterstock.com
© Excellent Backgrounds/www.Shutterstock.com

Library of Congress Control Number: 2012937827

ISBN-13: 978-1-111-30910-7

ISBN-10: 1-111-30910-8

Delmar
5 Maxwell Drive
Clifton Park, NY 12065-2919
USA

Cengage Learning is a leading provider of customized learning solutions with office locations around the globe, including Singapore, the United Kingdom, Australia, Mexico, Brazil, and Japan. Locate your local office at: **international.cengage.com/region**

Cengage Learning products are represented in Canada by Nelson Education, Ltd.

To learn more about Delmar, visit **www.cengage.com/delmar**

Purchase any of our products at your local college store or at our preferred online store **www.cengagebrain.com**

Printed in the United States of America
1 2 3 4 5 6 7 16 15 14 13 12

This text is dedicated to our chapter contributors. Each of you has generously shared your expertise, wisdom, and time to stimulate the thinking of our next generation of speech-language pathologists and audiologists. We and our readers thank you for your commitment to a lifetime of professionalism.

Contents

SECTION II Employment Issues 157

10 Building Your Career 202

Marva Mount, MA
Melanie W. Hudson, MA

11 Professional Autonomy and Collaboration 221

Janet E. Brown, MA
Jaynee A. Handelsman, PhD

16 Service Delivery Issues in Early Intervention 335

Corey Herd Cassidy, PhD

17 Service Delivery Issues in Private Practice 356

Kenneth E. Wolf, PhD

18 Strategically Promoting Access to Speech-Language Pathology and Audiology Services 375

Brooke Hallowell, PhD
Bernard P. Henri, PhD

23 Child Abuse and Elder Mistreatment 477

Rosemary Lubinski, EdD

24 Service Delivery for Culturally and Linguistically Diverse Populations 491

Hortencia Kayser, PhD

25 Supervision and Mentoring 509

Melanie W. Hudson, MA

Foreword

With this fourth edition of *Professional Issues in Speech-Language Pathology and Audiology*, the authors introduce you to a new way of looking at information pertinent to these dynamic fields. Information is all around us; however, understanding that information within its appropriate context can often be what is most crucial. The professions of speech-language pathology and audiology have long been affected by internal, external, societal, technological, and regulatory influences. It is through a detailed understanding of these factors that we are able to make decisions and ultimately discuss the "why" of our actions. *Professional Issues in Speech-Language Pathology and Audiology, Fourth Edition* helps the reader understand the background, significance, and necessary future perspective for issues surrounding clinical practice in both speech-language pathology and audiology.

In this edition, many chapters will serve as current and future resource tools for practitioners and academics alike. The book provides foundational information on ethics, evidence-based practice, and professional organizations. In addition, the authors include updates on work settings and employment issues, such as supervision, for both the new and seasoned clinician. This edition contains information on emerging and other growing areas of practice as well. In fact, many of these issues could not have been envisioned even 10 short years ago. These issues include telepractice and technology, private practice, updates in documentation, and the future of the practice of our science as we envision it today. These areas of practice continue to shape the future of our professions, and this book provides the context from which the professions have emerged and continue to grow.

Many view the start of our discipline and subsequent professions as dating back to the early decades of the 1900s. Those before us could likely not have imagined where we are today, with the many challenges and rewards we face from both practical and academic perspectives. The current edition of this book helps you to understand who we are, where we came from, and where we are going. It serves as a "must read" for students, professionals, and academics both in classroom and professional settings.

Mark DeRuiter, MBA, PhD, CCC-A/SLP

Mark DeRuiter is the Director of Graduate Studies and Clinical Programs at the University of Minnesota, Twin Cities. He teaches coursework in counseling and professional issues and has research interests in speech perception as well as clinical practice within the professions. He is certified by the American Speech-Language-Hearing Association (ASHA) as both an audiologist and a speech-language pathologist, and he is a Fellow of the American Academy of Audiology (AAA). Mark has a history of service on ASHA's Council for Clinical Certification and Special Interest Group 11, Administration and Supervision.

Preface

It has been almost 20 years since the first edition of *Professional Issues in Speech-Language Pathology and Audiology* was published. With each edition, our professions become more sophisticated and complex. We are expected to work with more difficult cases, work with clients from a wide diversity of backgrounds, and achieve goals in less time using evidence-based approaches. In addition, we must keep abreast of all the issues that affect how we practice. These challenges make our professions vibrant and stimulating.

This fourth edition of *Professional Issues in Speech-Language Pathology and Audiology* is intended to be a primary text and a resource for faculty, students, and practicing clinicians seeking a comprehensive introduction to contemporary issues that affect our professions and our service delivery across settings. We hope that students and practitioners will better understand that what you do clinically is influenced by political, social, educational, health care, and economic concerns. Your professional identity is enhanced when you understand the myriad factors that define what you do, with whom, for how long, and at what cost. With this information and insight, you can assume a more proactive, rather than passive, view of your profession.

How to Use This Text

You are probably reading this text because you are taking a course in Contemporary Professional Issues or Ethics. Table A shows how you can meet the ASHA standards for audiology and speech-language pathology in various chapters. What you should notice in this table is that certain topics are repeated. Yes, we deliberately built in repetition so that you will realize that issues, such as ethics and liability, are not stand-alone topics but are relevant to our professional organizations, all work settings, documentation, technology, and so forth. Another example of this intentional repetition is the topic of technology. You will read about technology as one of the important megatrends in Chapter 1 and again in chapters devoted to documentation, ethics, securing employment, and more. This topic is so important that we also have a chapter devoted specifically to it. Yet one more topic that you will read about time and again is that of research, specifically evidence-based practice. The importance of research is a recurring theme throughout the text. So as you read, look for these persistent issues.

Consider reading the text and setting up class topics around such themes as ethics, documentation, demographics and cultural diversity, economic issues, legal bases for what we do, technology, research, getting and keeping a job, working productively in specific settings, and advocacy. We have placed a special emphasis in this edition on how to secure employment and, once you have gotten a job, how to build your job into a satisfying career.

New to the Fourth Edition

With each edition of this text, we have asked the continuing authors to update their chapters to reflect new issues and concerns in our professions. Several new chapters appear in this edition, including Professional Issues: A View from History by Judith Felson Duchan. This chapter provides her unique perspective on how our professions developed through the years. Another new chapter is titled Documentation Issues by Barbara Moore. Few issues affect our service delivery more than documentation, and in this chapter Dr. Moore covers both the laws affecting documentation as well as strategies for effective documentation. One of the themes in this book is how to secure employment, and in this issue we created a follow-up chapter, Building Your Career, which provides useful information once you have gotten a job. In this chapter, Marva Mount and Melanie Hudson discuss specific and practical strategies for making your first and subsequent employment productive and satisfying.

We also have authors new to the text. These include Gail Brook and Ingrida Lusis of ASHA; Judith Duchan, professor emeritus of the University of Buffalo; Carol Dudding, who does research in technology and communication disorders; Perry Flynn and Charlette Green, both with years of public school experience; Cory Herd, who specializes in early intervention; Alex Johnson, Provost and Vice President at the MGH Institute of Health Professions; and Barbara Moore, Director of Special Youth Services in the Anaheim School District. We thank them for adding their currency and expertise to this text.

In reading the chapters and writing our own, we realized that there was a sea of acronyms that might appear daunting. New to this edition is a list of acronyms. We placed this at the beginning of the book so that you can use it to decode what may appear as an alphabet soup. Some authors have also added appendices to their chapters to define specialized terms.

No graduate class inspires discussion as much as one focused on professional issues. To help you and your professors instigate discussions, we have added even more Critical Thinking questions at the end of each chapter. Many of these are "What would you do?" or "What are the advantages and disadvantages of?" types of questions. We are also providing your professors with some multiple-choice questions and essay questions for each chapter that they might use to assess your knowledge base. We encourage you to add more discussion questions and launch some lively debates in and out of class. This process of class discussion will provide you with the ability to articulate strong arguments and advocate for your profession and your clients.

Also Available

Also available is an Instructor Companion Website to accompany *Professional Issues in Speech-Language Pathology and Audiology* (ISBN-13: 978-1-111-30911-4).

This website includes additional materials to support the text, including essay questions and slide presentations to accompany each chapter. Contact your sales representative or log on to http://login.cengage.com to gain access to these free materials.

A Final Thought

We hope that by reading this text and engaging in class discussions you will become motivated to read other resources from your professional associations, become involved in professional committees, attend conferences on professional issues, and serve as professional activists to promote what we do. Listen to and read a variety of sources that keep you abreast of national and local issues that affect our clients and their clinical services. We encourage you to meld your clinical competence with your currency in professional issues.

About the Authors

Rosemary Lubinski received her BS from Bloomsburg University (PA) and her MA and EdD from Columbia University. She is Professor of Speech-Language Pathology in the Department of Communicative Disorders and Sciences at the University of Buffalo where she has spent her entire academic career. Dr. Lubinski has worked as a university professor and clinical supervisor as well as a clinician in the schools, a hospital outpatient rehabilitation center, a nursing home, private practice, and home health care. Her primary interests are in the communication problems of the elderly and those with dementia, aphasia, and traumatic brain injury as well as issues affecting the professions of audiology and speech-language pathology. She is a frequent presenter at international and national conferences, recipient of state and national grants, and the author of numerous articles and chapters. A Fellow of ASHA and active in Special Interest Group 15, Gerontology, Dr. Lubinski has published two books related to gerontology: *Dementia and Communication* and *Communication Technologies for the Elderly: Vision, Hearing and Speech*. She has also published the text *A Guide to Cultural Competence in the Curriculum: Speech-Language Pathology*. This is her fourth edition of *Professional Issues in Speech-Language Pathology and Audiology.*

Melanie W. Hudson received her BS from James Madison University (VA) and her MA from George Washington University. She has more than 30 years of experience in the profession, working in public schools, private practice, and as a guest lecturer at universities. She also served as an adjunct faculty member at Georgia State University. She presents nationally to school districts and at professional conferences on clinical supervision, best practices in school-based settings, and clinical practice related to autism spectrum disorders. She has served on ASHA's Speech-Language Advisory Council and currently serves as the coordinator for ASHA's Special Interest Group 11, Administration and Supervision. She is the past-president of the Georgia Speech-Language and Hearing Association and is the national director of EBS Healthcare.

Acknowledgments

Reviewers

The following professionals provided valuable feedback during the development of the fourth edition.

Kathleen R. Fahey
Professor, Audiology & Speech-Language Sciences
University of Northern Colorado
Greeley, Colorado

Susan Thomas Frank, MA (ABD)/CCC-SLP
Assistant Professor
Marshall University
Huntington, Australia

John Lowe III, PhD, CCC-SLP, L ASHA Fellow
Former Department Chair, Dean, and Professor
Former: University of Central Arkansas and three other universities
Former: Conway, Arkansas; Current: Hilliard, Ohio

Valeria Matlock
Associate Professor, Department of Speech Pathology and Audiology
Tennessee State University
Nashville, Tennessee

Sheree Reese, EdD, CCC-SLP, BRS-F
Professor, Director of Center for Communication Disorders
Kean University
Union, New Jersey

J. Stephen Sinclair, PhD
Chair and Professor
California State University Northridge
Northridge, California

Mark J. Witkind
Continuing Education Administrator & Clinical Specialist
The Bilingual Center of Miami
Miami, Florida

Contributors

Dolores E. Battle, PhD
Professor Emeritus
Buffalo State College
Speech-Language Pathology Department
Buffalo, New York

Fred H. Bess, PhD
Professor and Director, National Center for Childhood Deafness and Family Communication
Vanderbilt Bill Wilkerson Center
Vanderbilt University
Nashville, Tennessee

Gail Page Brook, BA
Research Analyst and Technical Writer
American Speech-Language-Hearing Association
Rockville, Maryland

Janet E. Brown, MA
Director, Health Care Services in Speech-Language Pathology
American Speech-Language-Hearing Association
Rockville, Maryland

Karen E. Brown, PhD
Assistant Professor
Eastern Kentucky University
Richmond, Kentucky

Judith Felson Duchan, PhD
Professor Emeritus
Department of Communicative Disorders and Sciences
University at Buffalo
Buffalo, New York

Carol C. Dudding, PhD
Assistant Professor, Director of SLP Graduate Program
Communication Sciences and Disorders
James Madison University
Harrisonburg, Virginia

Perry Flynn, MEd
Associate Professor, Department of Communicative Disorders and Sciences
University of North Carolina at Greensboro
Consultant to the North Carolina Department of Public Instruction in the Area of Speech-Language Pathology
Greensboro, North Carolina

Lee Ann C. Golper, PhD
Professor, Director of SLP Clinical Programs
Department of Hearing and Speech Sciences, School of Medicine
Vanderbilt University
Nashville, Tennessee

Charlette Green, MS
Director, Special Education
Cherokee County Schools
Canton, Georgia

Sue T. Hale, MCD
Director of Clinical Education
and Assistant Professor
Department of Hearing and Speech Sciences
Vanderbilt Bill Wilkerson Center
Vanderbilt University
Nashville, Tennessee

Brooke Hallowell, PhD
Professor and Director, Neurolinguistics
Laboratory
Ohio University
Athens, Ohio

Jaynee Handelsman, PhD
Assistant Director, Vestibular Testing Center
Department of Otolaryngology, University
of Michigan
Ann Arbor, Michigan

Bernard Henri, PhD
Executive Director
Cleveland Hearing and Speech Center
Cleveland, Ohio

Corey L. Herd Cassidy, PhD
Associate Professor
Waldron College of Health and Human Services
Communication Sciences and Disorders
Radford University
Radford, Virginia

Louise M.H. Hickson, PhD
Professor
School of Health and Rehabilitation Sciences
The University of Queensland
Brisbane, Australia

Jennifer Horner, PhD, JD
Professor and Associate Dean for Research
and Graduate Studies
College of Health Sciences and Professions
Ohio University
Athens, Ohio

Melanie W. Hudson, MA
National Director
EBS Healthcare
Woodstock, Georgia

Alex Johnson, PhD
Provost and Vice President for
Academic Affairs
MGH Institute of Health Professions
Boston, Massachusetts

Hortencia Kayser, PhD
Director EBS United, Multicultural, Bilingual,
and International Programs
Springfield, Missouri

Raymond D. Kent, PhD
Professor Emeritus
Department of Communicative Disorders
University of Wisconsin–Madison
Madison, Wisconsin

Ann W. Kummer, PhD
Senior Director, Division of Speech
Pathology, Cincinnati Children's Hospital
Medical Center
Professor of Clinical Pediatrics
and Professor of Otolaryngology,
Head & Neck Surgery
University of Cincinnati Medical Center
Cincinnati, Ohio

Rosemary Lubinski, EdD
Professor
Department of Communicative Disorders
and Sciences
University at Buffalo, SUNY
Buffalo, New York

Ingrida Lusis, BA
Director, Federal and Political Advocacy
American Speech-Language-Hearing Association
Washington, DC

Thomas D. Miller, PhD, JD
Professor
Department of Communication Sciences and Disorders
Nazareth College of Rochester
Rochester, New York

Barbara J. Moore, EdD
Director, Special Youth Services
Anaheim Union High School District
Anaheim Hills, California

Marva Mount, MA
National Director, Continuing Education
EBS Healthcare
Mansfield, Texas

Anna M. O'Callaghan, PhD
Charles Sturt University
Albury, New South Wales
Australia

Diane R. Paul, PhD
Director, Clinical Issues in Speech-Language Pathology
American Speech-Language-Hearing Association
Rockville, Maryland

Paul R. Rao, PhD
Vice President, Inpatient Operations and Compliance
National Rehabilitation Hospital
Washington, DC

Susan E. Sparks, MA
Speech-Language Pathologist
Sherwood Community Services
Lake Stevens, Washington

Steven C. White, PhD
Director, Health Care Economics and Advocacy
American Speech-Language-Hearing Association
Rockville, Maryland

Kenneth E. Wolf, PhD
Dean of the College of Science and Health,
William Paterson University
Wayne, New Jersey

Linda E. Worrall, PhD
Professor
School of Health and Rehabilitation Sciences
The University of Queensland
Brisbane, Australia

TABLE A Matrix of Chapter Content Relevant to the Council for Clinical Certification Standards for the Certificates of Clinical Competence

	Ch 1	Ch 2	Ch 3	Ch 4	Ch 5	Ch 6	Ch 7	Ch 8	Ch 9	Ch 10	Ch 11	Ch 12
Audiology Standards												
A9 Patient characteristics (ex. Demographics)	x							x				
A15 Assistive technology	x							x				
A16 Cultural diversity	x	x					x	x	x	x		x
A18 Principles of research	x		x		x	x					x	x
A19 Legal and ethical practices	x	x	x	x	x	x	x	x	x	x	x	x
A20 Health care and education delivery	x		x		x	x		x			x	x
A21 Universal precautions												
A22 Oral and written communication					x	x			x	x	x	
A28 Business practices								x				
A29 Working with related professionals				x	x	x	x	x		x	x	x
C10 Preparing a report												
C11 Referring to others												
D2 Develop culturally approp. rehab plan	x						x	x				x
D5 Collaboration EI, Schools, etc.	x										x	x
E1 Community education and advocacy											x	
E2 Consultation											x	x
E3 Promoting access to care	x							x			x	x
F1 Quality improvement					x	x						
F2 Research and evidence-based practice	x		x		x	x		x			x	x
F3 Implement research-based techniques	x				x	x		x			x	x
F4 Administration and supervision									x	x		x
F5 Program development											x	x
F6 Maintaining links with other programs				x			x				x	
Speech-Language Standards												
III-D Prevention, assessment, intervention												
III-E Ethical standards	x	x	x	x	x	x	x	x	x	x	x	x
III-F Research and evidence-based practice	x	x	x		x	x		x			x	x
III-G Contemporary professional issues	x	x	x	x	x	x	x	x	x	x	x	x
III-H Certification and licensure	x	x	x	x	x	x	x		x	x	x	x
IV-B Oral and written communication	x				x	x			x	x	x	x
IV-G.1f Reporting to support evaluation	x									x		
IV-G.1g Client referral										x		
IV-G.2f Reporting to support intervention										x		
IV-G.2g Client identification and referral										x		
IV-G.3a Communicate effectively	x								x	x	x	x

	Ch 13	Ch 14	Ch 15	Ch 16	Ch 17	Ch 18	Ch 19	Ch 20	Ch 21	Ch 22	Ch 23	Ch 24	Ch 25	Ch 26	Ch 27	Ch 28	Ch29
		x	x	x	x	x			x	x	x	x		x			
	x	x				x								x			
		x	x	x	x	x		x		x		x	x				
	x	x	x	x	x	x	x						x	x		x	x
	x	x	x	x	x	x	x	x	x	x	x	x	x	x	x	x	x
	x	x	x	x	x	x	x	x		x	x			x	x		
	x	x		x			x			x							
			x	x		x	x	x	x								
					x		x										
		x	x	x	x	x			x		x						
		x	x	x													
			x	x		x											
		x	x	x		x		x				x					
			x	x													
				x	x	x			x								
		x	x	x	x	x											
	x	x	x	x	x	x			x			x		x			
	x	x			x		x	x	x	x	x	x	x				
	x	x		x	x	x	x		x			x	x	x		x	x
													x			x	x
		x	x	x	x	x	x	x	x			x	x				
				x		x	x					x		x			
				x		x	x		x		x						
		x	x	x	x	x	x			x	x	x		x			
	x		x	x	x	x	x	x	x	x	x	x	x	x	x	x	x
	x	x	x	x	x	x		x	x			x	x	x		x	x
	x	x	x	x	x	x	x	x	x	x	x	x	x	x	x	x	x
		x	x		x	x			x		x	x	x	x			
		x	x	x	x	x	x	x	x					x			
		x	x	x				x	x								
		x	x	x	x												
		x	x	x				x	x								
		x	x	x					x			x					
	x	x	x	x	x	x	x	x	x	x	x	x	x	x			

Acronyms

AAA: American Academy of Audiology
AAC: Augmentative and Alternative Communication
AAE: African American English
AAO-HNS: American Academy of Otolaryngology – Head and Neck Surgery
AAPPSLPA: American Academy of Private Practice in Speech-Language Pathology and Audiology
AARP: American Association of Retired Persons
ABA: American Board of Audiology
ABC System: A (High Priority), B (Medium Priority), C (Low Priority)
ABER: Auditory Brainstem Evoked Response
ABIM: American Board of Internal Medicine
ABR: Auditory Brainstem Response
AC: Advisory Council
ACAE: Accreditation Commission for Audiology Education
ACE: Award for Continuing Education
ACEBP: Advisory Committee on Evidence-Based Practice
ACO: Accountable Care Organization
ACT: American College Testing Program
ADA: Americans with Disabilities Act
ADEA: Age Discrimination in Employment Act of 1967
ADL: Activity of Daily Living
AGREE: Appraisal of Guidelines for Research and Evaluation
AHRQ: Agency for Healthcare Research and Quality
AIDS: Acquired Immune Deficiency Syndrome
ALS: Amyotrophic Lateral Sclerosis
AMA: American Medical Association
ANCDS: Academy of Neurologic Communication Disorders and Sciences
APR: Annual Performance Report
APS: Adult Protective Services
ARRA: American Recovery and Reinvestment Act of 2009
ASD: Autism Spectrum Disorder
ASHA: American Speech-Language-Hearing Association
AT: Assistive Technology
ATC: Assistive Technology for Cognition
AuD: Doctor of Audiology
AYP: Adequate Yearly Progress
BAA: British Academy of Audiology
BAAS: British Association of Audiological Scientists
BAAT: British Association of Audiologists
BBA: Balanced Budget Act
BBP: Bureau of Business Practice
BBRA: Balanced Budget Refinement Act
BCBSA: Blue Cross Blue Shield Association
BIPA: Benefits Improvement and Protection Act
BLS: Bureau of Labor Statistics
BOD: Board of Directors
BSHAA: British Society of Hearing Aid Audiologists
BSHT: British Society of Hearing Therapists
CAA: Council on Academic Accreditation
CAOHC: Council for Accreditation in Occupational Hearing Conservation

CAP: Computerized Accreditation Program
CAPCSD: Council of Academic Programs in Communication Sciences and Disorders
CARF: Commission on Accreditation of Rehabilitation Facilities
CASLPA: Canadian Association of Speech-Language Pathologists and Audiologists
CCC: Certificate of Clinical Competence
CCC-A: Certificate of Clinical Competence in Audiology
CCC-SLP: Certificate of Clinical Competence in Speech-Language Pathology
CCI: Center for Cultural Interchange
CCI: Correct Coding Initiative
CCSPA: Council of University Supervisors in Speech-Language Pathology and Audiology
CCSS: Common Core State Standards
CCSSO: Council of Chief State School Officers
CDC: Centers for Disease Control and Prevention
CDCHU: Center on the Developing Child at Harvard University
CD-ROM: Compact Disc-Read-Only Memory
CDS: Communication Disorders and Sciences
CDSS: Clinical Decision Support System
CE: Continuing Education
CEC: Council for Exceptional Children
CF: Clinical Fellowship
CFCC: Council for Clinical Certification in Audiology and Speech-Language Pathology
CFR: Code of Federal Regulations
CFSI: Clinical Fellowship Skills Inventory
CFY: Clinical Fellowship Year
CHEA: Council on Higher Education Accreditation
CHIP: Children's Health Insurance Program
CI: Confidence Interval
CIC: Completely in Canal
CIRRIE: Center for International Rehabilitation Research Information and Exchange
CLD: Cultural and Linguistic Diversity
CMHs: Certification Maintenance Hours
CMS: Centers for Medicare & Medicaid Services
CMV: Cytomegalovirus
COBRA: Consolidated Omnibus Budget Reconciliation Act
COPs: Conditions of Participation
CORE: Collaboration, Observation, Reflection, and Evaluation
CORF: Comprehensive Outpatient Rehabilitation Facility
CoSN: Consortium for School Networking
CPLOL: Comité Permanent de Liaison des Orthophonistes/Logopèdes de l'Union Européenne
CPOP: Certificate Program for Otolaryngology Personnel
CPR: Cardiopulmonary Resuscitation
CPS: Child Protective Services
CPT: Current Procedural Terminology
CSC: Computer Sciences Corporation
CSD: Communication Sciences and Disorders
CSDCAS: Communication Sciences and Disorders Centralized Application Service for Clinical Education in Audiology and Speech-Language Pathology
CSEP: Center for the Study of Ethics in the Professions
CSSPA: Council of University Supervisors in Speech-Language Pathology and Audiology
CV: Curriculum Vitae
CWD: Child with a Disability
DDS: Doctor of Dentistry
DEU: Dedicated (Collaborative) Education Unit
DOE: U.S. Department of Education
DOTPA: Developing Outpatient Therapy Payment Alternatives
DPT: Doctor of Physical Therapy
DRA: Deficit Reduction Act
DRG: Diagnosis-Related Group
DSW: Doctor of Social Work
DTI: Diffusion Tensor Imaging
DVD: Digital Versatile/Video Disc
EBHC: Evidence-Based Health Care
EBP: Evidence-Based Practice
EBSR: Evidence-Based Systematic Review
ED: Department of Education
EdD: Doctor of Education
EDI: Electronic Data Interchange
EEO: Equal Employment Opportunity
EEOC: Equal Employment Opportunity Commission

EHA: Education for All Handicapped Children Act
EHDI: Early Hearing Detection and Intervention
EHR: Electronic Health Record
EI: Early Intervention
ELL: English Language Learner
EMR: Electronic Medical Record
EMTALA: Emergency Medical Treatment and Labor Act
ENG: Electronystagmography
ENT: Ear, Nose, and Throat
EPHI: Electronic Protected Health Information
EPSDT: Early Periodic Screening, Diagnosis, and Treatment
ERISA: Employee Retirement Income Security Act of 1974
ESEA: Elementary and Secondary Education Act
ESL: English as a Second Language
ETS: Educational Testing Service
FACS: Functional Assessment of Communication Skills for Adults
FAPE: Free Appropriate Public Education
FCM: Functional Communication Measure
FDA: Food and Drug Administration
FD&C Act: Federal Food, Drug and Cosmetic Act
FEES: Fiberoptic Endoscopic Evaluation of Swallowing
FERPA: Family Educational Rights and Privacy Act
FIM: Functional Independence Measure
FM: Frequency Modulated
fMRI: Functional Magnetic Resonance Imaging
FPCO: Family Policy Compliance Office
FRL: Free and Reduced Lunch
GAO: Government Accountability Office
GDP: Gross Domestic Product
GERD: Gastroesophageal Reflux Disease
GPA: Grade Point Average
GRE: Graduate Record Examination
HBV: Hepatitis B Virus
HCA: Hearing Conservation Amendment
HCEC: Health Care Economics Committee
HCFA: Health Care Financing Administration
HCPCS: Healthcare Common Procedures Coding System
HES: Higher Education Data System
HHA: Home Health Agency
HHS: Health and Human Services
HIE: Health Information Exchange
HIPAA: Health Insurance Portability and Accountability Act of 1996
HIT: Health Information Technology
HIV: Human Immunodeficiency Virus
HMO: Health Maintenance Organization
HR: Human Resources
HSV: Herpes Simplex Virus
IALP: International Association of Logopedics and Phoniatrics
IASLT: Irish Association of Speech and Language Therapists
ICC: Infection Control Committee
ICC: Interagency Coordinating Council
ICD: International Classification of Diseases
ICF: International Classification of Functioning, Disability and Health
ICRA: International Collegium of Rehabilitative Audiology
IDEA: Individuals with Disabilities Education Act
IDEIA: Individuals with Disabilities Education Improvement Act
IEP: Individualized Education Program
IFSP: Individualized Family Service Plan
IOM: Institute of Medicine
IOM: Internet-Only Manual
IP: Internet Protocol
IPA: Independent Practice Association
IPEC: Interprofessional Care Collaborative
IRB: Institutional Review Board
IRF-PAI: Inpatient Rehabilitation Facility-Patient Assessment Instrument
ISA: International Society of Audiology
ISA: Irish Society of Audiology
IST: Instructional Support Team
JD: Juris Doctorate (law degree)
KASA: Knowledge and Skills Assessment
KT: Knowledge Translation
LAN: Local Area Network
LAST: Liberal Arts and Sciences Test

LEA: Local Education Agency
LEP: Limited English Proficient
LLC: Limited Liability Company
LLD: Language Learning Disability
LOE: Levels of Evidence
LPAA: Life Participation Approach to Aphasia
LR: Likelihood Ratio
LRE: Least Restrictive Environment
LTACH: Long-Term Acute Care Hospital
LTC: Long-Term Care
LTCF: Long-Term Care Facility
MAC: Medicare Administrative Contractor
MARC: Mentoring for Academic-Research Careers
MAT: Miller Analogies Test
MBP: Munchausen by Proxy
MC: Managed Care
MCO: Managed Care Organization
MD: Doctor of Medicine
MDAT: Multidisciplinary Assessment Team
MDS: Minimum Data Set
MedPAC: Medicare Payment Advisory Committee
MIPPA: Medicare Improvements for Patients and Providers Act
MMA: Medicare Prescription Drug, Improvement, and Modernization Act
MOSAIC: Multiplying Opportunities for Services and Access to Immigrant Children
MPFS: Medicare Physician Fee Schedule
MPPR: Multiple Procedure Payment Reduction
MRI: Magnetic Resonance Imaging
MRSA: Methicillin-Resistant Staphylococcus Aureus
MSDS: Material Safety Data Sheet
MUE: Medically Unlikely Edits
NAEP: National Assessment of Educational Progress
NAFDA: National Association of Future Doctors of Audiology
NAFTA: North American Free Trade Agreement
NARF: National Association of Rehabilitation Facilities
NATS: National Association of Teachers of Speech
NCATE: National Council for Accreditation of Teacher Education
NCCP: National Center for Children in Poverty
NCELA: National Clearing House for English Language Acquisition
N-CEP: ASHA's National Center for Evidence-Based Practice in Communication Disorders
NCHS: National Center for Health Statistics
NCLB: No Child Left Behind Act
NEA: National Education Association
NGA: National Governors Association Center for Best Practices
NGS: National Governmental Services
NHS: National Health Service
NICHD: National Institute of Child Health & Human Development
NICU: Neonatal Intensive Care Unit
NIDCD: National Institute on Deafness and Other Communication Disorders
NIH: National Institutes of Health
NIRS: Near-Infrared Spectroscopy
NOMS: National Outcomes Measurement System
NPI: National Provider Identifier
NPO: Nothing by Mouth
NPV: Negative Predictive Value
NRH: National Rehabilitation Hospital
NSOME: Nonspeech Oral-Motor Exercises
NSSLHA: National Student Speech Language Hearing Association
NZAS: New Zealand Audiological Society
NZSTA: New Zealand Speech-language Therapists' Association
OAE: Otoacoustic Emission
OASIS: Outcome and Assessment Information Set
OBRA: Omnibus Reconciliation Act
OGET: Oklahoma General Education Test
OIG: Office of Inspector General
OPIM: Other Potentially Infectious Material
OPTE: Oklahoma Professional Teaching Exam
OSAT: Oklahoma Subject Area Test
OSEP: Office of Special Education Programs
OSERS: Office of Special Education and Rehabilitative Services
OSHA: Occupational Safety and Health Administration
OT: Occupational Therapy(ist)
OTD: Doctor of Occupational Therapy

OTO: Otologic Technician
P&P: Policy and Procedure
P2P: Peer-to-Peer File Sharing Program
PAC: Post-Acute Care
PASC: Pediatric Audiology Specialty Certification
PCP: Primary Care Physician
PEP: Personalized Education Plan
PharmD: Doctor of Pharmacy
PhD: Doctor of Philosophy
PHI: Protected Health Information
PHR: Personal Health Record
PI: Performance Improvement
PL: Public Law
PLOP: Present Level of Performance
PMPM: Per Member, Per Month Premium
PPACA: Patient Protection and Affordable Care Act
PPD: Purified Protein Derivative
PPE: Personal Protective Equipment
PPO: Preferred Provider Organization
PPS: Prospective Payment System
PQRI: Physician Quality Reporting Initiative
PQRS: Physician Quality Reporting System
PRI: Protected Research Information
PRN: Pro Re Nata—as the circumstances arise
PsyD: Doctor of Psychology
PT: Physical Therapy(ist)
PTA: Parent-Teacher Association
PV: Predictive Value
QCL: Quality of Communication Life
R01: Research Project Grant
RAC: Recovery Audit Contractor
RAI: Resident Assessment Instrument
RBRVS: Resource-Based Relative Value Scale
RCCP: Registration Council for Clinical Physiologists
RCR: Responsible Conduct of Research
RCSLT: Royal College of Speech and Language Therapists
RCT: Randomized Controlled Trial
RFA: Request for Applications
RPO: Related Professional Organization
RSAC: ASHA Research and Scientific Affairs Committee
RtI or RTI: Response-to-Instruction/Intervention
RUC HCPAC: Resource Update Health Care Professionals Advisory Committee
RUG: Resource Utilization Group
RVU: Relative Value Unit
SAA: Student Academy of Audiology
SALT: Systematic Analysis of Language
SASLHA: South African Speech-Language-Hearing Association
SAT: Scholastic Aptitude Test
ScD: Doctor of Science
SCHIP: State Children's Health Insurance Program
SD: Spasmodic Dysphonia
SD: Standard Deviation
SEA: State Education Agency
SED: Survey of Earned Doctorates
SERTOMA: Service to Mankind
SGD: Speech Generating Device
SHRM: Society of Human Resources Management
SIGN: Scottish Intercollegiate Guideline Network
SITE: Society for Information Technology and Teacher Education
SLP: Speech-Language Pathologist
SLPA: Speech-Language Pathology Assistant
SLPCF: Speech-Language Pathology Clinical Fellowship
SLPD: Speech-Language Pathology Doctorate
SNF: Skilled Nursing Facility
SnNout: Sensitivity high, Negative result—rule out
SOAP: Subjective, Objective, Assessment, Plan
SPA: Speech Pathology Australia
SPAI: Supervisee Performance Assessment Instrument
SPP: State Performance Plan
SpPin: Specificity high, Positive result—rule in
SR: Systematic Review
SSR: Single Subject Research
STAR: State Advocates for Reimbursement
STATS: Short-Term Alternatives for Therapy Services

STEP: Student to Empowered Professional
SWOT: Strength, Weakness, Opportunity, Threat
TB: Tuberculosis
TEFRA: Tax Equity and Fiscal Responsibility Act
TJC: The Joint Commission
TN: Trade NAFTA
TRHCA: Tax Relief and Health Care Act
TTY/TDD: Text Telephone/Telecommunications Device for the Deaf
UK: United Kingdom
USC: U.S. Code
VA: Veterans Administration
VNG: Videonystagmography
WASP: Waveforms Annotations Spectograms and Pitch
WHO: World Health Organization

SECTION I

Overview of the Professions

1

Professions for the Twenty-First Century

Rosemary Lubinski, EdD
Melanie W. Hudson, MA

SCOPE OF CHAPTER

We are in a time of rapid social, economic, and technological transformations in our country. These changes affect us as a society, individuals, and professionals. This chapter challenges you to think about the macro changes occurring in our society that affect the clinical milieu in which we provide services and the skills we need as audiologists and speech-language pathologists to respond to these changes. We challenge you to think creatively and critically so that you are in a leading, rather than a reactive, position. Today's clinicians must come equipped with state-of the-art clinical skills, positive workplace skills, and also professional foresight. This combination of skills and vision will help you serve clients with high-quality, innovative, and cost-effective services.

This chapter helps you understand many of the issues that are likely to affect your service delivery in the next few years. We begin with a discussion of six issues that influence our professional practice: changing demographics, the economy, new medical models, trends in education, technology, and globalization. This discussion leads to the skills you will need to practice effectively in today's professional world. Hopefully, reading this material and discussing it with peers and colleagues will help you to identify other emerging issues in your own community and work setting. Use this information as a springboard for analytical thinking and dialogue. We want you not only performing competently as a clinician but also thinking at a higher level.

As you read this chapter, consider our scopes of practice in audiology and speech-language pathology. (See the appendices at the end of the chapter for the most current Scopes of Practice in Audiology and Speech-Language Pathology.) Remember that these practices are dynamic. Ask yourself how the themes presented in this chapter influence your current and future scopes of practice as you progress through the twenty-first century.

TWENTY-FIRST-CENTURY INFLUENCES

The six issues that affect our profession discussed in this chapter are not discrete but are inextricably interrelated. For example, the aging of our society and the changing demographics in our schools are intertwined with the availability of funds to pay for services. Technology influences changes in medical and educational models, and the globalization of our professions challenges us to think across borders when serving our clients. You may even see other relationships once you start thinking in a systemic and critical way.

Changing Demographics

It is easy to observe that the U.S. population is changing. Two major changes have implications for us as audiologists and speech-language pathologists. The population is getting older and more diverse racially, ethnically, and linguistically. Keep in mind that these changes create not only a new client pool but also a new clinician demography.

Aging The aging of the population is at a critical juncture in our history. In 2011 the first baby boomers, born between 1946 and 1964, reached the age of 65. The proportion of elderly will increase from about 13 percent of the population in 2009 to 20 percent in 2030. This will result in around 72 million older people (American Medical Association, 2008). There will be not only more older people but also more very old among this group. The population over 75 years of age will eventually exceed the population between 65 and 74. By 2050 there should be at least 19 million people age 85 and older. Among these older groups, there is a higher number of women than men.

The increasing number of elderly is a global phenomenon. For example, by 2030 there is expected to be close to a billion elders across the world, accounting for 12 percent of the world's population (He, Sengupta, Velkoff, & DeBarros, 2005). A decrease in fertility and mortality rates accounts for this increase. Europe and North America have the highest proportions of elderly in the early twenty-first century. The most rapid increases in older populations, however, are expected in developing countries around the world, which will create new health care, economic, and social challenges to these emerging economies.

The older population will be different from previous generations of older people and will require more and different health services than younger cohorts. For example, it is expected that older people will be increasingly racially and ethnically diverse (Center for Health Workforce Studies, 2006). We can expect there to be more older Hispanic and Asian people in years to come in the United States. The new generation of older people will have more educational and socioeconomic resources, although there are inequalities between the sexes and among income, racial, and ethnic groups (Federal Interagency Forum on Aging-Related Statistics, 2010). Poverty in old age affects women more than men and Hispanics and African Americans more than whites. About 87 percent of older people indicate that Social Security is a major source of their income (Administration on Aging, 2010). Moreover, those approaching old age (50 to 64) may have been the most affected by the 2008 financial crisis due to a loss of savings from retirement accounts (Federal Interagency Forum on Aging-Related Statistics, 2010). These individuals may be in the workforce longer as they delay retirement, thereby affecting the availability of jobs for young people beginning employment.

With aging there will be an increase in functional limitations and the prevalence of chronic conditions, particularly among the very old (Bernstein et al., 2003). Major chronic conditions include hypertension, arthritis, heart disease, cancer, diabetes, and stroke (Federal Interagency Forum on Aging-Related Statistics, 2010). Again, these chronic diseases are distributed differently among major racial and ethnic groups. For example, non-Hispanic blacks report higher levels of hypertension and diabetes than non-Hispanic whites (Federal Interagency Forum on Aging-Related Statistics, 2010). Clinical depression affects at least 18 percent of older women and 10 percent of older men, with these percentages increasing with advancing age. About 42 percent of those over age 65 have functional disabilities, with women having higher levels of functional limitations than men. Hearing impairments affect at least 42 percent of older men and 30 percent of older women, with these percentages again increasing with age and institutionalization. The prevalence of vision loss increases with age, stroke, traumatic brain injury, and progressive neurological diseases. About 20 percent of elders in the community have trouble seeing, and this number also increases with age and institutionalization.

The vast majority of elders live in the community, with only about 4 percent residing in institutional settings such as nursing homes. This percentage increases with age to the point where about 15.4 percent of those over age 85 years reside in such a setting (Administration on Aging, 2010). More than 72 percent of older men in the community reside with a spouse while the percentage of older women is split between those who live with a spouse (42 percent) and those who live alone (39 percent). Remember that some community-based elders reside in housing that provides various meal preparation and housekeeping services. The availability of such community-based services may prevent relocation to a nursing home.

Interestingly, about 20 percent of older people live in multigenerational families in the community (Pew Research Center, 2010). This percentage increases for Hispanics, African Americans, and Asians. Older adults, particularly women, are likely to live with their middle-age children and their grandchildren. These extended families provide support and some financial assistance. Thus, you are likely to interact with several generations in the aging family.

Many of the new health care procedures and technologies are targeted at elderly patients. For example, knee and hip replacements have become more common among older people. There is also a trend for more aggressive treatment of the elderly (Bernstein et al., 2003). Some argue that these approaches forestall institutionalization and the need for more intense health or personal care; others argue that there should be limits on such procedures, especially for the very old.

Diversity The second major demographic societal change is the increasing number and percentage of racial, ethnic, and linguistic minorities. According to the U.S. Census Bureau (2010b), about 72 percent of the population is white, 12 percent black or African American, and 4.8 percent Asian. Hispanics or Latinos of any race constitute 16.3 percent of the population. In 2007 minorities comprised over one-third of the U.S. population, and this number is expected to increase to 54 percent by 2050 (U.S. Census Bureau, 2008). The greatest growth in minorities will be among Hispanics, who will triple from 47 million to 133 million during the period 2008 to 2050. There will also be significant growth among Asians, American Indians, and Alaska Natives, and those who consider themselves as being of two or more races. Much of the minority population is located along the periphery of the United States and in Hawaii. California and Texas alone account for one-third of the nation's minority populations (Minckler, 2008).

While today's school population is 44 percent minority, this will grow to 62 percent by 2050 (U.S. Census Bureau, 2008). Today, most minority students attend schools in central city locations, and the greatest percentage of these is Hispanic students (National Center for Education Statistics, 2007). About 37 percent of public school students in urban fringe communities are minorities. The percentage of minority students varies by state and area. For example, the District of Columbia has a 95 percent minority rate in its schools, New Mexico has 53 percent of its students considered Hispanic, and Hawaii has 73 percent of its students from an Asian/Pacific Islander background.

Other than English, the most commonly spoken language at home is Spanish (more than 29 million). Chinese has become the second most common non-English language, with about 2 million speakers. Other common languages spoken in the United States include French, German, Tagalog, Vietnamese, Italian, Korean, Russian, Polish, and Arabic (Vistawide, 2011). There is a disproportionate percentage of non-English speakers (about one-third) located in the western part of the United States. Areas adjacent to Mexico and the Atlantic and Pacific oceans have high proportions of linguistic diversity. It should also be noted that states such as Georgia, Utah, Arkansas, and Oregon have doubled their numbers of non-English speakers in the past 20 years (Vistawide, 2011). See Chapter 24 for a discussion of multicultural issues.

While the percentage of people in the United States who have disabilities is about 22 percent (38 percent among the elderly), the percentage of minorities with disabilities ranges from about 12 percent of Asians to 30 percent among American Indians and Alaska Natives (Centers for Disease Control and Prevention, 2010). Rates for severe disabilities that impact functional activities are highest among blacks (12 percent). The rates for disability increase with age across all minority groups (Bradsher, 1996). African Americans constitute the highest proportion of children and youth with disabilities (U.S. Office of Special Education Programs, 2002).

These statistics reflect not only our potential clients but also the communication disorders workforce. Speech-language pathologists and audiologists are growing older, too. This particularly affects academia. The graying of the academic faculty in communication sciences disorders has resulted in a shortage of available doctoral-level applicants to fill academic positions (Hull, 2007). There is an insufficient number of replacements in the pipeline, and few of these are minorities. The average age of faculty members is about 55 years old, and a mass retirement of faculty is expected within the next few years (Hull, 2007).

The number of minorities entering the professions is also less than expected. In 2008, the American Speech-Language-Hearing Association (ASHA) reported that about 6.8 percent of its members, nonmember certificate holders, and international affiliates are members of a racial minority as compared with about 25 percent of the U.S. population (American Speech-Language-Hearing Association, 2008). To promote greater inclusion of culturally and linguistically diverse individuals in our professions, ASHA has a special listing of members from racial/minority backgrounds who may be available for faculty positions.

Poverty A third demographic trend potentially affecting our delivery of audiology or speech-language pathology services is the prevalence of poverty in the United States. According to the U.S. Census Bureau (2010a), 43.6 million people (14.3 percent) lived in poverty in the United States. Much of the increase in poverty occurred following the Recession of 2008. The poverty rate among elders has remained about 10 percent, although there are higher rates among women and minorities. Older minority women who live alone have the highest poverty rates (American Association of Retired People, 2008).

According to the National Center for Children in Poverty (NCCP) (Chau, Thampi, & Wight, 2010), 36 percent of all those who live in poverty are children. Nineteen percent (14 million) of children under the age of 18 live in poverty in the United States, and 46 percent of infants and toddlers live in low-income families. This group defines poverty as an income of $22,050 for a family of four with two children. The percentage of children in poverty increases to 40 percent if the definition includes low-income families who earn up to $44,100. Many of the families living in poverty are made up of parents with less than a high school education (85 percent), have only one parent (52 percent), are black (61 percent), Hispanic (62 percent), American Indian (57 percent), or are immigrants (60 percent). More than half of poor children live in urban areas.

What are the implications of these demographic changes on our client and clinician pools? Without doubt, we are becoming an older society, at least for the next 40 years, and older clients will have special needs and require clinicians who have skills to meet those needs. Emerging professionals must be prepared with the knowledge and experience of how best to serve the complex client needs of older populations. Moreover, professionals must be prepared to justify to elders, other health professionals, and third-party payers the value of providing communication, hearing, and swallowing services in the presence of competing client needs, advancing age, and efforts to contain health care costs.

There will also be a more multicultural client base. Clinicians will need more expertise in working with clients from a variety of ethnic, racial, and linguistic backgrounds across all types of settings, from schools to home care to medical sites. Our preprofessional training and continuing education will need to focus on geriatric and diversity content. The need for more clinicians from a variety of cultural and linguistic backgrounds is also clear, and ways are needed to attract these individuals into our professions. Finally, the aging of academia poses challenges for the maintenance of college and university programs and the continued development of our professions that emanate from a strong science base.

The National Economy

Before 2008, few of us thought about the terms *depression*, *recession*, *unemployment*, and *foreclosures*. The Depression was something our grand- or great-grandparents experienced, and recessions were simply abstract downturns that usually did not affect us personally. The Recession of 2008 has been considered the worst downturn since the Great Depression. Professionals have become acutely aware of the national economy and its effects on our delivery of services, business practices, and our personal finances. Students wonder if there will be jobs, where those jobs might be located, and the salaries and benefits that might be offered. Faculty postpone retirement because of diminished retirement accounts. Research funding has become increasingly more competitive. Clients and third-party payers want the best-quality service for the most economical investment. Although the economy recovers slowly and without a robust increase in employment rates, clients and insurers are likely to be considering the absolute necessity of our services and the costs of reimbursement.

A national debate is occurring as to how best to manage our national expenses and the debt that our country has accrued. Continued national debt has major implications for each of us. Simply, the government must reduce its expenditures and/or increase its income, usually in the form of higher taxes. Cutting spending may involve reducing benefits programs (e.g., Medicare, Medicaid, Social Security) and student financial aid. Increasing taxes lowers the amount of money individuals and corporations have to spend, to hire employees, and to invest in the economy. Not addressing the national debt has far greater implications on our ability to attract investments, get loans at reasonable rates, and manage inflation because of the weakened dollar. The problems and their solutions are not simple and do affect us as individuals and professionals.

Cutbacks in spending have implications for our service delivery in all settings. For example, schools want to see positive educational outcomes for a larger number of students. Reductions in spending for Medicare and Medicaid also affect what and how much service we offer to older people and those of low income. Third-party insurers increase limitations on covered services. Both audiologists and speech-language pathologists have had to learn the best way to bill for services from third-party insurers, how to file claims, and how to appeal denials for services provided.

Without doubt, the aging of the population and the increasing costs of health care both affect the services we provide. Health care comprises 17.3 percent of the nation's gross domestic product (GDP) or more than $8,000 for every person in the United States per year (Blue Cross Blue Shield, 2010). In contrast, national defense and food each represent 5.5 percent of the GDP. Health care is expected to rise to 17.7 percent of the GDP by 2015. The United States spends more on health care as a percentage of its GDP than any other country in the world. Some would argue that this is without better outcomes than in those countries that spend less.

Health care costs are expected to continue to increase in the years to come, especially with the aging of the population. Older people use more health care than any other cohort, and health care costs increase with advancing age. In recent years, elders' health expenses went for physician outpatient hospital services (35 percent), inpatient hospital services (25 percent), prescription drugs (16 percent), and long-term care facilities (13 percent). Interestingly, there has been a decrease in inpatient hospital costs and long-term care while there has been an increase in costs for physicians and prescription drugs (Federal Interagency Forum on Aging-Related Statistics, 2010).

The national economic problems also have implications for education funding. Rising expenses mean that local school districts must increase class sizes, reduce program offerings, lay off staff, increase taxes, or look to their state governments for aid. Federal subsidies for college student financial aid directly affect the ability of our students to pay for their undergraduate and graduate education. Increasing costs of higher education result in many students graduating with greater debt. In 2008, the average undergraduate owed at least $23,200 of debt at graduation (Project on Student Debt, 2009). For those with additional years of graduate study, the amount is far greater, and graduates will be mired in debt for many years to come. Repayment of such debt minimizes their purchasing power for homes, goods, services, and investments.

The Recession of 2008 has also affected state and local economies. In 2011, 24 states projected budget shortfalls through 2013 (McNichol, Oliff, & Johnson, 2011). These deficiencies affect monies available for Medicaid and education, both areas that include some of the most vulnerable families and individuals. Many states received assistance through the American Recovery Act of 2009, but this funding ends, and many states will face shortfalls. According to the Center on Budget and Policy Priorities (McNichol, Oliff, & Johnson, 2011), "States are likely to respond with spending cuts and tax increases seen larger than those that have already been enacted"

(p. 8). Lack of funding from the state level trickles down to local communities, which must increase property and school taxes in a time of lower employment and decreasing property values and/or reduce services and cut jobs. These are difficult decisions that affect you as a professional and as a citizen taxpayer.

The solutions for the national debt, increasing health costs especially for elders, and reductions in education funding are interrelated and have direct implications for us as professionals and individuals. Our first obligation is to become better informed about national economic issues and work arduously to ensure that speech-language and hearing services are mandated and maintained at reasonable rates. We need evidence-based studies that prove that what we do makes quantitative and qualitative differences in students' lives and improves their ability to participate productively in education and employment. For elders, we need to prove that what we do enhances their ability to live independently as long as possible, access the care they need, participate in decision making regarding their lives and care, and have a positive quality of life as long as possible. We need to be not only skilled and efficient clinicians but also ready to employ our skills in advocacy, communication, and leadership. For more discussion on each of the topics discussed thus far, see Chapters 18 and 21.

New Medical Models

Patient-Centered Medical Homes One way to provide better-quality and less expensive medical service is through the advent of new medical models of service delivery. Several trends are evident. First is the creation of patient-centered medical homes (sometimes called medical homes or advanced medical homes). Originating in 1967 by the American Academy of Pediatrics, the concept includes several principles. Each patient has a personal physician and that person leads a team of qualified professionals to collectively care for patients. There is a whole-person orientation across the life span. Care is coordinated and integrated especially through Health Information Exchanges (HIEs), and patients and families are encouraged to participate in care decisions. Evidence-based practice and clinical decision support tools guide decision making. Access is facilitated through new options for communication and expanded service hours. And finally, payment should include all aspects of care, communication, and quality improvement for all types of patients (American Academy of Family Physicians et al., 2007). Note the important role of the primary care physician in creating teams of professionals to serve patients, the role of patients and families in decision making, and the need for evidence-based methods.

Retail Clinics Another trend is the creation of retail and worksite clinics. The number of retail medical clinics has quadrupled between 2006 and 2008, though they still represent a small percentage of sites of care (8 percent versus 79 percent of individuals who visit a physician's office) (Blue Cross Blue Shield Association, 2010). Retail clinics are located outside traditional physicians' offices either as freestanding walk-in clinics or within drugstores or discount chain stores. They tend to be staffed by nurse practitioners and focus on common illnesses and preventive care. Patients with more serious illnesses are referred to emergency rooms or their own physician. Critical to this type of health care is the use of technology for documentation, collaboration, and billing. Note also that some of these new clinics are staffed by physician assistants and nurse practitioners who may not be familiar with our services and thus not make referrals to us as needed. Thus, we have an obligation to provide continuing education to these professionals to keep them informed about what we do, for whom, and with what benefits, especially to health care.

Health Information Technology Health Information Technology (HIT) is at the core of the new medical models. Technology is used for e-prescribing and electronically enabled care coordination. According to the Office of the National Coordinator for Health Information Technology (2011), Health Information Technology enhances patient care management through secure use and sharing of health information, particularly the use of Electronic Health Records (EHRs). HIT facilitates coordination of care and patient participation in decision making and improves efficient and accurate diagnosis. It is predicted that HIT will reduce both errors and costs and improve access to quality care. The use of Health Information Exchanges facilitates the transfer of information electronically across medical organizations within a medical system or across a community or region. Not only does exchange of information encourage greater continuity in care across a number of health care providers and more analysis of the health of a community, it also reduces expenses. Further, more than 40 percent of physicians are using EHR systems to record patient visits, results, and recommendations. All professionals using such technologies will face ethical issues related to the transfer of information across the Internet. (Technology is discussed in more depth later in this chapter and in Chapter 26.)

Customer Service Speech-language pathologists and audiologists should also be aware of the emphasis on "customer service" in new health care models. The advent of health care offered in retail centers focused awareness of the need for "service delivered with a smile" (Carroll, 2011). Quality of care is intimately linked with how satisfied patients are with the service they receive in a medical setting. Jablonski (2004) states "... satisfied customers will tell five or seven others of their experiences, while dissatisfied customers will tell their stories to as many as 20 people. Customer satisfaction is, at the very least, a public relations imperative." Improving service includes better access to services during the week, reduction in redundancies especially in information intake, personalization of service from point of entry to discharge, and reduction in waiting time.

Audiologists and speech-language pathologists will need to fit into the new medical models. We will need to be part of patients' medical homes and ensure that other practitioners know what we do and its value to patients and caregivers. Remember that you will need to educate service providers in retail clinics of patients' communication, hearing, and swallowing needs so that they can make appropriate referrals to you. You will be documenting your assessments and interventions and providing that information electronically to others. Undoubtedly, our documentation skills will need to change so that information is easily and quickly understood by a variety of other professionals. Finally, how we communicate with patients and caregivers will continue to be critical to patients' perceptions of our skills and value to them. Positive public relations are not discretionary when patients have options of whether and where they will use our services.

Transforming Education

With a new century comes a new need for better education of our children to prepare them to lead productive and meaningful lives. Students must learn how to use their knowledge of core subjects and to think analytically so that they can compete not only with the child next door but also with the children in Asia and Europe. To meet the increasing and changing standards for academic performance, educational programs are reconsidering the outcomes that must be achieved if students are to enter higher education and the workforce with the skills that make them skilled and competitive.

Tony Wagner (2008) in his book *The Global Achievement Gap* hypothesizes that there are seven "survival skills" that students must acquire. These include critical thinking and problem solving; collaboration across networks and leading by influence; agility and adaptability; initiative and entrepreneurship; effective oral and written communication; accessing and analyzing information; and curiosity and imagination. To achieve these skills, there is less emphasis on test scores and more focus on the higher levels of thinking as portrayed in Bloom's Taxonomy of Educational Objectives. Students are encouraged to develop through active and collaborative learning and improved thinking skills such as synthesis, analysis, and evaluation. The National Academy of Sciences (1997) also stresses the need for improved education in science, mathematics, engineering, and technology. It, too, identifies higher-level thinking skills as core to improved educational outcomes and the ability to succeed in the workplace.

The 21st Century Workforce Commission (North Central Regional Educational Laboratory, 2003) identifies four areas in which schools need to prioritize their educational efforts. First is digital-age literacy including technological literacy, visual and information literacy, and cultural literacy. A second priority should be the development of inventive thinking that encompasses adaptability and self-direction, curiosity, creativity and risk taking, and higher-order thinking. Its third focus is on interactive communication and the development of social and personal skills. Finally, schools need to develop students who are highly productive and can prioritize, plan, and use real-world tools.

Thus, schools of the twenty-first century need to balance teaching for local, state, and national test results and creating a learning environment that produces students who have high-level thinking skills, can use technology effectively, and can interact with coworkers in the workplace and globally. Speech-language pathologists and audiologists need to think creatively about how their knowledge base and services can help students with communication disorders achieve these new learning goals and also serve as a resource for classroom teachers, students, and parents. Our knowledge base about literacy development, higher-level thinking skills, social communication, and technology can be an asset within the educational environment for students with and without communication disorders.

Technology

Every aspect of our daily lives is influenced by technology, particularly information technology. This revolution transforms the way we connect and collaborate with others, think, provide and receive health care, teach and learn, conduct research, do business, and entertain ourselves. Those who are "knowledge workers" and can use technology to analyze and evaluate information are likely to find jobs (Brown, 1999). Technology itself has become a major industry in the United States. More than 77 percent of people in the United States use the Internet. Sixty percent of American workers view technology as key to having a competitive advantage in the workplace (Intercall, 2010). Thus, technology literacy is vital to our prosperity as a nation and our ability to innovate, create jobs, and provide higher-quality services across industries and disciplines.

Educational changes must also incorporate technology skills from a child's first educational experiences. In fact, today's three-year-old is likely to come to preschool with a Leapfrog computer in his backpack. Schools, however, must not only provide computer access but also teach the higher-level thinking skills that underlie creative and reasoned use of technology. Schools must also train teachers in the variety of technologies available and how their use enhances educational outcomes and communication with other teachers, parents, and students. Technology can bring teachers together to share information and teaching strategies.

Technological advances in medicine are numerous and fast changing. Technologies have been developed that help physicians and others better understand the body's anatomy and physiology, diagnose diseases and disorders, and provide more objective data and timely care. Transfer of patient information to other specialists and to databases can be done with a few strokes on a keyboard and reach all parts of the world quickly. Consultations have become easier and faster.

Advances in technology are also evident in training of medical students with the use of patient virtual reality. Of particular interest to speech-language pathologists is the use of telepractice to treat and communicate with patients in their homes. Use of personal technology may also help researchers link with subjects and clinicians to gather data and provide immediate feedback regarding a diagnosis or progress.

Technology also enables patients themselves to access a variety of information sources available on the Internet about their health care. Popular sites include WebMD, Microsoft Health Vault, Google Health, and individual insurance plans. Individuals may also make their public health records (PHRs) accessible through electronic means to qualified practitioners.

Speech-language pathologists and audiologists have also been on the forefront of the technological revolution. Portable and accessible computerized technology can facilitate communication for expressively impaired individuals, from young children in schools to older people in their homes or long-term care facilities. Computer technologies are being used to compensate for cognitive impairments (Sohlberg, 2011). Software has been developed to treat many disorders including aphasia, traumatic brain injury, autism, and attention difficulties. Our older clients may reside in "smart homes" based in technology and universal and transgenerational design that assist them with limitations in activities of daily living. There are even "apps" available for the iPhone and iPod Touch for those with expression difficulties. Our ability to assist with a swallowing evaluation is a result of the development of fiber-optic endoscopic and radiologic technologies. Speech science research is served by sophisticated technology to study speech production and perception. Technology also facilitates research collaboration and creation of multisite databases that will serve to improve our scientific evidence base. Telepractice, in which you serve clients in distant sites, is likely to be one way to serve clients more easily and more quickly.

Technology is also at the core of audiology. Audiologists use an array of sophisticated technology to assess hearing and balance including audiometers, tympanometers, auditory brainstem response equipment, electronystagmography, oto-acoustic emission equipment, and balance technology. In addition, audiologists assess and prescribe a variety of assistive listening devices including the latest developments in digital hearing aids, other assistive listening devices, and environmental technologies such as infrared and frequency modulated (FM) systems. Recently, audiologists have been involved in the assessment and programming of cochlear implants for individuals with severe hearing impairment.

Communication disorders specialists will find that every aspect of their professional lives involves some type and use of technology. Many clients will have "Googled" their concerns before visiting you and arrive with a different knowledge base than clients in previous years. More of your clients will be computer savvy and expect you to use technology in working with them. Thus, you will need to keep current on rapid developments in this area. You will also be expected to use technology to document your results, bill for services, and communicate and collaborate with other professionals and clients. It is likely that some of you will use telepractice to serve clients outside your regular office. Keep in mind, however, that technology is not an end in itself, but a tool to facilitate your work and your client's ability to hear and communicate. Finally, issues related to information accuracy on the Internet and privacy when communicating through the Internet must be considered. Read more about telepractice and technology in Chapter 26.

Globalization

At first you may not realize that you are part of a global profession or that what happens in other parts of the world affects you. Globalization is defined as a "process in which geographic distance becomes a factor of diminishing importance in the establishment and maintenance of cross-border economic, political, and socio-cultural relations" (Organisation for Economic Co-operation and Development, 2000, p. 173). At some time in your career, you will interact in person or via the Internet with a professional from another country. Networking with international colleagues enhances the development of our professions worldwide and also allows us to access expertise being developed globally.

Speech-language pathology is an established or growing profession in North and South America, Europe, Asia, Africa, and Australia. There are more than 50,000 speech-language pathologists or logopedists in the European Union alone (Standing Liaison Committee of Speech and Language Therapists and Logopedists, 2010). Audiology is also growing throughout the world, and there are numerous international associations in the United States and Canada, the United Kingdom, Europe, Asia, Australia, Africa, and the Middle East. You may want to attend international conferences or invite colleagues to visit your program.

Increased mobility may motivate you to seek professional employment in other countries. It is important to check with local, provincial/state, and national licensing agencies for certification or licensing and employment regulations. You may also want to collaborate with colleagues in other countries for clinical or research purposes. Computer technology provides an excellent mechanism to transfer scientific or clinical information, facilitate face-to-face interaction with colleagues and clients, and observe or supervise clinical work. Always check that your transfer of digital information meets the confidentiality requirements of your setting and state. Computer technology also facilitates continuing education from international sources that you may never have been able to access. Through computer technology, you may network with professionals and capitalize on their expertise or provide information to them. For more information on international alliances, see Chapter 7.

SKILLS NEEDED TOMORROW

The U.S. Secretary of Labor appointed a commission in 1999 to define skills and workplace competencies young people need to be successful in the work world (U.S. Department of Labor, 1999). Foundational skills include being able to communicate receptively and expressively in oral and written forms, do basic computations, and use a variety of mathematical techniques. Other skills include the use of higher-level thinking such as problem solving and creative reasoning. Positive personal skills consist of responsibility, self-esteem, sociability, self-management, integrity, and honesty (U.S. Department of Labor, 1991). The competencies that contribute to success in the workplace include being able to use all the resources available in the workplace and being able to work effectively with others on a team or in a leadership role. Successful workers also know how to acquire and evaluate information, especially through the use of information technology. Achievement in the workplace involves understanding the complexity and organization of the setting. Finally, all workers must be able to use a variety of technologies.

Several themes emanate from the earlier discussion of twenty-first-century influences and basic and foundational work skills listed earlier. First is the need to be able to communicate effectively in writing and in speech. It is through communication that you will be able to interact competently on a team and with individual clients, caregivers, and colleagues. You will need to communicate with older clients and those from diverse backgrounds. You are likely to communicate with colleagues worldwide. Each of these takes special communication skills. Leadership also derives from polished written and oral communication skills.

Tomorrow's communication disorders specialists also need to have advanced thinking skills. You will be more successful if you think innovatively and analytically and can communicate your ideas to others persuasively. Tomorrow's creativity will likely involve the use of technology to serve clients and boost our scientific base.

You will need enhanced people skills that reflect your commitment to your setting and your clients. You may be your client's most important advocate. Clients are becoming more sophisticated and will also expect greater client service. Expect them to communicate their degree of satisfaction to others, to you, and via the Internet. Every clinical interaction is a potential public relations opportunity for you and our professions.

You must also be able to access information quickly and effectively to provide the best quality clinical services. Thus, you will need to use technology as part of your everyday skills and for planning, service, documentation, billing, research, and advocacy. You can use technology to help you understand the cultural and age-related characteristics your clients bring to the clinical situation. You may be expected to provide research-based evidence to support the techniques you use and data that illustrate client improvement.

Not only do you need specific skills, but you need to bring positive attitudes to your workplace. These attitudes will underscore your success in the future. The first is flexibility. Many of you will not work in settings that provide employment or benefits security. Some of you by choice or circumstances will work part time, be contracted by a central employer, or be self-employed. Some of you will work in one setting in the morning and another in the afternoon. You will also need to bring an attitude of self-motivation and adaptability. Employers will expect you to come with a "can-do" attitude, able to assume responsibility and self-assess and modify on the spot. In addition, your employer will want you to participate as a productive team member and advocate for the setting's goals. Much is expected of you, and much you will do. See Chapter 10 for a discussion of employer expectations.

SUMMARY

Success in our professions in the twenty-first century has become increasingly dependent on understanding how macro-level social and economic issues affect our skills and services. For audiologists and speech-language pathologists to thrive in the current socioeconomic environment, professionals must have a keen eye focused on how these issues affect our professions. Uncertainty in the workplace is likely to be part of employment for years to come. Thus, only those who have excellent basic and foundational skills, in addition to high-level professional knowledge and competencies in communication disorders, will be employed or employable. Our clientele is likely to be more diverse as are our colleagues. Use of technology will be central to how we provide services and interact with colleagues around the world. Our value will emanate from a professional culture that is based in science, leadership, sensitivity to diversity, interpersonal skills, and vision.

CRITICAL THINKING

1. Twenty-five years from now, what will professional historians say about the professions of audiology or speech-language pathology? What factors do you think will affect our development and our provision of services across settings and client groups?
2. Think about the geographical area in which you work or are likely to work. What comprises the demographics of this area? How have the demographics changed in the past 10 years? How should you prepare to work with the variety of client groups in your geographic area?
3. What technology do you use now in your clinical practice? How does it facilitate the quality and efficiency of what you do? What advances would you like to see in technology to help you provide better science for our professions or service to our clients?

4. How should our preprofessional and continuing education focus on social and economic changes in our society? How does knowledge about these areas improve your delivery of speech-language, swallowing, or hearing services?
5. What opportunities have you had for serving older clients, those from diverse backgrounds, and those in poverty? How well prepared do you feel to do this? What can you do to enhance your skills?
6. Read a recent national newspaper (print or online). What topics are represented and how do these affect you as a professional and a citizen? Why does keeping up on current events help you as a professional audiologist or speech-language pathologist?
7. How does globalization affect you as a clinician? What opportunities have you had to interact with professionals around the world? What might you do to develop such interactions?

REFERENCES

Administration on Aging. (2010). *A profile of older Americans: 2009.* Washington, DC: Department of Health and Human Services.

American Academy of Family Physicians et al. (2007). *Joint principles of the patient-centered medical home.* Retrieved from http://www.medicalhomeinfo.org/downloads/pdfs/jointstatement.pdf

American Association of Retired People. (2008). *Poverty and aging in America.* Washington, DC: Author.

American Medical Association. (2008). *Health care trends 2008.* Retrieved from http://www.ama-assn.org/go/healthcaretrends

American Speech-Language-Hearing Association. (2008). *2008 ASHA member counts.* Retrieved from http://www.asha.org/uploadedfiles/2008-member-counts.pdf

Bernstein, A., Hing, E., Moss, A., Allen, K., Siller, A., & Tiggle, R. (2003). *Health care in America: Trends in utilization.* Hyattsville, MD: National Center for Health Statistics.

Blue Cross Blue Shield Association. (2010). *Keeping healthcare affordable.* Available from http://www.bcbs.com/employers/healthcare-trends-report/

Bradsher, J. (1996). *Disability among racial and ethnic groups.* Washington, DC: Disability Statistics Center.

Brown, B. (1999). *Knowledge workers.* Retrieved from http://www.calpro-online.org/eric/docs/tia00072.pdf

Carroll, J. (2011). *It's January 15, 2020. What have we learned about healthcare in the last decade?* Available from http://www.jimcarroll.com/2008/11/its-january-15-2020-what-have-we-learned-about-healthcare-in-the-last-decade/

Center for Health Workforce Studies, University at Albany. (2006). *The impact of the aging population on the health workforce in the United States: Summary of findings.* Rensselaer, NY: Author.

Centers for Disease Control and Prevention. (2010). *Disability and health.* Retrieved from http://www.cdc.gov/ncbddd/disabilityandhealth/data.html

Chau, M., Thampi, K., & Wight, V. (2010). *Basic facts about low-income children, 2009.* National Center for Children in Poverty. Available from http://www.nccp.org/publications/pub_971.html

Federal Interagency Forum on Aging-Related Statistics. (2010). *Older Americans 2010: Key indicators of well-being.* Washington, DC: Government Printing Office.

He, W., Sengupta, M., Velkoff, V., & DeBarros, K. (2005). *65+ in the United States: 2005.* Washington, DC: Department of Health and Human Services.

Hull, R. (2007). *Addressing the national shortage of PhD-level faculty/scholars in the fields of speech-language pathology and audiology.* Retrieved from https://www.osep-meeting.org/2007conf/Presentations/Monday/5_CommunityOfPracticeAffinity_4.45%20to%205.45pm/4_AddressingTheNationalShortageOfPhD.ppt

Intercall. (2010). *Technology in the workplace.* Retrieved from http://www.intercall.com/files/ic_study-summary_final.pdf

Jablonski, R. (2004). *Customer focus: The cornerstone of quality management.* Retrieved from http://findarticles.com/p/articles/mi_m3257/is_n11_v46/ai_14176753/

McNichol, E., Oliff, P., & Johnson, N. (2011). *States continue to feel recession's impact.* Retrieved from http://www.cbpp.org/cms/?fa=view&id=711

Minckler, D. (2008). *U.S. minority population continues to grow.* Retrieved from http://iipdigital.usembassy.gov/st/english/article/2008/05/20080513175840zjsredna0.1815607.html#axzz1vFQeABA8

National Academy of Sciences. (1997). *Preparing for the 21st century: The education imperative.* Retrieved from http://www.nas.edu/21st/education/

National Center for Education Statistics. (2007). *Status and trends in the education of racial and ethnic minorities.* Retrieved from http://nces.ed.gov/pubs2007/minoritytrends/ind_2_7.asp

North Central Regional Educational Laboratory. (2003). *enGauge 21st century skills.* Naperville, IL: NCREL and Metiri Group.

Office of the National Coordinator for Health Information Technology. (2011). Retrieved from http://healthit.hhs.gov/portal/server.pt/community/healthit_hhs_gov__home/1204

Organisation for Economic Co-operation and Development. (2000). *The creative society of the 21st century.* Paris, France: Author.

Pew Research Center. (2010). *The return of the multi-generational family household.* Retrieved from http://www.pewsocialtrends.org/2010/03/18/the-return-of-the-multi-generational-family-household/

The Institute for College Access & Success. (2009). *The project on student debt.* Retrieved from http://projectonstudentdebt.org

Sohlberg, M. (2011). Assistive technology for cognition. *The ASHA Leader,* 16.

Standing Liaison Committee of Speech and Language Therapists and Logopedists. (2010). *The organization.* Available from http://www.cplol.eu/eng/organization.htm

U.S. Census Bureau. (2008). *An older and more diverse nation by midcentury.* Retrieved from http://www.census.gov/newsroom.releases/archives/population/ cb08-123.html

U.S. Census Bureau. (2010a). *About poverty.* Retrieved from http://www.census.gov/hhes/www/poverty/about/overview/index.html

U.S. Census Bureau. (2010b). *State and county quickfacts.* Retrieved from http://quickfacts.census.gov/qfd/states/00000.html

U.S. Department of Labor. (1991). *What work requires of schools: A SCANS report for America 2000.* Washington, DC: Author.

U.S. Department of Labor. (1999). *Futurework: Trends and challenges for work in the 21st century.* Washington, DC: Author.

U.S. Office of Special Education Programs. (2002). *Facts from OSEP's National Longitudinal Studies.* Retrieved from http://www.nlts2.org/fact_sheets/nlts2_fact_sheet_2004_11.pdf

Vistawide. (2011). *World languages and cultures.* Retrieved from http://www.vistawide.com/languages/us_languages2.htm

Wagner, T. (2008). *The global achievement gap.* New York, NY: Basic Books.

Appendix 1-A

ASHA Scope of Practice in Audiology

STATEMENT OF PURPOSE

The purpose of this document is to define the scope of practice in audiology in order to (a) describe the services offered by qualified audiologists as primary service providers, case managers, and/or members of multidisciplinary and interdisciplinary teams; (b) serve as a reference for health care, education, and other professionals, and for consumers, members of the general public, and policy makers concerned with legislation, regulation, licensure, and third party reimbursement; and (c) inform members of ASHA, certificate holders, and students of the activities for which certification in audiology is required in accordance with the ASHA Code of Ethics.

Audiologists provide comprehensive diagnostic and treatment/rehabilitative services for auditory, vestibular, and related impairments. These services are provided to individuals across the entire age span from birth through adulthood; to individuals from diverse language, ethnic, cultural, and socioeconomic backgrounds; and to individuals who have multiple disabilities. This position statement is not intended to be exhaustive; however, the activities described reflect current practice within the profession. Practice activities related to emerging clinical, technological, and scientific developments are not precluded from consideration as part of the scope of practice of an audiologist. Such innovations and advances will result in the periodic revision and updating of this document. It is also recognized that specialty areas identified within the scope of practice will vary among the individual providers. ASHA also recognizes that credentialed professionals in related fields may have knowledge, skills, and experience that could be applied to some areas within the scope of audiology practice. Defining the scope of practice of audiologists is not meant to exclude other appropriately credentialed postgraduate professionals from rendering services in common practice areas.

Audiologists serve diverse populations. The patient/client population includes persons of different race, age, gender, religion, national origin, and sexual orientation. Audiologists' caseloads include individuals from diverse ethnic, cultural, or linguistic backgrounds, and persons with disabilities. Although audiologists are prohibited from discriminating in the provision of professional services based on these factors, in some cases such factors may be relevant to the development of an appropriate treatment plan. These factors may be considered in treatment plans only when firmly grounded in scientific and professional knowledge.

This scope of practice does not supersede existing state licensure laws or affect the interpretation or implementation of such laws. It may serve, however, as a model for the development or modification of licensure laws.

The schema in Figure 1A–1 depicts the relationship of the scope of practice to ASHA's policy documents that address current and emerging audiology practice areas; that is, preferred practice patterns, guidelines, and position statements. ASHA members and ASHA-certified professionals are bound by the ASHA Code of Ethics to provide services that are consistent with the scope of their competence, education, and experience (ASHA, 2003). There are other existing legislative and regulatory bodies that govern the practice of audiology.

FRAMEWORK FOR PRACTICE

The practice of audiology includes both the prevention of and assessment of auditory, vestibular, and related

SOURCE: Reprinted with permission from Scope of Practice in Audiology. Available from http://www.asha.org/policy.

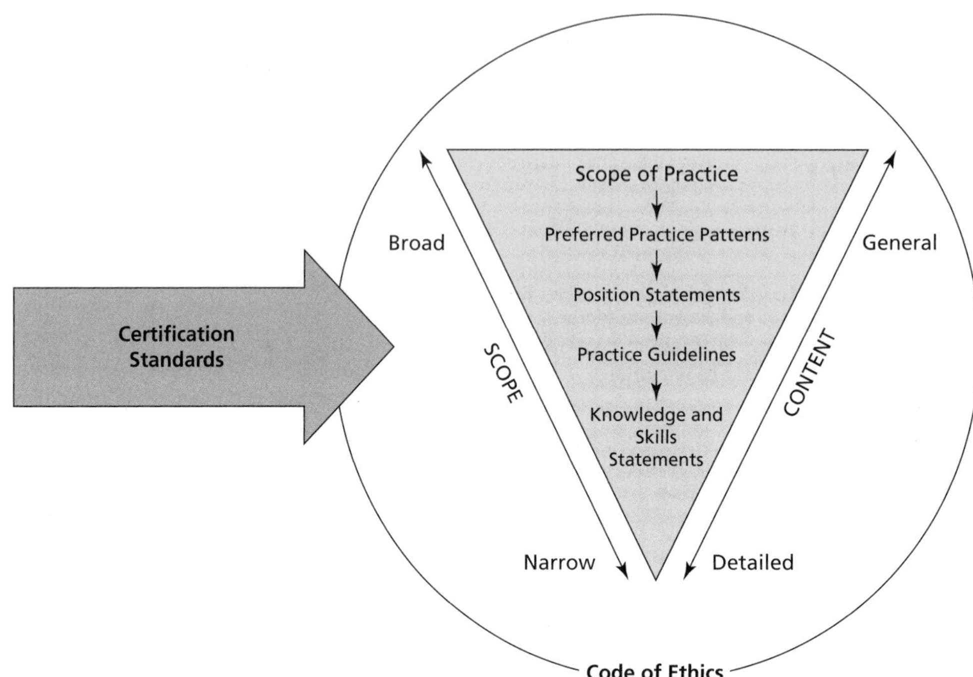

FIGURE 1A–1 Conceptual framework of ASHA standards and policy statements.
Reprinted with permission from Scope of Practice in Audiology. Available from http://www.asha.org/policy. Copyright 2004 by American Speech-Language-Hearing Association. All rights reserved.

impairments as well as the habilitation/rehabilitation and maintenance of persons with these impairments. The overall goal of the provision of audiology services should be to optimize and enhance the ability of an individual to hear, as well as to communicate in his/her everyday or natural environment. In addition, audiologists provide comprehensive services to individuals with normal hearing who interact with persons with a hearing impairment. The overall goal of audiologic services is to improve the quality of life for all of these individuals.

The World Health Organization (WHO) has developed a multipurpose health classification system known as the International Classification of Functioning, Disability, and Health (ICF) (WHO, 2001). The purpose of this classification system is to provide a standard language and framework for the description of functioning and health. The ICF framework is useful in describing the role of audiologists in the prevention, assessment, and habilitation/rehabilitation of auditory, vestibular, and other related impairments and restrictions or limitations of functioning.

The ICF is organized into two parts. The first part deals with Functioning and Disability while the second part deals with Contextual Factors. Each part has two components. The components of Functioning and Disability are:

- **Body Functions and Structures:** Body Functions are the physiological functions of body systems and Body Structures are the anatomical parts of the body and their components. Impairments are limitations or variations in Body Function or Structure such as a deviation or loss. An example of a Body Function that might be evaluated by an audiologist would be hearing sensitivity. The use of typanometry to access the mobility of the tympanic membrane is an example of a Body Structure that might be evaluated by an audiologist.

SOURCE: Reprinted with permission from Scope of Practice in Audiology. Available from http://www.asha.org/policy. Copyright 2004 by American Speech-Language-Hearing Association. All rights reserved.

- **Activity/Participation:** In the ICF, Activity and Participation are realized as one list. Activity refers to the execution of a task or action by an individual. Participation is the involvement in a life situation. Activity limitations are difficulties an individual may experience while executing a given activity. Participation restrictions are difficulties that may limit an individual's involvement in life situations. The Activity/Participation construct thus represents the effects that hearing, vestibular, and related impairments could have on the life of an individual. These effects could include the ability to hold conversations, participate in sports, attend religious services, understand a teacher in a classroom, and walk up and down stairs.

The components of Contextual Factors are:

- **Environmental Factors:** Environmental Factors make up the physical, social, and attitudinal environment in which people live and conduct their lives. Examples of Environmental Factors, as they relate to audiology, include the acoustical properties of a given space and any type of hearing assistive technology.
- **Personal Factors:** Personal Factors are the internal influences on an individual's functioning and disability and are not a part of the health condition. These factors may include but are not limited to age, gender, social background, and profession.

Functioning and Disability are interactive and evolutionary processes. Figure 1A–2 illustrates the interaction of the various components of the ICF.

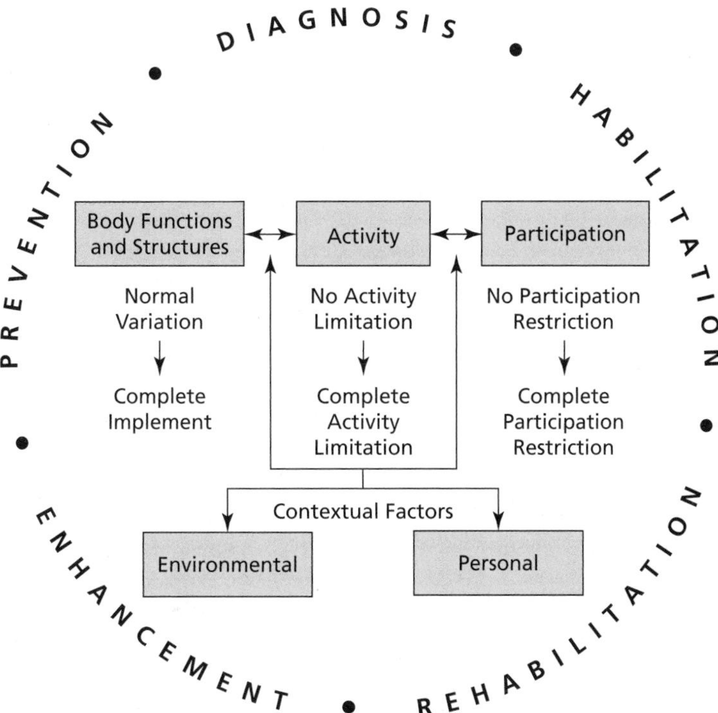

FIGURE 1A–2 Application of WHO (2001) framework to the practice of audiology.

Each component of the ICF can be expressed on a continuum of function. On one end of the continuum is intact functioning. At the opposite end of the continuum is completely compromised functioning. Contextual Factors (Environmental and Personal Factors) may interact with any of the components of functioning and disability. Environmental and Personal Factors may act as facilitators or barriers to functioning.

The scope of practice in audiology encompasses all of the components of the ICF. During the assessment phase, audiologists perform tests of Body Function and Structure. Examples of these types of tests include otoscopic examination, pure-tone audiometry, tympanometry, otoacoustic emissions measurements, and speech audiometry. Activity/Participation limitations and restrictions are sometimes addressed by audiologists through case history, interview, questionnaire, and counseling. For example, a question such as "Do you have trouble understanding while on the telephone?" or "Can you describe the difficulties you experience when you participate in a conversation with someone who is not familiar to you?" would be considered an assessment of Activity/Participation limitation or restriction. Questionnaires that require clients to report the magnitude of difficulty that they experience in certain specified settings can sometimes be used to measure aspects of Activity/Participation. For example: "Because of my hearing problems, I have difficulty conversing with others in a restaurant." In addition, Environmental and Personal Factors also need to be taken into consideration by audiologists as they treat individuals with auditory, vestibular, and other related impairments. In the above question regarding conversation in a restaurant, if the factor of "noise" (i.e., a noisy restaurant) is added to the question, this represents an Environmental Factor. Examples of Personal Factors might include a person's background or culture that influences his or her reaction to the use of a hearing aid or cochlear implant. The use of the ICF framework (WHO, 2001) may help audiologists broaden their perspective concerning their role in evaluating a client's needs or when designing and providing comprehensive services to their clients. Overall, audiologists work to improve quality of life by reducing impairments of body functions and structures, Activity limitations/Participation restrictions and Environmental barriers of the individuals they serve.

DEFINITION OF AN AUDIOLOGIST

Audiologists are professionals engaged in autonomous practice to promote healthy hearing, communication competency, and quality of life for persons of all ages through the prevention, identification, assessment, and rehabilitation of hearing, auditory function, balance, and other related systems. They facilitate prevention through the fitting of hearing protective devices, education programs for industry and the public, hearing screening/conservation programs, and research. The audiologist is the professional responsible for the identification of impairments and dysfunction of the auditory, balance, and other related systems. Their unique education and training provides them with the skills to assess and diagnose dysfunction in hearing, auditory function, balance, and related disorders. The delivery of audiologic (re)habilitation services includes not only the selecting, fitting, and dispensing of hearing aids and other hearing assistive devices, but also the assessment and follow-up services for persons with cochlear implants. The audiologist providing audiologic (re) habilitation does so through a comprehensive program of therapeutic services, devices, counseling, and other management strategies. Functional diagnosis of vestibular disorders and management of balance rehabilitation is another aspect of the professional responsibilities of the audiologist. Audiologists engage in research pertinent to all of these domains.

Audiologists currently hold a master's or doctoral degree in audiology from a program accredited by the Council on Academic Accreditation in Audiology and Speech-Language Pathology (CAA) of the American Speech-Language-Hearing Association. ASHA-certified audiologists complete a supervised postgraduate professional experience or a similar supervised professional experience during the completion of the doctoral degree as described in the ASHA certification standards. Beginning January 1, 2012, all applicants for the Certificate of Clinical Competence in Audiology must have a doctoral degree from a CAA-accredited university program. Demonstration of continued professional development is mandated for the maintenance of the Certificate of Clinical Competence in Audiology. Where required, audiologists are licensed or registered by the state in which they practice.

PROFESSIONAL ROLES AND ACTIVITIES

Audiologists serve a diverse population and may function in one or more of a variety of activities. The practice of audiology includes:

A. Prevention
   1. Promotion of hearing wellness, as well as the prevention of hearing loss and protection of hearing function by designing, implementing, and coordinating occupational, school, and community hearing conservation and identification programs;
   2. Participation in noise measurements of the acoustic environment to improve accessibility and to promote hearing wellness.

B. Identification
   1. Activities that identify dysfunction in hearing, balance, and other auditory-related systems;
   2. Supervision, implementation, and follow-up of newborn and school hearing screening programs;
   3. Screening for speech, orofacial myofunctional disorders, language, cognitive communication disorders, and/or preferred communication modalities that may affect education, health, development or communication and may result in recommendations for rescreening or comprehensive speech-language pathology assessment or in referral for other examinations or services;
   4. Identification of populations and individuals with or at risk for hearing loss and other auditory dysfunction, balance impairments, tinnitus, and associated communication impairments as well as of those with normal hearing;
   5. In collaboration with speech-language pathologists, identification of populations and individuals at risk for developing speech-language impairments.

C. Assessment
   1. The conduct and interpretation of behavioral, electroacoustic, and/or electrophysiologic methods to assess hearing, auditory function, balance, and related systems;
   2. Measurement and interpretation of sensory and motor evoked potentials, electromyography, and other electrodiagnostic tests for purposes of neurophysiologic intraoperative monitoring and cranial nerve assessment;
   3. Evaluation and management of children and adults with auditory-related processing disorders;
   4. Performance of otoscopy for appropriate audiological management or to provide a basis for medical referral;
   5. Cerumen management to prevent obstruction of the external ear canal and of amplification devices;
   6. Preparation of a report including interpreting data, summarizing findings, generating recommendations and developing an audiologic treatment/management plan;
   7. Referrals to other professions, agencies, and/or consumer organizations.

D. Rehabilitation
   1. As part of the comprehensive audiologic (re) habilitation program, evaluates, selects, fits and dispenses hearing assistive technology devices to include hearing aids;
   2. Assessment of candidacy of persons with hearing loss for cochlear implants and provision of fitting, mapping, and audiologic rehabilitation to optimize device use;
   3. Development of a culturally appropriate, audiologic rehabilitative management plan including, when appropriate:
      a. Recommendations for fitting and dispensing, and educating the consumer and family/caregivers in the use of and adjustment to sensory aids, hearing assistive devices, alerting systems, and captioning devices;
      b. Availability of counseling relating to psycho social aspects of hearing loss, and other auditory dysfunction, and processes to enhance communication competence;
      c. Skills training and consultation concerning environmental modifications to facilitate development of receptive and expressive communication;
      d. Evaluation and modification of the audiologic management plan.

SOURCE: Reprinted with permission from Scope of Practice in Audiology. Available from http://www.asha.org/policy.

4. Provision of comprehensive audiologic rehabilitation services, including management procedures for speech and language habilitation and/or rehabilitation for persons with hearing loss or other auditory dysfunction, including but not exclusive to speechreading, auditory training, communication strategies, manual communication and counseling for psychosocial adjustment for persons with hearing loss or other auditory dysfunction and their families/caregivers;
5. Consultation and provision of vestibular and balance rehabilitation therapy to persons with vestibular and balance impairments;
6. Assessment and non-medical management of tinnitus using biofeedback, behavioral management, masking, hearing aids, education, and counseling;
7. Provision of training for professionals of related and/or allied services when needed;
8. Participation in the development of an Individual Education Program (IEP) for school-age children or an Individual Family Service Plan (IFSP) for children from birth to 36 months old;
9. Provision of in-service programs for school personnel, and advising school districts in planning educational programs and accessibility for students with hearing loss and other auditory dysfunction;
10. Measurement of noise levels and provision of recommendations for environmental modifications in order to reduce the noise level;
11. Management of the selection, purchase, installation, and evaluation of large-area amplification systems.

E. Advocacy/ Consultation

1. Advocacy for communication needs of all individuals that may include advocating for the rights/funding of services for those with hearing loss, auditory, or vestibular disorders;
2. Advocacy for issues (i.e., acoustic accessibility) that affect the rights of individuals with normal hearing;
3. Consultation with professionals of related and/or allied services when needed;
4. Consultation in development of an Individual Education Program (IEP) for school-age children or an Individual Family Service Plan (IFSP) for children from birth to 36 months old;
5. Consultation to educators as members of interdisciplinary teams about communication management, educational implications of hearing loss and other auditory dysfunction, educational programming, classroom acoustics, and large-area amplification systems for children with hearing loss and other auditory dysfunction;
6. Consultation about accessibility for persons with hearing loss and other auditory dysfunction in public and private buildings, programs, and services;
7. Consultation to individuals, public and private agencies, and governmental bodies, or as an expert witness regarding legal interpretations of audiology findings, effects of hearing loss and other auditory dysfunction, balance system impairments, and relevant noise-related considerations;
8. Case management and service as a liaison for the consumer, family, and agencies in order to monitor audiologic status and management and to make recommendations about educational and vocational programming;
9. Consultation to industry on the development of products and instrumentation related to the measurement and management of auditory or balance function.

F. Education/Research/Administration

1. Education, supervision, and administration for audiology graduate and other professional education programs;
2. Measurement of functional outcomes, consumer satisfaction, efficacy, effectiveness, and efficiency of practices and programs to maintain and improve the quality of audiologic services;
3. Design and conduct of basic and applied audiologic research to increase the knowledge base, to develop new methods and programs, and to determine the efficacy, effectiveness, and efficiency of assessment and treatment paradigms; disseminate research findings to other professionals and to the public;

SOURCE: Reprinted with permission from Scope of Practice in Audiology. Available from http://www.asha.org/policy.

4. Participation in the development of professional and technical standards;
5. Participation in quality improvement programs;
6. Program administration and supervision of professionals as well as support personnel.

PRACTICE SETTINGS

Audiologists provide services in private practice; medical settings such as hospitals and physicians' offices; community and university hearing and speech centers; managed care systems; industry; the military; various state agencies; home health, subacute rehabilitation, long-term care, and intermediate-care facilities; and school systems. Audiologists provide academic education to students and practitioners in universities, to medical and surgical students and residents, and to other related professionals. Such education pertains to the identification, functional diagnosis/assessment, and non-medical treatment/management of auditory, vestibular, balance, and related impairments.

REFERENCES

American Speech-Language-Hearing Association. (1996, Spring). Scope of practice in audiology. *ASHA, 38*(Suppl. 16), 12–15.

American Speech-Language-Hearing Association. (2003). Code of ethics (revised). *ASHA Supplement, 23*, 13–15.

World Health Organization (WHO). (2001). *ICF: International classification of functioning, disability and health*. Geneva, Switzerland: Author.

RESOURCES

General

American Speech-Language-Hearing Association. (1979, March). Severely hearing handicapped. *ASHA, 21*.

American Speech-Language-Hearing Association. (1985, June). Clinical supervision in speech-language pathology and audiology. *ASHA, 27*, 57–60.

American Speech-Language-Hearing Association. (1986, May). Autonomy of speech-language pathology and audiology. *ASHA, 28*, 53–57.

American Speech-Language-Hearing Association. (1987, June). Calibration of speech signals delivered via earphones. *ASHA, 29*, 44–48.

American Speech-Language-Hearing Association. (1988). *Mental retardation and developmental disabilities curriculum guide for speech-language pathologists and audiologists*. Rockville, MD: Author.

American Speech-Language-Hearing Association. (1989, March). Bilingual speech-language pathologists and audiologists: Definition. *ASHA, 31*, 93.

American Speech-Language-Hearing Association. (1989, June/July). AIDS/HIV: Implications for speech-language pathologists and audiologists. *ASHA, 31*, 33–38.

American Speech-Language-Hearing Association. (1990). The role of speech-language pathologists and audiologists in service delivery for persons with mental retardation and developmental disabilities in community settings. *ASHA, 32* (Suppl. 2), 5–6.

American Speech-Language-Hearing Association. (1990, April). Major issues affecting delivery of services in hospital settings: Recommendations and strategies. *ASHA, 32*, 67–70.

American Speech-Language-Hearing Association. (1991). Sound field measurement tutorial. *ASHA, 33* (Suppl. 3), 25–37.

SOURCE: Reprinted with permission from Scope of Practice in Audiology. Available from http://www.asha.org/policy.

American Speech-Language-Hearing Association. (1992). 1992 U.S. Department of Labor definition of speech-language pathologists and audiologists. *ASHA, 4*, 563–565.

American Speech-Language-Hearing Association. (1992, March). Sedation and topical anesthetics in audiology and speech-language pathology. *ASHA, 34* (Suppl. 7), 41–42.

American Speech-Language-Hearing Association. (1993). National health policy: Back to the future (technical report). *ASHA, 35* (Suppl. 10), 2–10.

American Speech-Language-Hearing Association. (1993). Position statement on national health policy. *ASHA, 35* (Suppl. 10), 1.

American Speech-Language-Hearing Association. (1993). Professional performance appraisal by individuals outside the professions of speech-language pathology and audiology. *ASHA, 35* (Suppl. 10), 11–13.

American Speech-Language-Hearing Association. (1994, January). The protection of rights of people receiving audiology or speech-language pathology services. *ASHA, 36*, 60–63.

American Speech-Language-Hearing Association. (1994, March). Guidelines for the audiologic management of individuals receiving cochleotoxic drug therapy. *ASHA, 36* (Suppl. 12), 11–19.

American Speech-Language-Hearing Association. (1995, March). Guidelines for education in audiology practice management. *ASHA, 37* (Suppl. 14), 20.

American Speech-Language-Hearing Association. (1997). *Preferred practice patterns for the profession of audiology*. Rockville, MD: Author.

American Speech-Language-Hearing Association. (1997, Spring). Position statement: Multiskilled personnel. *ASHA, 39* (Suppl. 17), 13.

American Speech-Language-Hearing Association. (1998). Position statement and guidelines on support personnel in audiology. *ASHA, 40* (Suppl. 18), 19–21.

American Speech-Language-Hearing Association. (2001). *Scope of practice in speech-language pathology*. Rockville, MD: Author.

American Speech-Language-Hearing Association. (2002). *Certification and membership handbook: Audiology*. Rockville, MD: Author.

American Speech-Language-Hearing Association. (2003). Code of ethics (revised). *ASHA Supplement 23*, 13–15.

Joint Audiology Committee on Clinical Practice. (1999). *Clinical practice statements and algorithms*. Rockville, MD: American Speech-Language-Hearing Association.

Joint Committee of the American Speech-Language-Hearing Association (ASHA) and the Council on Education of the Deaf (CED). (1998). Hearing loss: Terminology and classification: Position statement and technical report. *ASHA, 40* (Suppl. 18), 22.

Paul-Brown, Diane. (1994, May). Clinical record keeping in audiology and speech pathology. *ASHA, 36*, 40–43.

Amplification

American Speech-Language-Hearing Association. (1991). Amplification as a remediation technique for children with normal peripheral hearing. *ASHA, 33* (Suppl. 3), 22–24.

American Speech-Language-Hearing Association. (1998). Guidelines for hearing aid fitting for adults. *American Journal of Audiology, 7*(1), 5–13.

American Speech-Language-Hearing Association. (2000). Guidelines for graduate education in amplification. *ASHA Supplement, 20*, 22–27.

American Speech-Language-Hearing Association. (2002). Guidelines for fitting and monitoring FM systems. *ASHA Desk Reference, 2*, 151–172.

American Speech-Language Hearing Association. (2004). Technical report: Cochlear implants in press. *ASHA Supplement, 24*.

Audiologic Rehabilitation

American Speech-Language-Hearing Association. (1981, April). On the definition of hearing handicap. *ASHA, 23*, 293–297.

American Speech-Language-Hearing Association. (1984, May). Definition of and competencies for aural rehabilitation. *ASHA, 26*, 37–41.

American Speech-Language-Hearing Association. (1990). Aural rehabilitation: An annotated bibliography. *ASHA, 32* (Suppl. 1), 1–12.

SOURCE: Reprinted with permission from Scope of Practice in Audiology. Available from http://www.asha.org/policy.

American Speech-Language-Hearing Association. (1992, March). Electrical stimulation for cochlear implant selection and rehabilitation. *ASHA, 34* (Suppl. 7), 13–16.

American Speech-Language-Hearing Association. (2001). *ARBIB: Audiologic rehabilitation—basic information bibliography*. Rockville, MD: Author.

American Speech-Language-Hearing Association. (2001). *Knowledge and skills required for the practice of audiologic/aural rehabilitation*. Rockville, MD: Author.

Audiologic Screening

American Speech-Language-Hearing Association. (1988, November). Telephone hearing screening. *ASHA, 30*, 53.

American Speech-Language-Hearing Association. (1994, June/July). Audiologic screening (Executive summary). *ASHA, 36*, 53–54.

American Speech-Language-Hearing Association Audiologic Assessment Panel 1996. (1997). *Guidelines for audiologic screening*. Rockville, MD: Author.

(Central) Auditory Processing Disorders

American Speech-Language-Hearing Association. (1979, December). The role of the speech-language pathologist and audiologist in learning disabilities. *ASHA, 21*, 1015.

American Speech-Language-Hearing Association. (1990). Audiological assessment of central auditory processing: An annotated bibliography. *ASHA, 32* (Suppl. 1), 13–30.

American Speech-Language-Hearing Association. (1996, July). Central auditory processing: Current status of research and implications for clinical practice. *American Journal of Audiology, 5*(2), 41–54.

Business Practices

American Speech-Language-Hearing Association. (1987, March). Private practice. *ASHA, 29*, 35.

American Speech-Language-Hearing Association. (1991). Business, marketing, ethics, and professionalism in audiology: An updated annotated bibliography (1986–1989). *ASHA, 33* (Suppl. 3), 39–45.

American Speech-Language-Hearing Association. (1991). Considerations for establishing a private practice in audiology and/or speech-language pathology. *ASHA, 33* (Suppl. 3), 10–21.

American Speech-Language-Hearing Association. (1991). Report on private practice. *ASHA, 33* (Suppl. 6), 1–4.

American Speech-Language-Hearing Association. (1994, March). Professional liability and risk management for the audiology and special-language pathology professions. *ASHA, 36* (Suppl. 12), 25–38.

Diagnostic Procedures

American Speech-Language-Hearing Association. (1978). Guidelines for manual pure-tone threshold audiometry. *ASHA, 20*, 297–301.

American Speech-Language-Hearing Association. (1988, March). Guidelines for determining threshold level for speech. *ASHA*, 85–89.

American Speech-Language-Hearing Association. (1988, November). Tutorial: Tympanometry. *Journal of Speech and Hearing Disorders, 53*, 354–377.

American Speech-Language-Hearing Association. (1990). Guidelines for audiometric symbols. *ASHA, 32* (Suppl. 2), 25–30.

American Speech-Language-Hearing Association. (1991). Acoustic-immittance measures: A bibliography. *ASHA, 33* (Suppl. 4), 1–44.

American Speech-Language-Hearing Association. (1992, March). External auditory canal examination and cerumen management. *ASHA, 34* (Suppl. 7), 22–24.

Educational Audiology

American Speech-Language-Hearing Association. (1991). Utilization of Medicaid and other third party funds for covered services in the schools. *ASHA, 33* (Suppl. 5), 51–59.

American Speech-Language-Hearing Association. (1995, March). Acoustics in educational settings: Position statement and guidelines. *ASHA, 37* (Suppl. 14), 15–19.

American Speech-Language-Hearing Association. (1997). Trends and issues in school reform and their effects on speech-language pathologists, audiologists, and students with communication disorders. *ASHA Desk Reference, 4, 317–326.*

American Speech-Language-Hearing Association. (1997, Spring). Position statement: Roles of audiologists and speech-language-pathologists working with persons with attention deficit hyperactivity disorder: Position statement and technical report. *ASHA, 39* (Suppl. 17), 14.

American Speech-Language-Hearing Association. (2002). *Guidelines for audiology service provision in and for schools.* Rockville, MD: Author.

American Speech-Language-Hearing Association. (2002). Appropriate school facilities for students with speech-language-hearing disorders: Technical report. *ASHA Supplement 23,* 83–86.

Electrophysiological Assessment

American Speech-Language-Hearing Association. (1987). *Short latency auditory evoked potentials.* Rockville, MD: Author.

American Speech-Language-Hearing Association. (1992, March). Neurophysiologic intraoperative monitoring. *ASHA, 34* (Suppl. 7), 34–36.

American Speech-Language-Hearing Association. (2003). Guidelines for competencies in auditory evoked potential measurement and clinical applications. *ASHA Supplement 23,* 35–40.

Geriatric Audiology

American Speech-Language-Hearing Association. (1988, March). Provision of audiology and speech-language pathology services to older persons in nursing homes. *ASHA,* 772–774.

American Speech-Language-Hearing Association. (1988, March). The roles of speech-language pathologists and audiologists in working with older persons. *ASHA, 30,* 80–84.

American Speech-Language-Hearing Association. (1997, Spring). Guidelines for audiology service delivery in nursing homes. *ASHA, 39* (Suppl. 17), 15–29.

Occupational Audiology

American Speech-Language-Hearing Association. (1996, Spring). Guidelines on the audiologist's role in occupational and environmental hearing conservation. *ASHA, 38* (Suppl. 16), 34–41.

American Speech-Language-Hearing Association. (1997, Spring). Issues: Occupational and environmental hearing conservation. *ASHA, 39* (Suppl. 17), 30–34.

American Speech-Language-Hearing Association. (2004). The audiologist's role in occupational hearing conservation and hearing loss prevention programs in press. *ASHA Supplement 24.*

American Speech-Language-Hearing Association. (2004). The audiologist's role in occupational hearing conservation and hearing loss prevention programs: Technical report in press. *ASHA Supplement 24.*

Pediatric Audiology

American Speech-Language-Hearing Association. (1991). Guidelines for the audiological assessment of children from birth through 36 months of age. *ASHA, 33* (Suppl.5), 37–43.

American Speech-Language-Hearing Association. (1991). The use of FM amplification instruments for infants and preschool children with hearing impairment. *ASHA, 33* (Suppl. 5), 1–2.

American Speech-Language-Hearing Association. (1994, August). Service provision under the Individuals with Disabilities Education Act-Part H, as amended (IDEA-Part H) to children who are deaf and hard of hearing—ages birth to 36 months. *ASHA, 36,* 117–121.

Joint Committee on Infant Hearing. (2000). JCIH year 2000 position statement: Principles and guidelines for early hearing detection and intervention programs. *American Journal of Audiology, 9,* 9–29.

Vestibular

American Speech-Language-Hearing Association. (1992, March). Balance system assessment. *ASHA, 34* (Suppl. 7), 9–12.

American Speech-Language-Hearing Association. (1999, March). Role of audiologists in vestibular and balance rehabilitation: Position statement, guidelines, and technical report. *ASHA, 41* (Suppl. 19), 13–22.

SOURCE: Reprinted with permission from Scope of Practice in Audiology. Available from http://www.asha.org/policy.

Appendix 1-B

ASHA Scope of Practice in Speech-Language Pathology

INTRODUCTION

The *Scope of Practice in Speech-Language Pathology* includes a statement of purpose, a framework for research and clinical practice, qualifications of the speech-language pathologist, professional roles and activities, and practice settings. The speech-language pathologist is the professional who engages in clinical services, prevention, advocacy, education, administration, and research in the areas of communication and swallowing across the life span from infancy through geriatrics. Given the diversity of the client population, ASHA policy requires that these activities are conducted in a manner that takes into consideration the impact of culture and linguistic exposure/acquisition and uses the best available evidence for practice to ensure optimal outcomes for persons with communication and/or swallowing disorders or differences.

As part of the review process for updating the *Scope of Practice in Speech-Language Pathology*, the committee made changes to the previous scope of practice document that reflected recent advances in knowledge, understanding, and research in the discipline. These changes included acknowledging roles and responsibilities that were not mentioned in previous iterations of the *Scope of Practice* (e.g., funding issues, marketing of services, focus on emergency responsiveness, communication wellness). The revised document also was framed squarely on two guiding principles: evidence-based practice and cultural and linguistic diversity.

STATEMENT OF PURPOSE

The purpose of this document is to define the *Scope of Practice in Speech-Language Pathology* to

1. delineate areas of professional practice for speech-language pathologists;
2. inform others (e.g., health care providers, educators, other professionals, consumers, payers, regulators, members of the general public) about professional services offered by speech-language pathologists as qualified providers;
3. support speech-language pathologists in the provision of high-quality, evidence-based services to individuals with concerns about communication or swallowing;
4. support speech-language pathologists in the conduct of research; and
5. provide guidance for educational preparation and professional development of speech-language pathologists.

This document describes the breadth of professional practice offered within the profession of speech-language pathology. Levels of education, experience, skill, and proficiency with respect to the roles and activities identified within this scope of practice document vary among individual providers. A speech-language pathologist typically does not practice in all areas of the field. As the ASHA Code of Ethics specifies, individuals may practice only in areas in which they are competent (i.e., individuals' scope

SOURCE: Reprinted with permission from Scope of Practice in Speech-Language Pathology. Available from http://www.asha.org/policy.

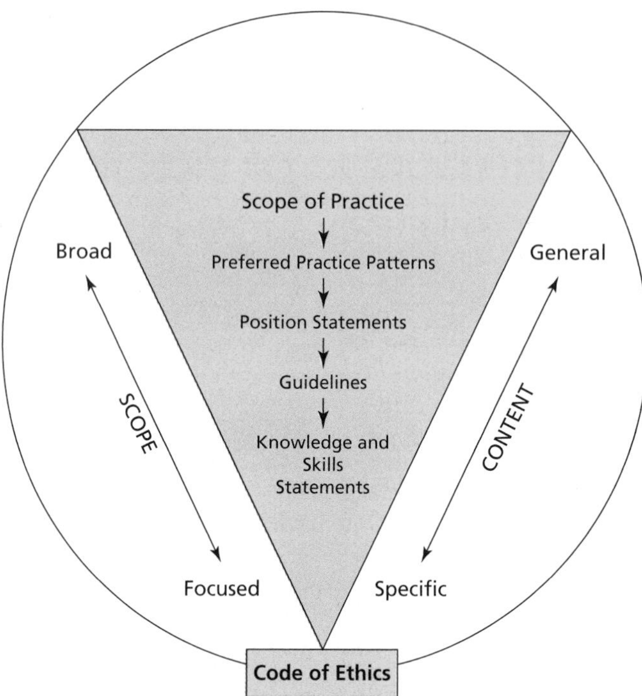

FIGURE 1B–1 Conceptual framework of ASHA practice documents

Reprinted with permission from Scope of Practice in Speech-Language Pathology. Available from http://www.asha.org/policy. Copyright 2007 by American Speech-Language-Hearing Association. All rights reserved.

of competency), based on their education, training, and experience.

In addition to this scope of practice document, other ASHA documents provide more specific guidance for practice areas. Figure 1B–1 illustrates the relationship between the ASHA Code of Ethics, the *Scope of Practice*, and specific practice documents. As shown, the ASHA Code of Ethics sets forth the fundamental principles and rules considered essential to the preservation of the highest standards of integrity and ethical conduct in the practice of speech-language pathology.

Speech-language pathology is a dynamic and continuously developing profession. As such, listing specific areas within this Scope of Practice does not exclude emerging areas of practice. Further, speech-language pathologists may provide additional professional services (e.g., interdisciplinary work in a health care setting, collaborative service delivery in schools, transdisciplinary practice in early intervention settings) that are necessary for the well-being of the individual(s) they are serving but are not addressed in this Scope of Practice. In such instances, it is both ethically and legally incumbent upon professionals to determine whether they have the knowledge and skills necessary to perform such services.

This scope of practice document does not supersede existing state licensure laws or affect the interpretation or implementation of such laws. It may serve, however, as a model for the development or modification of licensure laws.

FRAMEWORK FOR RESEARCH AND CLINICAL PRACTICE

The overall objective of speech-language pathology services is to optimize individuals' ability to communicate and swallow, thereby improving quality of life.

As the population profile of the United States continues to become increasingly diverse (U.S. Census Bureau, 2005), speech-language pathologists have a responsibility to be knowledgeable about the impact of these changes on clinical services and research needs. Speech-language pathologists are committed to the provision of culturally and linguistically appropriate services and to the consideration of diversity in scientific investigations of human communication and swallowing. For example, one aspect of providing culturally and linguistically appropriate services is to determine whether communication difficulties experienced by English language learners are the result of a communication disorder in the native language or a consequence of learning a new language.

Additionally, an important characteristic of the practice of speech-language pathology is that, to the extent possible, clinical decisions are based on best available evidence. ASHA has defined evidence-based practice in speech-language pathology as an approach in which current, high-quality research evidence is integrated with practitioner expertise and the individual's preferences and values into the process of clinical decision making (ASHA, 2005). A high-quality basic, applied, and efficacy research base in communication sciences and disorders and related fields of study is essential to providing evidence-based clinical practice and quality clinical services. The research base can be enhanced by increased interaction and communication with researchers across the United States and from other countries. As our global society is becoming more connected, integrated, and interdependent, speech-language pathologists have access to an abundant array of resources, information technology, and diverse perspectives and influence (e.g., Lombardo, 1997). Increased national and international interchange of professional knowledge, information, and education in communication sciences and disorders can be a means to strengthen research collaboration and improve clinical services.

The World Health Organization (WHO) has developed a multipurpose health classification system known as the International Classification of Functioning, Disability and Health (ICF; WHO, 2001). The purpose of this classification system is to provide a standard language and framework for the description of functioning and health. The ICF framework is useful in describing the breadth of the role of the speech-language pathologist in the prevention, assessment, and habilitation/rehabilitation, enhancement, and scientific investigation of communication and swallowing. It consists of two components:

1. Health Conditions
   a. Body Functions and Structures: These involve the anatomy and physiology of the human body. Relevant examples in speech-language pathology include craniofacial anomaly, vocal fold paralysis, cerebral palsy, stuttering, and language impairment.
   b. Activity and Participation: Activity refers to the execution of a task or action. Participation is the involvement in a life situation. Relevant examples in speech-language pathology include difficulties with swallowing safely for independent feeding, participating actively in class, understanding a medical prescription, and accessing the general education curriculum.
2. Contextual Factors
   a. Environmental Factors: These make up the physical, social, and attitudinal environments in which people live and conduct their lives. Relevant examples in speech-language pathology include the role of the communication partner in augmentative and alternative communication, the influence of classroom acoustics on communication, and the impact of institutional dining environments on individuals' ability to safely maintain nutrition and hydration.
   b. Personal Factors: These are the internal influences on an individual's functioning and disability and are not part of the health condition. These factors may include, but are not limited to, age, gender, ethnicity, educational level, social background, and profession. Relevant examples in speech-language pathology might include a person's background or culture that influences his or her reaction to a communication or swallowing *disorder.*

The framework in speech-language pathology encompasses these health conditions and contextual factors. The health condition component of the ICF can be expressed on a continuum of functioning. On one end of the continuum is intact functioning. At the opposite end of the continuum is completely compromised functioning. The

SOURCE: Reprinted with permission from Scope of Practice in Speech-Language Pathology. Available from http://www.asha.org/policy.

contextual factors interact with each other and with the health conditions and may serve as facilitators or barriers to functioning. Speech-language pathologists may influence contextual factors through education and advocacy efforts at local, state, and national levels. Relevant examples in speech-language pathology include a user of an augmentative communication device needing classroom support services for academic success, or the effects of premorbid literacy level on rehabilitation in an adult post brain injury. Speech-language pathologists work to improve quality of life by reducing impairments of body functions and structures, activity limitations, participation restrictions, and barriers created by contextual factors.

QUALIFICATIONS

Speech-language pathologists, as defined by ASHA, hold the ASHA Certificate of Clinical Competence in Speech-Language Pathology (CCC-SLP), which requires a master's, doctoral, or other recognized postbaccalaureate degree. ASHA-certified speech-language pathologists complete a supervised postgraduate professional experience and pass a national examination as described in the ASHA certification standards. Demonstration of continued professional development is mandated for the maintenance of the CCC-SLP. Where applicable, speech-language pathologists hold other required credentials (e.g., state licensure, teaching certification).

This document defines the scope of practice for the field of speech-language pathology. Each practitioner must evaluate his or her own experiences with preservice education, clinical practice, mentorship and supervision, and continuing professional development. As a whole, these experiences define the scope of competence for each individual. Speech-language pathologists may engage in only those aspects of the profession that are within their scope of competence.

As primary care providers for communication and swallowing disorders, speech-language pathologists are autonomous professionals; that is, their services are not prescribed or supervised by another professional. However, individuals frequently benefit from services that include speech-language pathologist collaborations with other professionals.

PROFESSIONAL ROLES AND ACTIVITIES

Speech-language pathologists serve individuals, families, and groups from diverse linguistic and cultural backgrounds. Services are provided based on applying the best available research evidence, using expert clinical judgments, and considering clients' individual preferences and values. Speech-language pathologists address typical and atypical communication and swallowing in the following areas:

- speech sound production
    - articulation
    - apraxia of speech
    - dysarthria
    - ataxia
    - dyskinesia
- resonance
    - hypernasality
    - hyponasality
    - cul-de-sac resonance
    - mixed resonance
- voice
    - phonation quality
    - pitch
    - loudness
    - respiration
- fluency
    - stuttering
    - cluttering
- language (comprehension and expression)
    - phonology
    - morphology
    - syntax
    - semantics
    - pragmatics (language use, social aspects of communication)
    - literacy (reading, writing, spelling)

SOURCE: Reprinted with permission from Scope of Practice in Speech-Language Pathology. Available from http://www.asha.org/policy.

  - prelinguistic communication (e.g., joint attention, intentionality, communicative signaling)
  - paralinguistic communication
- cognition
  - attention
  - memory
  - sequencing
  - problem solving
  - executive functioning
- feeding and swallowing
  - oral, pharyngeal, laryngeal, esophageal
  - orofacial myology (including tongue thrust)
  - oral-motor functions

Potential etiologies of communication and swallowing disorders include:

- neonatal problems (e.g., prematurity, low birth weight, substance exposure);
- developmental disabilities (e.g., specific language impairment, autism spectrum disorder, dyslexia, learning disabilities, attention deficit disorder);
- auditory problems (e.g., hearing loss or deafness);
- oral anomalies (e.g., cleft lip/palate, dental malocclusion, macroglossia, oral-motor dysfunction);
- respiratory compromise (e.g., bronchopulmonary dysplasia, chronic obstructive pulmonary disease);
- pharyngeal anomalies (e.g., upper airway obstruction, velopharyngeal insufficiency/incompetence);
- laryngeal anomalies (e.g., vocal fold pathology, tracheal stenosis, tracheostomy);
- neurological disease/dysfunction (e.g., traumatic brain injury, cerebral palsy, cerebral vascular accident, dementia, Parkinson's disease, amyotrophic lateral sclerosis);
- psychiatric disorder (e.g., psychosis, schizophrenia); and
- genetic disorders (e.g., Down syndrome, fragile X syndrome, Rett syndrome, velocardiofacial syndrome).

The professional roles and activities in speech-language pathology include clinical/educational services (diagnosis, assessment, planning, and treatment), prevention and advocacy, and education, administration, and research.

CLINICAL SERVICES

Speech-language pathologists provide clinical services that include the following:

- prevention and pre-referral
- screening
- assessment/evaluation
- consultation
- diagnosis
- treatment, intervention, management
- counseling
- collaboration
- documentation
- referral

Examples of these clinical services include:

1. using data to guide clinical decision making and determine the effectiveness of services;
2. making service delivery decisions (e.g., admission/eligibility, frequency, duration, location, discharge/dismissal) across the lifespan;
3. determining appropriate context(s) for service delivery (e.g., home, school, telepractice, community);
4. documenting provision of services in accordance with accepted procedures appropriate for the practice setting;
5. collaborating with other professionals (e.g., identifying neonates and infants at risk for hearing loss, participating in palliative care teams, planning lessons with educators, serving on student assistance teams);
6. screening individuals for hearing loss or middle ear pathology using conventional pure-tone air conduction methods (including otoscopic inspection), otoacoustic emissions screening, and/or screening tympanometry;
7. providing intervention and support services for children and adults diagnosed with speech and language disorders;

SOURCE: Reprinted with permission from Scope of Practice in Speech-Language Pathology. Available from http://www.asha.org/policy.

8. providing intervention and support services for children and adults diagnosed with auditory processing disorders;
9. using instrumentation (e.g., videofluoroscopy, electromyography, nasendoscopy, stroboscopy, endoscopy, nasometry, computer technology) to observe, collect data, and measure parameters of communication and swallowing or other upper aerodigestive functions;
10. counseling individuals, families, coworkers, educators, and other persons in the community regarding acceptance, adaptation, and decision making about communication and swallowing;
11. facilitating the process of obtaining funding for equipment and services related to difficulties with communication and swallowing;
12. serving as case managers, service delivery coordinators, and members of collaborative teams (e.g., individualized family service plan and individualized education program teams, transition planning teams);
13. providing referrals and information to other professionals, agencies, and/or consumer organizations;
14. developing, selecting, and prescribing multimodal augmentative and alternative communication systems, including unaided strategies (e.g., manual signs, gestures) and aided strategies (e.g., speech-generating devices, manual communication boards, picture schedules);
15. providing services to individuals with hearing loss and their families/caregivers (e.g., auditory training for children with cochlear implants and hearing aids; speechreading; speech and language intervention secondary to hearing loss; visual inspection and listening checks of amplification devices for the purpose of troubleshooting, including verification of appropriate battery voltage);
16. addressing behaviors (e.g., perseverative or disruptive actions) and environments (e.g., classroom seating, positioning for swallowing safety or attention, communication opportunities) that affect communication and swallowing;
17. selecting, fitting, and establishing effective use of prosthetic/adaptive devices for communication and swallowing (e.g., tracheoesophageal prostheses, speaking valves, electrolarynges; this service does not include the selection or fitting of sensory devices used by individuals with hearing loss or other auditory perceptual deficits, which falls within the scope of practice of audiologists; ASHA, 2004); and
18. providing services to modify or enhance communication performance (e.g., accent modification, transgender voice, care and improvement of the professional voice, personal/professional communication effectiveness).

PREVENTION AND ADVOCACY

Speech-language pathologists engage in prevention and advocacy activities related to human communication and swallowing. Example activities include:

1. improving communication wellness by promoting healthy lifestyle practices that can help prevent communication and swallowing disorders (e.g., cessation of smoking, wearing helmets when bike riding);
2. presenting primary prevention information to individuals and groups known to be at risk for communication disorders and other appropriate groups;
3. providing early identification and early intervention services for communication disorders;
4. advocating for individuals and families through community awareness, health literacy, education, and training programs to promote and facilitate access to full participation in communication, including the elimination of societal, cultural, and linguistic barriers;
5. advising regulatory and legislative agencies on emergency responsiveness to individuals who have communication and swallowing disorders or difficulties;
6. promoting and marketing professional services;
7. advocating at the local, state, and national levels for improved administrative and governmental policies affecting access to services for communication and swallowing;
8. advocating at the local, state, and national levels for funding for research;

SOURCE: Reprinted with permission from Scope of Practice in Speech-Language Pathology. Available from http://www.asha.org/policy.

9. recruiting potential speech-language pathologists into the profession; and
10. participating actively in professional organizations to contribute to best practices in the profession.

EDUCATION, ADMINISTRATION, AND RESEARCH

Speech-language pathologists also serve as educators, administrators, and researchers. Example activities for these roles include:

1. educating the public regarding communication and swallowing;
2. educating and providing in-service training to families, caregivers, and other professionals;
3. educating, supervising, and mentoring current and future speech-language pathologists;
4. educating, supervising, and managing speech-language pathology assistants and other support personnel;
5. fostering public awareness of communication and swallowing disorders and their treatment;
6. serving as expert witnesses;
7. administering and managing clinical and academic programs;
8. developing policies, operational procedures, and professional standards; and
9. conducting basic and applied/translational research related to communication sciences and disorders, and swallowing.

PRACTICE SETTINGS

Speech-language pathologists provide services in a wide variety of settings, which may include but are not exclusive to:

1. public and private schools;
2. early intervention settings, preschools, and day care centers;
3. health care settings (e.g., hospitals, medical rehabilitation facilities, long-term care facilities, home health agencies, clinics, neonatal intensive care units, behavioral/mental health facilities);
4. private practice settings;
5. universities and university clinics;
6. individuals' homes and community residences;
7. supported and competitive employment settings;
8. community, state, and federal agencies and institutions;
9. correctional institutions;
10. research facilities; or
11. corporate and industrial settings.

REFERENCES

American Speech-Language-Hearing Association. (2004). *Scope of practice in audiology*. Available from http://www.asha.org/policy

American Speech-Language-Hearing Association. (2005). *Evidence-based practice in communication disorders* [Position statement]. Available from http://www.asha.org/policy

Lombardo, T. (1997, Spring). The impact of information technology: Learning, living, and loving in the future. *The Labyrinth: Sharing Information on Learning Technologies. 5*(2). Available from http://www.mcli.dist.maricopa.edu/LF/Spr97/spr97L8.html

U.S. Census Bureau. (2005). *Population profile of the United States: Dynamic version. Race and Hispanic origin in 2005*. Available from http://www.census.gov

World Health Organization. (2001). *International classification of functioning, disability and health*. Geneva, Switzerland: Author

SOURCE: Reprinted with permission from Scope of Practice in Speech-Language Pathology. Available from http://www.asha.org/policy.

RESOURCES

ASHA Cardinal Documents

American Speech-Language-Hearing Association. (2003). *Code of ethics (Revised)*. Available from http://www.asha.org/policy

American Speech-Language-Hearing Association. (2004). *Preferred practice patterns for the profession of speech-language pathology*. Available from http://www.asha.org/policy

American Speech-Language-Hearing Association. (2005). *Standards for the certificate of clinical competence in speech-language pathology*. Available from http://www.asha.org/about/membership-certification/handbooks/slp/slp_standards.htm

General Service Delivery Issues

Admission/Discharge Criteria

American Speech-Language-Hearing Association. (2004). *Admission/discharge criteria in speech-language pathology* [Guidelines]. Available from http://www.asha.org/policy

Autonomy

American Speech-Language-Hearing Association. (1986). *Autonomy of speech-language pathology and audiology* [Relevant paper]. Available from http://www.asha.org/policy

Culturally and Linguistically Appropriate Services

American Speech-Language-Hearing Association. (2002). *American English dialects* [Technical report]. Available from http://www.asha.org/policy

American Speech-Language-Hearing Association. (2004). *Knowledge and skills needed by speech-language pathologists and audiologists to provide culturally and linguistically appropriate services* [Knowledge and skills]. Available from http://www.asha.org/policy

Definitions and Terminology

American Speech-Language-Hearing Association. (1982). *Language* [Relevant paper]. Available from http://www.asha.org/policy

American Speech-Language-Hearing Association. (1986). *Private practice* [Definition]. Available from http://www.asha.org/policy

American Speech-Language-Hearing Association. (1993). *Definition of communication disorders and variations* [Definition]. Available from http://www.asha.org/policy

American Speech-Language-Hearing Association. (1998). *Terminology pertaining to fluency and fluency disorders* [Guidelines]. Available from http://www.asha.org/policy

Evidence-Based Practice

American Speech-Language-Hearing Association. (2004). *Evidence-based practice in communication disorders: An introduction* [Technical report]. Available from http://www.asha.org/policy

American Speech-Language-Hearing Association. (2005). *Evidence-based practice in communication disorders: An introduction* [Position statement]. Available from http://www.asha.org/policy

Private Practice

American Speech-Language-Hearing Association. (1990). *Considerations for establishing a private practice in audiology and/or speech-language pathology* [Technical report]. Available from http://www.asha.org/policy

American Speech-Language-Hearing Association. (1991). *Private practice* [Technical report]. vailable from http://www.asha.org/policy

American Speech-Language-Hearing Association. (1994). *Professional liability and risk management for the audiology and speech-language pathology professions* [Technical report]. Available from http://www.asha.org/policy

American Speech-Language-Hearing Association. (2002). *Drawing cases for private practice from primary place of employment* [Issues in ethics]. Available from http://www.asha.org/policy

Professional Service Programs

American Speech-Language-Hearing Association. (2005). *Quality indicators for professional service programs in audiology and speech-language pathology* [Quality indicators]. Available from http://www.asha.org/policy

SOURCE: Reprinted with permission from Scope of Practice in Speech-Language Pathology. Available from http://www.asha.org/policy.

Speech-Language Pathology Assistants

American Speech-Language-Hearing Association. (2001). *Knowledge and skills for supervisors of speech-language pathology assistants* [Knowledge and skills]. Available from http://www.asha.org/policy

American Speech-Language-Hearing Association. (2004). *Guidelines for the training, use, and supervision of speech-language pathology assistants* [Guidelines]. Available from http://www.asha.org/policy

American Speech-Language-Hearing Association. (2004). *Support personnel* [Issues in ethics]. Available from http://www.asha.org/policy

American Speech-Language-Hearing Association. (2004). *Training, use, and supervision of support personnel in speech-language pathology* [Position statement]. Available from http://www.asha.org/policy

Supervision

American Speech-Language-Hearing Association. (1985). *Clinical supervision in speech-language pathology and audiology* [Position statement]. Available from http://www.asha.org/policy

American Speech-Language-Hearing Association. (2004). *Clinical fellowship supervisor's responsibilities* [Issues in ethics]. Available from http://www.asha.org/policy

American Speech-Language-Hearing Association. (2004). *Supervision of student clinicians* [Issues in ethics]. Available from http://www.asha.org/policy

Clinical Services and Populations

Apraxia of Speech

American Speech-Language-Hearing Association. (2007). *Childhood apraxia of speech* [Position statement]. Available from http://www.asha.org/policy

American Speech-Language-Hearing Association. (2007). *Childhood apraxia of speech* [Technical report]. Available from http://www.asha.org/policy

Auditory Processing

American Speech-Language-Hearing Association. (1995). *Central auditory processing: Current status of research and implications for clinical practice* [Technical report]. Available from http://www.asha.org/policy

American Speech-Language-Hearing Association. (2005). *(Central) auditory processing disorders* [Technical report]. Available from http://www.asha.org/policy

American Speech-Language-Hearing Association. (2005). *(Central) auditory processing disorders—the role of the audiologist* [Position statement]. Available from http://www.asha.org/policy

Augmentative and Alternative Communication (AAC)

American Speech-Language-Hearing Association. (1998). *Maximizing the provision of appropriate technology services and devices for students in schools* [Technical report]. Available from http://www.asha.org/policy

American Speech-Language-Hearing Association. (2001). *Augmentative and alternative communication: Knowledge and skills for service delivery* [Knowledge and skills]. Available from http://www.asha.org/policy

American Speech-Language-Hearing Association. (2004). *Roles and responsibilities of speech-language pathologists with respect to augmentative and alternative communication* [Position statement]. Available from http://www.asha.org/policy

American Speech-Language-Hearing Association. (2004). *Roles and responsibilities of speech-language pathologists with respect to augmentative and alternative communication* [Technical report]. Available from http://www.asha.org/policy

Aural Rehabilitation

American Speech-Language-Hearing Association. (2001). *Knowledge and skills required for the practice of audiologic/aural rehabilitation* [Knowledge and skills]. Available from http://www.asha.org/policy

Autism Spectrum Disorders

American Speech-Language-Hearing Association. (2006). *Guidelines for speech-language pathologists in diagnosis, assessment, and treatment of autism spectrum disorders across the life span* [Guidelines]. Available from http://www.asha.org/policy

American Speech-Language-Hearing Association. (2006). *Knowledge and skills needed by speech-language pathologists for diagnosis, assessment, and treatment of autism spectrum disorders across the life span* [Knowledge and skills]. Available from http://www.asha.org/policy

SOURCE: Reprinted with permission from Scope of Practice in Speech-Language Pathology. Available from http://www.asha.org/policy.

American Speech-Language-Hearing Association. (2006). *Principles for speech-language pathologists in diagnosis, assessment, and treatment of autism spectrum disorders across the life span* [Technical report]. Available from http://www.asha.org/policy

American Speech-Language-Hearing Association. (2006). *Roles and responsibilities of speech-language pathologists in diagnosis, assessment, and treatment of autism spectrum disorders across the life span* [Position statement]. Available from http://www.asha.org/policy

Filipek, P. A., Accardo, P. J., Ashwal, S., Baranek, G. T., Cook, E. H., Dawson, G., et al. (2000). Practice parameter: Screening and diagnosis of autism—report of the Quality Standards Subcommittee of the American Academy of Neurology and the Child Neurology Society *Neurology, 55*, 468–479

Cognitive Aspects of Communication

American Speech-Language-Hearing Association. (1990). *Interdisciplinary approaches to brain damage* [Position statement]. Available from http://www.asha.org/policy

American Speech-Language-Hearing Association. (1995). *Guidelines for the structure and function of an interdisciplinary team for persons with brain injury* [Guidelines]. Available from http://www.asha.org/policy

American Speech-Language-Hearing Association. (2003). *Evaluating and treating communication and cognitive disorders: Approaches to referral and collaboration for speech-language pathology and clinical neuropsychology* [Technical report]. Available from http://www.asha.org/policy

American Speech-Language-Hearing Association. (2003). *Rehabilitation of children and adults with cognitive-communication disorders after brain injury* [Technical report]. Available from http://www.asha.org/policy

American Speech-Language-Hearing Association. (2005). *Knowledge and skills needed by speech-language pathologists providing services to individuals with cognitive-communication disorders* [Knowledge and skills]. Available from http://www.asha.org/policy

American Speech-Language-Hearing Association. (2005). *Roles of speech-language pathologists in the identification, diagnosis, and treatment of individuals with cognitive-communication disorders: Position statement.* Available from http://www.asha.org/policy

Deaf and Hard of Hearing

American Speech-Language-Hearing Association. (2004). *Roles of speech-language pathologists and teachers of children who are deaf and hard of hearing in the development of communicative and linguistic competence* [Guidelines]. Available from http://www.asha.org/policy

American Speech-Language-Hearing Association. (2004). *Roles of speech-language pathologists and teachers of children who are deaf and hard of hearing in the development of communicative and linguistic competence* [Position statement]. Available from http://www.asha.org/policy

American Speech-Language-Hearing Association. (2004). *Roles of speech-language pathologists and teachers of children who are deaf and hard of hearing in the development of communicative and linguistic competence* [Technical report]. Available from http://www.asha.org/policy

Dementia

American Speech-Language-Hearing Association. (2005). *The roles of speech-language pathologists working with dementia-based communication disorders* [Position statement]. Available from http://www.asha.org/policy

American Speech-Language-Hearing Association. (2005). *The roles of speech-language pathologists working with dementia-based communication disorders* [Technical report]. Available from http://www.asha.org/policy

Early Intervention

American Speech-Language-Hearing Association. *Roles and responsibilities of speech-language pathologists in early intervention* (in preparation). [Position statement]

American Speech-Language-Hearing Association. *Roles and responsibilities of speech-language pathologists in early intervention* (in preparation). [Technical report]

American Speech-Language-Hearing Association. *Roles and responsibilities of speech-language pathologists in early intervention* (in preparation). [Guidelines]

American Speech-Language-Hearing Association. *Roles and responsibilities of speech-language pathologists in early intervention* (in preparation). [Knowledge and skills]

SOURCE: Reprinted with permission from Scope of Practice in Speech-Language Pathology. Available from http://www.asha.org/policy.

National Joint Committee on Learning Disabilities. (2006). *Learning disabilities and young children: Identification and intervention.* Available from http://www.ldonline.org/article/11511?theme=print

Fluency

American Speech-Language-Hearing Association. (1995). *Guidelines for practice in stuttering treatment* [Guidelines]. Available from http://www.asha.org/policy

Hearing Screening

American Speech-Language-Hearing Association. (1997). *Guidelines for audiologic screening* [Guidelines]. Available from http://www.asha.org/policy

American Speech-Language-Hearing Association. (2004). *Clinical practice by certificate holders in the profession in which they are not certified* [Issues in ethics]. Available from http://www.asha.org/policy

Language and Literacy

American Speech-Language-Hearing Association. (1981). *Language learning disorders* [Position statement]. Available from http://www.asha.org/policy

American Speech-Language-Hearing Association and the National Association of School Psychologists (1987). *Identification of children and youths with language learning disorders* [Position statement]. Available from http://www.asha.org/policy

American Speech-Language-Hearing Association. (2000). *Roles and responsibilities of speech-language pathologists with respect to reading and writing in children and adolescents* [Guidelines]. Available from http://www.asha.org/policy

American Speech-Language-Hearing Association. (2000). *Roles and responsibilities of speech-language pathologists with respect to reading and writing in children and adolescents* [Position statement]. Available from http://www.asha.org/policy

American Speech-Language-Hearing Association. (2000). *Roles and responsibilities of speech-language pathologists with respect to reading and writing in children and adolescents* [Technical report]. Available from http://www.asha.org/policy

American Speech-Language-Hearing Association. (2002). *Knowledge and skills needed by speech-language pathologists with respect to reading and writing in children and adolescents* [Knowledge and skills]. Available from http://www.asha.org/policy

Mental Retardation/Developmental Disabilities

American Speech-Language-Hearing Association. (2005). *Knowledge and skills needed by speech-language pathologists serving persons with mental retardation/developmental disabilities* [Knowledge and skills]. Available from http://www.asha.org/policy

American Speech-Language-Hearing Association. (2005). *Principles for speech-language pathologists serving persons with mental retardation/developmental disabilities* [Technical report]. Available from http://www.asha.org/policy

American Speech-Language-Hearing Association. (2005). *Roles and responsibilities of speech-language pathologists serving persons with mental retardation/developmental disabilities* [Guidelines]. Available from http://www.asha.org/policy

American Speech-Language-Hearing Association. (2005). *Roles and responsibilities of speech-language pathologists serving persons with mental retardation/developmental disabilities* [Position statement]. Available from http://www.asha.org/policy

Orofacial Myofunctional Disorders

American Speech-Language-Hearing Association. (1989). *Labial-lingual posturing function* [Technical report]. Available from http://www.asha.org/policy

American Speech-Language-Hearing Association. (1991). *The role of the speech-language pathologist in assessment and management of oral myofunctional disorders* [Position statement]. Available from http://www.asha.org/policy

American Speech-Language-Hearing Association. (1993). *Orofacial myofunctional disorders* [Knowledge and skills]. Available from http://www.asha.org/policy

Prevention

American Speech-Language-Hearing Association. (1987). *Prevention of communication disorders* [Position statement]. Available from http://www.asha.org/policy

SOURCE: Reprinted with permission from Scope of Practice in Speech-Language Pathology. Available from http://www.asha.org/policy.

American Speech-Language-Hearing Association. (1987). *Prevention of communication disorders tutorial* [Relevant paper]. Available from http://www.asha.org/policy

Severe Disabilities

National Joint Committee for the Communication Needs of Persons With Severe Disabilities. (1991). *Guidelines for meeting the communication needs of persons with severe disabilities.* Available from http://www.asha.org/docs/html/GL1992-00201.html

National Joint Committee for the Communication Needs of Persons With Severe Disabilities (2002). *Access to communication services and supports: Concerns regarding the application of restrictive "eligibility" policies* [Technical report]. Available from http://www.asha.org/policy

National Joint Committee for the Communication Needs of Persons With Severe Disabilities. (2003). *Access to communication services and supports: Concerns regarding the application of restrictive "eligibility" policies* [Position statement]. Available from http://www.asha.org/policy

Social Aspects of Communication

American Speech-Language-Hearing Association. (1991). *Guidelines for speech-language pathologists serving persons with language, socio-communicative and/or cognitive-communicative impairments* [Guidelines]. Available from http://www.asha.org/policy

Swallowing

American Speech-Language-Hearing Association. (1992). *Instrumental diagnostic procedures for swallowing* [Guidelines]. Available from http://www.asha.org/policy

American Speech-Language-Hearing Association. (1992). *Instrumental diagnostic procedures for swallowing* [Position statement]. Available from http://www.asha.org/policy

American Speech-Language-Hearing Association. (2000). *Clinical indicators for instrumental assessment of dysphagia* [Guidelines]. Available from http://www.asha.org/policy

American Speech-Language-Hearing Association. (2001). *Knowledge and skills needed by speech-language pathologists providing services to individuals with swallowing and/or feeding disorders* [Knowledge and skills]. Available from http://www.asha.org/policy

American Speech-Language-Hearing Association. (2001). *Knowledge and skills for speech-language pathologists performing endoscopic assessment of swallowing functions* [Knowledge and skills]. Available from http://www.asha.org/policy

American Speech-Language-Hearing Association. (2001). *Roles of speech-language pathologists in swallowing and feeding disorders* [Position statement]. Available from http://www.asha.org/policy

American Speech-Language-Hearing Association. (2001). *Roles of speech-language pathologists in swallowing and feeding disorders* [Technical report]. Available from http://www.asha.org/policy

American Speech-Language-Hearing Association. (2004). *Guidelines for speech-language pathologists performing videofluoroscopic swallowing studies.* [Guidelines]. Available from http://www.asha.org/policy

American Speech-Language-Hearing Association. (2004). *Knowledge and skills needed by speech-language pathologists performing videofluoroscopic swallowing studies.* Available from http://www.asha.org/policy

American Speech-Language-Hearing Association. (2004). *Role of the speech-language pathologist in the performance and interpretation of endoscopic evaluation of swallowing* [Guidelines]. Available from http://www.asha.org/policy

American Speech-Language-Hearing Association. (2004). *Role of the speech-language pathologist in the performance and interpretation of endoscopic evaluation of swallowing* [Position statement]. Available from http://www.asha.org/policy

American Speech-Language-Hearing Association. (2004). *Role of the speech-language pathologist in the performance and interpretation of endoscopic evaluation of swallowing* [Technical report]. Available from http://www.asha.org/policy

American Speech-Language-Hearing Association. (2004). *Speech-language pathologists training and supervising other professionals in the delivery of services to individuals with swallowing and feeding disorders* [Technical report]. Available from http://www.asha.org/policy

SOURCE: Reprinted with permission from Scope of Practice in Speech-Language Pathology. Available from http://www.asha.org/policy.

Voice and Resonance

American Speech-Language-Hearing Association. (1993). *Oral and oropharyngeal prostheses* [Guidelines]. Available from http://www.asha.org/policy

American Speech-Language-Hearing Association. (1993). *Oral and oropharyngeal prostheses* [Position statement]. Available from http://www.asha.org/policy

American Speech-Language-Hearing Association. (1993). *Use of voice prostheses in tracheotomized persons with or without ventilatory dependence* [Guidelines]. Available from http://www.asha.org/policy

American Speech-Language-Hearing Association. (1993). *Use of voice prostheses in tracheotomized persons with or without ventilatory dependence* [Position statement]. Available from http://www.asha.org/policy

American Speech-Language-Hearing Association. (1998). *The roles of otolaryngologists and speech-language pathologists in the performance and interpretation of strobovideolaryngoscopy* [Relevant paper]. Available from http://www.asha.org/policy

American Speech-Language-Hearing Association. (2004). *Evaluation and treatment for tracheoesophageal puncture and prosthesis* [Technical report]. Available from http://www.asha.org/policy

American Speech-Language-Hearing Association. (2004). *Knowledge and skills for speech-language pathologists with respect to evaluation and treatment for tracheoesophageal puncture and prosthesis* [Knowledge and skills]. Available from http://www.asha.org/policy

American Speech-Language-Hearing Association. (2004). *Roles and responsibilities of speech-language pathologists with respect to evaluation and treatment for tracheoesophageal puncture and prosthesis* [Position statement]. Available from http://www.asha.org/policy

American Speech-Language-Hearing Association. (2004). *Vocal tract visualization and imaging* [Position statement]. Available from http://www.asha.org/policy

American Speech-Language-Hearing Association. (2004). *Vocal tract visualization and imaging* [Technical report]. Available from http://www.asha.org/policy

American Speech-Language-Hearing Association. (2005). *The role of the speech-language pathologist, the teacher of singing, and the speaking voice trainer in voice habilitation* [Technical report]. Available from http://www.asha.org/policy

American Speech-Language-Hearing Association. (2005). *The use of voice therapy in the treatment of dysphonia* [Technical report]. Available from http://www.asha.org/policy

Health Care Services

Business Practices in Health Care Settings

American Speech-Language-Hearing Association. (2002). *Knowledge and skills in business practices needed by speech-language pathologists in health care settings* [Knowledge and skills]. Available from http://www.asha.org/policy

American Speech-Language-Hearing Association. (2004). *Knowledge and skills in business practices for speech-language pathologists who are managers and leaders in health care organizations* [Knowledge and skills]. Available from http://www.asha.org/policy

Multiskilling

American Speech-Language-Hearing Association. (1996). *Multiskilled personnel* [Position statement]. Available from http://www.asha.org/policy

American Speech-Language-Hearing Association. (1996). *Multiskilled personnel* [Technical report]. Available from http://www.asha.org/policy

Neonatal Intensive Care Unit

American Speech-Language-Hearing Association. (2004). *Knowledge and skills needed by speech-language pathologists providing services to infants and families in the NICU environment* [Knowledge and skills]. Available from http://www.asha.org/policy

American Speech-Language-Hearing Association. (2004). *Roles and responsibilities of speech-language pathologists in the neonatal intensive care unit* [Guidelines]. Available from http://www.asha.org/policy

American Speech-Language-Hearing Association. (2004). *Roles and responsibilities of speech-language pathologists in the neonatal intensive care unit* [Position statement]. Available from http://www.asha.org/policy

American Speech-Language-Hearing Association. (2004). *Roles and responsibilities of speech-language pathologists in the neonatal intensive care unit* [Technical report]. Available from http://www.asha.org/policy

SOURCE: Reprinted with permission from Scope of Practice in Speech-Language Pathology. Available from http://www.asha.org/policy.

Sedation and Anesthetics

American Speech-Language-Hearing Association. (1992). *Sedation and topical anesthetics in audiology and speech-language pathology* [Technical report]. Available from http://www.asha.org/policy

Telepractice

American Speech-Language-Hearing Association. (2004). *Speech-language pathologists providing clinical services via telepractice* [Position statement]. Available from http://www.asha.org/policy

American Speech-Language-Hearing Association. (2004). *Speech-language pathologists providing clinical services via telepractice* [Technical report]. Available from http://www.asha.org/policy

American Speech-Language-Hearing Association. (2005). *Knowledge and skills needed by speech-language pathologists providing clinical services via telepractice* [Technical report]. Available from http://www.asha.org/policy

School Services

Collaboration

American Speech-Language-Hearing Association. (1991). *A model for collaborative service delivery for students with language-learning disorders in the public schools* [Relevant paper]. Available from http://www.asha.org/policy

Evaluation

American Speech-Language-Hearing Association. (1987). *Considerations for developing and selecting standardized assessment and intervention materials* [Technical report]. Available from http://www.asha.org/policy

Facilities

American Speech-Language-Hearing Association. (2003). *Appropriate school facilities for students with speech-language-hearing disorders* [Technical report]. Available from http://www.asha.org/policy

Inclusive Practices

American Speech-Language-Hearing Association. (1996). *Inclusive practices for children and youths with communication disorders* [Position statement]. Available from http://www.asha.org/policy

Roles and Responsibilities for School-Based Practitioners

American Speech-Language-Hearing Association. (1999). *Guidelines for the roles and responsibilities of the school-based speech-language pathologist* [Guidelines]. Available from http://www.asha.org/policy

"Under the Direction of" Rule

American Speech-Language-Hearing Association. (2004). *Medicaid guidance for speech-language pathology services: Addressing the "under the direction of" rule* [Position statement]. Available from http://www.asha.org/policy

American Speech-Language-Hearing Association. (2004). *Medicaid guidance for speech-language pathology services: Addressing the "under the direction of" rule* [Technical report]. Available from http://www.asha.org/policy

American Speech-Language-Hearing Association. (2005). *Medicaid guidance for speech-language pathology services: Addressing the "under the direction of" rule* [Guidelines]. Available from http://www.asha.org/policy

American Speech-Language-Hearing Association. (2005). *Medicaid guidance for speech-language pathology services: Addressing the "under the direction of" rule* [Knowledge and skills]. Available from http://www.asha.org/policy

Workload

American Speech-Language-Hearing Association. (2002). *Workload analysis approach for establishing speech-language caseload standards in the schools* [Guidelines]. Available from http://www.asha.org/policy

American Speech-Language-Hearing Association. (2002). *Workload analysis approach for establishing speech-language caseload standards in the schools* [Position statement]. Available from http://www.asha.org/policy

American Speech-Language-Hearing Association. (2002). *Workload analysis approach for establishing speech-language caseload standards in the schools* [Technical report]. Available from http://www.asha.org/policy

SOURCE: Reprinted with permission from Scope of Practice in Speech-Language Pathology. Available from http://www.asha.org/policy.

2

Professional Issues: A View from History

Judith Felson Duchan, PhD

SCOPE OF CHAPTER

One way to obtain a deeper perspective on the professional issues that are in this book is to step back in time. A historical view will show you that the matters covered in this book are dynamic and ever-changing. It is mistaken to think that today's professional practices arrived on the scene full-blown, with little struggle, or tweaking. Rather, our professional ancestors worked long and hard to develop today's professional practices in communication disorders. They deliberated, tried certain approaches that they then abandoned, and tried other approaches that they then changed to fit the times. A long-term view of practices also helps one appreciate the role that social circumstances play in the formulation of professional practices. Indeed, today's professionals in the areas of speech-language pathology and audiology are still fine-tuning established practices and creating new ones to meet contemporary needs and circumstances. Professional practices within this historical perspective are rendered as processes rather than products. In this vein, our hopes for our professional progeny should be that you will continue to redo, replace, or add to what we take as today's givens.

This venture back in time tracks but a small segment of today's taken-for-granted practices in communication disorders. It begins with conditions leading to the formation of the American Academy of Speech Correction in 1925. This was the organization that a half-century later, in 1978, took on the name we know today, the American Speech-Language-Hearing Association (ASHA). The chapter also describes changes in ASHA's organization over time with a particular focus on changes in its membership and certification requirements, and on changes in scope of practices. You will also read about the creation of the American Academy of Audiology (AAA), a second professional organization wholly devoted to professional issues in audiology. The chapter ends by identifying some trends occurring today, such as the move toward evidence-based practices that are likely to lead to significant changes that will be included in tomorrow's historical accounts.

This is not the first history to be written about the field of communication disorders and the two professional areas associated with it—speech-language pathology and audiology. One can, with some digging in obvious as well as more obscure places, find other historical renderings of various aspects of both professions. Most such depictions are short and specific, geared to a particular domain of practice, such as childhood language disorders (Aram & Nation, 1982; Leonard, 2000), phonological disorders (Bowen, 2009), voice disorders (Boone, 2010; Von Leden, 1990;), stuttering (Bobrick, 1995; Wingate, 1999), aphasia (Howard & Hatfield, 1987; Lorch, 2005; Tesak & Code, 2008), public school practices (Black, 1966; Duchan, 2009; Schoolfield, 1938), hearing aids (Deafness in Disguise, 2010), diagnostic audiology (Jerger, 2009), and aural rehabilitation (Hull, 2001; Ross, 1997). Some histories can be found tucked into larger texts or articles about a particular domain of practice. For example, a history on language disorders in children can be found in Aram and Nation (1982), Chapman (2007), and Leonard (2000); Hull (2001) contains a history on aural rehabilitation; histories on diagnostic audiology can be found in Newby (1980) and Stach (1998); and Bowen (2009) has a history of phonological disorders in children. Many histories are recollections and memorials that provide biographical and professional information about the contributions of individuals and professional programs that have made their mark on the discipline and/or the profession (e.g., Berry, 1965; Duchan, 2011c; Malone, 1999; Moeller, 1975).

There have been but few detailed histories of professional issues such as membership and certification, professional organizations and journals, and trends in clinical practice in the United States (Jerger, 2009; Malone, 1999; Paden, 1970; Van Riper, 1981). Perhaps the best known of these is Elaine Pagel Paden's 1970 history of the American Speech and Hearing Association. In her history, Paden describes the founding of ASHA in 1925; the organization's publications over the years; and the changes in membership qualifications, ethics, and relationships between ASHA and other organizations. The period covered in her book, *A History of the American Speech and Hearing Association,* is from 1925 to 1958.

A second history of professional issues is a 2009 publication devoted to the growth of audiology in the United States. In it the author, James Jerger, describes the U.S. origins of audiology covering the years from 1922, when the first commercial audiometer appeared on the market, to 2009, when his book was published. Jerger's book begins by describing the circumstances and major players involved in the establishment of the audiology profession just after the Second World War. He then presents milestones in diagnosis and rehabilitation, with separate sections dedicated to advances in pediatric audiology, auditory processing disorders, tinnitus, and hearing conservation. Jerger's book ends with a section on professional considerations. In that section he includes the medical connection, the education requirements of audiology, the origin and nature of professional organizations devoted to different aspects of audiology, and research support that has been available to audiologists over the years.

A third history of the profession is from my own website (Duchan, 2011b). There I have tried to show, among other things, how the profession of speech correction grew out of the progressive movement, between 1870 and 1914—a time in which people in this country made considered efforts to improve the lives of the disenfranchised, the impoverished, and those with disabilities.

This chapter draws from these previous histories, as well as other primary and secondary sources. The aim is to create a picture of how the professional areas of speech-language pathology and audiology in the United States have developed over the years, with a focus on milestones since 1925 when the group declared itself a profession in the United States. The areas covered are the historical changes in the professional organization, its membership and credentialing requirements, and changes in its scope of practices. See the appendix for an outline summary of significant historical milestones.

THE PROFESSION'S ORGANIZATION: 1918–1990

Just prior to the establishment of the early professional organizations made up of people interested in research and practices in speech correction, the country was experiencing social upheaval. The industrial revolution produced overcrowding and slums in the major cities. In addition, a large group of immigrants was settling in cities, people who arrived from southern and eastern Europe following the disruptions of the First World War.

In response to these social needs, there was a movement in America called *progressivism* (McGerr, 2003). The aim of those involved in the movement was to create new societal structures to improve conditions for the poor, disabled, and disenfranchised. They were called *progressives* because they believed that social reforms could produce a better future. Labor unions were formed to improve wages and working conditions. Child labor laws were passed to protect children who were in the workforce. Women campaigned for the vote. Asylums for the blind, deaf, and mentally retarded were founded. Settlement houses were formed in the inner cities to provide food, clothing, education, and a sense of community to new immigrants. And compulsory education became law.

A number of professions were organized in the United States at this time to respond to these social needs and progressive ideals. Indeed, before that time there was no official professional class of people in this country. A first agenda was for the various specialty groups to establish membership qualification requirements. Another issue that the new professions faced was creating a scope of practice for their members. One way this was done was to identify terminology and diagnostic categories for which they were responsible. College and university programs were instituted, conventions were held, and journals were created so that the newly formed professions could identify their own areas of expertise and exclude others. In this way, they could also promulgate what they considered to be best practices.

Many of the founders of the newly defined speech correction profession were members of already established professions such as medicine, education, psychiatry, psychology, and public speaking (then called elocution). Smiley Blanton, who in 1914 developed the first graduate-level program in speech pathology, was strongly affiliated with the professions of psychiatry and elocution; Walter Babcock Swift, who organized a group of public school speech therapists in 1918, was a physician and public school administrator; and Carl Seashore, who promoted the founding of ASHA around 1925, was one of the first psychologists in America (see Duchan, 2011c, for biographies of these three founders).

While coming from different professional and disciplinary backgrounds, these early founders had a common interest in topics related to speech correction. They began to develop alliances with one another, sometimes meeting in one another's homes. Informal gatherings also took place at national meetings of the National Education Association (NEA) and of the National Association of Teachers of Speech (NATS). The NEA group was led by Walter Swift and consisted mostly of public school clinicians from the eastern United States. They called themselves the National Society for the Study and Correction of Speech Disorders. The second group, associated with NATS, was led by a small cadre of professionals whose names are among our declared founders: Lee Edward Travis, Robert West, Sara Stinchfield, and Paula Camp. This group dubbed its organization the American Academy of Speech Correction. It was the better organized of the two groups and the one that was to eventually take hold in 1925 and grow into what we call today the American Speech-Language-Hearing Association.

Some 15 years later, during the Second World War, aural rehabilitation centers were established by medical departments in the armed forces to provide hearing services for military personnel (Doerfler, 1981; Jerger, 2009; Ross, 1997). The military called upon training programs in speech correction and otology to staff the centers. The personnel tested the hearing of members of the armed services, fitted them with hearing aids, and provided lip reading and counseling to military personnel with hearing losses.

Following World War II, these same hearing specialists returned to civilian life and lobbied for the founding of their new area of specialty, one that they called *audiology*. The field grew. Audiologists were employed by Veterans Administration hospitals and in private practices of otolaryngologists, community hearing centers, and university speech clinics. Many of these newly minted audiologists or hearing researchers remained affiliated with the academic discipline of speech pathology, as evidenced by the 1947 renaming of the national organization to include hearing in its association title, and by the 1948 addition of *hearing* to the name of its professional journal.

Audiologists continued to expand their services. In 1988, under the leadership of James Jerger, they formed their own organization, the American Academy of Audiology (AAA). The group held its first national convention in 1999 and in that same year began to issue the *Journal of the American Academy of Audiology*. This publication is devoted to research and practices related to hearing and its disorders. Many audiologists belong to both AAA and ASHA and attend both national conventions. Hearing research is published in the AAA journal as well as in ASHA journals, especially the relatively new ASHA journal dedicated to audiology with an emphasis on clinical and professional issues, *The American Journal of Audiology*.

Between World War I and World War II, the fields of speech correction and audiology in the United States became well established. The two fields considered themselves as part of a single professional organization—the American Speech and Hearing Association, or ASHA. The national organization by 1948 was working from a well-oiled constitution and set of bylaws, was meeting annually, and as of 1936, was communicating with and among its members through its own professional journal, the *Journal of Speech Disorders*. In the years that have followed, the organization and the two professional areas within it have continued to grow, creating specialty publications, increasing their membership exponentially, and expanding those domains considered to be within their scopes of practice.

MEMBERSHIP AND PROFESSIONAL QUALIFICATION REQUIREMENTS: 1926 TO TODAY

In 1926, two years after it declared itself an entity within a larger parent organization, the charter members of the American Academy of Speech Correction wrote a constitution laying out its organizational structure and its membership requirements. The constitution was approved by its host organization, the National Association of Teachers of Speech, and was published in its journal, called the *Quarterly Journal of Speech,* in 1927 (American Academy of Speech Correction, 1927, pp. 312–313). The goals laid out in the group's constitution were to provide a leadership role for stimulating interest and securing recognition of speech correction as a profession. It also aimed to raise clinical standards and encourage scholarly research (American Academy of Speech Correction, 1927, p. 312).

The bylaws of the constitution set the following criteria for membership:

i. Active present participation either in actual clinical work in speech correction or in administrative duties immediately concerned with supervision and direction of such work.

ii. Possession of an M.D., Ph.D., D.D.S., or of a Master's degree, in the securing of which degree important work shall have been done in speech correction or some closely allied field such as psychology, phonetics, modern languages, mental hygiene, psychiatry, or medicine.

iii. Publication of original research in the form of a monograph, magazine article, or book.

iv. Possession of a professional reputation untainted by a past record (or present record) of unethical practices such as blatant commercialization of professional services, or guaranteeing of "cures" for stated sums of money.

v. A bonafide interest in speech made manifest by continued membership in the National Association of Teachers of Speech. (American Academy of Speech Correction, 1927, p. 313)

The 1926 bylaws also stipulated that "no more than five new members can be inducted into the academy any one year" (American Academy of Speech Correction, 1927, p. 312). The membership committee was further instructed not to elect anyone "who is not known personally to at least two members of the membership committee or to 10 members of the academy at large" (Malone, 1999, p. 75).

These restrictive criteria reveal that the Academy did not see itself as a group that represented or policed practitioners in the field. Nor did it see itself as a group that required practitioners to pass qualification requirements in order to practice. Rather, it regarded itself as a learned or honorary society. The 25 members in 1930 were essentially the same group of people who served as charter members in 1925.

In 1930, members of the Academy opened their doors to practitioners by creating a new kind of associate membership with a less rigorous set of membership qualifications for clinicians. Associates were required to have a bachelor's degree and three years of employment in the field of speech correction. They were also required to have "adequate education in the physiology of speech and its disorders" (Paden, 1970, p. 65). To become an associate, one also had to be approved by a 10-member panel made up of Fellows of the organization. This was reduced to the requirement of two members for approval in 1936.

Unlike for Fellows, members at the associate level were not required to have a publication or outstanding achievement. Nor were they required to have an advanced degree. This group was to eventually form the bulk of the membership in the organization.

This shift in focus from a strictly academic, scholarly, honorary organization to one that included practitioners is reflected in the name changes made in 1927 and 1934. In 1927 the organization changed its designation of *Academy* to *Society*, and in 1934 it changed its title from *Society* to *Association*. Both *Society* and *Association* have meanings that are broader and more inclusive than *Academy*, reflecting a change in how the leaders saw the role of the organization. Another part of the name change in 1934 was to remove the word *Study*. This, too, indicated that the organization was opening up to practitioners and shifting from a purely academic to a more clinical-based identity. See Table 2–1.

TABLE 2–1 Name Changes of the National Association

American Academy of Speech Correction (1925)
American Society for the Study of Disorders of Speech (1927)
American Speech Correction Association (1934)
American Speech and Hearing Association (1947)
American Speech-Language-Hearing Association (1978)

A more substantive move toward a democratic organization occurred in 1942 when the organization changed its bylaws to invite practicing speech correctionists to become members of the professional organization. In keeping with this shift, three new levels of membership were established as additions to the fellow and associate (American Speech Correction Association, 1943, pp. 41–51). One, also called associate, was for students studying to become speech pathologists. Students could receive the *Journal of Speech Disorders* by becoming a paying member of the organization. A second addition was an advanced level of clinical membership, called a professional member, which differentiated members with experience from those who were beginners in the profession. Professional members were required to have master's degrees.

Another level of membership was also instituted in 1942, one designed to honor outstanding members of the association. This was a precursor to today's Honors of the Association award that recognizes those who have made outstanding contributions to the profession. The first Honors was given to Carl Seashore in 1944 for his contributions to the profession and to his research in the field (American Speech Correction Association, 1945, pp. 1–2). See Duchan (2011c) for more on Seashore and his contributions.

As the organization approached its thirtieth birthday in the 1950s, it went through social changes that led to further revisions in its membership and credentialing policies. Elaine Paden (1970) in her history of ASHA identified two of those social changes: an increase in specialized knowledge and a growing group of nonpracticing scientists seeking membership. Here is Paden's description of the knowledge explosion during the 1950s that led to a differentiation in curricula between speech pathology and audiology:

> Increased knowledge, based both on experience and on research, spawned more course offerings, and few individuals could be expected to cover the entire span. Specialization became an accepted necessity. The most apparent partition was between the areas of speech and hearing. Although the profession had always included both aspects of communication disorders, persons were now being trained who were

> experts in hearing but who had only basic knowledge of the rest of the general field. Meantime, the typical speech pathologist had not had time in his academic training to become equally prepared in the area of hearing (Paden, 1970, p. 68).

This proliferation of information and courses in each of the two subareas of the profession led the 1952 executive council of the professional organization to create two separate career paths, one for speech pathology, another for audiology (American Speech and Hearing Association, 1952). This separation of certification requirements was made available at basic (clinical) and advanced (professional and fellow) levels. Some applicants received certification in both speech pathology and audiology, having fulfilled the qualification requirements in both professional tracks.

Behind the proliferation of information was a new group of research scientists in the field who did not have the clinical coursework or clinical experience required for membership. In 1952 this led to a one-way separation between membership and credentialing requirements in the organization. That is, a researcher or someone with interest in the field could become a member without having to meet clinical requirements for certification. But it was not a full separation. It allowed membership without certification, but not certification without membership. Those who wanted certification were still required to be members and to continue their membership throughout the time they held their certification status.

This second half of the separation between membership and certification was not to take place until 1978 following a lawsuit against ASHA by a member, Dale Bogus Lieberman (Malone, 1999, pp. 73–75; Mylott, 2010). Lieberman's lawyers contended that ASHA was violating the Sherman Antitrust Act because it had a monopoly over professional certification and in that role required that those applying for certification pay their dues as members. ASHA argued that people could practice without certification, thereby showing that it was not a monopoly that was misusing its power. The case was settled out of court. Shortly thereafter, ASHA separated its membership from certification, no longer requiring that professionals seeking certification be dues-paying members of the organization.

In 1952 ASHA required completion of at least 30 semester hours in the major and 275 hours of clinical practicum for basic-level certification. Also required was one year of sponsored clinical experience (American Speech and Hearing Association, 1952). Neither a graduate degree nor a national examination was required for certification at this point. Advanced certification under the 1952 rules required 60 semester hours in the major, 400 hours of clinical practicum, and four years of professional experience. Those applying for advanced certification in audiology had to pass a nationally administered written and oral examination on science and practices associated with hearing and hearing loss.

Membership and certification requirements continued to change through the 1960s. In 1965 the organization returned to offering a single type of certification for both audiology and speech pathology—the Certificate of Clinical Competence (CCC), known in today's parlance as "the Cs." The new certificate merged the earlier two-tiered system of basic and advanced levels of membership into one. To qualify for certification, one had to be a graduate of a master's degree speech pathology or audiology program. The master's degree required completion of 60 semester hours in specified areas and 275 hours of clinical practicum. Certification in speech pathology and audiology also required nine months of supervised full-time professional employment, a letter from the candidate's academic program director, and a passing score on a national examination in the field of either speech pathology or audiology.

Over the next two decades, between 1965 and 1985, the professions continued to expand their knowledge base. Both wings of the profession felt the need to increase their professional requirements to accommodate the burgeoning scientific information, which was accomplished by increasing the course and practicum requirements in preprofessional training programs. In 1973 the number of clinical hours required for certification increased from 275 to 300 hours, and the academic content requirements became more specific. Coursework in the professional areas increased to 75 hours (including basic sciences).

The 1993 certification and degree requirements included coursework in language disorders for the first time. For the speech-language pathology track, six hours were required in the area of language disorders, and for audiologists three hours of language disorders were required. This emphasis on language disorders led to yet another name change in 1978. The American Speech and Hearing Association became the American Speech-Language-Hearing Association.

Leaders in ASHA have long debated about what has come to be called the entry-level degree requirement. The founders required a graduate degree for membership, a requirement that was changed when the organization opened its doors to practicing clinicians. In 1965, there were contentious debates again, but this time it was about whether to move from a bachelor's to master's level requirement for basic membership and certification. Duane Spriestersbach, ASHA president at the time, remembers that "a lot of training programs... were threatened and were not at all convinced that this was necessary or appropriate" (Malone, 1999, p. 87). Both Charles Van Riper and Bryng Bryngelson argued against the upgrade for fear that current practitioners without master's degrees would be disenfranchised (Malone, 1999, p. 87). The entry-level degree for clinicians in hospitals and agencies was changed from a bachelor's to a master's level in 1968.

In a similar vein are the recent proposals to move from a master's level to a doctoral entry-level requirement for clinical practice in speech-language pathology. As early as 1958, Virgil Anderson, a researcher in voice disorders at Stanford University and an active member of ASHA, proposed a professional doctorate in speech-language pathology, to the dismay of most of his colleagues in the organization. Here is a report from that time of how Anderson's idea was received:

> Some startled, some anxious, and some enthusiastic listeners made up the group to whom Virgil Anderson proposed a new degree, clinically oriented, at the November convention. This degree was tossed about with a great deal of speculation as to its name, its place among the time-honored MA, MS, and PhD. It was evident that its proponent was interested primarily in giving those with extensive clinical experience an opportunity to get recognition other than certification for their particular skills—especially those who might not choose to follow the path of PhD study (Nelson, 1958, p. 81).

The idea of a clinical track toward doctoral-level degrees finally took hold for audiologists some 40 years after Anderson first proposed it (Academy of the Doctors of Audiology, 2010). In 1997 ASHA approved a professional doctoral requirement for audiologists. The degree requirements went into effect in 2012 and include a strong clinical component of at least 75 hours of postbaccalaureate study and 12 months of full-time, supervised experience. The credentialing can be fulfilled by having a specialized doctorate in audiology (AuD), a PhD, or another kind of doctorate, such as a Doctorate of Science (ScD). Some professionals are now arguing for a doctoral requirement to provide services in speech-language pathology (Bernthal, 2007; Lubinski, 2003). As for all histories, the full story cannot yet be told, because the events being described are still unfolding.

School Certification

In the first half of the twentieth century, except in a few instances (Carrell, 1946; Gifford, 1925; Irwin, 1955), ASHA was the only organization that issued an official credential to practice as a speech-language pathologist and audiologist in any setting. In the late 1940s, individual states began establishing certification requirements for public school teachers (Carrell, 1946). Speech-language pathologists working in public school settings in the three decades between 1925 and 1955 were required to meet the same standards as public school teachers (Irwin, 1953, 1959), and, for some states, clinicians were required to have additional coursework and experience in working with "speech handicapped school children" (Irwin, 1959). Students enrolled in curricula specializing in speech pathology needed to take additional coursework in education to work in public schools. State departments of education later in the 1950s began to require that teachers of "speech handicapped school children" have basic speech certification from ASHA. By 1955, 15 states required ASHA's basic certification for practicing in schools, and by 1959 the number had increased to 32 (Irwin, 1959). Today most of the 50 state departments of education require specialized training in the field to practice in public as well as private school settings, with requirements varying from state to state. See details in American Speech-Language-Hearing Association, 2009.

State Licensure

In 1969 the state of Florida began a second movement at the state level to credential people. This one provided state licensure for those working in noneducational settings. Professionals working in settings that receive third-party payments, such as Medicaid, insurance coverage, and health department monies, must now have a state license to practice. All states now have established agencies (boards) in their state health departments to review and monitor practices and issue licenses in speech-language pathology and audiology.

Continuing Education

Another requirement for professionals, one involving postgraduate certification standards, has recently been put into place by ASHA. In 1999 ASHA added a continuing education requirement. To maintain their certification status, members are now mandated to pay annual membership fees and to accumulate 30 certification maintenance hours of continuing education credits over a period of three years (American Speech-Language-Hearing Association, 2011). Individual states also incorporate continuing education as a requirement for state licensure as does the American Academy of Audiology. See Chapter 3 for more discussion of credentialing issues.

SCOPE OF PRACTICE AND PRACTICE FRAMEWORKS: 1926 TO TODAY

It was not clear to the founders of the profession in the United States what services they should be providing and to whom. For example, should they be responsible for diagnosing and treating those whose communication disorders are secondary to other disorders, such as intellectual disabilities? Should they provide services to those who wanted to improve their speech, but who had no speech problems? Should they be the ones responsible for testing and rehabilitating those with hearing losses or should they focus exclusively on the speech problems accompanying those losses? Much of the activity of the early practitioners and founders of the profession involved establishing a taxonomy and complete listing of conditions that should fall within their professed scope of practice.

A nomenclature committee, set up in 1927 by the American Speech Correction Association, worked to provide an outline and descriptions of the various conditions that speech correctionists should know about and be responsible for. In the words of Sara Stinchfield, member and primary mover of the nomenclature committee:

> The attempt is made in this arrangement to give the student an outline of practically all of the commonly found disorders of speech, such as appear in home, school, and speech clinic, and to so group them that they may come under one of seven main headings: dysarthria, dyslalia, dyslogia, dysphasia, dysphemia, dysphonia, or dysrhythmia.... It was necessary for the committee on terminology to coin a number of new terms having old prefixes, frequently defining the older and better-known terms as synonymous with the coined ones (Stinchfield, 1933, p. 29).

The charter members and early officers of ASHA put forth considerable effort to come up with a logical scheme and labels naming different kinds of speech disorders. Following is an example of exchanges on this topic in a letter written in 1929 by Robert West to Elmer Kenyon, then the president of the organization, about what to call late developing speech:

> I rather balk at "normolalia" for infantile speech. We are not concerned with the baby talk of a baby; rather we are concerned with the baby talk of a child who has in other respects passed out of babyhood so that he has a type of speech that would be normal were he an infant. We must then choose some word that shows that it is not a normal condition. Why not then use a term translation of our phrase baby talk, such as "pedolalia"?

SOURCE: From West, R. (1929, February 2). Unpublished personal letter to Elmer Kenyon. Washington, DC: American Speech-Language-Hearing Association Archives. Reprinted with permission.

While the stated purpose for the taxonomy was to provide students with an outline of the disorders of speech, the members of the national organization saw the listing as a key to their newly forming professional identity. In a letter from Sara Stinchfield to the council members of the American Society for the Study of Disorders of Speech, Stinchfield recommended that Walter Swift and his followers not have access to the taxonomy for fear that the others would "hurt" their effort to come up with a definitive taxonomy (Stinchfield, 1929).

The eventual listing of major types and subtypes of speech disorders classified by the nomenclature committee was extensive. It included over 100 different diagnostic categories with Greek and Latin names (Duchan, 2011a). The categories were grouped into six main types, some of which have withstood the tests of time (e.g., dysarthria, dysphasia). Our ancestors' predilection for Greek and Latin-based terminology has changed considerably over time in the United States, being replaced by the use of accessible English phraseology such as language disorders, voice disorders, or hearing loss. However, one can still find traces

TABLE 2–2 Comparison of Diagnostic Terminology between 1931 and Today

Main Diagnostic Categories and Their Definitions (Stinchfield & Robbins, 1931)	Today's Names for 1931 Categories
Dysarthria: Defects of articulation due to lesions of the nervous system	Dysarthria and motor speech disorders
Dyslalia: Functional and organic defects in articulation	Articulation and phonological disorders
Dyslogia: Difficulty in the expression of ideas by speech, due to psychoses	Pragmatic disorders
Dysphasia: Impairment of language due to weakened mental imagery through disease, shock, or injury	Aphasia
Dysphemia: Variable disorders of speech due to psychoneuroses	Fluency disorders
Dysphonia: Defects of voice	Voice disorders
Dysrhythmia: Defects of rhythm other than stuttering	Intonation problems

of our earlier preference for classical medical terms as evidenced by the diagnostic category names such as dysarthria, echolalia, aphasia, dyslexia, and dysphagia. Table 2–2 offers a comparison of some of the terms used then and now. It translates the six main categories that served as a conceptual organizing structure some 80 years ago into today's parlance. It also includes the 1931 definitions, some of which contain theories about causality that have become outmoded (weakened mental states, psychoses).

The scope of practice laid out by the nomenclature committee in 1931 changed dramatically following World War II. Around 1942, the term *audiology* was coined to describe the services provided to military personnel with suspected and actual hearing losses. Specialists involved in hearing testing and aural rehabilitation of military personnel during the war lobbied for the creation of a new field of audiology, one that they had been practicing in the military hospitals. Audiology was seen then, as it is now, as a field that was separate but closely allied with speech correction. Also following the war new attention was paid to the veterans with speech and language problems such as aphasia resulting from war-induced head injuries (Sheehan, 1948).

While services to those with aphasia and hearing impairment were provided before the war, the increase in need and funding during the war led to major upgrades in these areas of practice. Hearing loss in the Stinchfield-Robbins 1931 taxonomy was treated as an etiology for speech problems (deaf mutism), and aphasia was seen then as but a small domain that speech correctionists were trained to handle. The main focus of professionals in those very early years, judging from their writings and paper presentations, was on stuttering. However, practitioners and academics alike typically saw themselves as generalists rather than specialists. Faculty members in speech pathology typically taught courses in all areas of the field, as is evidenced from the many programs that had only one faculty member specializing in all areas of speech correction.

During and following World War II, the areas of audiology and aphasia grew in importance, becoming established areas of professional specialization. This was particularly true in the newly established veteran's hospitals where specialized hearing and aphasia clinics and research centers were funded by the government and served as a source for research studies and for experimentation and advancements in clinical methods. These Veterans Administration (VA) clinics became epicenters of research and clinical activity in aphasia and audiology for many subsequent generations of students and professionals.

In the 1950s, professionals in both speech pathology and audiology began creating conceptual frameworks to guide their clinical practices and add coherence to their practice. These frameworks were psycholinguistic models that differentiated perceptual-motor problems from higher-order ones (Kirk & McCarthy, 1961; Myklebust, 1954; Wepman, Jones, Bock, & Van Pelt, 1960). Areas such as hearing loss and aphasia that had been treated as separate areas of practice became conceptually associated within these psycholinguistic processing models. The effort for diagnosticians, then, was not only to identify and isolate disorders from one another but also to determine how that disorder impacts other areas in the psycholinguistic processing system.

These models helped lead to the growth in the 1960s of new areas of specialization, considerably expanding professional practice areas. While each new specialty has its own historical origins and milestones, one can see some general growth trends when examining them together.

The specialty fields often begin as a research and practice subarea within a more general category of practice. This was true, for example, for autism, which was first categorized as a subtype of emotional disturbance. Some of the fringe areas were later able to stand on their own, breaking off from their host categories. This happened, for example, for audiology during and after World War II and for autism spectrum disorders more recently.

The degree of independence of new areas depended upon their developing a research base as well as on creating diagnostic and therapeutic practices dedicated to their area of practice. National committees were created to carve out the details of the scope and practices for those areas able to gain traction. The committees specified what clinical skills were needed to serve the new population and what rules, regulations, and guidelines were needed to monitor those providing services in that area. In the past 20 years, the credibility of a new area of practice has been based on how well the therapy associated with the area meets the standards of evidence-based practices (American Speech-Language-Hearing Association, 2004).

Milestones for acquiring full and robust independence occurred when areas formed their own interest groups in ASHA, published their own specialty journal, formulated their own certification standards, and developed their own evidence-based guidelines. For the area of multiculturalism and disability rights, the final milestone has been to infuse all areas of practice with new practice sensibilities about their area of specialty.

Table 2–3 shows the origins and early developmental progression of eight specialty areas that have evolved in the past 50 years. Included in the table are indicators of the primary force driving the expansion of the area, references to some of the earliest work in the area, information about when professionals in speech-language pathology and audiology first laid claim to the area, some references to early rules and regulations governing practices in the area, and information about whether and when the group became a special interest group and/or created a journal devoted to its area of specialty.

The specialty areas listed in Table 2–3 established themselves in the profession in a variety of ways. Among the most influential forces driving their growth were social reforms, technological advances, and changes in conceptual frameworks. As can be seen from Table 2–3, different specialty areas came about as a result of different driving forces.

Specialties Arising from Social Reform Movements

Reverberations from the civil rights movements in the 1960s were deeply felt in speech-language pathology. The first wave of changes was to remove clinical practice biases toward those who spoke in dialects other than Standard American English. African Americans in the profession, such as Orlando Taylor, Ron Williams, and Vicki Deal-Williams, lobbied for clinicians to treat dialect differences as legitimate and normal departures from Standard English and to differentiate them from errors arising from language disorders (Deal-Williams, 2009; Moore, 2009; Taylor, 1969; Williams, 1975).

TABLE 2–3 Stages of Growth in a Group of Eight Specialty Professional Areas Emerging in the Half-Century from 1960 to 2010

Diagnostic Category	Force behind Expansion	Early Work	Practice Domain	Regulations	SIG	Journal
1. Auditory processing disorders	Information processing framework	Myklebust, 1954; Katz, 1968; Keith, 1977	ASHA 1993 Task force on central auditory processing ASHA 2002 Working group on auditory processing disorders	ASHA, 1996a		
2. Augmentative and alternative communication	Technology advances	McDonald & Schultz, 1973; Vanderheiden, 1976	ASHA 1981 Ad hoc committee on augmentative communication	ASHA, 1981 Position statement	1997	AAC 1984
3. Autism spectrum disorders	Shift from emotional problem to communication or behavioral problem	Kanner, 1943; Lovaas, 1987	ASHA 2003 Ad hoc committee on autism spectrum disorders	ASHA, 2006 Position statement		
4. Cochlear implant services	Technology advances	House & Berliner, 1991	First cochlear implant performed in 1958	ASHA, 2004 Technical report		
5. Dysphasia: Swallowing	Technology	Larsen, 1972; Logemann, 1983	Ad hoc committee on dysphasia ASHA, 1987	ASHA, 1987 Report	1997	Dysphagia

(*Continues*)

TABLE 2–3 Stages of Growth in a Group of Eight Specialty Professional Areas Emerging in the Half-Century from 1960 to 2010 (*Continued*)

6. Inclusive practices	Social reform—disability movement		Participation and engagement as intervention goals	Rehabilitation Act, 1973; Education for All Handicapped Children Act, 1975; Americans with Disabilities Act, 1990; IDEA, 1990; ASHA, 1996b		
7. Language/ learning disabilities	Information processing	Strauss & Lehtinen, 1947	National Joint Committee on Learning Disabilities 1975 (see Abrams, 1987)	ASHA, 1976	1997	*Topics in Learning Disabilities* (1967); *Topics in Language Disorders* (1980)
8. Multiculturalism	Social reform	Baratz, 1969; Taylor, 1969; Williams, 1975	ASHA, 1969 Office of Multicultural Affairs	ASHA, 1983 Position paper	1997	

The civil rights movement in the profession has grown steadily over the past 50 years, leading to new ASHA mandates and guidelines for best practices, ASHA's Office of Multicultural Affairs (established 1969), and one of ASHA's 18 special interest groups titled Communication Disorders and Sciences in Culturally and Linguistically Diverse (CLD) Populations. See Chapter 24 for more discussion of this issue.

The disability rights movement sparked a second wave of social changes in the 1970s. New legislation growing out of the movement included Public Law 94-142 in 1975, its reenactment as the Individuals with Disabilities Education Act (IDEA) in 1990, and the Americans with Disabilities Act of 1990. These have all strongly affected professional practices. The school inclusion movement, for example, is based on the concepts arising in the disability movement that children with severe communication needs have the right to regular education. The service emphasis within this view is to find ways to support children so they can access and participate in regular classroom activities (American Speech-Language-Hearing Association, 1996b). Similarly, the focus on altering environments to include adults with disabilities has led to new interventions and clinical responsibilities that promote participation and engagement in everyday life activities (for example, Language Participation Approach to Aphasia [LPAA] Project Group, 2011). Chapter 15 discusses school-related legislation and issues.

The disability rights movement required that clinicians reframe their services by shifting from a traditional medically based model, with its focus on remediation of individual disabilities, to a socially based one that works to reduce barriers and promote communication access (Duchan, 2001; Language Participation Approach to Aphasia Project Group, 2011; Lubinski, 2008; Simmons-Mackie, 2000). The model is variously referred to as the social model (Byng & Duchan, 2005; Simmons-Mackie, 2000), the life participation model (Language Participation Approach to Aphasia Project Group, 2011), the communication access model (Connect, 2011), or the environmental approach (Lubinski, 2008). Social model practices have had a strong impact on scope of practices for children as well as adults, creating new types of interventions, such as training in conversational skills for family members of children with communication disabilities (Hanen, 1975) and adults (Kagan, Black, Duchan, Simmons-Mackie, & Square, 2001; McVicker, Parr, Pound, & Duchan, 2009), developing competence-based approaches for service personnel (Jorgensen, McSheehan, & Sonnenmeier, 2009), adapting the curriculum and delivery systems to accommodate children in regular classrooms (Erickson, Koppenhaver, Yoder, & Nance, 1997), and using the principles of universal design to create communicatively accessible environments in public institutions (Lubinski, 2008; Parr, Pound, & Hewitt, 2006 ; Pound, Duchan, Penman, Hewitt, & Parr, 2007).

Specialty Areas Arising from Technological Advances

The development of computer technology has also dramatically altered research and clinical practice in all areas of professional practice. Among the areas most affected are three specialty areas that owe their very existence to advances in computer technology: augmentative-alternative communication (AAC), cochlear implantation, and the specialty of swallowing or dysphagia. The techniques involved in augmenting communication often involve computer devices and computer-generated speech. Indeed, Greg Vanderheiden, one of the primary founders of the field of AAC, was an engineer whose main efforts were to design and tailor electronic devices to augment or provide alternatives to speaking for nonspeaking individuals at the Trace Center in Madison, Wisconsin (Vanderheiden, 2002).

Similarly, the practices involving cochlear implants for those with severe hearing losses grew out of the invention of the device around 1958. The implant involves the integral workings of various electronic parts, including a microphone, a speech processor, a transmitter, and a receiver. It also contains an electrode array that collects the auditory impulses from the stimulator and transmits them to different regions of the auditory nerve. Audiologists have designed a new set of clinical practices to train those with implants to use them effectively, and specialty certification is now attainable for providing cochlear implant services (American Board of Audiology, 2011).

The field of swallowing therapies also depends heavily on technology for evaluating patients. The two main assessments of swallowing functioning, the videofluoroscopic swallowing study (VFSS) and the videoendoscopic evaluation, both involve specialized training in the use of assessment instruments (American Speech-Language-Hearing Association, 2004). Dysphagia assessment and intervention has enhanced the visibility and showcased the skills of speech-language pathologists, particularly in medically based settings.

Evolution and Creation of Conceptual Frameworks

The past 50 years of our history have seen a number of changes in practices that have come about as a result of new ways of looking at disabilities and their etiologies. The area of autism offers a sterling example of how shifts in conceptual frameworks have altered our scope of practice. Leo Kanner first portrayed autism in 1943 as a kind of emotional disorder (Kanner, 1943). The disorder, in his view as a psychoanalyst, was caused by lack of parental affection. Following Kanner, the entire medical establishment in the United States considered the communication difficulties of those with autism as being secondary to their emotional disability. Therapies began with work on the emotional problem, in hopes that the communication disabilities would then take care of themselves. The most blatant version of this view was that of Bruno Bettelheim, who advocated removing children from their homes to give them the love that they were deprived of by their "refrigerator mothers" (Bettelheim, 1950). Physicians and psychologists, not communication specialists, were the professionals who were seen as having the needed expertise in emotional rehabilitation. Another prevailing framework adding to the problem came from within the profession of speech-language pathology. It was the information processing depiction of communication, the so-called box-and-arrow models that had no place for emotional content in the communication process (Baker, Croot, McLeod, & Paul, 2001; Duchan, in progress).

But this all changed with the 1987 work of Ivar Lovaas, a behavioral psychologist who published a study showing that nonverbal children with autism could learn to speak. Thus began a shift in thinking about the disorder. Once speech-language pathologists agreed that autism was a social-communicative disability, other frameworks in the field of speech-language pathology were brought to bear on research and practice in the area. Clinicians and researchers focused on intentionality, social skill building, and providing augmentative and alternative communication opportunities to children with autism, thereby creating what is now an important area in our scope of practice.

Another and even broader tectonic shift in the scope of clinical and research practices for the field of speech pathology occurred in the 1970s. It was a time, following Chomsky's linguistic revolution, when a new discipline was emerging in the social sciences, one grounded in theories and research in the fields of psychology and linguistics. The combined discipline came to be called psycholinguistics. The psycholingistic framework that focused on language structure and processing shifted the thinking and practice in areas such as delayed speech, articulation problems, and aphasia. The shifts led to name changes of the well-worn categories, with delayed speech becoming childhood language disorders and articulation problems changing to phonological disorders. Linguistic analyses became substituted for or added to diagnostic testing methods and newly devised language therapies targeted linguistic rules or psychological processes such as memory and attention (Duchan, 2011d).

In the 1970s, the psycholinguistic model provided clinicians with a framework for the construction of yet another diagnostic group, children with language-learning disabilities (LLD). The psycholinguistic focus on researching, identifying, and treating LLD children was so influential that leaders in the profession, such as Kay Butler, started a movement to have the term *language* added to ASHA's title and to change the professionals' name from *speech pathologist* to *speech-language pathologist*. These changes were acted upon in 1978 when professionals in the field added *language* to their titles.

This emphasis on language learning and processing positioned clinicians in public schools to play a key role in identifying and providing services to children with language-learning problems. Fred Spahr, the managing director of ASHA from 1980 to 2003, commented on the impact of adding language and LLD to ASHA's scope of practices in schools:

> There have been big changes also in speech-language pathology in the schools. When I first began at ASHA almost 90% of the caseloads of school-based clinicians were made up of children with articulation disorders. Today 90% of their caseloads are children with language-based disorders. This change is owing to the foresight of leaders in the late 1970s and early 1980s who recognized that the education and training of speech pathologists (as they were known then) would allow us to deal with issues related to language and language training in children. And today this training has allowed clinicians to enter the important area of literacy.

SOURCE: Uffen, E. (2003, October 07). Goodbye, Fred: And our best wishes for a happy and productive retirement. *The ASHA Leader.* Retrieved from http://www.asha.org/Publications/leader/2003/031007/031007e.htm. Reprinted with permission.

In audiology, one can also see the influence of an elaborately detailed information-processing conceptual framework. Audiologists who had previously focused on peripheral aspects of hearing began to emphasize stages of processing of auditory information including what came to be called central auditory processing. Tests measuring different kinds of processing have evolved, research has been conducted to locate the source of the auditory processes in the neurological system, and therapies have been devised to remediate central auditory processing disorders (American Speech-Language-Hearing Association, 1996a; Keith, 1977; Masters, Stecker, & Katz, 1992). Audiologists have also expanded their diagnostic and intervention services into tinnitus, vestibular disorders, and cochlear implants. Developments in hearing aid technology and the license to dispense hearing aids greatly enhanced audiologists' scope of practice.

RECENT TRENDS

The new millennium brings with it its own set of professional issues, adding to and continuing with those that came before. As outlined in Chapter 1 by Lubinski and Hudson, many sea changes are taking place in our society. These involve upheavals in population demographics, the economy, educational and medical practices, information technology, and globalization. To accommodate this changing world, speech-language pathologists and audiologists have already been changing how they go about their business. The Internet, for example, has resulted in major changes in how clients get information and how clinicians carry out diagnostic and therapeutic tasks (e.g., Lubinski & Higginbotham, 1997; Mullennix & Stern, 2010).

The various changes have impacted professional activities in a number of ways. For example, two new special interest groups have been created in ASHA. Division 17 is dedicated to dispensing information and dealing with issues related to globalization, and Division 18 is dedicated to dealing with the impact of technology on professional practices, or what the founders of the division have called telepractice. See Chapter 26 for further discussion of technology and telepractices.

Among the most robust and far-reaching changes affecting professional practices are those coming from the evidence-based practice movement. This movement began in our field in the late 1990s following the lead of medical researchers in Canada and England (Dollaghan, 2007; Sackett, Straus, Richardson, Rosenberg, & Haynes, 2000). An important catalyst for the movement was the writings of David Sackett and his colleagues in the *British Journal of Medicine*. While the movement as such is a twentieth- and twenty-first-century one, Sackett and others have traced its philosophical origins to the late nineteenth century (Sackett, Rosenberg, Gray, Haynes, & Richardson, 1996, p. 71). It was then, in France, that positivism first took root (Comte, 1907). The positivist view of the world and of how science is best carried out is one that favors sense experience over subjective experience and positive, measurable data over derived or inferential (deep structure) information. Positivism has led to other movements in the profession, including the standardized testing movement beginning in the 1970s and the profession's effort to obtain measurable outcomes for therapy practices that took hold in the 1990s (Fratalli, 1998). Evidence-based practice builds upon these earlier movements by favoring standardized and well-controlled data collection to evaluate therapy efficacy and efficiency.

This positivist bias of the evidence-based movement is reflected in its focus on large research studies, especially those using randomized, experimentally controlled trials. The studies tend to be about the usefulness of a particular kind of treatment within a particular domain of practice. Evidence-based studies have been done to evaluate the effectiveness or efficacy of many areas of practice, such as augmentative communication intervention (Schlosser, 2000) and auditory processing disorder therapies (Fey et al., 2010). Areas that have received particular attention in the evidence-based literature are those whose practices have been controversial (e.g., Lof & Watson, 2008, on nonspeech oral motor exercises).

Besides focusing primarily on randomized controlled studies, the evidence-based practice movement has given rise to a healthy literature comparing the findings from different studies. These research studies involving what has been called meta-analyses have been done in different areas of practice, including, for example, treatments for developmental speech and language delay and aphasia (Law, Garrett, & Nye, 2004; Robey, 1998).

The emphasis on empirical, measurable research outcomes from controlled studies has tended to result in inattention to significant and helpful areas of evidence, such as the voice of the client (Kovarsky & Curran, 2007; Kovarsky, 2008), the degree of client engagement in the therapeutic activity (Simmons-Mackie & Kovarsky, 2009), and the quality of the relationship between those involved in the clinical interaction (Fourie, 2011). Some have argued that the experiment itself can bias the results being obtained (Duchan, 1993, 1995). Indeed, the major figures in the evidence-based practices field, including Sackett et al. (1996) and Dollaghan (2007), have bemoaned the narrow, positivist view that has come to dominate the evidence-based literature. These authors have argued for enriching and expanding on the definition of evidence in typical evidence-based discussions to include phenomenological or subjective evidence as well as results of qualitative research. Those promoting a broader view of evidence have also argued that clinicians should base their decision making not only on research evidence but also on evidence gathered from their own clinical experience and from their clients' values, goals, and preferences (Dollaghan, 2007; Sackett et al., 2000). Sackett and his colleagues have observed that:

> Without clinical expertise, practice risks becoming tyrannized by evidence, for even excellent external evidence may be inapplicable to or inappropriate for an individual patient. Without current best evidence, practice risks becoming rapidly out of date, to the detriment of patients (Sackett et al., 1996, p. 72).

Read Chapters 29 and 30 for further discussion of the state of science in our professions and evidence-based practice as professional issues.

SUMMARY

In this short history of the profession of communication disorders, I have tried to show how professional practices in both speech-language pathology and audiology have changed considerably over the years and how they continue to change. My aim has been to capture the dynamics and direction of growth by focusing on three areas of professional change—the founding of the organization, changes in membership and certification requirements, and growth and specialization in areas of service delivery.

In the early days of the professional organization, leaders worked to establish an honorary academy, to create bylaws that included goals and membership requirements, and to carve out a scope of practice. Later the organization opened its doors to clinicians. Still later, it began credentialing its members, creating criteria for providing services in speech pathology and audiology. ASHA increased its training and credentialing requirements in response to the burgeoning information associated with different areas of practice. In its latest stages, the organization began to expand into new areas of specialty including autism, central auditory processing disorders, and swallowing. These new specialty areas have their own histories, with different driving forces, modes of independence, and growth patterns. The areas that were most successful in establishing professional autonomy within the organization were ones that were associated with social changes going on in the society (multicultural and inclusionary practices following a social model), ones that took advantage of technological advances (AAC, cochlear implants, and swallowing), and ones that were consistent with newly emerging conceptual frameworks (autism, language and learning disabilities, and auditory processing disorders). Together, these shifts in practices and functions of the organization illustrate the complexity and dynamic nature of professional issues in the field. The historical events described in this chapter have been offered as a context for understanding how today's practices came about as well as a context for understanding that today's practices are about to become tomorrow's history.

CRITICAL THINKING

1. What are several examples of how professional issues of today are a continuation of those of the past?
2. How have the histories of audiology and speech pathology differed over the years?
3. How have social attitudes and changes in society affected professional practices of the past?
4. What are some other societal trends, besides ones mentioned in this chapter, that have had an impact on professional practices?

5. What are some pros and cons of evidence-based practices?
6. What aspects of today's professions need changing and why do you think they should be changed?
7. What avenues are available to you to bring about changes in the profession?
8. How might a historical perspective help one's understanding and enactment of professional practices?

REFERENCES

Abrams, J. (1987). National Joint Committee on Learning Disabilities: History, mission, process. *Journal of Learning Disabilities, 20*(2), 102–106.

Academy of the Doctors of Audiology. (2010). *Au.D. history.* Retrieved from http://www.audiologist.org/aud-history.html

American Academy of Speech Correction. (1927). Association news. *Quarterly Journal of Speech, 12,* 311–317.

American Academy of Speech Correction. (1927). Association news. *Quarterly Journal of Speech, 12,* 311–317.

American Board of Audiology. (2011). *Cochlear implants specialty certification.* Retrieved from http://www.americanboardofaudiology.org/specialty/ci.html

American Speech Correction Association. (1943). Membership regulation. *Journal of Speech Disorders, 8*(1) 41–51.

American Speech Correction Association. (1945). The American Speech Correction Association presents the honors of the association to Carl Emil Seashore. *Journal of Speech Disorders, 10,* 1–2.

American Speech and Hearing Association. (1952). Clinical certification requirements of the American Speech and Hearing Association. *Journal of Speech and Hearing Disorders, 17,* 249–254.

American Speech and Hearing Association. (1969). *Office of Multicultural Affairs.* Retrieved from http://www.asha.org/practice/multicultural/about.htm

American Speech and Hearing Association. (1976, May). Learning disabilities. *ASHA, 18,* 282–290.

American Speech-Language-Hearing Association. (1981). Report of ad hoc committee on communication processes and nonspeaking persons. Position statement on nonspeech communication. *ASHA, 23*(8), 577–581.

American Speech-Language-Hearing Association. (1983). Social dialects and implications of the positions on social dialects [Position paper]. *ASHA, 25*(9), 23–27.

American Speech-Language-Hearing Association. (1987). Dysphasia. *ASHA, 29,* 57–58.

American Speech-Language-Hearing Association. (1996a). Central auditory processing: Current status of research and implications for clinical practice. *American Journal of Audiology, 5,* 41–54.

American Speech-Language-Hearing Association. (1996b). *Inclusive practices for children and youths with communication disorders* [Position statement]. Retrieved from http://www.asha.org/docs/html/PS1996-00223.html

American Speech-Language-Hearing Association. (2004). *Guidelines for speech-language pathologists performing videofluoroscopic swallowing studies* [Guidelines]. Retrieved from http://www.asha.org/docs/html/GL2004-00050.html#sec1.2

American Speech-Language-Hearing Association. (2006). *Roles and responsibilities of speech-language pathologists in diagnosis, assessment, and treatment of autism spectrum disorders across the life span* [Position statement]. Retrieved from http://www.asha.org/docs/html/PS2006-00105.html

American Speech-Language-Hearing Association (2009). *State teacher credentialing requirements.* Retrieved from http://www.asha.org/advocacy/state/StateTeacherCredentialingRequirements.htm

American Speech-Language-Hearing Association. (2011). *A chronology of changes in ASHA's certification standards.* Retrieved from http://www.asha.org/certification/CCC_history.htm

Aram, D., & Nation, J. (1982). Historical heritage of child language disorders. In D. Aram & J. Nation (Eds.), *Child language disorders* (pp. 7–31). St. Louis, MO: C.V. Mosby.

Baker, E., Croot, K., McLeod, S., & Paul, R. (2001). Psycholinguistic models of speech development and their application to clinical practice. *Journal of Speech-Language and Hearing Research, 44*, 685–702.

Baratz, J. (1969). Language and cognitive assessments of Negro children: Assumptions and research needs. *ASHA, 11*, 87–91.

Bernthal, J. (2007, May 29). Looking back and to the future of professional education in speech-language pathology. *The ASHA Leader.* Retrieved from http://www.asha.org/Publications/leader/2007/070529/070529c.htm

Berry, M. (1965). Historical vignettes of leadership in speech and hearing: III Stuttering. *ASHA, 7*, 78–79.

Bettelheim, B. (1950). *Love is not enough: The treatment of emotionally disturbed children.* Glencoe, IL: Free Press.

Black, M. (1966). The origins and status of speech therapy in the schools. *ASHA, 8*, 419–425.

Bobrick, B. (1995). *Knotted tongues: Stuttering in history and a quest for a cure.* New York, NY: Simon & Schuster.

Boone, D. (2010). A historical perspective of voice management: 1940–1970. *Perspectives on Voice and Voice Disorders, 20*, 47–55.

Bowen, C. (2009). *Children's speech sound disorders.* New York, NY: Wiley.

Byng, S., & Duchan, J. (2005). Social model philosophies and principles: Their applications to therapies for aphasia. *Aphasiology, 19*, 906–922.

Carrell, J. (1946). State certification of speech correctionists. *Journal of Speech Disorders, 11*(2), 91–95.

Chapman, R. (2007). Children's language learning: An interactionist perspective. In R. Paul (Ed.), *Language disorders from a developmental perspective* (pp. 3–53). Mahwah, NJ: Lawrence Erlbaum Associates.

Comte, A. (1907). *A general view of positivism.* London, England: Routledge and Sons.

Connect, the Communication Disability Network. (2011). *Communication, collaboration, roles, disability, access.* Retrieved from http://www.ukconnect.org/opinion_384.aspx

Deafness in Disguise. (2010). *Concealed hearing devices of the 19th century.* St. Louis, MO: Washington University School of Medicine. Retrieved from http://beckerexhibits.wustl.edu/did/19thcent/index.htm

Deal-Williams, V. (2009). The roots of our experience: Trials and triumphs. *The ASHA Leader, 24.* Retrieved from http://www.asha.org/Publications/leader/2009/090324/090324d/

Doerfler, L. (1981). A short history of audiology and aural rehabilitation. *ASHA, 23*, 858.

Dollaghan, C. (2007). *The handbook for evidence-based practice in communication disorders.* Baltimore, MD: Paul H. Brookes.

Duchan, J. (1993). Issues raised by facilitated communication for theorizing and research on autism. *Journal of Speech and Hearing Research, 36*, 1108–1119.

Duchan, J. (1995). The role of experimental research in validating facilitated communication. *Journal of Speech and Hearing Research, 38*, 207–210.

Duchan, J. (2001). Impairment and social views of speech-language pathology: Clinical practices re-examined. *Advances in Speech-Language Pathology, 3*(1), 37–45.

Duchan, J. (2009). The early years of speech-language and hearing services in U.S. schools. *Language, Speech and Hearing Services in Schools.* Retrieved from http://lshss.asha.org/cgi/content/abstract/41/2/152

Duchan, J. (2011a). *Diagnostic taxonomy of Stinchfield and Robbins.* Retrieved from http://www.acsu.buffalo.edu/~duchan/history_subpages/stinchfieldtaxonomy.html

Duchan, J. (2011b). *Emergence of professionalism in late 19th and early 20th century America.* Retrieved from http://www.acsu.buffalo.edu/~duchan/new_history/hist19c/professionalism.html

Duchan, J. (2011c). *Pioneers of speech-language pathology and audiology*. Retrieved from http://www.acsu.buffalo.edu/~duchan/biographies.html

Duchan, J. (2011d). The linguistic era, 1965–1975. In *Getting here: A short history of speech-language pathology in America*. Retrieved from http://www.acsu.buffalo.edu/~duchan/1965-1975.html

Duchan, J. (in progress). *Emotional peek-a-boo in clinical relationships: Examples from today and yesterday*.

Erickson, K., Koppenhaver, D., Yoder, D., & Nance, J. (1997). Integrated communication and literacy instruction for a child with multiple disabilities. *Focus on Autism and Other Developmental Disabilities, 12*(3), 142–150.

Fey, M., Richard, G., Geffner, G., Kamhi, A., Medwetsky, L., Paul, D., et al. (2010, September 15) Auditory processing disorders and auditory/language interventions: An evidence-based systematic review. *Language, Speech and Hearing Services in Schools.* Available from http://lshss.asha.org/

Fourie, R. (Ed.). (2011). *Therapeutic processes for communication disorders.* New York, NY: Psychology Press.

Frattali, C. (1998). Outcomes measurement: Definitions, dimensions and perspectives. In C. Frattali (Ed.), *Measuring outcomes in speech-language pathology* (pp. 1–27). New York, NY: Thieme.

Gifford, M. F. (1925). Speech correction work in the San Francisco Public Schools. *Quarterly Journal of Speech Education, 11*, 377–381.

Hanen, A. (1975). *It takes two to talk.* Toronto, CA: Hanen Centre.

House, W., & Berliner, K. (1991). Cochlear implants: From idea to clinical practice. In H. Cooper (Ed.), *Cochlear implants: A practical guide* (pp. 9–33). Clifton Park, NY; Delmar Cengage Learning.

Howard, D., & Hatfield F. (1987). *Aphasia therapy: Historical and contemporary issues*. London, England: Erlbaum.

Hull, R. (Ed.). (2001). *Aural rehabilitation: Serving children and adults* (4th ed.). Clifton Park, NY; Delmar Cengage Learning.

Irwin, R. (1953). State certification in speech and hearing therapy. *The Speech Teacher, 2*, 124–128.

Irwin, R. (1955). State programs in speech and hearing therapy. Part II: Certification. *The Speech Teacher, 4*, 253–258.

Irwin, R. (1959). Speech therapy in the public schools: State legislation and certification. *Journal of Speech and Hearing Disorders, 24*(2), 127–143.

Jerger, J. (2009). *Audiology in the USA*. San Diego, CA: Plural Publishing.

Jorgensen, C., McSheehan, M., & Sonnenmeier, R. (2009). *The Beyond Access Model: Promoting membership, participation and learning for students with disabilities in the general education classroom.* Baltimore, MD: Paul H. Brookes.

Kagan, A., Black, S., Duchan, J., Simmons-Mackie, N., & Square, P. (2001). Training volunteers as conversation partners using "Supported Conversation for Adults with Aphasia" (SCA): A controlled trial. *Journal of Speech, Language and Hearing Research, 44*(3), 610–623.

Kanner, L. (1943). Autistic disturbances of affective contact. *Nervous Child, 2*, 217–250.

Katz, J. (1968). The SSW Test: An interim report. *Journal of Speech and Hearing Disorders, 33*, 132–146.

Keith, R. (Ed.). (1977). *Central auditory dysfunction*. New York, NY: Grune & Stratton.

Kirk, S., & McCarthy, J. (1961). *Illinois Test of Psycholinguistic Abilities.* Urbana, IL: University of Illinois Press.

Kovarsky, D. (2008). Representing voices from the life-world in evidence-based practice. *International Journal of Language and Communication Disorders, 43*, S1, 47–57.

Kovarsky, D., & Curran, M. (2007). The missing voice in the discourse of evidence-based practice. *Topics in Language Disorders, 27*(1), 50–61.

Language Participation Approach to Aphasia (LPAA) Project Group. (2011). *Life participation approach to aphasia*. Retrieved from http://www.asha.org/public/speech/disorders/LPAA.htm

Larsen, G. (1972). Rehabilitation for dysphagia paralytica. *Journal of Speech and Hearing Disorders, 37*, 187–194.

Law, J., Garrett, Z., & Nye, C. (2004). The efficacy of treatment for children with developmental speech and language delay/disorder: A meta-analysis. *Journal of Speech-Language-Hearing Research, 47*, 924–943.

Leonard, L. (2000). *Children with specific language impairment.* Boston, MA: MIT Press.

Lof, G., & Watson, M. (2008). A nationwide survey of nonspeech oral motor exercise use: Implications for evidence-based practice. *Language, Speech, and Hearing Services in Schools, 39*, 392–407.

Logemann, J. (1983). *Evaluation and treatment of swallowing disorders.* San Diego, CA: College-Hill Press.

Lorch, M. (Ed.). (2005). The history of aphasiology [Special issue]. *Journal of Neurolinguistics. 18*, 4.

Lovaas, O. (1987). Behavioral treatment and normal educational and intellectual functioning in young autistic children. *Journal of Consulting and Clinical Psychology, 55*, 3–9.

Lubinski, R. (2003). Revisiting the professional doctorate in medical speech-language pathology. *Journal of Medical Speech-Language Pathology, 11,* lix–lxii.

Lubinski, R. (2008). Environmental approach to adult aphasia. In R. Chapey (Ed.), *Language intervention strategies in aphasia and related neurogenic communication disorders* (5th ed.). Baltimore, MD: Williams and Wilkins.

Lubinski, R., & Higginbotham, J. (Eds.). (1997). *Communication technologies for the elderly: Vision, hearing and speech.* Clifton Park, NY; Delmar Cengage Learning.

Malone, R. (1999). *The first 75 years: American Speech-Language-Hearing Association.* Rockville, MD: American Speech-Language-Hearing Association.

Masters, M., Stecker, N., & Katz, J. (1992). *Central auditory processing disorders: Mostly management.* New York, NY: Allyn & Bacon.

McDonald, E., & Schultz, A. (1973). Communication boards for cerebral palsied children. *Journal of Speech Hearing Disorders, 38*, 72–88.

McGerr, M. (2003). *A fierce discontent: The rise and fall of the progressive movement in America, 1870–1920.* New York, NY: Free Press.

McVicker, S., Parr, S., Pound, C., & Duchan, J. (2009). The Communication Partner Scheme: A project to develop long term, low cost access to conversation for people living with aphasia. *Aphasiology, 23*(1), 52–71.

Moeller, D. (1975). *Speech pathology and audiology: Iowa origins of a discipline.* Iowa City, Iowa: University of Iowa.

Moore, M. (2009, March 4). 1968: Orlando Taylor looks back. *The ASHA Leader*. Retrieved from http://www.asha.org/Publications/leader/2009/090324/090324d1.htm

Mullennix, J., & Stern, S. (Eds.). (2010). *Computer synthesized speech technologies: Tools for aiding impairment.* Hershey, PA: Medical Information Science Reference.

Myklebust, H. (1954). *Auditory disorders in children.* New York, NY: Grune & Stratton.

Mylott, K. (2010). *1978: SLP sues ASHA; Case raised issue: Did ASHA act like a monopoly?* Retrieved from http://ashawatch.blogspot.com/2010/08/1974-asha-member-sues-asha-case-raised.html

Nelson, S. (1958). News and announcements. *Journal of Speech and Hearing Disorders, 23*(1) 81–92.

Newby, H. (1980). *Audiology*. New York, NY: Appleton-Century-Crofts.

Paden, E. (1970). *A history of the American Speech and Hearing Association.* Washington, DC: American Speech and Hearing Association.

Parr, S., Pound, C., & Hewitt, A. (2006). Communication access to health and social services. *Topics in Language Disorders, 26*(3), 189–198.

Pound, C., Duchan, J., Penman, T., Hewitt, A., & Parr, S. (2007). Communication access to organisations. *Aphasiology, 21*, 23–38.

Robey, R. (1998). A meta-analysis of clinical outcomes in the treatment of aphasia. *Journal of Speech, Language, and Hearing Research, 41,* 172–187.

Ross, M. (1997). A retrospective look at the future of aural rehabilitation. *Journal of the Academy of Rehabilitative Audiology,* 30, 11–20. Retrieved from http://www.hearingresearch.org/ross/aural_rehabilitation/a_retrospective_look_at_the_future_of_aural_rehabilitation.php

Sackett, D., Rosenberg, W., Gray, J., Haynes, R., & Richardson, W. (1996). Evidence-based medicine. What it is and what it isn't. *British Medical Journal, 312*, 71–72.

Sackett, D., Straus, S., Richardson, W., Rosenberg, W., & Haynes, R. (2000). *Evidence-based medicine: How to practice and teach EBM.* Edinburgh, Scotland: Churchill Livingstone.

Schlosser, R. W. (2000). *The efficacy of augmentative and alternative communication intervention: Toward evidence-based practice.* San Diego, CA: Academic Press.

Schoolfield, L. (1938). The development of speech correction in America in the 19th century. *Quarterly Journal of Speech, 24,* 101–116.

Sheehan, V. (1948). Techniques in the management of aphasia. *Journal of Speech and Hearing Disorders, 13,* 241–246.

Simmons-Mackie, N. (2000). Social approaches to the management of aphasia. In L. Worrall & C. Frattali (Eds.), *Neurogenic communication disorders: A functional approach* (pp. 162–168). New York, NY: Thieme.

Simmons-Mackie, N., & Kovarsky, D. (Eds.). (2009). Engagement in clinical practice. *Seminars in Speech and Language, 30,* 1.

Stach, B. (1998). *Clinical audiology: An introduction.* Clifton Park, NY: Delmar Cengage Learning.

Stinchfield, S. (1929). Personal letter to Robert West. Unpublished material in the ASHA Archives. Washington, DC: American Speech-Language-Hearing Association.

Stinchfield, S. (1933). Speech disorders. New York, NY: Harcourt Brace.

Stinchfield, S., & Robbins, S. (1931). *A dictionary of terms dealing with disorders of speech.* Boston, MA: Expression Company.

Strauss, A., & Lehtinen, L. (1947). *Psychopathology and the education of the brain-injured child.* New York, NY: Grune & Stratton.

Taylor, O. (1969). Social and political involvement of the American Speech and Hearing Association. *ASHA, 11,* 216–218.

Tesak, J., & Code, C. (2008). *Milestones in the history of aphasia: Theories and protagonists.* New York, NY: Psychology Press.

Uffen, E. (2003, October 7). Goodbye Fred. *The ASHA Leader.* Retrieved from http://www.asha.org/Publications/leader/2003/031007/031007e.htm

United States Congress. (1973). Rehabilitation Act. Available from http://mastercodeprofessional.com/accessibility_files/Rehabilitation_Act_of_1973.pdf.

United States Congress. (1975). Education for All Handicapped Children Act (PL 94-142). Available from http://www.scn.org/~bk269/94-142.html

United States Congress. (1990). Individuals with Disabilities Education Act (IDEA). Reauthorized in 2004. Available from http://idea.ed.gov/explore/view/p/%2Croot%2Cstatute%2C

United States Congress. (1990). Americans with Disabilities Act. Available from http://www.ada.gov

Vanderheiden, G. (1976). Providing a child with a means to indicate. In G. Vanderheiden & K. Grilley (Eds.), *Non-vocal communication techniques and aids for the severely physically handicapped.* Baltimore, MD: University Park Press.

Vanderheiden, G. (2002). A journey through early augmentative communication and computer access. *Journal of Rehabilitation Research and Development, 39*(6 Suppl.), 39–53. Retrieved from http://www.rehab.research.va.gov/jour/02/39/6/sup/vanderheiden.html

Van Riper, C. (1981). An early history of ASHA. *ASHA, 23,* 855–858.

Von Leden, H. (1990). Pioneers in the evolution of voice care and voice science in the United States of America. *Journal of Voice, 4,* 99–106.

Wepman, J., Jones, L., Bock, D., & Van Pelt, D. (1960). Studies in aphasia: Background and theoretical formulations. *Journal of Speech and Hearing Disorders, 25,* 323–332.

West, R. (1929, February 2). Unpublished personal letter to Elmer Kenyon. Washington, DC: American Speech-Language-Hearing Association Archives.

Williams, R. (1975). *Ebonics: The true language of black folks.* St. Louis, MO: Institute of Black Studies.

Wingate, M. (1999). *Stuttering: A short history of a curious disorder.* Westport, CT: Bergin & Garvey.

Appendix 2-A

Milestones in the History of Speech-Language Pathology and Audiology in the United States

- **1870–1914** Period of progressive movement in the United States, one that promoted values that provided a context for development of the helping professions.
- **1914** Establishment of the first graduate-level program in speech pathology, organized by Smiley Blanton at the University of Wisconsin.
- **1918** Walter Babcock Swift organized public school clinicians in the Northeast. Their group, affiliated with the National Education Association, was called the National Society for the Study and Correction of Speech Disorders.
- **1922** First commercial audiometer made available.
- **1925** Formation of the American Academy of Speech Correction.
- **1926–1927** Formation and approval of the constitution of the American Academy of Speech Correction, including bylaws.
- **1927** American Academy of Speech Correction renamed American Society for the Study of Disorders of Speech.
- **1930** American Academy of Speech Correction created an associate level of membership, allowing practitioners to become members.
- **1934** American Society for the Study of Disorders of Speech renamed the American Speech Correction Association.
- **1945** Establishment of audiology as a profession, following World War II.
- **1947** American Speech Correction Association renamed the American Speech and Hearing Association.
- **1952** Two sets of membership requirements were created by American Speech and Hearing Association, one for speech pathology and one for audiology.
- **1952** ASHA separated its membership and credentialing requirements—one could become a member but not be certified as a clinician.
- **1965** Certificate of Clinical Competence was established for both speech pathologists and audiologists.
- **1968** Master's-level degree was required to practice in hospitals and agencies.
- **1969** State of Florida began a movement for state certification of professionals in speech pathology to work in noneducational settings.
- **1970** American Speech and Hearing Association published Elaine Pagel Paden's book tracing its history from its 1925 origins.
- **1978** American Speech and Hearing Association renamed the American Speech-Language-Hearing Association.
- **1978** Certification and membership requirements were separated. One could become certified without being a member of the association (this has since been reversed).

- **1988** Formation of the American Academy of Audiology (AAA).
- **1993** Language requirements were instituted for certification.
- **1997** The professional doctorate in audiology was established. It went into effect in 2012.
- **1999** First national convention of AAA was held.
- **1999** First issue of the *Journal of the American Academy of Audiology* was published.
- **1999** Continuing education requirement was established for continued membership in ASHA.
- **2009** James Jerger's book on the *history of audiology* was published.

3

Establishing Competencies in Professional Education, Certification, and Licensure

Dolores E. Battle, PhD

SCOPE OF CHAPTER

Speech-language pathologists and audiologists must have the professional skills and knowledge to ensure their services are of high quality and do no harm to the consumer. Preparation for careers in speech-language pathology and audiology begins at the undergraduate level and continues through the graduate degree. Professional education continues throughout the career to maintain competence and currency in the area of practice.

On completion of a graduate degree in communication sciences and disorders, speech-language pathologists and audiologists can begin independent practice of their professions. They are also eligible to obtain clinical certification and licensure in their profession. The Certificate of Clinical Competence (CCC), which identifies speech-language pathologists and audiologists as meeting the standards for entry into their profession, is established by the Council for Clinical Certification (CFCC) of the American Speech-Language-Hearing Association (ASHA). The American Board of Audiology (ABA) also provides certification for audiologists. Licensure is also available in most states for audiology and speech-language pathology. Integration of education and credentialing for practice of the professions is necessary to ensure that services are delivered by qualified personnel according to the highest ethical standards of the professions. This chapter provides an overview of the components of the standards for professional education, certification, and licensure necessary for entry into the professions of speech-language pathology and audiology.

PROFESSIONAL EDUCATION

Accreditation

An academic degree is a title conferred on an individual by a college or university in recognition of completion of a course of study or for attainments in research or in a profession (Knowles, 1977). The process of accreditation ensures the quality of academic programs. Educational institutions are accredited by external agencies to ensure that the education provided by institutions of higher education meets acceptable levels of quality. Accreditation is intended to protect the interests of students; benefit the public; and improve the quality of teaching, learning, research, and professional practice (ASHA, 2011a). It offers assurance that the academic program meets established standards in at least six areas: (1) administrative structure and governance; (2) faculty and instructional staff; (3) curriculum, including both academic and clinical education; (4) students; (5) assessment; and (6) program resources. The Council of Academic Accreditation (CAA) of the American Speech-Language-Hearing Association accredits master's degree programs in speech-language pathology and eligible clinical doctoral programs in audiology. The Accreditation Commission for Audiology Education (ACAE) of the American Academy of Audiology also accredits AuD educational programs. See the Resources section at the end of this chapter for additional information on accreditation.

Undergraduate Preprofessional Education

There are more than 280 colleges and universities that provide undergraduate or preprofessional education in communication sciences and disorders in the United States and in at least 51 other countries around the world. Approximately 75 percent of the programs also provide graduate education. Undergraduate education in communication sciences and disorders is considered preprofessional education because graduates do not qualify for independent practice, certification by ASHA, or state licensure. The purpose of preprofessional programs is to provide students with a foundation in the liberal arts and sciences, some exposure to the discipline of communication sciences, and an introduction to communication disorders. They also prepare for graduate study those students who desire to continue in the discipline. All undergraduate programs are in institutions that have regional accreditation and recognition by the U.S. Department of Education, and some undergraduate programs are in institutions that are accredited by the National Council for Accreditation of Teacher Education (NCATE). There is, however, no specialized accreditation for undergraduate programs in communication sciences and disorders.

Admission to Undergraduate Programs Applicants to undergraduate programs in communication sciences and disorders are usually required to provide evidence of a strong college preparatory high school program that includes laboratory sciences, computational mathematics, and some exposure to a language other than English. Many programs require a satisfactory performance on the Scholastic Aptitude Test (SAT), the American College Testing Program (ACT), or similar standardized test used to predict success in college. In addition, programs often prefer students who have had some volunteer or work experience in human services, such as working with young children, adults or older adults, or people with disabilities. Prospective students are urged to check with the program in which they plan to enroll for specific admission requirements.

Undergraduate Curriculum Although the Certificate of Clinical Competence (CCC) is not awarded until the applicant has a graduate degree, preparation usually begins at the undergraduate level. The standards for the ASHA CCC specify that applicants must have prerequisite knowledge of the biological sciences, physical sciences, mathematics, and the social/behavioral sciences. Although the specific coursework in an undergraduate program is defined by the degree-granting institution, undergraduate coursework in the discipline usually includes a minimum of 30 semester credit hours in courses such as anatomy and physiology of the speech and hearing mechanism, articulatory and acoustic phonetics and/or linguistics, physics of sound or speech acoustics, development of speech and language, instrumentation or technology in communication science, the neural basis of communication, hearing sciences, and introduction to the nature and prevention of communication disorders. More clinically focused coursework is also typically included, such as the nature of hearing and hearing disorders, aural rehabilitation, clinical methods, and observation. In addition, many programs require coursework in statistics.

Because they are preprofessional in nature, most undergraduate programs do not provide students with practicum experience other than 25 hours of supervised observation. Programs that do offer supervised clinical practice usually limit the experience to 25 hours in the senior year. A few programs, however, may offer more extensive clinical practicum through a student teaching experience at the undergraduate level.

Many undergraduate students increase their understanding of cultural and linguistic diversity and their fluency in a language other than English by engaging in community service or study-abroad programs either for a full semester or a short-term or summer program. Students who wish to engage in study abroad or international study should coordinate their academic program with their advisor before their junior year so they will be able to fulfill the requirements for the bachelor's degree and transition to graduate school. Some international study programs are in English-speaking countries and are able to offer courses or observational opportunities for speech-language pathology for undergraduate students.

Transition to Graduate School Undergraduate students who wish to pursue a graduate education in communication sciences and disorders usually prepare for the transition early in their senior year. Because most graduate programs require the Graduate Record Examination (GRE) for admission, students should take the examination early in their senior year. Letters of recommendation from faculty who are able to attest to their ability to succeed in graduate school and a personal statement or letter of intent are also frequently required. Because graduate programs vary, students should also work with their advisor to identify the graduate schools that will serve their individual needs. Information about graduate programs can be found online at EdFind, ASHA's online, on-demand academic program search engine. EdFind provides current, accurate, and comprehensive information on graduate academic programs in communication sciences and disorders. See the Resources section for information on EdFind.

The Council on Academic Programs in Communication Sciences and Disorders (CAPCSD) has established a Communication Sciences and Disorders Centralized Application Service (CSDCAS) for clinical education in audiology and speech-language pathology. CSDCAS is a state-of-the-art, web-based application that offers applicants a convenient way to apply to multiple clinical education programs in audiology and speech-language pathology by completing one single application. Approximately 50 of the 241 graduate programs in communication sciences and disorders are participating in the program. See the Resources section for more information on CSDCAS.

Graduate Education

The major objective of graduate education in communication sciences and disorders is to prepare students for the independent practice of the professions, careers in speech and hearing science, or advancement to doctoral programs. The first master's degrees in speech-language pathology and audiology were awarded in the 1920s. Today, there are more than 300 graduate degree programs in communication sciences and disorders in the United States including more than 50 doctoral programs in speech-language pathology/speech and hearing sciences and 76 doctoral programs in audiology.

A graduate degree is usually the minimal degree required for the practice of speech-language pathology. The minimal requirement for practice of speech-language pathology and audiology varies across the states; however, in all but a few states, a graduate degree in speech-language pathology and a license are required for the practice of speech-language pathology in all settings including the public schools. For example, in four states (Florida, Georgia, Maine, and New York), one can practice for a limited period of time with a bachelor's degree in the public schools, and in three states (Arizona, Oregon, and Nevada) one can practice with a full teaching license with a bachelor's degree. A graduate or doctoral degree is required for the practice of audiology in most states, including practice in the public schools. The Resources section contains information on credential requirements by state.

Admission to the Graduate Program Admission to graduate programs in communication sciences and disorders requires a strong undergraduate record in liberal arts and sciences in addition to 18 to 30 semester hours of preprofessional coursework in the basic sciences and the communications sciences. Although there is considerable variability in the requirements for admission to graduate study in communication sciences and disorders, programs usually require applicants to submit the following: (1) scores on the verbal, quantitative, and/or analytic writing sections of the GRE or Millers Analogies Test (MAT); (2) official transcripts indicating successful completion of the bachelor's degree and required coursework; (3) three letters of recommendation from people knowledgeable about the student's ability to be successful in graduate or doctoral study; (4) a written personal statement expressing the applicant's interest in the chosen career or other topic offered by the program; and (5) a personal interview. Interviews are usually optional but are highly recommended.

Graduate Curriculum According to the standards for academic accreditation, the curriculum of graduate programs must be sufficient to permit students to meet recognized national standards for entry into the practice of the profession (Council for Clinical Certification, 2011).

The curricula of individual graduate programs often reflect the interests and strengths of the individual members of the program faculty as well as meet the national standards. All programs accredited by the Council for Academic Accreditation (CAA) provide coursework and clinical practicum for those who are seeking the ASHA CCC as well as state licensure and teacher certification for those who desire the credentials. A few programs offer a program in speech and hearing science; however, these programs do not lead to clinical certification.

Graduate programs for speech-language pathology and audiology have different curricula because the preparation is for two separate professions. Preparations for both professions have the following similar features for completion: (1) academic coursework; (2) clinical practicum; and (3) a culminating activity such as a comprehensive examination, research project, or thesis.

Speech Language Pathology Curriculum The graduate curriculum for speech-language pathology usually requires 36 or more semester credit hours that encompass the current scope of practice with children and adults and a minimum of 400 hours of supervised practice. Most programs require four full-time semesters and at least one summer beyond the bachelor's degree. Some programs permit students to complete some coursework as part-time students or through distance education.

The curricular sequence introduces the development of the knowledge base in the professional discipline, followed by the application of that knowledge to the assessment and treatment of communication disorders and/or to speech-language science. Graduate curricula often include advanced coursework in basic communication sciences such as neuroscience and linguistics as well as coursework in specific disorders such as aphasia, dysphagia, neurological disorders, motor speech disorders, fluency disorders, voice and resonance disorders, craniofacial anomalies and associated communication disorders, cognitive and language disorders, augmentative and alternative communication, hearing disorders, and aural rehabilitation. Coursework also usually includes instruction related to cultural and linguistic diversity, research methodology, professional issues, and ethics.

Most graduate programs require students to obtain initial clinical practicum in a university on-campus clinic followed by clinical experience in other settings where they may obtain experience with both children and adults with a variety of communication disorders. Most programs require at least one semester of full-time or part-time supervised experience in an off-campus school, hospital, clinic, and/or rehabilitation center.

Throughout the program, there is ongoing formative assessment of knowledge and skills necessary for independent practice. At the culmination of the program, a summative assessment ensures that the learning outcomes for professional preparation have been achieved. The summative assessment is usually a comprehensive examination administered by the department that assesses the student's ability to synthesize academic knowledge obtained in the graduate program to solve clinical problems.

Post-degree, there is a 36-week paid clinical fellowship with a mentor that ensures that the fellow progresses toward meeting established goals and achievement of the clinical skills necessary for independent practice.

Audiology Curriculum Effective 2012, graduate students seeking clinical certification by ASHA and/or the American Academy of Audiology (AAA) in audiology are required to complete a minimum of 75 semester credit hours of postbaccalaureate study that culminates in a doctoral degree. However, some states continue to require the master's degree in audiology for the professional license. Students should check with their states to determine the specific requirements for the practice of audiology.

Applicants to doctoral programs in audiology usually hold a bachelor's degree in communicative disorders or speech and hearing sciences. They have a strong background in basic course sequences in speech and hearing sciences and in behavioral sciences along with significant work in disorders of communication. The doctoral program may be either a clinical doctorate (e.g., AuD) that prepares individuals for clinical practice, administration, and clinical track faculty positions or a research doctorate (e.g., PhD or EdD) that prepares individuals for an academic or research career with the expectation of contributing to the science of the discipline as well as to the preparation of future professionals and scientists.

Because there are few, if any, preprofessional or undergraduate programs in audiology, many students interested in audiology graduate programs complete coursework in basic and communication sciences in undergraduate communication sciences disorders or speech-language pathology programs. Students interested in audiology graduate programs may complete additional coursework related to audiology and hearing. Although the requirements vary by the program, prerequisite coursework at the undergraduate level often includes coursework such as anatomy and physiology of the hearing mechanism, hearing science, physics of sound, physical acoustics, acoustics of speech, electrophysiology, statistics, research design, introduction to audiology, and aural rehabilitation.

The graduate or doctoral professional coursework related to audiology includes courses such as amplification, diseases and disorders of the hearing mechanism, pharmacology, vestibular functioning and balance, counseling, central auditory testing, central auditory processing, evaluation and fitting of hearing aids, real ear measurements, pediatric audiology, cochlear implants, and specific diagnostic testing such as auditory brainstem response (ABR) and evoked oto-acoustic emissions (OAE). In addition, the program includes coursework in ethical standards, research principles, and current professional issues.

The course of study prior to awarding the doctoral degree must include a minimum of 12 months of full-time supervised clinical practicum sufficient in depth and breadth to achieve the knowledge and skills necessary for independent professional practice. A clinical fellowship is not required for the doctoral degree in audiology. In states that do not require the doctoral degree, there may continue to be a 36-week clinical fellowship requirement for the state license to practice.

Culminating Activity The graduate degree usually requires a culminating activity designed to show that the student has acquired an appropriate knowledge base in the discipline and can use that knowledge in an integrated manner to address problems in the discipline. The culminating activity is usually undertaken in the last semester or final year of the graduate program and is the final step toward completion of the degree. The specific options vary with the institution and/or the program. They usually consist of a comprehensive examination, a research project, or a thesis.

Comprehensive Examination Comprehensive examinations are designed to allow the student to demonstrate the ability to synthesize knowledge gained during the academic program and to apply that knowledge to solve clinical or theoretical problems. Comprehensive examinations may be oral, written, or a combination of both. They may be questions or problems developed by the faculty that are related to the curriculum and clinical experiences of the program. They measure the outcomes of the specific program. Some programs use a national examination such as the Praxis II Examination in Speech-Language Pathology or Audiology developed by the Educational Testing Service for the comprehensive examination. Such examinations are not directly related to the specific program, but to the general scope of practice of the profession.

The Master's or AuD Projects A master's or AuD project is an independent task developed by the student with the guidance of a faculty member. AuD projects are often termed *capstone projects*. These projects are usually case studies, research projects of a limited scale, literature reviews to answer a specific question or to review a particular topic area, or a similar activity that requires the student to integrate knowledge obtained in the course of study. There may be an expectation that the project is presented before the faculty or student peers. The project is usually retained in the department.

Thesis or Dissertation A thesis or dissertation is original research that attempts to present the answer to a research or clinical question or hypothesis following a prescribed method of inquiry. A thesis is usually research of a limited scale in a master's program developed with the guidance of a faculty member in consultation with a committee of faculty scholars. A dissertation is a document prepared in support of candidature for a doctoral degree presenting the result of original research using a systematic scientific method to solve new or existing problems or to develop new theories. For both the thesis and dissertation, the product is a written document that presents the literature reviewed to develop the hypothesis, the methodology, an analysis of the results, and a discussion of the results including application to the discipline. The student may be required to defend or present the thesis or dissertation to a group of faculty and/or student peers. Students who intend to pursue doctoral education are strongly encouraged to complete the master's degree thesis as their culminating activity as preparation for doctoral research and study.

Doctoral Education

The doctoral degree is the highest degree granted by educational institutions (Knowles, 1977). The University of Paris awarded the first doctorates in religion in

1150. The Doctor of Philosophy (PhD) was first conferred in Paris in the mid-thirteenth century. The doctoral degree, as granted in the United States and several other nations, is a relatively modern development. Until well into the nineteenth century, the bachelor's degree was the highest degree awarded in the United States. German institutions, famed for their development of scientific method, began to attract American students to study for the doctoral degree. Possession of the German doctorate became so prestigious that steps were taken to create similar programs in the United States.

The first American doctoral degree in speech-language pathology was awarded to Sara M. Stinchfield at the University of Wisconsin in 1921 (Neidecker & Blosser, 1993). Currently, there are several hundred institutions in the United States awarding the doctoral degree, including more than 75 in speech-language pathology and audiology.

Doctoral education is more than an extension of the master's degree program. Fundamental to the meaning of a doctoral degree is demonstrated achievement in three broad areas: (1) mastery of the essential theory and knowledge in the field in which the degree is awarded, (2) completion of pertinent research or scholarship relevant to the field, and (3) a dissertation or scholarly work that is an original contribution to the knowledge base in the particular field (Council of Graduate Schools in the United States, 1990). Potential doctoral students choose the program because of the opportunity to study with a particular senior researcher or because of a specialty field of study available at the institution.

Types of Doctoral Degrees There are two types of doctoral degrees awarded in the United States—honorary degrees and earned degrees. Earned degrees may be research, first-professional, or professional degrees.

Honorary degrees, known as *honoris causa ad gradum,* are granted by universities to recognize outstanding professional attainment or public service. Honorary degrees require no academic work. Those holding the honorary doctorate do not use the title of "doctor."

Earned degrees require significant academic work in a discipline. Doctoral degrees are not merely extensions of the master's degree. Rather, they represent a significant advancement in the discipline with a specialization in a specific area of research and scholarship or clinical practice. Three types of earned doctoral degrees are awarded in the United States—the research doctorate, the professional doctorate, and the clinical doctorate.

The *research doctorate* is a mark of highest academic achievement in a particular field (Council of Graduate Schools in the United States, 1990). It prepares students for careers as faculty in colleges and universities, researchers, and scholars. Research doctorates usually involve study in the discipline as well as interdisciplinary areas to prepare the individual for specialization and contributions to the knowledge base of the discipline through original research.

The *professional doctorate* is a type of research doctorate. The professional doctorate is defined as "the highest university award given in a particular field in recognition of completion of academic preparation for professional practice" (Council of Graduate Schools in the United States, 1990, p. 1). The aim of the professional doctorate is to integrate professional and academic knowledge. Those pursuing a professional doctorate are expected to make a contribution to both theory and practice in the field and to develop professional practice by making a contribution to professional knowledge.

The *clinical doctorate* places emphasis on clinical practice. The clinical doctorate, like the research doctorate, is a mark of high achievement in a particular field; however, the intention is to prepare knowledgeable, competent clinicians. The clinical doctorate is not a replacement for the research doctorate. Rather, it refers to specialized preparation for those who wish to do clinical or applied research and/or to become direct service providers to the public or to other professions. Preparation in applied or clinical research and the completion of a research project related to a clinical problem is usually required for the completion of a clinical doctorate. Those holding the clinical doctorate often seek employment in university or college clinics, teaching hospitals, or rehabilitation or other health care programs. They may enter private practice.

The Doctor of Audiology (AuD) is considered either a clinical or professional doctorate. The AuD places emphasis on clinical education, with a major component of the program being clinical practice in a variety of settings and with a variety of clients whose hearing impairments require a high degree of expertise for appropriate evaluation and treatment. Some programs also require clinical research as a component of the degree program.

Although only in existence since the early 1990s, the number of academic programs that offer the AuD degree continues to grow. There are currently 76 AuD programs in the United States. ASHA has identified the doctoral degree, with AuD as the preferred title, for entry into the practice of the profession of audiology.

The doctoral degree became required for clinical certification in audiology on January 1, 2012. People holding the AuD often are employed in hospitals, rehabilitation facilities, private practice, or industry.

Doctoral Curriculum Doctoral programs in speech-language pathology or speech-language sciences require at least three years of full-time study beyond the master's degree or four years beyond the bachelor's degree without any intervening master's degree. There is no set time limit for gaining the doctorate; however, some universities set a maximum time of six to seven years to prevent students from extending their work indefinitely.

Most candidates for the doctoral degree in speech-language pathology enter the program after completion of the master's degree and the clinical fellow experience. Some may choose to be employed for several years before beginning the doctoral program. Most candidates for the doctorate in audiology or AuD degree enter the program after completing an undergraduate program in communication sciences and disorders or a related field.

Academic Coursework in Doctoral Programs In addition to advanced work in the discipline, coursework in doctoral programs in speech-language pathology may include study in related areas such as special education, reading, linguistics, neurology, neuroscience, pharmacology, rehabilitation science, psychology, human development, statistics, or other interdisciplinary areas related to the area of interest. If the program is a research doctorate, there must be sufficient curriculum to provide a firm basis in the development and analysis of research and laboratory science, including research design, scientific inquiry, and statistics. For the clinical doctorate, there must be a sufficient knowledge base and analytical skills to develop and analyze the results of clinical inquiry.

For the professional doctorate, such as the AuD, there must be a sufficient knowledge base to ensure the development of expertise necessary for the development of clinical skills that are robust both in depth and breadth of clinical practice. In addition, individuals must be able to interpret pertinent research and apply it to clinical practice. To ensure that the chosen program of study is robust and consistent with the university standards for awarding the degree, all doctoral candidates must file a plan of study with the university early in their course of study.

Preliminary and Qualifying or Comprehensive Examinations Most doctoral programs require that preliminary examinations be taken early in the degree program to assess the student's knowledge of the field so that an appropriate plan of study can be designed. At or near the end of the formal coursework portion of the program, doctoral students take qualifying or comprehensive examinations to verify they have the necessary foundation in the discipline on which to develop individual research or advanced clinical practice. The examinations usually require the candidate to integrate knowledge from various areas of the discipline. On completion of the comprehensive examination, the individual is admitted to candidacy and is referred to as a doctoral candidate.

Residency or Full-Time Study Most doctoral programs recognize that, to develop the intensity of involvement in doctoral study, at least one year of the doctoral program must be completed on a full-time basis. This is called the residency period. It allows the candidate the opportunity to engage fully in interaction with faculty and others in scholarly and clinical pursuits. Interaction with scholars and practitioners is essential in the development of the approach to problem solving, research, and critical thinking necessary for completion of the degree.

Dissertation or Culminating Activity All graduate programs require the completion of a culminating activity for the degree. In doctoral programs, this is usually a dissertation, an independent research project, or advanced clinical study, depending on the type of degree to be earned. The culminating activity is usually begun during the year of residency after the completion of the academic curriculum and the qualifying or comprehensive examination. Doctoral candidates usually develop an original hypothesis or clinical problem and design a study or project to test the hypothesis or solve the problem using methods of scientific inquiry. A primary faculty advisor directs the culminating activity, assisted by a committee of scholars, researchers, or practitioners.

After completion of the project, the research doctoral candidate prepares or writes the dissertation. The formal, extended, written document describes the basis of the research or problem, research questions or hypotheses, methodology, results, and conclusions. It also includes a discussion of the implications of the results for the profession, clinical practice, or future research (Blake, 1995). Because the dissertation or culminating activity is intended to make a contribution to the field of knowledge, the dissertation is usually evaluated by at least one external reviewer or scholar familiar with the field of inquiry from outside the department or university. Doctoral programs usually require that the candidate defend the dissertation or the culminating activity before a body of scholars, researchers, and practitioners.

The oral defense allows the doctoral candidate to demonstrate mastery of the knowledge and skills required for the degree to ensure the degree was earned according to the standards established by the granting university.

Postdoctoral Study

Postdoctoral study, usually referred to as "post doc," is highly specialized study taken by an individual usually within five years of completion of a doctoral degree. It is usually one to three years of advanced study in a specialized area of research or clinical study in collaboration with a known scholar or expert in a particular field. Government grants such as those from the National Institutes of Health and the National Institute for Deafness and Other Communication Disorders (NIDCD); foundations, such as the American Speech-Language Hearing Foundation; or private agencies in a particular area of demonstrated need often fund postdoctoral study for individuals with the highest potential to develop into successful independent scientists through research training and career development opportunities. Post docs may also be supported through an appointment as temporary or visiting faculty with a stipend or sponsorship award. See NIDCD in the Resources section at the end of the chapter for further information on postdoc career opportunities.

Distance Education

Distance education is instruction that occurs when the instructor and student are separated by distance, time, or both. Distance education programs are used by individuals who are unable to attend a typical university program either because they are not geographically close to the university or to a particular instructor or because they are not able to attend the college courses at the time when they are offered, or both. The instruction may be synchronous (i.e., live at the same time) or asynchronous (i.e., delayed or received at a later time from the original instruction).

Distance education is not new. In the nineteenth century, education was obtained by correspondence courses, with coursework provided by mail. As technology improved, education is now available to people in remote geographical areas through audio recordings, Skype, podcasts, chats, videotapes, telephone, and tele-courses. Advances in technology and the need for new models of education that function with changes in lifestyle have made distance education available for continuing education, specific academic coursework, and some academic degrees.

According to the Council on Academic Accreditation (CAA), a distance education program is one in which 50 percent or more of the required graduate academic credit hours, excluding clinical practicum, are accrued when the learner is separate from the instructor. Distance education programs must be accredited by the CAA and meet the same standards as other programs accredited by the CAA. To ensure that the same academic standards apply, there must be regular substantive interaction between the students enrolled in the program and the instructor. The interaction may be synchronous or asynchronous. Synchronous instruction is live, real-time instruction through videoconference or other live instruction. Asynchronous distance instruction is provided at a different time through web-based or CD-ROM or other instruction that is not live but rather is viewed at a time selected by the student. The interaction must use interactive technology, which may include web-based technology, the Internet, closed circuit, cable, broadband lines, fiber optics, satellite, wireless, audio conferencing, prerecorded video cassette, DVD or DC-ROM, or other available technology to ensure appropriate interaction during instruction. The program must provide students with academic and theoretical knowledge, clinical education, virtual clients, directed readings, online discussions, as well as class and individual projects and secure examinations. Most of the programs offer graduate coursework; however, several programs offer prerequisite courses for students with bachelor's degrees in other disciplines who are completing coursework for admission to graduate programs (Boswell, 2007; Page, Amster, Gil, & Griffiths, 2010).

The CAA has been accrediting academic programs with distance education components since 1998. At least 35 academic programs currently provide some academic courses and/or degrees through distance education in speech-language pathology and/or audiology. According to ASHA EdFind (American Speech-Language-Hearing Association, 2011a), several programs offer all academic coursework required for the degree through distance learning. Of the 241 accredited master's degree programs in speech-language pathology, only 20 are specifically accredited as distance education programs; that is, they offer 50 percent or more of their graduate academic coursework through distance education. Currently, none of the 71 accredited audiology programs are specifically accredited for distance education.

Students completing courses or degree programs through distance education are expected to meet the same academic standards of the degree-granting institution as students attending the regular on-site program

(Dudding & Purcell-Robertson, 2003). To ensure that the student who is enrolled in the distance program is actually the student receiving academic credit, the CAA requires that programs document, implement, and consistently apply their institutional policies regarding verification of a student's identity and privacy.

PROFESSIONAL LICENSURE

The purpose of regulation of the practices of speech-language pathology and audiology is to protect the consumer from harm resulting from unscrupulous or incompetent practice and from improper diagnosis and treatment. It also assures the consumer that services are being provided in a manner that meets professional standards for ethical practice. Regulation may be in the form of licensure, certification, or registration.

The Professional License

Licensing is the process by which a state government grants an individual the right to practice a given profession in a defined scope of practice. Licensure is based on the belief that stringent entry requirements and ongoing scrutiny by the state will protect the public health, safety, and welfare of consumers from unscrupulous or incompetent practice. Permission to practice the profession is granted when the applicant can demonstrate that the minimal degree of competence has been attained. Professional licenses issued by governmental agencies are usually required for practice in areas where the agency has legal jurisdiction, such as the public schools or health care agencies.

All states require that speech-language pathologists and audiologists be licensed or otherwise regulated (i.e., registration or certification). States have different eligibility requirements, fees, and continuing education requirements. As shown in Table 3–1, all states, including the District of Columbia, regulate one or both professions.

In most states, the requirements for the license are identical to the requirements for the ASHA CCC. However, although the doctorate is required for certification in audiology by the ASHA CFCC, the doctorate is required for the license by only 24 states. Currently, 18 states permit the license with either a doctorate or a master's degree.

Licensing laws contain broad provisions governing the practice of the professions. Because they are the laws of the state, licensure laws can be changed only by legislative act. Rules or regulations are established by authorized agencies in the state to implement the provisions established in the law. Regulations, or what is referred to as *regs*, may be changed by the authorized agency.

Components of Licensure Laws Although the specific content of the licensure laws varies from state to state, each law has the following basic components: a statement of intent, definition of the area of practice, prohibited acts, requirements, provisions for discipline, and identification of the regulatory body. The law may also have special provisions about transferability, exemptions, or other matters particular to the state.

Intent Licensure laws usually include a statement that explains the purpose of the statute.

Definition of Practice Licensure laws, also referred to as *practice acts*, usually establish a "scope of practice"; that is, they define what the person covered by the act is allowed to do in the practice of the profession. The scope of practice or permitted acts varies with each state. For example, according to New York State Education Law (1974), the practice of speech-language pathology includes the application of principles, methods and procedures of measurement, prediction, nonmedical diagnosis, testing, counseling, consultation, rehabilitation, and instruction related to the development and disorders of speech, voice, swallowing, and/or language. In some states, speech-language pathologists are permitted to do endoscopic swallowing evaluations, albeit with some restrictions, but in others they are not.

Prohibited Act Many state licensure laws prohibit the use of the professional title by individuals not holding the license. This prohibition assures the public that anyone using the title has met the standards established by the law and regulatory agency.

State Regulatory Board of Examiners Licensure laws usually establish a board of examiners or an advisory council that is appointed by the regulatory agency. The boards are made up of licensed professionals. They usually include at least one consumer or public member to ensure that consumer needs are protected and represented in board activity.

General Requirements Most states have general requirements that apply to all licensed professions in the state. For example, to be licensed in New York as a speech-language

TABLE 3–1 States Regulating Speech-Language Pathologists (SLP), Audiologists (A), and Support Personnel (SP) (as of December 2010)

(L=License R=Registration O=Other Regulation X=None C=Certification)

State	SLP	A	SP	State	SLP	A	SP
Alabama	L	L	R	Nebraska	L	L	R
Alaska	L	L	R	Nevada	L	L	O
Arizona	L	L	L	New Hampshire	L	L*	C
Arkansas	L	L	R	New Jersey	L	L	X
California	L	L	R	New Mexico	L*	L*	L
Colorado	L	L	X	New York	L	L	X
Connecticut	L*	L*	O	North Carolina	L	L	R
Delaware	L*	L*	O	North Dakota	L	L	X
Florida	L	L	C	Ohio	L*	L*	L
Georgia	L	L	R	Oklahoma	L	L	L
Hawaii	L*	L*	X	Oregon	L	L	C
Idaho	L	L	L	Pennsylvania	L	L	R
Illinois	L	L	L	Rhode Island	L	L	R
Indiana	L*	L*	R	South Carolina	L	L	L
Iowa	L	L	X	South Dakota	L*	L*	X
Kansas	L*	L*	R	Tennessee	L	L	R
Kentucky	L	L	L	Texas	L*	L*	L
Louisiana	L*	L*	L	Utah	L	L	R
Maine	L	L	R	Vermont	L	L	X
Maryland	L	L*	L	Virginia	L	L	C
Massachusetts	L*	L*	L	Washington	L	L	C
Michigan	L	L	X	Washington, DC	L	L	X
Minnesota	L	L	O	West Virginia	L	L	R
Mississippi	L	L	R	Wisconsin	L	L	X
Missouri	L	L	R	Wyoming	L	L	R
Montana	L*	L*	R				

* Indicates school-based personnel are required to be licensed.

Source: Table compiled using data from ASHA's State Support Personnel Trends and 2010 Quarterly Report IV documents. Retrieved from http://www.asha.org/uploadedFiles/SupportPersonnelTrends.pdf and from http://dev2010.asha.org/uploadedFiles/2010QuarterlyReportIV.pdf

pathologist or audiologist, you must be of good moral character; be at least 21 years of age; and meet education, examination, and experience requirements.

Education In addition to the general requirements, the person holding the license must meet specific education requirements. All state laws regulating speech-language pathologists and audiologists specify the master's degree or a graduate degree or equivalent as the minimum for receipt of the license. In most states, the education requirements for obtaining a license in speech-language pathology and audiology were developed after a model provided by ASHA. Consequently, the requirements are similar across the states. Some states refer directly to the ASHA standards for the CCC so that the state requirements are identical to those of the CCC, including all revisions. Most states, however, identify the requirements independent of the CCC and are thus unaffected by changes in the CCC unless specific modifications are made in the state laws or regulations. For example, although ASHA certification requires the doctorate in audiology for certification, only 24 states require a doctorate degree for practice.

Some states require coursework in addition to that required by ASHA certification. For example, Florida requires one hour of training in HIV/AIDS and two hours in prevention of medical errors (Florida Department of Health, 2011).

Experience Most states require applicants for the license to have completed a minimum of 325 clock hours at the graduate level or 400 supervised clock hours. Most require the equivalent of a nine-month or 36-week, full-time supervised clinical experience after awarding of the degree.

Examination All state licensure laws require applicants to demonstrate their professional knowledge in the area of practice by passing an examination such as the Praxis II Examination in Speech-Language Pathology. This is the same examination required for ASHA's CCC; however, states may set their own passing score for satisfying the knowledge requirement.

Exemptions Many state licensure laws have provisions that exempt certain people, such as federal employees, from holding the license to practice the professions. Some states have provisions that exempt people holding teacher certification by the state department of education from holding the professional license for practice in schools.

Continuing Education The right to continue to practice after initial entry into the profession is usually regulated by a requirement to periodically demonstrate continued competence. Of the 50 states that regulate or license the practice of audiology or speech-language pathology or both, 47 states require a prescribed program of continuing education for renewal of the license. As shown in Table 3–2, there is considerable variation in the requirement for the demonstration of continued competence across states.

Professional Discipline Licensure laws contain provisions for people who violate the professional code of conduct. The sanctions for violations of a state license may include probation, suspension or revocation of the license, and/or payment of a fine. The individual may also be referred to the attorney general if a felony is alleged to have been committed. See Chapters 5 and 6 for further discussion of professional ethics and liability.

Transferability and Reciprocity A license to practice in one state is not directly transferable to another state. There are no reciprocal agreements among the states. Individuals must apply for a license in each state in which they wish to practice.

Interim Practice or Temporary Licenses Interim practice provisions allow a person to practice for a period of time before the actual license is issued or while a license is pending. Provisions for interim practice or temporary licenses vary across the states.

PROFESSIONAL CERTIFICATION

Whereas a professional license is permission granted by state law to do something that is otherwise forbidden, certification is a statement that one has completed a particular course of study, passed an examination, or met other qualifications for the certification. It is not a permission to act; rather, it is a statement of qualification. Professional certification is issued by a private organization. For example, the Clinical Certification Board of the American Speech-Language-Hearing Association issues the Certificates of Clinical Competence in speech-language pathology and audiology. The American Board of Audiology issues certification in audiology. Professional certification does not involve the power of state or law. Teacher certification may be specified in the education laws of a particular state such as New York State Education Law.

TABLE 3–2 Continuing Competence Requirements by States

State	No. of CE Hours	Time (Years)	ASHA CEU Preapproved	Comments
Alabama	12	1		
Alaska	NA*			
Arizona	10	1		
Arkansas	10	1		At least 5 hours in specified content area
California	24	2	X	
Colorado	NA			
Connecticut	20	2		
Delaware	30	2		Minimum 14 hours focusing on clinical skills; approved continuing education courses per licensure period listed on state website
Florida	30	2	X	18 hours clinical skills, 2 hours prevention of medical errors
Georgia	20	2		CEU credit must be directly related to scope of practice
Hawaii	NA			
Idaho	10	1		
Illinois	20	2	X	
Indiana	36	2		Up to 6 hours of self-study permitted
Iowa	30	2		
Kansas	20	2		
Kentucky	15	1	X	May carry over up to 5 hours
Louisiana	10	1	X	At least 5 hours must be in area of licensure
Maine	25	2	X	May carry over unlimited number of hours
Maryland	20	2		Up to 5 hours of self-study permitted
Massachusetts	20	2	X	Minimum 10 hours in area of licensure
Michigan	20 (AuD)	2		
Minnesota	30	2	X	At least 20 hours directly related to area of licensure

(*Continues*)

TABLE 3–2 Continuing Competence Requirements by States *(Continued)*

State	No. of CE Hours	Time (Years)	ASHA CEU Preapproved	Comments
Mississippi	20	2	X	Minimum 10 hours directly related to clinical practicum
Missouri	30	2	X	Minimum 20 hours from approved sponsors
Montana	40	2	X	At least 25 hours from approved sponsors
Nebraska	20	2	X	Up to 3 hours of self-study permitted
Nevada	15	1		Maximum 8 hours in practice management
New Hampshire (A)	20	2	X	May carry over up to 10 hours
New Hampshire	30 (SLP)	2	X	
	20 (AuD)	2		
New Jersey	20	2	X	Minimum 15 hours directly related to practice
New Mexico	10	1	X	May carry over up to 10 hours
New York	30	3		At least 20 hours directly related to area of licensure
North Carolina	30	3		
North Dakota	10	1		
Ohio	20	2	X	Minimum 10 hours related to clinical practice
Oklahoma	20	2		
Oregon	40	2	X	
Pennsylvania	20	2		
Rhode Island	20	2	X	
South Carolina	16	1	X	Minimum 8 hours in clinical practice
South Dakota	12	1		Audiology only
Tennessee	10	1		
Texas	10	1		May carry over up to 20 hours
Utah	20	2		
Vermont	30	3		
Virginia	30	2	X	Minimum 15 hours related to area of licensure
Washington	30	3		

(Continues)

(*Continued*)

West Virginia	20	2	
Wisconsin	20	2	
Wyoming	12	1	X
Washington, DC	NA		

*NA- Not Applicable

Source: Table compiled using data from ASHA's State Licensure Trends document. Retrieved from http://www.asha.org/uploadedFiles/StateLicensureTrends.pdf

ASHA Certificates of Clinical Competence

The credentials issued by professional associations, such as ASHA or AAA, are voluntary unless required by an agency where there is no governmental jurisdiction. The credential issued by ASHA is the Certificate of Clinical Competence. ASHA developed its first standards for the practice of the profession in 1942. The CCC permits the holder to provide independent clinical services and to supervise the clinical practice of student trainees, other clinicians who do not hold the certification, and support personnel.

Requirements for the Certificates of Clinical Competence

The Council for Clinical Certification (CFCC) is responsible for the ASHA Certificates of Clinical Competence in both speech-language pathology and audiology (2011). The standards for the CCCs follow the same model as those for the professional license, that is, a required academic degree, coursework in basic communication sciences and disorders, a supervised clinical practicum, a period of supervised professional experience, and an examination.

The standards for the CCCs are revised periodically to ensure that the standards are consistent with the scopes of practice of the professions. They are developed following a rigorous validation study of the knowledge and skills necessary for entry into independent practice of the particular profession. Validation studies are conducted periodically by an independent organization to determine whether the standards continue to meet the needs of independent practice. Changes in the requirements are made if necessary. The implementation language is also revised periodically to ensure there is clarity and consistency in the application and interpretation of the standards.

CCC in Speech-Language Pathology The salient features of the current standards for the CCC in speech-language pathology include the following:

1. A graduate degree (master's or doctorate) in speech-language pathology, speech language and hearing science, or an allied discipline.
2. The graduate education in speech-language pathology must have been initiated and completed in a program accredited in speech-language pathology by the Council of Academic Accreditation in Audiology and Speech-Language Pathology (CAA) of the American Speech-Language-Hearing Association.
3. A minimum of 36 graduate credit hours of academic credit that reflect a well-integrated program of study dealing with biological/physical sciences and mathematics; behavioral and or social sciences, including normal aspects of human behavior and communication; and prevention, evaluation, and treatment of speech-language, hearing, and related disorders. Some coursework must deal with issues pertaining to normal and abnormal development and behavior across the life span and to culturally diverse populations.
4. A minimum of 400 clock hours of supervised clinical practicum, of which at least 375 clock

hours are direct client/patient contact and 25 are supervised observation hours.

5. A passing score on the Praxis II Examination in Speech-Language Pathology.
6. Completion of a full-time supervised speech-language pathology clinical fellowship of at least 36 weeks that establishes collaboration between the clinical fellow and a mentor.
7. A maintenance of certification requirement.

CCC in Audiology The scope of practice of the profession of audiology has changed rapidly in the past decade in response to data presented by audiologists and an extensive skills validation study. The salient features of the standards for the CCC in audiology include the following:

1. Completion of an academic program that includes a minimum of 75 graduate semester credit hours of postbaccalaureate study that culminates in a doctoral degree.
2. A graduate degree granted by a program accredited by the CAA.
3. The program of study must include academic coursework and a minimum of 1,820 hours of supervised clinical practicum sufficient in depth and breadth to achieve the knowledge and skills outcome as defined by the CFCC.
4. The knowledge and developed skills must be obtained in six areas: foundations of practice, prevention/identification, assessment, (re)habilitation, advocacy/consultation, and education/research/administration.
5. There must be a passing score on a comprehensive examination at the culmination of the educational preparation.
6. A maintenance of certification requirement.

Specialty Recognition

Specialty recognition is a voluntary program that allows recognition of individual practitioners who have obtained advanced knowledge and experience in a given specialty area, such as child language disorders, fluency, or swallowing and swallowing disorders, following earning the CCC. Specialty recognition identifies individuals who have specific experience and knowledge beyond that held by the standards established for the CCC. It is a means for consumers to identify practitioners who choose to meet established educational and experience criteria and who focus all or part of their practice in a particular specialty area recognized by ASHA.

Certification by the American Board of Audiology

The American Academy of Audiology (AAA) is a professional organization for audiologists. The AAA has established a certification program for audiologists administered by the American Board of Audiology (ABA). Individuals seeking certification by the ABA must demonstrate evidence of initial mastery of the core elements of audiologic knowledge. To be eligible for certification, audiologists must have earned a doctoral degree in audiology from a regionally accredited college or university. In addition, applicants for the certification must have obtained a passing score on a national examination as required by the ABA and have completed 2,000 hours of mentored professional practice within a three-year time period after completion of academic coursework. AuD students may apply for provisional board certification once they have completed all coursework and 375 hours of direct patient care but have not completed their fourth-year internship.

Audiologists certified by the ABA must be recertified every three years by completing 60 clock hours of continuing education in audiology including at least three hours in professional ethics. The recertification hours may be obtained in approved conferences, courses, seminars, or workshops or by authoring audiology articles in peer-reviewed journals, chapters, or professional books.

ABA Specialty Certification The American Board of Audiology has a specialty certification program in cochlear implants and is in the process of developing a specialty in pediatric audiology. Information about these programs can be found at the ABA's website, provided in the Resources section of this chapter.

Teacher Certification

A certified teacher is an educator who has earned credentials from an authoritative source, such as the government, department of education, a higher education institution, or a private source. Teacher certification allows educators to teach in schools that require authorization in general such as the public schools. In addition, it allows educators to teach particular content areas such as mathematics and related service areas such as speech-language pathology.

The teacher certification rules vary with each state. Teacher certification often requires an examination that is different from the examinations required for the ASHA CCC or state licensure. For example, New York State requires the New York State Teacher Certification Examination—Liberal Arts and Sciences Test (LAST) and the Elementary Assessment of Teaching Skills (ATS-W). Oklahoma requires passage of the Oklahoma General Education Test (OGET). California requires passage of the California Basic Educational Skills Test (California State Legislature, 2007). Be sure to check the specific requirements for your state.

Some states have teacher certification requirements that are not related to the professional discipline. For example, New York State requires applicants for certification as a Teacher of Students with Speech and Language Disabilities to take state-approved workshops in the needs of students with autism, child abuse identification, and school violence intervention. Several states also require applicants to pass a criminal background review or obtain fingerprint clearance.

In at least 24 states and many local school districts, those who hold both the Certificate of Clinical Competence and the teaching certificate for employment in the schools receive a supplement of from $100 to $5,000 to their annual salary (Boswell, 2007). The salary supplements are offered to assist the district in recruiting qualified speech-language pathologists to work in the districts because of personnel shortages.

It is imperative that individuals consult the laws for the individual state in which they are seeking employment. The ASHA website provides an overview of each state's certification requirements. See the Resources section at the end of this chapter.

REGISTRATION

Registration is similar to certification. It may not involve the government. However, persons engaged in some occupations must hold registration to engage in certain activities. Dietitians, for example, are registered in most states. The registering organization, the American Dietetic Association, is a private group. The government is not involved.

Certain support personnel or paraprofessionals, such as speech pathology assistants, audiology assistants, or hearing aid dispensers, must be registered to practice in a state. In some states, licensed professionals must also register to indicate to the public that they continue to meet the licensure requirements established for the profession. For example, in New York State, professionals are licensed in speech-language pathology or audiology, but to practice, they must also be registered with the New York State Education Department. Registration must be renewed every three years to assure the public that the standards for entry into practice are met and that competence has continued.

SUPPORT PERSONNEL

Because of increased demand, a more diverse client base, and an expanding scope of practice, more personnel are needed to provide speech-language and audiology services. Some tasks performed by speech-language pathologists and audiologists can be performed by personnel with less training than the licensed or certified professional. The use of speech-language pathology assistants or communication aides as support personnel in speech-language pathology has emerged as a viable way to both reduce costs and provide more services.

ASHA does not credential support personnel in speech-language pathology or audiology. However, ASHA has had guidelines for the use of support personnel since 1969. According to guidelines from ASHA, support personnel may be used to perform activities adjunct to the primary clinical efforts of speech-language pathologists (ASHA, 2004). The guidelines call for assistants to complete a minimum of an associate degree or equivalent course of study. Because the guidelines are national in scope, they may serve to bring about more uniformity in the terms used to identify speech-language pathology support personnel, training requirements, and supervisory responsibilities. A new level of ASHA membership for associates became available in 2011. Read Chapter 12 for a discussion of support personnel.

TELEPRACTICE

Issues related to telepractice have had an impact on state licensure (ASHA, 2011b). Telepractice means the use of advanced telecommunications and information technologies for the exchange of information from one site to another for the provision of services through a hardwire or Internet connection. Several state licensure laws currently have provisions regarding the use of telepractice. Most state that the provision of speech pathology or audiology services in the particular state through telephonic, electronic, or other means, regardless of the location of the speech pathologist or audiologist, shall constitute the practice of speech pathology or audiology and shall require a license to practice in the state. Because the laws change rapidly in this growing area of practice, consult your individual licensure boards to determine the status of telepractice laws in your state. See Chapter 26 for more discussion of telepractice.

INTERNATIONAL ISSUES

There are professional preparation programs for speech-language pathologists and audiologists in many countries around the world. Each country has its own educational requirements and standards for professional practice. Many countries follow the general format for education and training in the United States; however, while in some countries speech-language pathology and audiology are doctoring professions, in others the professions are specialties practiced at the bachelor's level. Several countries also require certification and licenses for practice. While the requirements are generally similar, they may differ in the required coursework, the amount and type of supervised clinical practicum, experience, and examinations. Speech-language pathologists or audiologists who wish to work in a country in which they are not a citizen must meet that country's visa, work permit, education, licensing, and regulatory requirements.

ASHA has a multilateral agreement with six English-speaking countries. These agreements relate to professional organizations including the Canadian Association of Speech-Language Pathologists and Audiologists (CASLPA), the Royal College of Speech Therapists in the United Kingdom, the Irish Association of Speech and Language Therapists, the New Zealand Speech-Language Therapists' Association (Incorporated), and the Speech Pathology Association of Australia Limited. The credentials in these countries, while similar to those of ASHA, are not considered essentially equivalent. This agreement recognizes common standards in academic and clinical practice and streamlines the recognition process for SLPs credentialed by the associations who seek accreditation of another association in the agreement. It is not a program of reciprocity; rather, it recognizes the areas of similarity and thus simplifies the application and credentialing process.

Approximately 2,000 certified ASHA members live outside the United States. To address international issues as they affect the professions, ASHA has established an International Issues Board. The board has been charged to develop, monitor, and recommend Association policies and actions related to international issues and facilitate ASHA's strategic planning and engagement with speech, language, and hearing organizations worldwide to promote scientific and resource exchange to improve the science and practice of the professions. In addition, Special Interest Group 17, Global Issues in Communication Sciences and Related Disorders, provides international leadership related to audiology and speech-language pathology services by promoting research, networking, collaboration, education, and mentoring for its affiliates, students, and other service providers in the global marketplace.

Members of the profession who reside abroad and who are not exclusively citizens of the United States may become international affiliates of ASHA. As international affiliates, they have access to ASHA online journals and special benefits for continuing education and other ASHA services and programs. ASHA has also recently established a special recognition award for Outstanding Contribution in International Achievement that was designed to recognize distinguished achievements and significant contributions in the area of communication disorders revealing great international impact.

ASHA maintains a relationship as an affiliated society with the International Association of Logopedics and Phoniatrics (IALP), a worldwide association of professionals and scientists interested in communication, speech-language pathology, voice, swallowing, and audiology. The IALP does not credential logopedists; however, it produces guidelines for the initial education of logopedists to give guidance to programs around the world that are starting educational programs (International Association of Logopedics and Phoniatrics, 1998, 1999; Cheng, 2010). The guidelines were used to assist in the development of newly established programs in Uganda, Sri Lanka, Malaysia, Vietnam, Korea, and Turkey as well as for improvements in programs in other countries. See Chapter 7 for more discussion of this topic.

CODE OF ETHICS

The preservation of the highest standards of integrity and ethical principles is vital to the responsible discharge of obligations in the professions of speech-language pathology and audiology. Speech-language pathologists and audiologists who hold the ASHA CCC must abide by the Code of Ethics to assure the public they hold paramount the welfare of the people they serve professionally, achieve and maintain the highest level of professional competence, and honor their responsibility to the public and to the professions. The Ethical Practices Board, which consists of members of the profession as well as consumers, reviews violations of the code. Violations of the code may result in probation or revocation of the CCC. People who are certified by the American Board of Audiology must abide by the Code of Ethics of the American Academy of Audiology. Those who hold state licensure must also abide by the code of professional conduct for their particular state. See Chapters 5 and 6 for further discussion of ethics and liability.

SUMMARY

Communication is a complex human behavior. The study of communication sciences and disorders and the practice of the professions of speech-language pathology and audiology are changing to meet the challenges of advancing knowledge of the complexities of speech, language, swallowing, and hearing impairment. The standards for practice must be current to assure the public that no harm will occur from improper evaluation or treatment. The assessment and treatment of communication disorders and the investigation of the nature of speech, language, swallowing, and hearing require a highly skilled professional. The practice of speech-language pathology requires a graduate degree and continuing education. The practice of audiology requires a doctoral degree as a minimum standard for entry into the practice of the profession in many states. The public must also feel confident that professionals follow standards of clinical and ethical practice. This promise is met by regulation through professional certification and/or professional licensure. By adhering to codes of professional conduct and ethical standards, speech-language pathologists and audiologists can assure the public that the services they provide are trustworthy.

CRITICAL THINKING

1. Review the licensure laws for speech-language pathologists and audiologists in your state. How do the requirements differ from the requirements for the ASHA CCC?
2. What harm could result from the delivery of speech-language pathology or audiology services by an unlicensed or uncertified person?
3. What has been the impact of the required doctoral degree in audiology on the profession of audiology? What would be the advantages or disadvantages of a doctoral entry degree for speech-language pathologists?
4. What are the advantages and disadvantages of professional standards for support personnel? Do you think that professional associations should certify support personnel? Why or why not?
5. How do you envision training for speech-language pathologists or audiologists changing in the next 10 years? Why might these changes be needed?
6. Why is continuing education a critical part of our professional preparation? If you are a practicing clinician, describe how you meet continuing education requirements for ASHA or ABA certification or licensure. If you are a student, what areas do you think will be of interest to you in continuing education?
7. Why is specialty certification or recognition valuable in our professions? Would you work toward specialty certification? Why?
8. Suppose your state was considering "sunsetting" licensure in your profession (i.e., eliminating it). What would be your reaction to this? What does licensure do for our professions' viability and identity?
9. You are a Canadian citizen who is about to complete degree requirements in either speech-language pathology or audiology. You plan on returning to Canada to practice. What is your plan of action to meet requirements in one of the provinces of your choice?
10. You have worked for several years and are now considering returning for a doctoral degree. What should you think about as you consider this academic program? What would you look for in a doctoral program? What do you think a doctoral program will achieve for you versus pursuing a consistent program of continuing education?

REFERENCES

American Speech-Language-Hearing Association. (2004). *Guidelines for credentialing, use, and supervision of speech-language pathology assistants.* Available from http://www.asha.org

American Speech-Language-Hearing Association. (2011a). *Standards for accreditation of graduate education programs in audiology and speech-language pathology.* Retrieved from http://www.asha.org/Academic/accreditation/accredmanual/section3.htm

American Speech-Language-Hearing Association. (2011b). *State licensure telepractice provisions.* Retrieved from http://www.asha.org/Practice/telepractice/telepractice-licensure

Blake, D. (1995). *The dictionary of educational terms.* Brookfield, VT: Ashgate Publishing.

Boswell, S. (2007, September 4). School salary supplements on the rise: Districts in New York, California are the latest to boost clinicians' salaries. *The ASHA Leader.*

California State Legislature. (2007). *California Speech-Language, Pathology, and Audiology Board Practice Act.* Chapter 5.3, Article 1, General provisions, 2530.2 (4)(f). Available from http://www.slpab.ca.gov/board_activity/laws_regs/lawsregs.pdf

Cheng, L. (Ed.). (2010). Education for speech and language pathology [Special issue]. *Folia Phoniatrica et Logopaedica, 62*(5), 205–262.

Council for Clinical Certification in Audiology and Speech-Language Pathology of the American Speech-Language-Hearing Association. (2011). *2011 Standards for the certificate of clinical competence in audiology.* Available from http://dev2010.asha.org/certification/aud2011standards

Council of Graduate Schools in the United States. (1990). *The doctor of philosophy degree.* Washington, DC: Author.

Dudding, C. C., & Purcell-Robertson, R. M. (2003, June 10). Beyond the technology: How to navigate distance education. *The ASHA Leader, 8*(11), 6–7, 16.

Florida Department of Health. (2011). Licensure requirements for speech-language pathology, Florida Board of Speech-Language Pathology and Audiology. Available from http://www.doh.state.fl.us/mqa/speech/sa_lic_req.html

International Association of Logopedics and Phoniatrics. (1998). Guidelines for the initial education in logopedics. *Folia Phoniatrica et Logopaedica, 50,* 230–234.

International Association of Logopedics and Phoniatrics. (1999). Guiding principles of training of support workers in communication disabilities in unserved areas. *Folia Phoniatrica et Logopaedica, 51,* 239–242.

Knowles, A. (Ed.). (1977). Degrees, diplomas, and certificates. In *International encyclopedia of higher education* (Vol. 4, pp. 1230–1241). San Francisco, CA: Jossey-Bass.

Neidecker, E., & Blosser, J. (1993). *School programs in speech language: Organization and management.* Englewood Cliffs, NJ: Prentice Hall.

New York State Education Department. (1974). Laws, rules & regulations. Education law. Article 159. Speech-language pathologists and audiologists: 8203, 1974, c.1055; 8202 amended L. 1983, c.43.1. Available from http://www.op.nysed.gov/prof/slpa/speechlaw.htm

Page, J., Amster, B., Gil, G., & Griffiths, S. (2010, April). *Distance education programs: Myth vs. reality.* Paper presented at the annual meeting of the Council of Academic Programs in Communication Sciences and Disorders, Austin, Texas. Retrieved from http://www.capcsd.org/proceedings/2010/toc2010.html

RESOURCES

Accreditation Commission for Audiology Education

The purpose of ACAE accreditation is to recognize, reinforce, and promote high-quality performance in AuD educational programs through a rigorous verification process. This process will produce evidence that AuD programs have prepared graduates who are qualified to be doctoral-level audiologists. It also will assure communities of interest that graduates will be able to function according to the national scope of practice, as defined by the professional organization.

Website: http://www.acaeaccred.org

American Academy of Audiology

The American Academy of Audiology is the world's largest professional organization of, by, and for audiologists. The active membership of more than 10,000 is dedicated to providing quality hearing care services through professional development, education, research, and increased public awareness of hearing and balance disorders.

Website: http://www.audiology.org

American Board of Audiology

The American Board of Audiology (ABA), an autonomous organization, is dedicated to enhancing audiologic services to the public by promulgating universally recognized standards in professional practice. The ABA encourages audiologists to exceed these prescribed standards, thereby promoting a high level of professional development and ethical practice.

Website: http://www.americanboardofaudiology.org

American Speech-Language-Hearing Association

The American Speech-Language-Hearing Association (ASHA) is the professional, scientific, and credentialing association for 145,000 members and affiliates who are audiologists; speech-language pathologists; and speech, language, and hearing scientists.

American Speech-Language-Hearing Association resources are available from ASHA, 2200 Research Boulevard, Rockville, MD 20850-3289.

Website: http://www.asha.org

Council for Clinical Certification in Audiology and Speech-Language Pathology (CFCC)

The CFCC defines the standards for clinical certification and applies those standards to the certification of individuals; it may also develop and administer a credentialing program for speech-language pathology assistants.

Website: http://www.asha.org/About/governance/committees/Council-for-Clinical-Certification-in-Audiology-and-Speech-Language-Pathology

Council of Academic Programs in Communication Sciences and Disorders (CAPCSD)

Founded in 1979, CAPCSD supports more than 260 programs worldwide that educate undergraduate and graduate students in the communication sciences and disorders. The Council keeps its membership ahead of the challenges that face academic programs, faculty, staff, and students engaged in the study of communicative sciences and disorders. The Council has established a Communication Sciences and Disorders Centralized Application Service (CSDCAS) for clinical education in audiology and speech-language pathology. CSDCAS is a state-of-the-art, web-based application that offers applicants a convenient way to apply to multiple clinical education programs in audiology and speech-language pathology by completing a single application.

Website: http://www.capcsd.org

Council on Academic Accreditation in Audiology and Speech-Language Pathology (CAA)

The purpose of the CAA is to formulate standards for the accreditation of graduate education programs that provide entry-level professional preparation in audiology and/or speech-language pathology.

CAA is the only accrediting agency for audiology and speech-language pathology education programs recognized by the Council on Higher Education Accreditation (CHEA) and the U.S. Department of Education.

Website: http://www.asha.org/academic/accreditation/CAA_overview.htm

EdFind

EdFind provides current, accurate, and comprehensive academic program information about master's and doctoral programs in speech-language pathology and speech language and hearing science and doctoral programs in audiology.

Website: http://www.asha.org/edfind

HES

The Higher Education Data System (HES) was developed by ASHA in collaboration with the Council of Academic Programs in Communication Sciences and Disorders (CAPCSD) and the Council on Academic Accreditation in Audiology and Speech-Language Pathology (CAA) to collect and report critical communication sciences and disorders (CSD) program data in a consistent and usable manner.

Website: http://www.asha.org/academic/HES/default.htm

International Association of Logopedics and Phoniatrics (IALP)

The IALP is the oldest international organization working on scientific, educational, and professional issues affecting people with communication, language, voice, speech, hearing, and swallowing disorders worldwide. IALP's mission is to provide a network that enables those concerned with communication sciences and disorders to work together and enrich their understanding by providing an opportunity to situate their work within broad multicultural perspectives. Its members, scientists, physicians, speech-language pathologists, and practitioners work in more than 57 countries and come from every continent around the world. The organization also has consultative status with the World Health Organization of the United Nations and works in association with the United Nations Department of Public Information.

Website: http://www.ialp.info

National Academy of Preprofessional Programs in Communication Sciences and Disorders (NAPP)

The National Academy of Preprofessional Programs in Communication Sciences and Disorders (NAPP) represents undergraduate programs in speech-language pathology and audiology. Member institutions are approved by state, regional, or national accrediting agencies and have an identifiable unit with the institution and do not offer graduate level studies. Check their website at http://www.calvin.edu/~jvwoude.

National Institute on Deafness and Other Communication Disorders (NIDCD)

The National Institute on Deafness and Other Communication Disorders (NIDCD) is one of the National Institutes of Health (NIH) within the U.S. Department of Health and Human Services (HHS) and is the federal focal point for research on human communication. The NIDCD funds research and research training in the normal and disordered processes of hearing, balance, smell, taste, voice, speech, and language. It also funds research and research training in more than two dozen disciplines, such as molecular genetics, physiology, cellular biology, linguistics, psychoacoustics, molecular genetics, epidemiology, bioengineering, nanotechnology, toxicology, computational biology, immunology, and structural biology—the full range of the biological and behavioral sciences.

Website: http://www.nidcd.nih.gov/Pages/default.aspx

National Student Speech Language Hearing Association

The National Student Speech Language Hearing Association (NSSLHA) is a preprofessional membership association for students interested in the study of communication sciences and disorders. Membership is available to undergraduate, graduate, or doctoral students enrolled full or part time in a communication sciences program or related major.

Website: http://www.nsslha.org

Overview of State Credential Requirements

The ASHA advocacy team provides a state-by-state overview of licensing laws, regulations, and teacher certification requirements for speech-language pathology and audiology.

Website: http://www.asha.org/advocacy/state/default.htm

FINANCIAL AID AND SCHOLARSHIPS

Information on scholarships available from ASHA can be obtained from the American Speech-Language-Hearing Foundation, 2200 Research Blvd., Rockville, MD 20850-3289.

Information on federal scholarships and assistantships through federally funded grants and contracts can be obtained through individual colleges and universities or the U.S. Department of Education, Office of Special Education and Rehabilitative Services, Division of Personnel Preparation, Washington, DC 20202.

Specific information on financial assistance, including privately funded scholarships for graduate study in communication sciences and disorders, is available from the financial aid office at the college or university you wish to attend.

Information on funding predoctoral, doctoral, and postdoctoral studies can be obtained from the National Institutes of Health website at http://www.asha.org/research/grants-funding/FundingStudents.htm.

4

Professional Organizations

Sue T. Hale, MCD
Fred H. Bess, PhD

SCOPE OF CHAPTER

This chapter introduces you to opportunities for affiliating with professional organizations. The benefits of membership are highlighted, but the more important objective is to help you discover the service, leadership, and learning opportunities these organizations present. Scenarios in the opening section set the stage for what associations can do for their members. A brief review of the construct of professional organizations is provided. The American Speech-Language-Hearing Association (ASHA) and the American Academy of Audiology (AAA) are highlighted as the two primary organizations for our professions. Related professional organizations, state associations, and student organizations are also described.

PRACTICAL DILEMMAS AND AFFILIATION

Consider the following:

- The only speech-language pathologist working in a rural school district has concerns about the size of the caseload the school district requires to be served. Unlike the predecessor in this position, this clinician serves a number of children who exhibit multiple and severe handicaps. How does the speech-language pathologist demonstrate that the current caseload/workload with fewer children is equivalent in effort to that of the previous clinician who saw greater numbers of children with less severe disorders?
- An audiologist is approached by a hearing aid manufacturer who offers an all-expense-paid educational opportunity regarding a new product line the manufacturer sells. The conference will take place for two hours a day during a five-day stay at an exclusive ski resort. The company representative also encourages the audiologist to invite a family member or spouse to come along. How should the audiologist respond?
- A speech-language pathologist in a medical setting is assigned to provide intervention for patients who require systems for alternative/augmentative communication, an area of practice with which the clinician has had little experience or education. How can the clinician locate relevant educational events and materials to assist in developing the necessary skills and knowledge to provide services in this area?
- An audiologist wants to communicate with other audiologists who are researching hearing aid products and cochlear implants. Where can the audiologist locate colleagues with similar interests?
- A speech-language pathologist is concerned that the arbitrary cap on reimbursement for services provided to hospital outpatients will soon be reinstated if legislation is not passed to eliminate the therapy cap. How can the speech-language pathologist maximize the value of advocacy efforts for legislation of this nature?

In each instance, affiliation with a professional association and taking advantage of the member benefits of that association will assist the professionals facing these practical dilemmas. Professional associations available to speech-language pathologists and audiologists support members in dealing with all of the instances listed previously: clarifying caseload versus workload issues to employers, handling ethical dilemmas in the workplace, accessing continuing education opportunities, affiliating with other professionals who have similar interests, and participating in grassroots and coordinated advocacy efforts. These are just a few of the benefits available to speech-language pathologists and audiologists who are members of professional associations.

Students in training who affiliate with organizations targeted to their interests and needs gain firsthand knowledge of the structure and benefits of these associations prior to entering the workforce. Student organizations provide opportunities for leadership development and volunteer service as well as educational materials and scholarly and professional publications. These organizations facilitate the transition of students to the workplace in regard to standards and credentialing, ethics, and networking. Two organizations available to students in communication sciences and disorders are the National Student Speech Language Hearing Association (NSSLHA), which is affiliated with ASHA, and the Student Academy of Audiology (SAA), which is affiliated with AAA. These organizations will be described in more detail later in the chapter.

HOW DO PROFESSIONAL ASSOCIATIONS WORK?

Professional associations offer an array of services and benefits to members as well as provide support and advocate on behalf of consumers served by those members. Professional associations have a targeted scope of activity, typically related to a particular discipline. Individuals who wish to affiliate with the association often have to meet requirements that relate to degrees held and other educational and professional qualifications.

Professional associations have a number of common characteristics. These organizations often take responsibility for providing members with educational programs and materials, scientific and professional publications, targeted legislative advocacy activities, standards and scopes of practice, marketing resources, and public information. An important characteristic of most professional organizations is a requirement that members agree to abide by a Code of Ethics, a set of standards for professional conduct that delineate responsibilities of the members to consumers, colleagues, and the profession. Professional associations are usually nonprofit organizations governed by a Board of Directors and operated with publicly accessible bylaws. The bylaws, which contain the organization's mission and goals, also describe the governance structure and how the work of the association is conducted. Most professional organizations operate with a combination of volunteer leaders, who often assume positions on the Board of Directors or other policy-making groups, and paid staff members who engage in day-to-day operations and support member services.

Professional organizations derive a large portion of the operating budget from member dues, but additional fiscal resources are often generated by conventions and continuing education activities, publications and product sales, affiliations with commercial entities (affinity credit cards, professional and casualty insurers, convention exhibitors), corporate sponsors, and investments. These sources of income support the member benefits and consumer advocacy goals of the organization.

ASHA and AAA are two national organizations with members from the professions of speech-language pathology and audiology. ASHA has members from both professions, while AAA has members from the profession of audiology.

ASHA: A NATIONAL PROFESSIONAL ORGANIZATION FOR SPEECH-LANGUAGE PATHOLOGISTS AND AUDIOLOGISTS

The American Speech-Language-Hearing Association is the largest and oldest scientific and professional organization representing the professions of speech-language pathology and audiology. ASHA began with a meeting in May 1925 in the home of Lee Edward Travis. There were fewer than 25 individuals at that first meeting, and they came together because they all held an interest in speech and its disorders. It was more than a decade before the number of members reached 60, and the organization began publishing its first scholarly journal. In 1947, the organization embraced the profession of audiology and was named the American Speech and Hearing Association. In the 1960s, the association established national standards for graduate training program accreditation and credentialing of service providers. In 1978, the organization changed its name once again to reflect the component of language in its research and clinical pursuits and became the American Speech-Language-Hearing Association. Throughout its history, the association has been characterized by enormous growth in membership and a corresponding need for greater staff support. In 2007 the association moved to its current headquarters in Rockville, Maryland, a 140,000-square-foot facility holding Gold LEED certification due to its environmentally focused construction and usage. About 250 staff members work in the ASHA National Office. See Chapter 2 for more on the founding of the professions.

Purpose

Bylaws address the purposes of an association. The purposes of ASHA, as stated in its bylaws (ASHA, 2008), are as follows:

1. To encourage basic scientific study of the processes of individual human communication with special reference to speech, language, hearing, and related disorders;
2. To promote high standards and ethics for the academic and clinical preparation of individuals entering the discipline of human communication sciences and disorders;
3. To promote the acquisition of new knowledge and skills for those within the discipline;
4. To promote investigation, prevention, and the diagnosis and treatment of disorders of human communication and related disorders;
5. To foster improvement of clinical services and intervention procedures concerning such disorders;
6. To stimulate exchange of information among persons and organizations, and to disseminate such information;
7. To inform the public about communication sciences and disorders, related disorders, and the professionals who provide services;
8. To advocate on behalf of persons with communication and related disorders; and
9. To promote the individual and collective professional interests of the members of the Association.

SOURCE: (Reprinted with permission from American Speech-Language-Hearing Association. (2012). *Bylaws of the American Speech-Language-Hearing Association* [Bylaws]. Available from http://www.asha.org/policy.)

The ASHA bylaws address many other issues and serve to provide information about all aspects of the operation and mission of the association, including governance, standards, the Code of Ethics, publications, and other key organizational components.

Membership

ASHA currently has more than 150,000 certified members, noncertified members, international affiliates, and nonmember certificate holders who are audiologists; speech-language pathologists; and speech, language, or hearing scientists. At the end of 2010, ASHA affiliates included more than 130,000 speech-language pathologists and 12,000 audiologists. Just fewer than 1,200 individuals were certified in both speech-language pathology and audiology (ASHA, 2011b). At the end of 2010, 94.3 percent of ASHA members were female, a continuation of a trend that has seen a gradual reduction in the percentage of males in the association. Also at the end of 2005, 7.15 percent of those affiliated with the association were members of racial/ethnic minority groups, and 24.7 percent of members were 55 years of age or older (ASHA, 2011b). Three of these demographic factors are concerning to the association.

Efforts have been initiated to recruit and retain males in the professions, but the numbers indicate that these efforts have not met with great success. The association has also worked to increase the number of professionals from racial and ethnic minorities, but the overall percentage in relation to the total membership has increased less than 1 percent since 2003. Success in the recruitment and retention of males and minority professionals is essential for a diverse workforce to be available to address the communication needs of all citizens. Finally, the large number of older members of the association suggests that retirement is on the horizon for many, particularly for the baby-boomer group. Many of the professionals in this group also have PhDs and fill the ranks of academia. The shortage of younger members who hold research and teaching degrees is concerning in regard to future training needs and, indeed, for the vitality of the knowledge base for the professions. ASHA in partnership with the Council of Academic Programs in Communication Sciences and Disorders is devoting large amounts of energy and resources to address the doctoral shortage. See Chapter 8 for further discussion of demographics of the profession.

It should be mentioned that the number of audiologists who are members of ASHA and hold the Certificate of Clinical Competence has held steady in recent years. While negligible changes in the total number of audiologists affiliated with ASHA have been observed and retention of audiology members/affiliates/certificate holders has held annually above 96 percent, the number of speech-language pathologists continues to increase annually. The result is that the percentage of audiology members in relation to the total ASHA membership has declined. These demographic trends will continue to engage the interest and attention of ASHA organizers for the foreseeable future.

ASHA is currently developing a program to create an opportunity for support personnel to affiliate with the association. See Chapter 12 for discussion of support personnel.

Standards

A key component of the American Speech-Language-Hearing Association is its standards program, which addresses issues of individual credentialing as well as accreditation of academic training. ASHA has offered the Certificate of Clinical Competence (CCC) in audiology and speech-language pathology for more than 40 years. These certificates have become nationally recognized credentials by governmental and educational agencies. The CCC standards have served as the model for the state licensure requirements in many states. Additionally, ASHA supports the accreditation of graduate programs in communication sciences and disorders through the Council on Academic Accreditation (CAA), the only accreditation program in the discipline that is recognized by the Council on Higher Education Accreditation of the U.S. Department of Education. Students who wish to receive the CCC must complete the requisite academic and clinical training in a CAA-accredited graduate training program. The newest CAA standards for graduate education and ASHA standards for professional credentialing in both audiology and speech-language pathology emphasize the attainment of knowledge and skills to address speech, language, and hearing needs across the life span and with a variety of disorders. See Chapter 3 for an in-depth discussion of CAA accreditation and ASHA certification, and see the list of resources at the end of this chapter for web addresses of ASHA certification and accreditation programs.

Governance

The governance structure of an association describes how policies are made, states who is responsible for certain work in the organization, and serves to guide a consumer or member in determining where to go for assistance with a certain problem or question. The governance structure of ASHA is described in detail in Article IV of the bylaws (ASHA, 2008, Article IV, 4.1–4.2). A visual display of the structure is presented in Figure 4–1 (ASHA, 2011a).

For ASHA, the work of governance is conducted by the Board of Directors (BOD), which holds the duties for policy making and fiscal responsibility. The BOD consists of 15 elected members. The President, President-elect, Past-president, and 10 Vice Presidents are elected by the membership in an electronic vote. The President, Vice President for Planning, Vice President for Government Relations and Public Policy, Vice President for Science and Research, and Vice President for Finance may be audiologists or speech-language pathologists. Audiologists are represented on the BOD by the Vice President for Academic Affairs in Audiology, Vice President for Standards and Ethics in Audiology, and Vice President for Audiology Practice. Similar vice presidential positions exist for speech-language pathology. The vice presidents who hold the positions associated with a specific profession are elected by a vote of ASHA members in that profession. The other members of BOD are the Executive Director of the association, who is a nonvoting member, and the Chairs of two advisory bodies, the Audiology Advisory Council and the Speech-Language Pathology Advisory Council.

The Advisory Councils are two bodies composed of ASHA members from each of the 50 states and the District of Columbia and representatives from the National Student Speech Language Hearing Association and ASHA's International Affiliates. The states and the two representative groups elect one speech-language pathologist and one audiologist to serve in each of the Advisory Councils (ACs) and to consider matters of importance to the association. Through electronic discussions and face-to-face meetings, the ACs provide guidance and input to the BOD. The Chair of each AC is elected by that body and serves on the Board of Directors as a full voting member.

The National Office

In addition to the volunteer leadership of the association, a national office staff of more than 250 members works in the day-to-day operation of the Association. The Executive Director works closely with Chief Operating Officers in speech-language pathology, audiology, science and research, multicultural affairs, communications, and operations to conduct the work of the National Office. These executives, referred to as the Facilitating Team, guide the work clusters in the National Office. The work clusters include academic affairs, certification, ethics; audiology practices; speech-language pathology practices; multicultural affairs; governmental relations and public policy; governance and operations; professional education; marketing and sales; public relations; publishing; the Action Center; the National Center for Evidence Based Practice; and other administrative and operational groups.

The administrators and staff in the National Office work to accomplish association purposes, develop and implement work plans to achieve association objectives, and monitor long-term operations. The National Office relates to members directly through the Action Center call line and other forms of person-to-person communication. ASHA has recently added social media to its member outreach efforts and is active on Facebook, Twitter, and the ASHAsphere Blog. Additionally, staff within the office maintain and update the website to maximize its benefit to members, students, and consumers. ASHA now distributes all of its journals to members electronically and through its website, and all articles in ASHA journals are archived on the site and available to members. Working with the volunteer leadership, the national office staff members are often the most direct link between the association and the members, and the work of the national office is essential to the association.

The Future

ASHA's future is dependent on many issues, many of which are tied to the ability to remain responsive and effective in a world where information must be gained and shared instantaneously and across national borders. Members will value services that meet their expectations for immediacy, accuracy, and currency. The ASHA website provides information regarding web-based seminars and dialogues and telecommunications of all types, which are association activities that address those expectations.

In addition, ASHA has developed a strategic plan to address concerns and issues that are considered central to the continuing mission of the association and its service to consumers and members. The Strategic Pathway to Excellence suggests a means for addressing key issues for the future. The vision of the Association is "making effective communication, a human right, accessible and

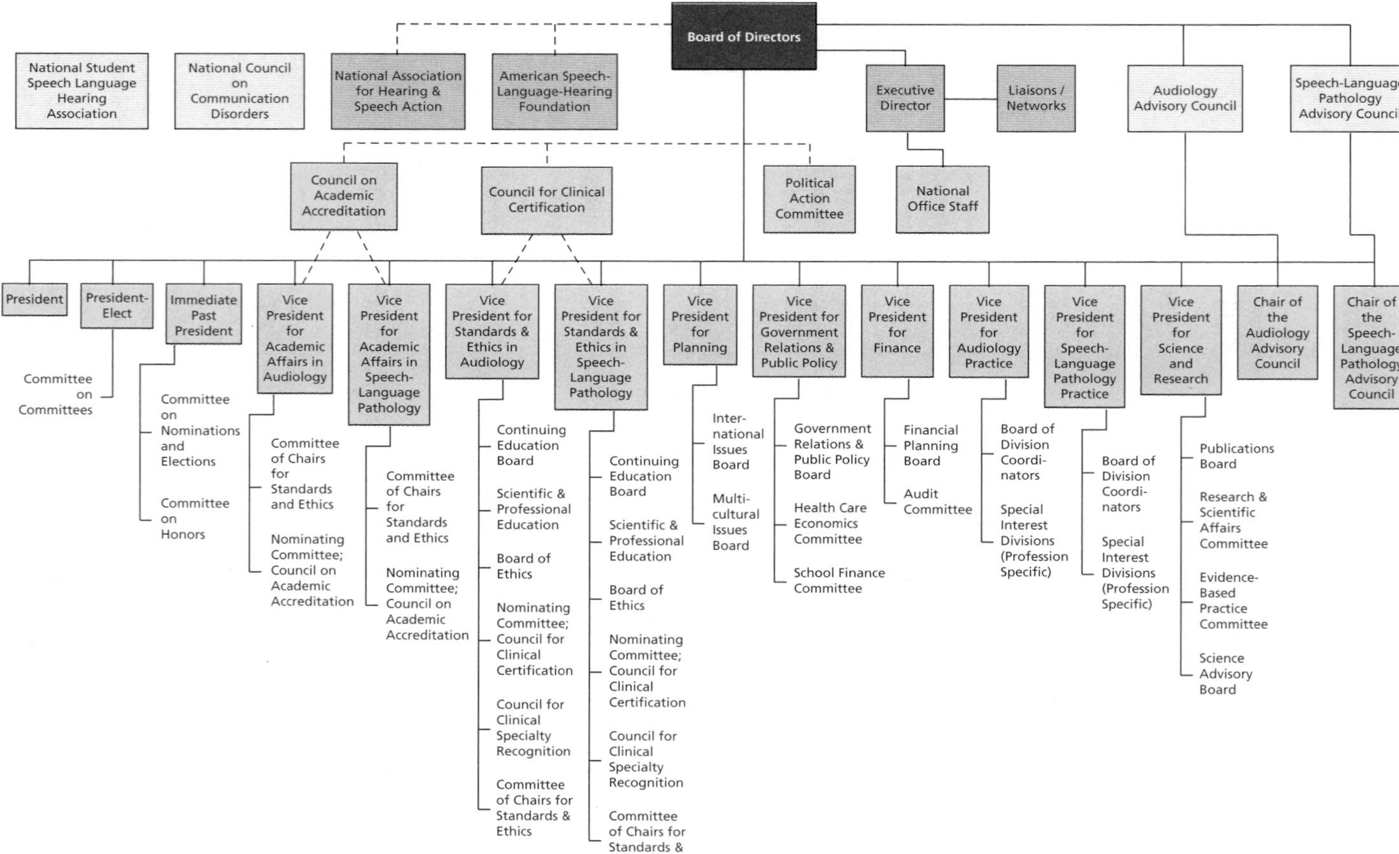

FIGURE 4–1 Association governance structure.

Reprinted with permission from ASHA Governance Structure. Available from http://www.asha.org/uploadedFiles/about/governance/ASHAGovStructure.pdf. Copyright 2009 by American Speech-Language Hearing Association.

achievable for all." (ASHA, 2011d). This vision rests on the mission of empowering the members and the professions to advocate on behalf of people with communication and related disorders, advance the science of the discipline, and promote effective human communication. ASHA has also identified strategic themes within the pathway: two professions, one discipline; scientifically based, professional practice; advocacy; and the member experience. Through the Strategic Pathway to Excellence, ASHA continues its commitment to the global professional community while maintaining a focus on the research, educational, legislative, and practice needs of its current members.

Special Interest Groups

Special Interest Groups were established within ASHA to promote knowledge and skills in specialized areas. ASHA members may join one or more of the Special Interest Groups and have access to educational programs, research, publications, and dialogue with members with similar interests. The Groups, which are closely aligned with the ASHA structure, have their own coordinating committees and have the opportunity to determine what programs and issues are most germane to the members of the Group at any given time. This model provides members with an opportunity to gain leadership experience and influence practice patterns within an area of specialization.

Eighteen Special Interest Groups address the diverse areas of language learning, neurogenic disorders, voice disorders, fluency disorders, orofacial disorders, hearing research and diagnostics, aural rehabilitation, hearing conservation, hearing disorders in childhood, issues in higher education, administration and supervision, augmentative and alternative communication, swallowing and swallowing disorders, communication issues in culturally and linguistically diverse populations, gerontology, school-based issues, global issues, and telepractice (ASHA, 2011c).

AAA: A NATIONAL PROFESSIONAL ORGANIZATION FOR AUDIOLOGISTS

The American Academy of Audiology (AAA) is the world's largest professional organization of, by, and for audiologists. The impetus for AAA dates back to the 1987 ASHA convention in New Orleans when a mini-seminar was presented on "The Future of Audiology." Richard Talbott chaired the session and recruited five well-known audiologists to discuss such critical issues as future needs and potential employment of audiologists, the knowledge base required to meet the future needs, the level of academic training needed to achieve the knowledge base, and the university faculty/supervisory personnel needs for training audiologists. One of the panel members, James Jerger, concluded his presentation by noting that it was now time for a new professional organization of, by, and for audiologists. Jerger's comments were met with an enthusiastic response. As a follow-up to the ASHA session, 32 audiology leaders met in Houston, Texas, in early 1988 at the invitation of James Jerger (Baylor College of Medicine). The purpose of the study group was to establish an independent, freestanding, national organization for audiologists. The group voted unanimously to develop a new organization for audiologists, to be called the American College of Audiology, and the first National Office was established at Baylor College of Medicine. In addition, an ad hoc steering committee was appointed to develop bylaws. Finally, before leaving the Houston meeting, each member of the founders group contributed $20 to establish the organization's first budget (Stach, 1998).

In the few short months to follow, remarkable progress was made. The newly developed bylaws for the organization were approved, the organization was renamed the American Academy of Audiology, the Academy was incorporated under the laws of the state of Tennessee, an organizational structure was established and officers elected, dues were established, committee assignments were made, dates for the first annual meeting were determined, and a major membership drive was launched. In 1989, the first AAA convention was held at Kiawah Island, South Carolina, and the response exceeded all expectations: Close to 600 participants, including 45 "charter" exhibitors, attended the meeting and literally overflowed the conference facilities.

Since 1989, the AAA has undergone significant growth in membership and development. By 1993, the AAA reached a point in membership size and fiscal responsibilities that it became necessary to move the National Office to Washington, DC, and contract staff to assist in the organization's management. Today, the AAA National Office is located in Reston, Virginia.

Purpose

According to the AAA bylaws (American Academy of Audiology, 2009), the Academy is a professional organization of individuals dedicated to providing quality hearing and balance care by advancing the profession of audiology through leadership, advocacy, education, public awareness, and support of research. The focus is to enhance the ability of AAA members to achieve career and practice objectives through professional development, education, research, and increased public awareness of hearing disorders and audiologic services.

Membership

AAA currently has close to 12,000 members, an impressive number given the relatively short time the organization has been in existence. Moreover, the number of new members added each year is growing substantially. The demographic breakdown of the AAA membership is similar to that of ASHA. In 2010, 79 percent of the membership of AAA was female, and 64 percent held doctoral degrees (this number will grow significantly now that the doctor of audiology degree will be required to practice in the profession.) Fifty-five percent of those with doctorates earned the AuD degree. Although AAA does not have data on the number of members representing racial/ethnic minority groups, the number is small and is probably similar to that of ASHA. Finally, 12 percent of audiologists are over age 55.

Both ASHA and AAA have been concerned about the inability to attract additional males and minorities into the profession despite the development of special recruitment initiatives. Equally disturbing is the number of professionals who are 55 years or older, most of whom will be retiring within the next 10 years. These demographic concerns have been discussed earlier in the membership section related to ASHA.

Standards

Similar to ASHA, the AAA has developed a standards program for certifying audiologists. The program, offered by the American Board of Audiology (ABA), certifies audiologists whose knowledge base and clinical skills are consistent with professionally established standards and who continue to add to their knowledge through various forms of continuing education. The ABA is working toward having states and government agencies recognize ABA certification. A goal of AAA has always been to serve as the professional home for all audiologists including those from other countries. Accordingly, the ABA Board recently approved a policy for certification of international audiologists. Eligibility requirements for international certification through AAA appear on the ABA website.

Finally, the ABA has begun to develop specialty certifications. The first specialty certification program offered by ABA was for cochlear implant audiologists, followed by a pediatric audiology specialty certification (PASC). To achieve specialty certification, specific requirements unique to a given specialty area must be met—details of the specialty certification programs offered by the ABA can also be found on the AAA website. See the Resources section for web addresses of organizations.

The AAA has also developed an accreditation process for universities offering AuD graduate training. Beginning in 2003, the Accreditation Commission for Audiology Education (ACAE) began developing education standards for AuD training programs. The purpose of ACAE accreditation is to recognize, reinforce, and promote high-quality performance in AuD educational programs through a rigorous verification process—a process designed to ensure that AuD programs prepare graduates who meet high standards and who demonstrate competencies considered essential for practice at the doctoral level. The ACAE Board of Directors adopted the completed standards in March 2005, following a rigorous peer review process. The standards can be found online at ACAE's website, which is listed in the Resources section of this chapter. In addition to ACAE, a technology company has been contracted for the development of a web-based accreditation system. This Computerized Accreditation Program (CAP) will be an innovative online accreditation system combining high-quality standards with state-of-the art technology. The result is accreditation *plus* an interactive, web-based process designed to facilitate ease in management and provide valuable information to program directors, faculty, students, and communities of interest. Some of the proposed features of the system include online participation, an interactive self-study process, and the ability to retrieve national trends and analyses from a data warehouse. The ACAE and CAP programs are expected to be launched in the near future.

Governance and the National Office

The governance structure of AAA is described in Article III of the bylaws (AAA, 2009). The structure is purposely designed to be streamlined so that the leadership can respond in a timely manner to its membership as well as to topical issues on the national front that arise from time to time throughout the year. To this end, the Academy is governed by a Board of Directors composed of 12 Fellows, including the President, President-elect, Past President, and nine Members at Large. Each member of the board is elected by the membership at large and possesses the power to vote on issues before the board. In addition to other duties, the Board of Directors is expected to (1) grant membership to those applicants whose qualifications, in the board's judgment, meet the requirements set forth by the bylaws; (2) establish boards, committees, and task forces, as necessary, to guide and assist the Academy in its mission, and appoint the Chair of such groups; (3) decide when and where the Annual Academy Meeting shall take place and elect a Program Chair for the meeting; and (4) transact all such other business in the interest of the membership.

The national office is composed of an Executive Director and an office staff of 34 who work closely with the President, other board members, and volunteers from the membership to facilitate operational activities of the Academy. Examples of such activities include government relations, credentialing, public relations, marketing, publications, continuing education, and professional education.

The Future

The AAA has experienced extraordinary growth and success during the first two decades of its existence. The future of AAA, however, will depend on the ability of the Academy leadership to continue to meet the ever-changing needs of audiologists and the profession as well as to develop effective tools to measure progress. Indeed, those organizations that fail to define their goals and critical success factors for the future and to communicate the goals to their members will not be successful. To this end, AAA leadership has developed a comprehensive strategic plan that sets the course for the future of the profession. Goals, strategies, and action plans have been developed to help ensure that the Academy will achieve its vision of advancing the science and practice of audiology and achieving public recognition of audiologists as experts in hearing and balance. Some of the specific goals in the AAA strategic plan include the following: (1) promote a member-driven environment that fosters involvement and provides services essential to their success; (2) partner with other organizations to advance hearing and balance initiatives; (3) shape the future of science and practice through effective leadership and advocacy; and (4) increase consumer and patient awareness of and access to optimal hearing and balance care.

RELATED PROFESSIONAL ORGANIZATIONS

Related professional organizations are available to individuals with research, clinical, or educational interests that may not be fully addressed within the scope of ASHA or AAA. Examples of these organizations are the Academy of Neurologic Communication Disorders and Sciences (ANCDS), an organization with professional, clinical, educational, scientific, and charitable interests directed toward the quality of life for adults and children with neurologic communication disorders; the Acoustical Society of America, an organization involved in the scientific pursuit of acoustics information, which includes members from diverse scientific professions, including physics, engineering, biology, psychology, and speech and hearing; and the Council for Exceptional Children (CEC), an organization dedicated to improving educational outcomes for students with exceptionalities such as developmental disabilities, learning disabilities, and communicative disabilities and deafness.

These are just a few of the many examples of related professional organizations that may engage the student or professional with special interests in a focused educational, clinical, or research area. A listing of some relevant related professional organizations is provided in the Resources section at the end of the chapter.

STATE ORGANIZATIONS

State organizations in speech-language pathology and audiology are often affiliated with a larger national organization and have similar purposes and structure when this is the case. For example, many state speech-language-hearing associations are recognized affiliates of ASHA. As such, they have access to ASHA's state-national relations resources, which provide informational and sometimes financial assistance with legislation, licensure, and other state-focused issues. The Council of State Association Presidents meets twice annually, once in the spring in conjunction with the ASHA State Policy Workshop and on the day prior to the annual ASHA convention. Contact information for state associations and other information pertinent to state licensing and teacher certification is found in the "ASHA State by State" section of the ASHA website. Audiology members in some states are also affiliated with AAA with similar benefits and connectivity.

State organizations have an opportunity to influence practice issues, regulations, funding decisions, and other aspects of the day-to-day practice of the professions within a locale. As such, these organizations offer students and professionals the opportunity to become engaged in activities of vital importance to their current or future livelihood.

Students are often provided reduced fees or even free memberships and convention registration if they assist with state activities. Assisting at the state association level is an excellent means to enter the volunteer workforce that is so essential to the viability of professional organizations. Students who affiliate with state associations while they are in their training programs have an opportunity to network with individuals who may ultimately be future employers or mentors when the students graduate.

STUDENT ORGANIZATIONS

Training programs in communication sciences and disorders typically have local chapters of the National Student Speech Language Hearing Association (NSSLHA) and the Student Academy of Audiology (SAA). Like the earlier model, NSSLHA, which is affiliated with ASHA, includes student members who are preparing for careers in audiology or in speech-language pathology. SAA, which is affiliated with AAA, includes student members preparing for careers in audiology.

NSSLHA

As the only student association formally recognized by ASHA, NSSLHA has representatives on the Audiology Advisory Council and the Speech-Language Pathology Advisory Council. Additionally, NSSLHA has representatives on a number of the ASHA councils and boards. The requirements for membership in NSSLHA are that an undergraduate or graduate student has an interest in the study of normal and disordered human communication behavior and is enrolled either part or full time in a training program in communication sciences. Local chapters in university settings allow students opportunities for leadership development, volunteerism, philanthropic work, professional networking, educational events, reduced ASHA convention registration, and a reduction in ASHA certification fees if membership is maintained throughout the graduate training program. ASHA and NSSLHA are working on a structure that will strengthen the relationship between the two organizations and create a more seamless transition from one organization to the other. The website for the NSSLHA organization is provided in the references at the end of the chapter. Under the new integrated model, NSSLHA will remain a student-led an separate 501 organization.

SAA

The Student Academy of Audiology is the national student division of the AAA that serves as a collective voice for students and advances the rights, interest, and welfare of students pursuing careers in audiology. The SAA essentially replaced a former student organization, the National Association of Future Doctors of Audiology (NAFDA). Founded in 1998 by an AuD doctoral student, NAFDA provided a number of benefits to students such as a student newsletter, an academic journal, and an online forum and chatroom.

For a brief period, both SAA and NAFDA existed as separate organizations but with similar objectives—SAA was the official student organization associated with AAA, and NAFDA was a student organization independent of AAA. In 2008, NAFDA and the AAA announced an agreement to merge NAFDA into AAA's SAA. The unified SAA has created new bylaws and has begun the business of fine-tuning a student organization for the profession of audiology. Some of the benefits of SAA include elected representatives with ties to AAA, educational opportunities, student publications/newsletters, and importantly, the opportunity for mentored leadership.

INTERNATIONAL PROFESSIONAL ORGANIZATIONS

For those who have an interest in international professional issues in speech-language pathology and audiology, affiliation with a number of professional organizations may be useful. For example, the International Society of Audiology and the International Association of Logopedics and Phoniatrics (IALP) provide membership and educational opportunities. In addition, you will read about professional organizations in other countries in Chapter 7, International Alliances. There you will read about associations in other English-speaking countries, including Australia, Canada, New Zealand, South Africa, and the United Kingdom.

SUMMARY

Students are encouraged to affiliate with national professional organizations as well as state organizations, special interest groups, and related professional organizations. Early involvement in these associations provides opportunities for volunteering, networking, advocacy, and learning. An excellent training ground for these experiences is active participation in a student organization affiliated with a national association, such as the National Student Speech Language Hearing Association or the Student Academy of Audiology. Being a member of a larger group makes it more likely that problems can be solved and answers to questions can be obtained in a coordinated, consistent, and effective manner. Being aware of the history and governance of associations will also help students as they choose to affiliate with those associations that will continue to be the most effective in representing member interests and in relating to the larger global community.

CRITICAL THINKING

1. What are the advantages of membership in a national professional organization?
2. Refer to the opening scenarios. What specific kinds of assistance could these individuals expect to get from their national professional organization(s)?
3. Create scenarios specific to your own area of interest or a problem you might encounter as a professional and discuss resources your professional organization might provide to address the issue.
4. What valuable experiences are likely to be gained from affiliation with a state organization, a special interest group, or a related professional organization?
5. Should a graduate student in audiology affiliate with NSSLHA, SAA, or both? Should a practicing audiologist hold membership in AAA, ASHA, or both?
6. After you graduate and hold a professional degree, you may be advised by a colleague that there is more value to belonging to a state organization and that using your limited resources to join a national professional organization is unwise. On what basis would your colleague make that argument? What support could you provide for joining a national organization?
7. Leadership in a student organization is often viewed as a resumé builder. In what way could you relate leadership experiences to a prospective employer so that the employer would value the experience and expect resulting transferable skills?
8. Professional organizations rely heavily on volunteer leadership, notably in committee service and board positions. What are the expected consequences, both positive and negative, if you volunteer as a leader for a professional organization?
9. When you graduate, you will join one or more professional organizations. Create a plan for 10 years postgraduation that will allow you to become a leader in one of those organizations.
10. Interview several audiologists about what they think about having two major professional

organizations devoted to hearing and its disorders (ASHA and AAA). What are the advantages and disadvantages of having these two professional organizations for practicing clinicians? With which organization(s) do you see yourself affiliating and why?

REFERENCES

American Academy of Audiology. (2009). *Bylaws of the American Academy of Audiology*. Available from http://www.audiology.org/

American Speech-Language-Hearing Association. (2008). *Bylaws of the American Speech-Language-Hearing Association* [Bylaws]. Available from http://www.asha.org/policy

American Speech-Language-Hearing Association. (2011a). *ASHA governance structure*. Rockville, MD: Author. Retrieved from http://www.asha.org/uploadedfilesabout/governance/ASHAGovStructure.pdf

American Speech-Language-Hearing Association. (2011b). *2010 ASHA member counts*. Rockville, MD: Author. Retrieved from http://www.asha.org/uploadedfiles/2010-member-counts.pdf

American Speech-Language-Hearing Association. (2011c). *Special interest groups*. Rockville, MD: Author. Retrieved from http://www.asha.org/SIG/Special-Interest-Group-Descriptions

American Speech-Language-Hearing Association. (2011d). *Strategic pathway to excellence*. Rockville, MD: Author. Retrieved from http://www.asha.org/about/pathway

Stach, B. (1998). In the beginning—1987–1988. *Audiology Today,* 6–11.

RESOURCES

National Organizations

Accreditation Commission for Audiology Education
http://www.audiology.org/education/accreditation

American Academy of Audiology
8300 Greensboro Drive, Suite 750
McLean, VA 22102
Phone: 702-790-8466, 800-AAA-2336
Website: http://www.audiology.org

American Board of Audiology
http://www.audiology.org/development/boardcertification

American Speech-Language-Hearing Association
10801 Rockville Pike
Rockville, MD 20852
Phone: 301-897-5700
Website: http://www.asha.org

Council for Clinical Certification
http://www.asha.org/certification/

Council on Academic Accreditation
http://www.asha.org/Academic/accreditation/AboutCAA

National Student Speech Language Hearing Association
10801 Rockville Pike
Rockville, MD 20852
Phone: 301-471-0481
Website: http://www.nsslha.org

Student Academy of Audiology
8300 Greensboro Drive, Suite 750
McLean, VA 22102
Phone: 702-790-8466, 800-AAA-2336
Website: http://www.audiology.org/education/students/SAA

State Professional Associations

For a complete list of state professional associations, see http://www.asha.org/advocacy/state/

Related Professional Organizations

Academy of Doctors of Audiology (ADA)
http://www.audiologist.org

Academy of Federal Audiologists and Speech-Language Pathologists (AFASLP)
http://afaslp.org/

Academy of Neurologic Communication Disorders and Sciences (ANCDS)
http://www.ancds.org

Academy of Rehabilitative Audiology (ARA)
http://www. audrehab.org

Acoustical Society of America (ASA)
http://www.acousticalsociety.org

Alexander Graham Bell Association for the Deaf and Hard of Hearing
http://www.agbell.org

American Academy of Private Practice in Speech Pathology & Audiology (AAPPSPA)
http://www.aappspa.org

American Auditory Society (AAS)
http://www.amauditorysoc.org

American Cleft Palate-Craniofacial Association (ACPA)
http://www.acpa-cpf.org

American Society for Deaf Children (ASDC)
http://www.deafchildren.org

American Tinnitus Association (ATA)
http://www.ata.org

Better Hearing Institute (BHI)
http://www.betterhearing.org

Brain Injury Association of America
http://www.biausa.org

Canadian Association of Speech-Language Pathologists and Audiologists (CASLPA)
http://www.caslpa.ca

Council for Exceptional Children (CEC)
http://www.cec.sped.org

Council of Academic Programs in Communication Sciences and Disorders (CAPCSD)
http://www.capcsd.org

Educational Audiology Association (EAA)
http://www.edaud.org

Hearing Loss Association of America (HLAA)
http://hearingloss.org/

International Association of Logopedics and Phoniatrics (IALP)
http://www.ialp.info/

International Association of Orofacial Myology (IAOM)
http://www.iaom.com

The International Dyslexia Association (IDA) (formerly Orton Dyslexia Society)
http://www.interdys.org

International Society for Augmentative and Alternative Communication (ISAAC)
http://www.isaac-online.org

International Society of Audiology (ISA)
http://www.isa-audiology.org

Linguistic Society of America (LSA)
http://www.lsadc.org

National Aphasia Association (NAA)
http://www.aphasia.org

National Black Association for Speech-Language and Hearing (NBASLH)
http://www.nbaslh.org

National Institute on Deafness and Other Communication Disorders (NIDCD)
http://www.nidcd.nih.gov

National Rehabilitation Association (NRA)
http://www.nationalrehab.org

National Stuttering Association (NSA)
http://www.nsastutter.org

Stuttering Foundation of America
http://www.stutteringhelp.org

5

Professional Ethics

Thomas D. Miller, PhD, JD

SCOPE OF CHAPTER

Have you ever wondered if your day-to-day professional activities met or exceeded the minimum standards established by your profession? No issue for audiologists and speech-language pathologists transcends more employment settings, levels of experience, or nature of clientele than ethical practice. The number of professionals in audiology, speech-language pathology, and speech and hearing sciences who intentionally commit unethical practice is extremely low. Professionals do, however, make mistakes, develop bad habits, or allow the motivations or constraints of their employment to lead them from preferred practice models. New technologies and practices may also challenge clinicians to review their ethical guidelines.

This chapter defines the role of professional ethics and explains regulation of the professions of audiology and speech-language pathology by professional organizations such as ASHA and AAA. Ethical standards of conduct are discussed and examples of unethical practice are presented. The chapter also suggests ways in which practicing professionals may decrease the risk of unethical practice complaints while improving the quality of their service. Legal liability is discussed in Chapter 6.

ROLE OF A PROFESSIONAL

The word *profession* comes from the Latin "bound by an oath" (Baker, 1999). Professionals render services to society as distinguished by their superior knowledge, training, and/or skill and have a special obligation to those they serve. Thus, they earn the respect of society for services provided. To maintain that respect, professionals are responsible for conforming to stated or implied minimum standards of conduct imposed by their particular profession. These standards are presented in a Code of Ethics that is designed by the profession itself. The professional assumes ethical responsibility for demonstration of the ability and competence of an ordinary member in good standing in the profession.

REGULATION OF THE PROFESSIONS

When society seeks to have input regarding the practice of a profession, one route is to license the profession through minimum standards, rules, and regulations established by legislators, appointed administrative bodies, or the courts.

In contrast, ethical principles and standards of conduct are established by members of a profession and are relative to given practices, procedures, and circumstances experienced by members of the profession. Although members of society benefit from professional ethics, they do not have direct input into the formation of those ethics. Ethical standards may be determined by professional organizations at the national, state, or regional levels; by accrediting agencies; or by employers. See the ASHA Code of Ethics and the AAA Code of Ethics in the appendices to this chapter.

One advantage (or, sometimes, disadvantage) of both legal and ethical regulation of a profession is that two distinct tracks are maintained. Each track performs a unique purpose and serves different professional needs. In some states, for example, it is legal to provide speech-language services in public schools with a bachelor's degree. Although legal, this violates the ASHA Code of Ethics, Principles of Ethics II, Rule A, which requires that "Individuals shall engage in the provision of clinical services only when they hold the appropriate Certificate of Clinical Competence or when they are in the certification process and are supervised by an individual who holds the appropriate Certificate of Clinical Competence" (American Speech-Language-Hearing Association, 2010). A professional may perform a task that is illegal but ethical or that may be perfectly legal but unethical. Ordinarily, conflicts involve the possession of appropriate credentials. For example, an audiologist who is otherwise ethical in holding certification to practice may be practicing illegally if he or she does not have a valid state license or registration. Likewise, speech-language pathologists (SLPs) may be practicing legally by holding a valid license but may be acting unethically if they are bound by a code of ethics that requires clinical certification to practice. However, many standards overlap or interact and resolution of the conflict is discretionary by the parties involved.

Audiologists and SLPs often seek practice advice from codes of professional ethics and/or from boards or committees that interpret and administer such codes. Codes of ethics generally try to strike a balance between presentation of proscriptions that may protect a professional from legal liability and proscriptions that set the highest internal standards for the profession (Boylan, 2000).

ETHICAL STANDARDS OF CONDUCT

Ethics are standards of conduct that guide your behavior as a professional. They define acceptable versus unacceptable behaviors and promote high and consistent standards of practice. Ethics are not feelings, are not law, are not religious, and are not scientific. Ethical standards across professions generally derive from five philosophical concepts (Santa Clara University, 2005).

1. The utilitarian approach: Do the most good and the least harm.
2. The right approach: Protect and respect the moral rights of those affected.
3. The fairness or justice approach: Treat all humans equally or fairly based on some defensible standard.
4. The common good approach: Our actions should enhance the community as a whole.
5. The virtue approach: Maintain the highest values, including truth, compassion, integrity, fairness, and prudence.

SOURCE: Reprinted with permission of the Markkula Center for Applied Ethics at Santa Clara University.

When standards reflective of these philosophies are compiled into a list by a professional organization, they are known as a professional code of ethics, a code of values, or a code of conduct. Baker (1999) in his history of ethics states that the first code of ethics for physicians and surgeons was proposed by Thomas Percival in Manchester, England, in 1794, followed by an expanded document in 1803. The first national professional association to adopt a code of ethics was the American Medical Association in 1847. Thousands of codes of ethics have been created by professions from accountants to zookeepers. Today's ethics codes derive from these early documents, define standards for minimally acceptable professional conduct, and provide for the following of sanctions that determine who is included in or excluded from a profession.

Codes of ethics generally have three components arranged in a top-down or general-to-specific framework: a prologue or preamble, principles, and rules or guidelines. The preamble, or the vision statement, describes why the code is important, for whom it is relevant, if it is mandatory, how it will be enforced, and which principles and rules are fundamental. Principles delineate the goals to be maintained. Principles generally emanate from the concepts of impartiality, full disclosure, confidentiality, due diligence, fidelity to professional responsibilities, and avoidance of conflict of interest (Colero, 2005). The rules of conduct are the specific do's and don'ts of each principle (Ethics Resource Center, 2005).

Codes of ethics are intended to be living documents that undergo periodic review and change as professions change. Codes must also be written to have some flexibility to meet changes in federal and state laws, scopes of practice, and new developments within the professions. In general, you will find that codes of ethics are user-friendly and avoid legal jargon. Remember that these are not laws, but professional guidelines. Useful resources for preparation or revision of codes of ethics can be found through the Center for the Study of Ethics in the Professions at Illinois Institute of Technology. This Center lists numerous national and international resources that study ethics across professions.

Speech-Language Pathology and Audiology Codes of Ethics

The establishment and maintenance of a code of ethics has been a major function of ASHA since its founding in 1925. The ASHA Code of Ethics, as provided for by Article III, §1C of the Association Bylaws, was first issued in 1930 as part of the bylaws and then as an independent document published in 1952. The code is binding for all members, certified nonmembers, applicants, and/or clinical fellows. It was last revised in March 2010. It can be found on the ASHA website, in the ASHA membership application booklet, and periodically in the *ASHA Leader* and other supplements. The American Academy of Audiology (AAA) also offers a code of ethics for its members. See Appendices 5–A and 5–B to this chapter for the latest ASHA and AAA Codes of Ethics.

The ASHA Code of Ethics is reviewed periodically by the Board of Ethics. This group of 12 members includes one public member and others across various occupational settings (clinicians, administrators, researchers, teachers, etc.). The Board analyzes current practice trends and violations to determine whether changes in the Code of Ethics are merited. Revisions are then circulated for peer review, finalization, and then approval by the Legislative Council. Thus, there are numerous levels of feedback to the Board of Ethics when revisions are proposed (Diefendorf, 2008).

Although the ASHA Code of Ethics provides standards relating to important ethical precepts, such as holding paramount the welfare of people served professionally, maintaining confidentiality, and professional competence, it is important to note a paragraph in the preamble that provides for ethical questions that may not be specifically covered by the Code:

> Any violation of the spirit and purpose of this Code shall be considered unethical. Failure to specify any particular responsibility or practice in this Code of Ethics shall not be construed as denial of the existence of such responsibilities or practices (ASHA, 2010).

State and regional professional associations also often have their own codes of ethics that may reflect variations in preferred practice models unique to the state or region. ASHA's policy recognizes the autonomy of these bodies and renders to them the responsibility for determining when or if violations of their codes occur. Only the ASHA Board of Ethics can make a determination of violations of the ASHA Code of Ethics (ASHA, 2008b).

If audiologists or speech-language pathologists are members of another professional organization (e.g., the Academy of Dispensing Audiologists, the American Academy of Audiology, the American Psychological Association, the Council for Exceptional Children), they should be aware these groups also have their own codes of ethics to which they may be bound. The Code of Ethics of the American Academy of Audiology is given in Appendix 5–B of this chapter. In addition, with the establishment of the Quadrilateral Mutual Recognition agreement among ASHA, the Canadian Association of Speech-Language Pathologists and Audiologists (CASLPA), the Royal College of Speech and Language Therapists (RCSLT) in the United Kingdom, and the Speech Pathology Association of Australia Limited (Boswell, 2004), it may be necessary to be familiar with these international codes of ethics. Once audiologists or SLPs sign the agreement to follow the ASHA Code of Ethics and hold a current Certificate of Clinical Competence, they must abide by the ASHA Code regardless of other certifications held or the location of services provided. See the ASHA website for membership certification and international rules.

The Center for the Study of Ethics in the Professions (CSEP) has been collecting codes of ethics of professional societies, corporations, governments, and academic institutions for more than 20 years. Currently, the CSEP has more than 850 codes of ethics in its archives (Center for the Study of Ethics in the Professions, 2005).

UNETHICAL PRACTICE COMPLAINT PROCESS

If you suspect that someone has violated a code of ethics, what should you do? The discussion here applies to violation of the ASHA Code of Ethics only. First, you should read the Code carefully, doing what is termed a *fair reading* whereby the evidence appears to suggest an ethical violation. Remember that the ASHA Code of Ethics applies to members, certificate holders, Clinical Fellows, and applicants for membership or certification only. Complete the Complaint of Alleged Violation of the ASHA Code of Ethics form available at the ASHA website and submit to ASHA's Director of Ethics. E-mail or faxed complaints are not accepted. The Board of Ethics will examine and weigh each complaint on its merits and adjudicate any violations (ASHA, 2009). Article III of the ASHA Bylaws establishes the Board of Ethics "to interpret, administer, and enforce the Code of Ethics of the Association" (ASHA, 1998, p. 46).

When a complaint of unethical practice is received by the ASHA Board of Ethics, the complaint is reviewed for subject matter and personal jurisdiction. The alleged offender (respondent) is notified of the complaint and is given 45 days to respond. The Board investigates the complaint and, if further proceedings are deemed warranted, prepares an Initial Determination, which includes its findings, proposed sanctions (if any), the proposed extent of disclosure of the findings, and notice to the parties to the complaint.

Following the Initial Determination, the respondent may request a Further Consideration hearing during which he or she may appear before the Board, present witnesses, and be represented by counsel. After the hearing, the Board issues its decision. The respondent may then appeal the decision in writing to the ASHA Executive Board. The Executive Board will issue a final decision.

The complaint process for AAA, while similar, varies in some ways. The Ethical Practice Board reviews the complaint and determines whether a Notification of Potential Ethics Concern is warranted. If warranted, the respondent receives notification and has 60 days to respond. The respondent may request a hearing before the Board. The Board may find that no violation existed or that a violation occurred. If a violation has occurred, the board determines appropriate sanctions. The respondent may appeal the finding to the AAA Board of Directors, whose decision is final.

Types of Complaints

Although the true nature of each complaint of unethical practice is, of necessity, kept confidential, common complaints have been found in the following categories:

- Practicing without appropriate certification
- Practicing beyond the scope of certification
- Providing supervision beyond the scope of certification
- Failure to refer
- Failure to file a report or filing a false report
- Advertising extremes (Miller, 1983; Miller & Lubinski, 1986)

Denton (2011) has reported the following trends in complaints received by ASHA:

- Unethical practice resulting from employer constraints or restrictions
- Training, use, and support of support personnel and assistants

- Questions regarding provision of services to culturally and linguistically diverse populations
- Dilemmas for audiologists and speech-language pathologists in private practices or groups who must provide ethical services *and* operate successful small businesses

Sanctions

Sanctions for unethical practice have three major purposes, according to Denton (2009). The first purpose is to penalize the person in violation of the Code. Second, sanctions serve as a means of educating and rehabilitating the individual in violation. Finally, sanctions serve to inform those professionals bound by the Code, and ASHA informs them of the Association's efforts to prevent future violations (Denton, 2009). ASHA sanctions for unethical practice may include a Cease and Desist Order, a Reprimand, Censure, and Withholding, Suspending, or Revoking Membership and/or Certification (ASHA, 2008a). AAA sanctions may include an Educative Letter, a Cease and Desist order, a Reprimand, Mandatory Continuing Education, Probation or Suspension, and Suspension or Revocation of Membership (American Academy of Audiology [AAA], 2009).

Disclosure

If the final decision of the ASHA Board of Ethics is a Censure or the Withholding, Suspension, or Revocation of Membership and/or Certificate(s) of Competence, this information will be published in an ASHA document that is distributed to its membership. When a Reprimand is given, only the following are notified of the decision: the respondent and counsel, the complainant, witnesses, and various ASHA staff members. This decision is strictly confidential (ASHA, 2008b). See the AAA website for further information on disclosure of ethical complaint decisions by that professional body.

Appeals

Respondents may appeal their board decision if they can demonstrate that the ASHA Board of Ethics did not follow process or the decision was "arbitrary and capricious and without any evidentiary basis" (ASHA, 2008a). The appeal may then go before the Executive Board. Guidelines regarding the process and timelines for this appeals process are outlined in the Statement of Practices and Procedures of the Board of Ethics (ASHA, 2008a).

PREPARING FOR FUTURE ETHICAL PRACTICE CONCERNS

The dynamic professions of audiology and speech-language pathology present constant changes and challenges for members to provide the best possible service to their clientele. Individuals working in health care settings continue to adapt to the transition from fee-for-service models to managed care. The scope of practice has expanded to the use of telepractice, multiskilling, and intraoperative monitoring. The development of new technologies in both speech-language pathology and audiology creates ethical challenges. Emphasis on evidence-based practice and treatment outcomes requires objective measures of the value of services rendered. The increased delegation of services to speech-language pathology assistants and volunteers provides new opportunities as well as increased ethical concerns and possibly liability for supervising clinicians. The challenge to do a better job with fewer resources continues to increase. These factors would seem to present growing obstacles to the provision of ethical and professional quality service. Former ASHA President Kay Butler (1996) pointed out, however, that the changes may not actually present future ethical dilemmas since the ethical standards of conduct are already in place. The challenge is to apply the existing ethics principles the professions have developed to our efforts to provide new and cost-effective service.

The application of current standards of conduct also applies to the changing roles of audiologists and speech-language pathologists working in school settings. The emphasis on least restrictive environment has resulted in more severely disabled students receiving services in schools while increased federal and state regulation has often resulted in reduction of assessment and intervention contact with students. Increased use of paraprofessionals, inclusion models, and outcomes measurement can present new ethical questions regarding caseload, delegation of service, and supervision liability. The ethical standards of conduct currently held by the professions must be durable enough to address the changing nature of service delivery models.

Examples of Professional Ethics Questions

The following are actual questions received by the author from students and practitioners. The answers suggested are the author's and represent one interpretation of ethical practice. Sections of the ASHA and AAA Codes of Ethics are included to reference portions of the codes used to address the questions.

Q1. I am a speech-language pathologist and own a small but growing private practice. I have developed an inexpensive electronic listening aid for use in therapy. I plan to market the instrument and sell it to some of my clientele and am wondering if it would be ethical for me to do so.

A1. The ASHA Code of Ethics prohibits misrepresentation and/or fraud in dispensing of products or services (ASHA, Principle III, Rule D). If the device in question is used as a component of a comprehensive treatment program and is not the focus of the treatment program and if the program can still be implemented without purchase of the device, it has traditionally been acceptable.

Q2. As a certified audiologist serving a rural community, I was asked by a parent if I could treat some speech-sound production problems in her child in addition to the central auditory processing therapy already being provided. I have an undergraduate degree in communication disorders and agreed to the additional therapy but later wondered if it was ethical.

A2. Both ASHA and AAA Codes prohibit the provision of services that fall beyond the competence or experience of the professional or beyond the scope of practice of the credential held. ASHA Principle of Ethics II states that "Individuals shall honor their responsibility to achieve and maintain the highest level of professional competence." The profession has determined that this level of competence is attained only after satisfactory completion of all of the requirements for the Certificate of Clinical Competence (CCC). In this case, the treatment of speech-sound production disorders falls within the scope, training, and experience of one who holds the CCC in speech-language pathology and should be provided by one who holds that credential. The audiologist must make every effort to refer the parent to an SLP for that service. (ASHA, Principle II, Rules A and B; AAA, Principle 2, Rule 2a; and ASHA, 2004a).

Q3. I am a certified speech-language pathologist working in a rural area. The nearest audiologist is a two-hour drive away. I have nine graduate credits and more than 100 hours of supervised practicum in audiology. Would I be in trouble if I gave a few air/bone conduction threshold tests to my students?

A3. Once again, this clinician could not only be "in trouble" but, more important, could put the integrity of the profession and the welfare of his/her clientele in question. (ASHA Principle II, Rules A and B; see also ASHA, 1996).

Q4. My husband says he doesn't want me working with patients who are HIV positive or who have AIDS. Am I unethical if I refuse to work with these patients?

A4. Numerous legal standards, as well as the ASHA and AAA Codes of Ethics, prohibit discrimination on the basis of disability. However, if the welfare of this clinician's patients would be jeopardized by her lack of academic preparation or practicum or by her own personal biases, she might do well to refer her HIV/AIDS patients to a more competent clinician (ASHA, Principle I, Rule C; AAA, Principle 1, Rule 1b).

(*Continues*)

Examples of Professional Ethics Questions (*Continued*)

Q5. My administrator has hired another speech-language pathologist to help with the growing dysphagia caseload. The new person has had no coursework or practicum in feeding and swallowing disorders but has been told by my administrator to "wing it" until funds are available to obtain training. She really needs the job. What should I do?

A5. This speech-language pathologist should discuss with the administrator the ethical principle that limits practice to the scope of an individual's competence. Requiring a professional to "wing it" not only places the patient with dysphagia in danger but creates substantial exposure to legal liability of all involved in the event of an undesirable outcome (ASHA, Principle II, Rule B).

Q6. Current state and federal regulations continue to limit the amount of service my early intervention (EI) students receive. How can I provide competent service to these needy children if my time with them is decreasing?

A6. In times of fiscal downturns, we will face efforts to reduce services as a way of saving money. This can be an opportunity to use the intent and letter of Codes of Ethics as well as growing evidence-based practices to educate administrators and legislators of the value of EI service with reference to the greater cost of provision of services later in students' development. You could also point out the proven effects of EI on literacy.

Q7. My school district has replaced some speech-language pathologists with speech-language pathology assistants. I have been assigned to supervise six of them and feel that I cannot provide adequate supervision for their work with our students. Does the Code of Ethics address this?

A7. The Code permits delegation of duties to support personnel only when a certificate holder can provide "appropriate supervision." In this case, it would be reasonable to argue that supervision of six speech-language pathology assistants would exceed "appropriate" levels of effective supervision (ASHA, Principle II, Rule D; ASHA, 2004b).

Q8. I spoke with a fellow audiologist who also has her CCC about an incident during which she was clearly engaged in unethical conduct. She became indignant and threatened me with a lawsuit if I reported her. Should I just forget about it?

A8. Both ASHA and AAA Codes require professionals to inform the respective Board of Ethics of perceived violations of the Code. ASHA, Principle IV, Rule I and J, and AAA, Principle 8, Rules 8c and 8d also obligate individuals to cooperate with the boards in the investigation and adjudication of complaints of unethical practice.

Q9. A professional colleague submitted a paper for publication that contained entire sections of text lifted from other works that were neither quoted nor cited. Although the university has a plagiarism policy, do I have any ethical responsibility beyond the university policy?

A9. The Codes prohibit misrepresentation of research results and professional dishonesty. (ASHA Principles III, Rule D, and IV, Rule D; AAA, Principle 6, Rules 6a and 6b, and Principle 7, Rule 7b)

Q10. An individual who is severely hard-of-hearing has applied to our speech-language pathology graduate program. She has superior undergraduate grades and references, but

(*Continues*)

(Continued)

we have doubts about whether her hearing loss will limit her success in the profession. Any thoughts?

A10. The conflict here is between ASHA Principle of Ethics I, Rule C, which prohibits discrimination on the basis of disability, and Principle of Ethics I, Rule A, which requires all services to be provided competently. Since graduate academic coursework and practicum are a formative as well as a summative process, this might be a chance to explore limitations and opportunities with the student in an objective environment, giving the student options to satisfy career goals as well as maintaining competent service to clientele.

Q11. A hearing aid company offers incentives for the sales of particular models of hearing aids. Is it unethical for me to participate in the promotion of these aids?

A11. Any activity that could constitute a conflict of interest jeopardizes the professional's primary duty to hold paramount the welfare of people served (ASHA, Principle III, Rule B; AAA, Principle 4, Rule 4). See also *American Academy of Audiology Guidelines on Financial Incentives from Hearing Instrument Manufacturers* (2005).

Q12. I have some patients in my caseload who are really not benefiting from treatment. I need the clinical hours, so I'm not planning to dismiss them until the end of the semester. That's OK ethically, isn't it?

A12. The Code of Ethics supports the provision of professional services for clients only when benefit can reasonably be expected. Artificial time boundaries such as semesters, marking periods, or payment periods must not be used to determine the length of therapy programs (ASHA, Principle I, Rule G; AAA, Principle 1, Rule 1a).

ETHICAL PRACTICE RISK MANAGEMENT

Risk management involves routine, careful, and detailed evaluation of every component of assessment and therapeutic procedures used to determine whether they conform to established standards of ethical conduct. Most unethical practice complaints can be avoided through continued awareness of the quality of service provided in light of conduct standards. The following examples show inexpensive ways of reducing the risk of professional complaints.

1. Make every effort to ensure effective oral and written communication with your clientele, their parents, or their spouses. Explain, to the degree necessary, the rationale for the use of individual procedures and techniques. Describe the program of therapy in such a way that the client, parents, or spouse know where he or she is in the progression of treatment at any time.
2. Strive to obtain truly informed consent. Informed consent requires not only that consent be obtained from the client or his or her parent or spouse but that the consent be based on reasonable understanding of procedures to be used, rationale, and expected outcomes. This may require the use of an interpreter for those who are hearing impaired or who speak other languages. It may also involve using graphics or a video presentation to explain procedures.
3. Review periodically the Codes of Ethics of ASHA, AAA, and/or any other professional organization of which you are a member. Keep current on amended codes of ethics. ASHA, AAA, and state and regional associations are excellent resources for obtaining updated information regarding practice standards and trends through their publications, committees, and conference presentations. Volunteer to serve on an ethical practices committee.
4. Encourage your local associations to have informal discussions on ethical practices or formal presentations by leaders within the professions.

This is a good setting in which to discuss Issues in Ethics statements published by ASHA on a regular basis. Such discussions help professionals engage in self-guided, ethical decision making.

5. Learn how to develop your "emotional intelligence" so that you are more aware of stressors that may compromise your ethical practice. For example, pressure to meet quotas from your administrator would be better dealt with through discussion than unethical practice.
6. Establish an ethical practices discussion group in your workplace. This may help to identify issues that present ethical challenges before they become problematic. Sharing resources on ethical practices in this informal format may provide support and education.
7. When in doubt, ask yourself, "How does this action or practice affect the welfare of my client?"

WHAT TO DO IF YOU FACE AN ETHICAL DILEMMA

Most clinicians will experience ethical predicaments at some point in their careers. While careful consideration of one's own professional judgment may sometimes be adequate, the following suggestions also may be of help:

1. Consult the current codes of ethics that apply to you.
2. Check with the Boards of Ethics of your local, state, and/or national professional associations.
3. Talk with a trusted colleague, supervisor, or former professor who is knowledgeable and willing to give confidential advice.
4. Retain an attorney who is experienced in professional liability issues, malpractice, contracts, or labor law. Most local bar associations can help with referrals.

SUMMARY

This chapter defined ethics, codes of ethics, and the process of what to do if you or a colleague is faced with an ethical dilemma. Numerous examples of possible ethical dilemmas are given for review and further discussion. The ASHA and AAA Codes of Ethics are provided in the appendices for your review. Remember that these are living documents that undergo periodic revision as the professions change and face new challenges.

People do not usually set out to be unethical in their conduct. They are most often good people who have developed bad habits or have made poor decisions or who are faced with unreasonable constraints in their employment settings. Fellow professionals must routinely and vigilantly honor both ethical and legal standards of conduct. Former ASHA President Nancy Swigert (1998) reminded Association members, "Failing to follow the Code of Ethics puts patients in jeopardy because they are not receiving appropriate services. It puts our colleagues in jeopardy because it reflects badly on everyone in the professions" (p. 11). If we maintain a working knowledge of the ethical codes to which we are bound, the professions can only benefit in a time of reimbursement constraints and aggressive service delivery restructuring. Nothing will upgrade the professions more.

CRITICAL THINKING

1. What would you do if you faced an ethical dilemma that was not covered in your professional Code of Ethics? What steps are appropriate for reporting an ethical violation?
2. Suppose you have made an "honest mistake." Is this a violation of the Code of Ethics? What should you do?
3. How do the expanding scopes of practice in SLP and audiology affect our Codes of Ethics? How will you keep abreast of changes in ASHA and/or AAA Codes of Ethics?
4. After reading the next chapter on legal issues and professional liability, contrast the similarities and differences between ethics and liability. Why do we need both?

5. Read through the ASHA and/or AAA Codes of Ethics. Which principles are reflective of the philosophical concepts (a) do the most good and the least harm, (b) protect and respect the moral rights of those affected, (c) treat all equally, (d) enhance the community as a whole, and (e) maintain the highest values of truth, compassion, fairness, and prudence?
6. Go to ASHA's website and find the Issues in Ethics statements. Choose one to read and summarize. Why did you choose this statement to review? What relevance does it have to your current clinical practice?
7. Use of technology presents some unique ethical challenges. How will you protect your clients' confidentiality when you use electronic records? What other ethical challenges does the use or prescription of technology (including hearing aids and expressive assistive devices) present for clinicians?
8. After reading other chapters on such issues as documentation and technology, revisit this chapter to consider ethical issues across a variety of current clinical practices. For example, what ASHA Principle of Ethics is involved with maintaining or distributing client records?
9. One of your colleagues takes pride in the fact that she does only the minimum amount of continuing education to maintain her certification and state licensure. In fact, she says that she often signs up for conferences but "skips" out and goes shopping and forges the documentation regarding presentation attendance when she attends a national convention. She appears, however, to be a good clinician. Is her attitude toward continuing education unethical? What would you say to her, if anything?
10. Review the Codes of Ethics for ASHA and AAA. Make up several scenarios and ask your peers if they think there are ethical violations in them.

REFERENCES

American Academy of Audiology. (2005). *Ethical practice guidelines on financial incentives from hearing instrument manufacturers.* Retrieved from http://www.audiologyonline.com/management/uploads/news/aaa_5-20-03.pdf

American Academy of Audiology. (2009). *Code of Ethics.* Retrieved from http://www.audiology.org/resources/documentlibrary/Pages/codeofethics.aspx

American Speech-Language-Hearing Association. (1996). Issues in ethics: Clinical practice by certificate holders in the profession in which they are not certified. *ASHA Supplement 16,* 62–63.

American Speech-Language-Hearing Association. (1998). Statement of practices and procedures of the Board of Ethics. *ASHA, 40*(Suppl. 18), 46–49.

American Speech-Language-Hearing Association. (2004a). Clinical practice by certificate holders in the profession in which they are not certified. *ASHA Supplement 24,* 39–40.

American Speech-Language-Hearing Association. (2004b). *Guidelines for the training, use, and supervision of speech-language pathology assistants.* Available from http://www.asha.org/

American Speech-Language-Hearing Association. (2005). *Medicaid guidance for school-based speech-language pathology services: Addressing the "under the direction of" rule.* Available from http://www.asha.org/

American Speech-Language-Hearing Association. (2008a). *Statement of practices and procedures for appeals of Board of Ethics decisions.* Available from http://www.asha.org/policy

American Speech-Language-Hearing Association. (2008b). *Statement of practices and procedures of the Board of Ethics.* Available from http://www.asha.org/policy

American Speech-Language-Hearing Association. (2009). *Guidelines for responding to a complaint of an alleged violation of the ASHA* Code of Ethics. Retrieved from http://www.asha.org/Practice/ethics/CompResp.htm

American Speech-Language-Hearing Association. (2010). *Code of Ethics*. Available from http://www.asha.org/policy

Baker, R. (1999). Codes of ethics: Some history. *Perspectives on the Professions.*Retrieved from http://www.library.illinois.edu/archives/workpap/MaherNEA2007.pdf

Boswell, S. (2004, October 19). International agreement brings mutual recognition of certification. *The ASHA Leader,* 1, 22.

Boylan, M. (2000). *Basic ethics* (pp. 152–164). Upper Saddle River, NJ: Prentice Hall.

Butler, K. (1996). Managed care: Emerging issues in clinical ethics. *ASHA, 38,* 7.

Center for the Study of Ethics in the Professions. (2005). *Code of ethics introduction*. Retrieved from http://ethics.iit.edu/research/introduction

Colero, L. (2005). *A framework for universal principles of ethics*. Retrieved from http://www.ethics.ubc.ca/papers/invited/colero.html

Denton, D. (2009). *How ASHA's Board of Ethics sanctions individuals found in violation of the Code of Ethics*. Retrieved from http://www.asha.org/Practice/ethics/sanctions.htm

Denton, D. (2011). *Trends in ethics inquiries received by the ASHA National Office* [From the Director of Ethics]. Retrieved from http://www.asha.org/practice/ethics/ethtrends.htm

Diefendorf, A. (2008, March). The ASHA Board of Ethics: An update on roles, responsibilities, and educational resources. *ASHA's Perspectives on Administration and Supervision, 18*, 4–9.

Ethics Resource Center. (2005). *Code construction and content*. Available from http://www.ethics.org/

Miller, T. (1983). *Professional liability in speech-language pathology and audiology: Unprofessional conduct and unethical practice.* Unpublished doctoral dissertation, State University of New York at Buffalo.

Miller, T., & Lubinski, R. (1986). Professional liability in speech-language pathology and audiology. *ASHA, 28*(6), 45–47.

Santa Clara University. (2005). *A framework for thinking ethically*. Retrieved from http://www.scu.edu/ethics/practicing/decision/framework.html/

Swigert, N. (1998). Taking ethics seriously. *ASHA, 40*(3), 11.

RESOURCES

American Academy of Audiology Ethical Practices
http://www.audiology.org

American Speech-Language-Hearing Association Board of Ethics
http://www.asha.org

Applied Ethics Resources on the World Wide Web
http://www.ethicsweb.ca/resources/

Center for the Study of Ethics in the Professions (CSEP)
Illinois Institute of Technology
HUB Mezzanine, Room 204
3241 S. Federal Street
Chicago, IL 60616-3793
Phone: 312-567-3017
Website: http://ethics.iit.edu

Ethics Resource Center
1747 Pennsylvania Avenue, Suite 400
Washington, DC 20006
Phone: 202-737-7258
E-mail: ethics@ethics.org

Appendix 5-A

ASHA Code of Ethics

Preamble

The preservation of the highest standards of integrity and ethical principles is vital to the responsible discharge of obligations by speech-language pathologists, audiologists, and speech, language, and hearing scientists. This Code of Ethics sets forth the fundamental principles and rules considered essential to this purpose.

Every individual who is (a) a member of the American Speech-Language-Hearing Association, whether certified or not, (b) a nonmember holding the Certificate of Clinical Competence from the Association, (c) an applicant for membership or certification, or (d) a Clinical Fellow seeking to fulfill standards for certification shall abide by this Code of Ethics. Any violation of the spirit and purpose of this Code shall be considered unethical. Failure to specify any particular responsibility or practice in this Code of Ethics shall not be construed as denial of the existence of such responsibilities or practices.

The fundamentals of ethical conduct are described by Principles of Ethics and by Rules of Ethics as they relate to the responsibility to persons served, the public, speech-language pathologists, audiologists, and speech, language, and hearing scientists, and to the conduct of research and scholarly activities.

Principles of Ethics, aspirational and inspirational in nature, form the underlying moral basis for the Code of Ethics. Individuals shall observe these principles as affirmative obligations under all conditions of professional activity.

Rules of Ethics are specific statements of minimally acceptable professional conduct or of prohibitions and are applicable to all individuals.

Principle of Ethics I

Individuals shall honor their responsibility to hold paramount the welfare of persons they serve professionally or who are participants in research and scholarly activities, and they shall treat animals involved in research in a humane manner.

Rules of Ethics

A. Individuals shall provide all services competently.

B. Individuals shall use every resource, including referral when appropriate, to ensure that high-quality service is provided.

C. Individuals shall not discriminate in the delivery of professional services or the conduct of research and scholarly activities on the basis of race or ethnicity, gender, gender identity/gender expression, age, religion, national origin, sexual orientation, or disability.

D. Individuals shall not misrepresent the credentials of assistants, technicians, support personnel, students, Clinical Fellows, or any others under their supervision, and they shall inform those they serve professionally of the name and professional credentials of persons providing services.

E. Individuals who hold the Certificate of Clinical Competence shall not delegate tasks that require the unique skills, knowledge, and judgment that are within the scope of their profession to assistants, technicians, support personnel, or any nonprofessionals over whom they have supervisory responsibility.

Last revised January 1, 2010

SOURCE: Reprinted with permission from Code of Ethics. Available from the website of the American Speech-Language-Hearing Association: http://www.asha.org/policy.

F. Individuals who hold the Certificate of Clinical Competence may delegate tasks related to provision of clinical services to assistants, technicians, support personnel, or any other persons only if those services are appropriately supervised, realizing that the responsibility for client welfare remains with the certified individual.

G. Individuals who hold the Certificate of Clinical Competence may delegate tasks related to provision of clinical services that require the unique skills, knowledge, and judgment that are within the scope of practice of their profession to students only if those services are appropriately supervised. The responsibility for client welfare remains with the certified individual.

H. Individuals shall fully inform the persons they serve of the nature and possible effects of services rendered and products dispensed, and they shall inform participants in research about the possible effects of their participation in research conducted.

I. Individuals shall evaluate the effectiveness of services rendered and of products dispensed, and they shall provide services or dispense products only when benefit can reasonably be expected.

J. Individuals shall not guarantee the results of any treatment or procedure, directly or by implication; however, they may make a reasonable statement of prognosis.

K. Individuals shall not provide clinical services solely by correspondence.

L. Individuals may practice by telecommunication (e.g., telehealth/e-health), where not prohibited by law.

M. Individuals shall adequately maintain and appropriately secure records of professional services rendered, research and scholarly activities conducted, and products dispensed, and they shall allow access to these records only when authorized or when required by law.

N. Individuals shall not reveal, without authorization, any professional or personal information about identified persons served professionally or identified participants involved in research and scholarly activities unless doing so is necessary to protect the welfare of the person or of the community or is otherwise required by law.

O. Individuals shall not charge for services not rendered, nor shall they misrepresent services rendered, products dispensed, or research and scholarly activities conducted.

P. Individuals shall enroll and include persons as participants in research or teaching demonstrations only if their participation is voluntary, without coercion, and with their informed consent.

Q. Individuals whose professional services are adversely affected by substance abuse or other health-related conditions shall seek professional assistance and, where appropriate, withdraw from the affected areas of practice.

R. Individuals shall not discontinue service to those they are serving without providing reasonable notice.

Principle of Ethics II

Individuals shall honor their responsibility to achieve and maintain the highest level of professional competence and performance.

Rules of Ethics

A. Individuals shall engage in the provision of clinical services only when they hold the appropriate Certificate of Clinical Competence or when they are in the certification process and are supervised by an individual who holds the appropriate Certificate of Clinical Competence.

B. Individuals shall engage in only those aspects of the professions that are within the scope of their professional practice and competence, considering their level of education, training, and experience.

C. Individuals shall engage in lifelong learning to maintain and enhance professional competence and performance.

D. Individuals shall not require or permit their professional staff to provide services or conduct research

Last revised January 1, 2010

SOURCE: Reprinted with permission from Code of Ethics. Available from the website of the American Speech-Language-Hearing Association: http://www.asha.org/policy.

activities that exceed the staff member's competence, level of education, training, and experience.

E. Individuals shall ensure that all equipment used to provide services or to conduct research and scholarly activities is in proper working order and is properly calibrated.

Principle of Ethics III

Individuals shall honor their responsibility to the public by promoting public understanding of the professions, by supporting the development of services designed to fulfill the unmet needs of the public, and by providing accurate information in all communications involving any aspect of the professions, including the dissemination of research findings and scholarly activities, and the promotion, marketing, and advertising of products and services.

Rules of Ethics

A. Individuals shall not misrepresent their credentials, competence, education, training, experience, or scholarly or research contributions.

B. Individuals shall not participate in professional activities that constitute a conflict of interest.

C. Individuals shall refer those served professionally solely on the basis of the interest of those being referred and not on any personal interest, financial or otherwise.

D. Individuals shall not misrepresent research, diagnostic information, services rendered, results of services rendered, products dispensed, or the effects of products dispensed.

E. Individuals shall not defraud or engage in any scheme to defraud in connection with obtaining payment, reimbursement, or grants for services rendered, research conducted, or products dispensed.

F. Individuals' statements to the public shall provide accurate information about the nature and management of communication disorders, about the professions, about professional services, about products for sale, and about research and scholarly activities.

G. Individuals' statements to the public when advertising, announcing, and marketing their professional services; reporting research results; and promoting products shall adhere to professional standards and shall not contain misrepresentations.

Principle of Ethics IV

Individuals shall honor their responsibilities to the professions and their relationships with colleagues, students, and members of other professions and disciplines.

Rules of Ethics

A. Individuals shall uphold the dignity and autonomy of the professions, maintain harmonious interprofessional and intraprofessional relationships, and accept the professions' self-imposed standards.

B. Individuals shall prohibit anyone under their supervision from engaging in any practice that violates the Code of Ethics.

C. Individuals shall not engage in dishonesty, fraud, deceit, or misrepresentation.

D. Individuals shall not engage in any form of unlawful harassment, including sexual harassment or power abuse.

E. Individuals shall not engage in any other form of conduct that adversely reflects on the professions or on the individual's fitness to serve persons professionally.

F. Individuals shall not engage in sexual activities with clients, students, or research participants over whom they exercise professional authority or power.

G. Individuals shall assign credit only to those who have contributed to a publication, presentation, or product. Credit shall be assigned in proportion to the contribution and only with the contributor's consent.

H. Individuals shall reference the source when using other persons' ideas, research, presentations, or products in written, oral, or any other media presentation or summary.

Last revised January 1, 2010

SOURCE: Reprinted with permission from Code of Ethics. Available from the website of the American Speech-Language-Hearing Association: http://www.asha.org/policy.

I. Individuals' statements to colleagues about professional services, research results, and products shall adhere to prevailing professional standards and shall contain no misrepresentations.

J. Individuals shall not provide professional services without exercising independent professional judgment, regardless of referral source or prescription.

K. Individuals shall not discriminate in their relationships with colleagues, students, and members of other professions and disciplines on the basis of race or ethnicity, gender, gender identity/gender expression, age, religion, national origin, sexual orientation, or disability.

L. Individuals shall not file or encourage others to file complaints that disregard or ignore facts that would disprove the allegation, nor should the Code of Ethics be used for personal reprisal, as a means of addressing personal animosity, or as a vehicle for retaliation.

M. Individuals who have reason to believe that the Code of Ethics has been violated shall inform the Board of Ethics.

N. Individuals shall comply fully with the policies of the Board of Ethics in its consideration and adjudication of complaints of violations of the Code of Ethics.

Last revised January 1, 2010

SOURCE: Reprinted with permission from Code of Ethics. Available from the website of the American Speech-Language-Hearing Association: http://www.asha.org/policy.

Appendix 5-B

Code of Ethics of American Academy of Audiology (Revised 2009)

Preamble

The Code of Ethics of the American Academy of Audiology specifies professional standards that allow for the proper discharge of audiologists' responsibilities to those served, and that protect the integrity of the profession. The Code of Ethics consists of two parts. The first part, the Statement of Principles and Rules, presents precepts that members (all categories of members, including Student Members) effective January 1, 2009 of the Academy agree to uphold. The second part, the Procedures, provides the process that enables enforcement of the Principles and Rules.

PART I. Statement of Principles and Rules

PRINCIPLE 1: Members shall provide professional services and conduct research with honesty and compassion, and shall respect the dignity, worth, and rights of those served.

Rule la: Individuals shall not limit the delivery of professional services on any basis that is unjustifiable or irrelevant to the need for the potential benefit from such services.

Rule 1b: Individuals shall not provide services except in a professional relationship, and shall not discriminate in the provision of services to individuals on the basis of sex, race, religion, national origin, sexual orientation, or general health.

PRINCIPLE 2: Members shall maintain high standards of professional competence in rendering services.

Rule 2a: Members shall provide only those professional services for which they are qualified by education and experience.

Rule 2b: Individuals shall use available resources, including referrals to other specialists, and shall not accept benefits or items of personal value for receiving or making referrals.

Rule 2c: Individuals shall exercise all reasonable precautions to avoid injury to persons in the delivery of professional services or execution of research.

Rule 2d: Individuals shall provide appropriate supervision and assume full responsibility for services delegated to supportive personnel. Individuals shall not delegate any service requiring professional competence to unqualified persons.

Rule 2e: Individuals shall not permit personnel to engage in any practice that is a violation of the Code of Ethics.

Rule 2f: Individuals shall maintain professional competence, including participation in continuing education.

PRINCIPLE 3: Members shall maintain the confidentiality of the information and records of those receiving services or involved in research.

Rule 3a: Individuals shall not reveal to unauthorized persons any professional or personal information obtained from the person served professionally, unless required by law.

PRINCIPLE 4: Members shall provide only services and products that are in the best interest of those served.

Rule 4a: Individuals shall not exploit persons in the delivery of professional services.

Rule 4b: Individuals shall not charge for services not rendered.

Rule 4c: Individuals shall not participate in activities that constitute a conflict of professional interest.

Rule 4d: Individuals using investigational procedures with patients, or prospectively collecting research data, shall first obtain full informed consent from the patient or guardian.

PRINCIPLE 5: Members shall provide accurate information about the nature and management of communicative disorders and about the services and products offered.

Rule 5a: Individuals shall provide persons served with the information a reasonable person would want to know about the nature and possible effects of services rendered, or products provided or research being conducted.

Rule 5b: Individuals may make a statement of prognosis, but shall not guarantee results, mislead, or misinform persons served or studied.

Rule 5c: Individuals shall conduct and report product-related research only according to accepted standards of research practice.

Rule 5d: Individuals shall not carry out teaching or research activities in a manner that constitutes an invasion of privacy, or that fails to inform persons fully about the nature and possible effects of these activities, affording all persons informed free choice of participation.

Rule 5e: Individuals shall maintain documentation of professional services rendered.

PRINCIPLE 6: Members shall comply with the ethical standards of the Academy with regard to public statements or publication.

Rule 6a: Individuals shall not misrepresent their educational degrees, training, credentials, or competence. Only degrees earned from regionally accredited institutions in which training was obtained in audiology, or a directly related discipline, may be used in public statements concerning professional services.

Rule 6b: Individuals' public statements about professional services, products, or research results shall not contain representations or claims that are false, misleading, or deceptive.

PRINCIPLE 7: Members shall honor their responsibilities to the public and to professional colleagues.

Rule 7a: Individuals shall not use professional or commercial affiliations in any way that would limit services to or mislead patients or colleagues.

Rule 7b: Individuals shall inform colleagues and the public in a manner consistent with the highest professional standards about products and services they have developed or research they have conducted.

PRINCIPLE 8: Members shall uphold the dignity of the profession and freely accept the Academy's self-imposed standards.

Rule 8a: Individuals shall not violate these Principles and Rules, nor attempt to circumvent them.

Rule 8b: Individuals shall not engage in dishonesty or illegal conduct that adversely reflects on the profession.

Rule 8c: Individuals shall inform the Ethical Practices Committee when there are reasons to believe that a member of the Academy may have violated the Code of Ethics.

Rule 8d: Individuals shall cooperate with the Ethical Practices Committee in any matter related to the Code of Ethics.

PART II. Procedures for The Management of Alleged Violations

Introduction

Members of the American Academy of Audiology are obligated to uphold the Code of Ethics of the Academy in their personal conduct and in the performance of their professional duties. To this end it is the responsibility of each Academy member to inform the Ethical Practices Committee of possible Ethics Code violations. The processing of alleged violations of the Code of Ethics will follow the procedures specified below in an expeditious manner to ensure that violations of ethical conduct by members of the Academy are halted in the shortest time possible.

Procedures

1. Suspected violations of the Code of Ethics shall be reported in letter format giving documentation sufficient to support the alleged violation. Letters must be addressed to:

   Chair, Ethical Practices Committee
   c/o Executive Director
   American Academy of Audiology
   11730 Plaza America Dr., Suite 300
   Reston, VA 20190

2. Following receipt of a report of a suspected violation, at the discretion of the Chair, the Ethical Practices Committee will request a signed Waiver of Confidentiality from the complainant indicating that the complainant will allow the Ethical Practices Committee to disclose his/her name should this become necessary during investigation of the allegation.
   a. The Ethical Practices Committee may, under special circumstances, act in the absence of a signed Waiver of Confidentiality. For example, in cases where the Ethical Practices Committee has received information from a state licensure or registration board of a member having his or her license or registration suspended or revoked, then the Ethical Practices Committee will proceed without a complainant.
   b. The Chair may communicate with other individuals, agencies, and/or programs for additional information as may be required for review at any time during the deliberation.
3. The Ethical Practices Committee will convene to review the merit of the alleged violation as it relates to the Code of Ethics.
   a. The Ethical Practices Committee shall meet to discuss the case, either in person, by electronic means or by teleconference. The meeting will occur within 60 days of receipt of the waiver of confidentiality, or of notification by the complainant of refusal to sign the waiver. In cases where another form of notification brings the complaint to the attention of the Ethical Practices Committee, the Committee will convene within 60 days of notification.
   b. If the alleged violation has a high probability of being legally actionable, the case may be referred to the appropriate agency. The Ethical Practices Committee may postpone member notification and further deliberation until the legal process has been completed.
4. If there is sufficient evidence that indicates a violation of the Code of Ethics has occurred, upon majority vote, the member will be forwarded a Notification of Potential Ethics Concern.
   a. The circumstances of the alleged violation will be described.
   b. The member will be informed of the specific Code of Ethics rule that may conflict with member behavior.
   c. Supporting Academy documents that may serve to further educate the member about the ethical implications will be included, as appropriate.
   d. The member will be asked to respond fully to the allegation and submit all supporting evidence within 30 calendar days.
5. The Ethical Practices Committee will meet either in person or by teleconference:
   a. within 60 calendar days of receiving a response from the member to the Notification of Potential Ethics Concern to review the response and all information pertaining to the alleged violation, or
   b. within sixty (60) calendar days of notification to member if no response is received from the member to review the information received from the complainant.
6. If the Ethical Practices Committee determines that the evidence supports the allegation of an ethical violation, then the member will be provided written notice containing the following information:
   a. The right to a hearing in person or by teleconference before the Ethical Practices Committee;
   b. The date, time and place of the hearing;
   c. The ethical violation being charged and the potential sanction
   d. The right to present a defense to the charges.

At this time the member should provide any additional relevant information. As this is the final opportunity for a member to provide new information, the member should carefully prepare all documentation.

7. Potential Rulings.
   a. When the Ethical Practices Committee determines there is insufficient evidence of an ethical violation, the parties to the complaint will be notified that the case will be closed.
   b. If the evidence supports the allegation of a Code violation, the rules(s) of the Code violated will be cited and sanction(s) will be specified.
8. The Committee shall sanction members based on the severity of the violation and history of prior ethical violations. A simple majority of voting members is required to institute a sanction unless otherwise noted. Sanctions may include one or more of the following:
   a. Educative Letter. This sanction alone is appropriate when:
      1. The ethics violation appears to have been inadvertent.
      2. The member's response to Notification of Potential Ethics Concern indicates a new awareness of the problem and the member resolves to refrain from future ethical violations.
   b. Cease and Desist Order. The member signs a consent agreement to immediately halt the practice(s) which were found to be in violation of the Code of Ethics.
   c. Reprimand. The member will be formally reprimanded for the violation of the Code of Ethics.
   d. Mandatory continuing education.
      1. The EPC will determine the type of education needed to reduce chances of recurrence of violations.
      2. The member will be responsible for submitting documentation of continuing education within the period of time designated by the Ethical Practices Committee.
      3. All costs associated with compliance will be borne by the member.
   e. Probation of Suspension. The member signs a consent agreement in acknowledgement of the Ethical Practices Committee decision and is allowed to retain membership benefits during a defined probationary period.
      1. The duration of probation and the terms for avoiding suspension will be determined by the Ethical Practices Committee.
      2. Failure of the member to meet the terms for probation will result in the suspension of membership.
   f. Suspension of Membership.
      1. The duration of suspension will be determined by the Ethical Practices Committee.
      2. The member may not receive membership benefits during the period of suspension.
      3. Members suspended are not entitled to a refund of dues or fees.
   g. Revocation of Membership. Revocation of membership is considered the maximum punishment for a violation of the Code of Ethics.
      1. Revocation requires a two-thirds majority of the voting members of the EPC.
      2. Individuals whose memberships are revoked are not entitled to a refund of dues or fees.
      3. One year following the date of membership revocation the individual may reapply for, but is not guaranteed, membership through normal channels and must meet the membership qualifications in effect at the time of application.
9. The member may appeal the Final Finding and Decision of the Ethical Practices Committee to the Academy Board of Directors. The route of Appeal is by letter format through the Ethical Practices Committee to the Board of Directors of the Academy. Requests for Appeal must:
   a. be received by the Chair, Ethical Practices Committee, within 30 days of the Ethical Practices Committee's notification of the Final Finding and Decision,

b. state the basis for the appeal, and the reason(s) that the Final Finding and Decision of the Ethical Practices Committee should be changed,

c. not offer new documentation.

The EPC chair will communicate with the Executive Director of the Association to schedule the appeal at the earliest feasible Board of Director's meeting.

The Board of Directors will review the documents and written summaries, and deliberate the case.

The decision of the Board of Directors regarding the member's appeal shall be final.

10. In order to educate the membership, upon majority vote the Ethical Practices Committee, the circumstances and nature of cases shall be presented in Audiology Today and in the Professional Resource area of the Academy website. The member's identity will not be made public.

11. No Ethical Practices Committee member shall give access to records, act or speak independently, or on behalf of the Ethical Practices Committee, without the expressed permission of the members then active. No member may impose the sanction of the Ethical Practices Committee, or to interpret the findings of the EPC in any manner which may place members of the Ethical Practices Committee or Board of Directors, collectively or singly, at financial, professional, or personal risk.

12. The Ethical Practices Committee Chair shall maintain a Book of Precedents that shall form the basis for future findings of the Committee.

Confidentiality and Records

Confidentiality shall be maintained in all Ethical Practices Committee discussion, correspondence, communication, deliberation, and records pertaining to members reviewed by the Ethical Practices Committee.

1. Complaints and suspected violations are assigned a case number.
2. Identity of members involved in complaints and suspected violations and access to EPC files is restricted to the following:
   a. EPC Chair
   b. EPC member designated by EPC Chair when the chair recuses him or herself from a case
   c. Executive Director
   d. Agent/s of the Executive Director
   e. Other/s, following majority vote of EPC
3. Original records shall be maintained at the Central Records Repository at the Academy office in a locked cabinet.
   a. One copy will be sent to the Ethical Practices Committee chair or member designated by the Chair.
   b. Copies will be sent to members.
4. Communications shall be sent to the members involved in complaints by the Academy office via certified or registered mail, after review by Legal Counsel.
5. When a case is closed,
   a. The chair will forward all documentation to the Academy Central Records Repository.
   b. Members shall destroy all material pertaining to the case.
6. Complete records generally shall be maintained at the Academy Central Records Repository for a period of five years.
   a. Records will be destroyed five years after a member receives a sanction less than suspension, or five years after the end of a suspension, or after membership is reinstated.
   b. Records of membership revocations for persons who have not returned to membership status will be maintained indefinitely.

(AAA, 2009)

6

Professional Liability

Jennifer Horner, PhD, JD

SCOPE OF CHAPTER

The health professions, including speech-language pathology and audiology, govern themselves with relative autonomy (Frattali, 2001). Autonomy entails responsibilities and, in turn, duties and liabilities. According to *Black's Law Dictionary* (1990, p. 1312), a *responsibility* is "the state of being answerable for an obligation, and includes judgment, skill, ability, and capacity. The obligation to answer for an act done, and to repair or otherwise make restitution for any injury it may have caused." The corresponding legal terms are *duty* and *liability.* According to Keeton and colleagues, a *duty* is "...an obligation, to which the law will give recognition and effect, to conform to a particular standard of conduct toward another" (Keeton, Dobbs, Keeton, & Owen, 1984, in Dickson, 1995, p. 523). *Black's* (1990, p. 914) defines *liability* as a broad legal term referring to "all character of debts and obligations."

The liabilities of speech-language pathologists and audiologists arise from duties assumed by virtue of the promises they have made to abide by standards of practice and codes of ethics of their parent professional organization(s) such as the American Speech-Language-Hearing Association (ASHA, 2001, 2002, 2003, 2004, 2005a), the American Academy of Audiology (AAA, 2005), and the Academy of Neurologic Communication Disorders and Sciences (ANCDS, 2005). They also acquire duties (and liabilities) to society by accepting a license to practice in their respective states. Duties and liabilities also stem from the various codes of law (federal and state statutes)—general laws governing society-at-large, the provision of, or reimbursement for, health care services, and the implicit responsibility to respect civil rights as well as to adhere to the laws governing labor and commerce.

Lapses in professional judgment, carelessness when applying diagnostic or treatment methods, and/or failure to obey applicable laws all come with a cost. According to a Technical Report by ASHA (1994), a review of insurance liability claims between January 1982 and June 1993 found a total of 129 claims—58 percent against audiologists and 20 percent against speech-language pathologists. The most frequent type of claim (25) was for improper treatment procedures, and the second most frequent (23) involved hearing aids. Other types of claims involved physical injuries, improper diagnoses, errors during intraoperative monitoring, property damages, and false claims. Although the number of claims on average was only about 12 per year, the total dollars paid by the insurer for these claims over the 10-year period was $1,865,000. To the author's knowledge, there are no recent published reports summarizing the frequency of professional misconduct allegations, professional malpractice complaints, settlements, or litigated lawsuits regarding speech-language pathologists or audiologists; but see Tanner's work as an expert witness in cases involving "dysphagia malpractice" (2007, 2010).

If the conduct of speech-language pathologists or audiologists falls below the legal standard of care or violates any other applicable legal standard, they may be liable for *professional misconduct.* In contrast, conduct that violates professional codes of ethics renders professionals liable for *unethical practices* (Miller, 2001, p. 66). Importantly, the same conduct can lead to liability in both forums. As ASHA (2004) points out, "the final decision of any state, federal, regulatory, or judicial body may be considered sufficient evidence that the Code was violated" (p. 190). In turn, ASHA's Board of Ethics may send its final decision to "any state agency that licenses or credentials speech-language pathologists or audiologists" (p. 190). Although this chapter focuses on professional liability, readers should recognize that the same alleged wrongdoing may have both ethical and legal implications. For more detail, see Chapter 5, Professional Ethics.

The purposes of this chapter are to identify the sources of law that apply to our learned professions, to outline the correspondence between patients' rights and professional duties, to explain the duties of speech-language pathologists and audiologists under state licensure laws, and to identify an array of federal statutes that apply to our professional practices. Finally, the law of negligence is explained as it applies to both individual practitioners and health care institutions, and the wisdom of being covered by both institutional and individual insurance policies is explained to protect against the risk of professional liability.

SOURCES OF LAW

The main sources of law at both the federal and state levels of government are constitutions, statutes, common law (case law), and regulations promulgated by legislatively authorized administrative agencies.

United States Constitution

The United States Constitution was approved September 17, 1787. This vibrant document articulates the structure and duties of the federal government, the relationship between federal and state governments, and the limits of federal authority over the states and their citizens. Article VI contains the *supremacy clause*, which states that the United States Constitution and federal laws are superior to, and binding on, states and their citizens. Article VI of the United States Constitution states:

> This Constitution, and the Laws of the United States which shall be made in Pursuance thereof; and all Treaties made, or which shall be made, under the Authority of the United States, shall be the supreme Law of the Land; and the Judges in every state shall be bound thereby, any Thing in the Constitution or Laws of any State to the contrary notwithstanding.

Among the amendments to the United States Constitution, the Fourteenth Amendment, ratified in 1868, is especially important because it limits the authority of the *state governments* to infringe the rights of citizens:

> Section 1. All persons born or naturalized in the United States and subject to the jurisdiction thereof, are citizens of the United States and of the State wherein they reside. No State shall make or

> enforce any law which shall abridge the privileges or immunities of citizens of the United States; nor shall any State deprive any person of life, liberty, or property, without due process of law; nor deny to any person within its jurisdiction the equal protection of the laws.

As interpreted by the United States Supreme Court, *liberty*, or "liberty interests," conveys the right to make personal decisions, including medical decisions (*Cruzan v. Director, Missouri Department of Health,* 1990). The *due process* clause, among other things, implies the right to notice, an opportunity to be heard, and the opportunity to appeal decisions affecting life, liberty, or property (e.g., due process rights under the Individuals with Disabilities Education Improvement Act of 2004). The *equal protection* clause provides the basis for numerous civil rights laws, including ensuring the right of disabled people to access public accommodations, such as hospitals and clinics (e.g., Americans with Disabilities Act of 1990, as amended; see also U.S. Department of Justice, 2011), and ensuring the right of disabled children to participate in the least restrictive learning environment inclusively with nondisabled children (e.g., the Individuals with Disabilities Education Improvement Act of 2004), based on the principles established in the landmark case of *Brown v. Board of Education* (1954; see also U.S. Department of Justice, 2009).

State Government

State governments have the authority—by virtue of their general "police powers"—to protect the health, safety, and welfare of citizens within their geographic boundaries (jurisdictions). State legislatures enact laws, which are then administered by the executive (governor) and the executive branch administrative agencies (e.g., departments of health, education, labor). State laws ultimately are enforced by state attorneys general and subsidiary law enforcement officials. Laws of a general nature are also enforced by each state (e.g., laws against theft, fraud, and other crimes) and those regulating insurance, health care institutions, and providers engaged in practice (commerce) within its geographic borders. All state laws affect the practice of speech-language pathology and audiology.

Legal controversies involving state law are handled by executive administrative agencies and the courts. The judicial system is tiered, with multiple trial courts at the base, courts of appeal in the middle, and supreme courts at the top. On matters involving only state law, the supreme court of the state has final jurisdiction; however, if the matter in state court involves a question of federal law, the decision may be subject to review, but only by the U.S. Supreme Court (Meador, 1991).

Federal Government

A separate source of laws affecting speech-language pathologists and audiologists originates at the federal level of government. Congress has the constitutional authority to regulate interstate commerce as well as to impose federal law on the states through its "conditional spending power." The U.S. Constitution, Article I, Section 8 allows Congress to enact laws for the general welfare of citizens (e.g., civil rights laws, food and drug laws, labor laws). The President of the United States oversees the applicable executive offices and executive agencies of the federal government (e.g., U.S. Department of Commerce, U.S. Department of Labor, U.S. Federal Trade Commission).

For any agency or institution receiving federal funds through statutory entitlement programs (whereby the federal government functions as a buyer of health care services), Congress may enable executive branch administrative agencies (e.g., the U.S. Department of Health and Human Services) to establish "conditions of participation" (CoPs). CoPs demand that health care providers comply with specific laws to protect public monies (e.g., the False Claims Act as applied to Medicare and Medicaid providers).

Legal controversies arising out of federal law are handled by the U.S. Attorney General and the U.S. Department of Justice, subsidiary law enforcement officials, executive administrative agencies, and, of course, the federal courts. The judicial system in the federal government, as in the states, is tiered. There are 94 federal judicial districts, each with a federal district court (the trial court) supplemented by subordinate federal magistrate judges (Meador, 1991). In addition, there are 12 geographically defined federal judicial circuits, each with a U.S. Circuit Court of Appeals. The 13th federal circuit court is the U.S. Court of Appeals for the Federal Circuit, whose jurisdiction is defined by subject matter (e.g., international trade, patent laws, and damage suits against the federal government). When a dispute involves the constitutional legitimacy of federal statutes or the application of federal law, the U.S. Supreme Court has discretion to step in as the final arbiter.

> The Supreme Court has jurisdiction to review all decisions of the federal appellate courts. It also has jurisdiction over decisions of the highest state courts when those courts have decided a question of federal law. The power to review cases from both state and federal courts gives the Supreme Court a unique position in the American judiciary's firmament. (Meador, 1991, p. 27)

In some areas, such as professional malpractice litigation, the federal government historically has left the governing law entirely in the hands of state legislatures and state courts. In other areas (e.g., some criminal laws), state law may coexist peacefully with federal law. Alternatively, when there is a conflict between state and federal laws, federal law may completely "pre-empt" (supersede) state law (e.g., the law pertaining to the administration of employee benefit plans). Or, when there is a conflict between state and federal laws, federal law will preempt state law *unless* coexisting state law is more stringent (Meador, 1991). For example, states may enforce medical privacy rules more stringently than federal laws pertaining to medical privacy.

In summary, the term *federalism* refers to the "interrelationships among the states and [the] relationship between the states and the federal government" (Black, 1990, p. 612). In the United States, the state and federal governments—each with executive, legislative, and judicial branches—exist side by side. As citizens of both the United States and the state in which they reside, speech-language pathologists and audiologists are held to the standards of both federal and state law; in turn, patients in the health care system are protected by both federal and state law. The law is expressed in state and federal constitutions, state and federal statutes (codes of law), state and federal executive branch administrative regulations, and finally, judicial cases (common law) that decide legal controversies of all types—statutory, regulatory, and constitutional. When legal disputes involve questions of federal law (federal statutes [in the U.S. Code, U.S.C.], federal regulations [published in the Code of Federal Regulations, C.F.R.], or questions of due process or equal protection under the U.S. Constitution), the U.S. Supreme Court has discretion to review lower court cases, and the U.S. Supreme Court's decisions are binding on all jurisdictions.

Rights and Duties

One purpose of our legal system is to adjudicate disputes or controversies involving the obligations of health professionals relative to the rights of individuals they serve. To say people have "rights" implies that they have "claims" on others to behave in certain ways. In the health care arena, patients' *legal rights* place particular *legal duties* (obligations) on health professionals. Although there is no explicit right to health care under the United States Constitution (with the exception of prisoners, people institutionalized by the state, or men and women in active military service), patients are able to hold health professionals responsible for providing services and for maintaining a standard of care. The sources of law allowing legal restitution for injury include general laws (both federal and state), statutory health care entitlement programs, employee benefit plans, practitioners' contracts with health care institutions, and private contracts between practitioners and patients.

For example, if individuals are eligible for health care under a statute (e.g., the Social Security Act), then health professionals agreeing to participate have duties to provide health care under the terms of that statute. When individuals enroll in health plans through their employers (an employee benefit plan), this requires contracts between the employer and hospitals, health maintenance organizations, and other health care entities and providers. Health professionals employed by, or contractually related to, those health care entities accept legal obligations consistent with this web of contracts. These contracts confer responsibilities on health professionals, not only to third-party payers but also to patients whom they serve. Finally, once health professionals accept patients into their clinical practices, they form special legal relationships between themselves and their patients. Inherent in such a relationship is the patient's right to receive (and pay for) appropriate clinical services, and the right to continuity of care; in turn, health professionals are duty-bound under common law to provide an appropriate standard of care (or to refer patients to credentialed professionals with the appropriate knowledge and skills).

In summary, even though there is no general "right" to health care in the United States, most individuals will receive health care by virtue of statutory entitlements, employee benefit plans, and contracts established among health care institutions, patients, and professionals. Health professionals' obligations arise from their participation in these arrangements (Scheutzow, 2004).

As summarized in Table 6–1, patients enjoy numerous rights or privileges, each of which corresponds to a duty or obligation on the part of health professionals. The table gives examples of governing law.

TABLE 6–1 Duties of Health Professionals Corresponding with Rights of Patients

Rights	Legal Duties	Governing Law (Example)
Right to health care (prisoners, institutionalized persons, service members)	Duty to provide health care	Eighth Amendment, United States Constitution "cruel and unusual punishment"
Right to services, per statutory entitlements (e.g., Medicare, Medicaid)	Duty to provide health care per conditions of participation	Social Security Act of 1965, as amended, Titles XVIII and XIX
Right to receive treatment without discrimination	Duty to treat individuals without regard to age, race, religion, gender, sexual preference, or disability	Constitutional law (Fourteenth Amendment of United States Constitution); Civil Rights Act of 1964, Section 1983; Rehabilitation Act of 1973, Section 504; Americans with Disabilities Act of 1990
Right, per statutory entitlement, to special education or related services to ensure free and appropriate education	Duty to provide health care under the statute	Individuals with Disabilities Education Improvement Act of 2004 (IDEA)
Right to emergency care and to be stabilized before discharge or transfer	Duty to provide care in an emergency department	Emergency Medical Treatment and Active Labor Act of 1986 (EMTALA)
Right to employee benefit plan benefits	Duty to provide health care under the terms of the contract	Employee Retirement Income Security Act of 1974 (ERISA)
Right to complete an advance directive	Duty to offer opportunity to complete an advance directive and to explain consent/refusal rights under state law	Federal Patient Self-Determination Act of 1990
Right to medical privacy	Duty to safeguard confidential information	Health Insurance Portability and Accountability Act of 1996, as amended, (HIPAA) and state laws
Right by contract to health care (e.g., with a private practitioner or an insurer)	Duty to provide health care under the terms of the contract	State law, breach of contract

(*Continues*)

(*Continued*)

Right to continuing care	Duty to provide care or transfer to a qualified professional	Common law of "abandonment"; see continuity of care rule, Council on Ethical and Judicial Affairs, AMA. Code of Medical Ethics 10.01(5)
Right to privacy in personal decisions	Duty of noninterference by the government	Constitutional law (e.g., *Griswold v. Connecticut*, 1965; *Cruzan v. Director, Missouri Department of Health*, 1990)
Right to informed consent	Duty to disclose risks, benefits, and alternatives	Common law of informed consent (e.g., *Canterbury v. Spence*, 1972)
Right to refuse	Duty to respect competent refusal	Common law; right to be informed of risks of refusal (e.g., *Truman v. Thomas*, 1980)
Right to bodily integrity, self-determination	Duty to refrain from touching or threatening to touch without consent	Assault and battery for unauthorized surgery (e.g., *Schloendorff v. Society of New York Hospitals*, 1914)
Right to be free of harassment or discrimination in the workplace	Duty of employers and coworkers to avoid subjecting others to situations that would be considered by reasonable people to be intimidating, hostile, or offensive	Title VII of the Civil Rights Act of 1964; Age Discrimination in Employment Act (ADEA) of 1967; Americans with Disabilities Act (ADA) of 1990, as amended
Right to be free from restraints	Duty to use care in administering chemical or physical restraints	Social Security Act of 1965, as amended; Title XVIII and XIX
Right to receive a level of care that is reasonable, skilled, and prudent	Duty to provide the degree of care and skill expected of the average practitioner in the class to which he or she belongs, acting in the same or similar circumstances	Common law negligence (e.g., *Helling v. Carey*, 1974)
Right to personal security	Duty to warn of serious, imminent threat to health or safety	*Tarasoff v. Regents of University of California* (1976)
Right to accurate and truthful medical records	Duty to report timely, accurate, truthful, and legible clinical records in the regular course of business	Paul-Brown, 1994; Horner, 2004

Duties of Health Professionals under State Licensure Laws

The criteria for licensing speech-language pathologists and audiologists are determined by each state in which the professional practices. According to ASHA's Technical Report on Telepractices, the National Council of State Boards of Examiners in Speech-Language Pathology and Audiology urges clinicians to "be licensed in the state in which the consumer is receiving the service" (ASHA, 2005b, p. 6). In a 2003 issue of *Seminars in Speech and Language* devoted to ethical and legal issues, Denton (2003) cited barriers to interstate use of telepractice and wrote: "The bottom-line rule of thumb is that speech-language pathologists must be licensed in the state where their client is receiving services *and* in the state from which they are providing services" (p. 315).

Without the option of holding a federal practice license (which would require an interstate legal compact among the states), speech-language pathologists and audiologists must practice within the geographic boundaries of the state in which they hold a license to practice. The South Carolina Code of Laws (Unannotated), Section Title 40, Chapter 67, provides an exemplar of a licensure law (sometimes referred to as a "practice act"). This licensure law explains that the Board of Examiners in Speech-Language Pathology and Audiology in South Carolina is under the administration of the Department of Labor, Licensing and Regulation. Like comparable licensure laws in other states, South Carolina's requires applicants to hold a master's degree in the appropriate discipline, along with the ASHA CCC or its equivalent (§40-67-220).

The licensure law explains that the term *audiologist* "means an individual who practices audiology" (§40-67-20(2)), and the term *speech-language pathologist* "means an individual who practices speech-language pathology" (§40-67-20(11)). In each case, the scope of practice is defined. For example, *audiology* or *audiology service* is defined as:

> ...screening, identifying, assessing, diagnosing, habilitating, and rehabilitating individuals with peripheral and central auditory and vestibular disorders; preventing hearing loss; researching normal and disordered auditory and vestibular functions; administering and interpreting behavioral and physiological measures of the peripheral and central auditory and vestibular systems; selecting, fitting, programming, and dispensing all types of amplification and assistive listening devices including hearing aids, and providing training in their use; providing aural habilitation, rehabilitation, and counseling to hearing impaired individuals and their families; designing, implementing, and coordinating industrial and community hearing conservation programs; training and supervising individuals not licensed in accordance with this chapter who perform air conduction threshold testing in the industrial setting; designing and coordinating infant hearing screening and supervising individuals not licensed in accordance with this chapter who perform infant hearing screenings; performing speech or language screening, limited to a pass-fail determination; screening of other skills for the purpose of audiological evaluation; and identifying individuals with other communication disorders. (§40-67-20(3))

The scope of practice for speech-language pathologists in South Carolina involves:

> ...screening, identifying, assessing, interpreting, diagnosing, rehabilitating, researching, and preventing disorders of speech, language, voice, oral-pharyngeal function, and cognitive/communication skills; developing and dispensing augmentative and alternative communication systems and providing training in their use; providing aural rehabilitation and counseling services to hearing impaired individuals and their families; enhancing speech-language proficiency and communication effectiveness; screening of hearing, limited to a pass-fail determination; screening of other skills for the purpose of speech-language evaluation; and identifying individuals with other communication disorders. (§40-67-20(12))

No person may practice the professions without a license (§40-67-30), and the license "is a personal right and not transferable... [it] is the property of the State ..." (§40-67-240(A)). Acts warranting disciplinary actions under §40-67-110 of the South Carolina licensure law are listed in Table 6–2.

If applicants falsify information for the purpose of obtaining a license, they may be found guilty of a misdemeanor, entailing a fine and/or imprisonment (§40-67-200). If practitioners violate the licensure law, the board may impose monetary fines, refuse to issue a license, or demand surrender of the license (§§40-1-110 to 40-1-150). The Board has jurisdiction over licensees and prior licensees (§40-67-115). Individuals aggrieved by a Board decision have the right to appeal Board decisions (§40-67-160).

TABLE 6–2 Duties of Health Professionals under the South Carolina Practice Acts (Types of Actions Warranting Disciplinary Actions)

[T]he board may take disciplinary action against a licensee who:

(1) violates federal, state, or local laws relating to speech-language pathology or audiology;

(2) violates a provision of this chapter or an order issued under this chapter or a regulation promulgated under this chapter;

(3) fraudulently or deceptively attempts to use, obtain, alter, sell, or barter a license;

(4) aids or abets a person who is not a licensed audiologist or speech-language pathologist in illegally engaging in the practice of audiology or speech-language pathology within this State;

(5) participates in the fraudulent procurement or renewal of a license for himself or another person or allows another person to use his license;

(6) commits fraud or deceit in the practice of speech-language pathology or audiology including, but not limited to:

 (a) misrepresenting an educational degree, training, credentials, competence, or any other material fact;

 (b) using or promoting or causing the use of any misleading, deceiving, improbable, or untruthful advertising matter, promotional literature, testimonial guarantee, warranty, label, brand, insignia, or any other representation;

 (c) willfully making or filing a false report or record in the practice of audiology or speech-language pathology or in satisfying requirements of this chapter;

 (d) submitting a false statement to collect a fee or obtaining a fee through fraud or misrepresentation;

(7) commits an act of dishonest, immoral, or unprofessional conduct while engaging in the practice of speech-language pathology or audiology including, but not limited to:

 (a) engaging in illegal, incompetent, or negligent practice of speech-language pathology or audiology;

 (b) providing professional services while mentally incompetent or under the influence of alcohol or drugs;

 (c) providing services or promoting the sale of devices, appliances, or products to a person who cannot reasonably be expected to benefit from the services, devices, appliances, or products;

 (d) diagnosing or treating individuals for speech or hearing disorders by mail or telephone unless the individual had been previously examined by the licensee and the diagnosis or treatment is related to the examination;

(8) is convicted of or pleads guilty or nolo contendere [no contest] to a felony or crime involving moral turpitude or a violation of a federal, state, or local alcohol or drug law, whether or not an appeal or other proceeding is pending to have the conviction or plea set aside;

(9) is disciplined by a licensing or disciplinary authority of another state, country, or nationally recognized professional organization or convicted of or disciplined by a court of any state or country for an act that would be grounds for disciplinary action under this section;

(10) fails to obtain informed consent when performing an invasive procedure or fails to obtain informed written consent when engaging in an experimental procedure;

(11) violates the code of ethics promulgated in regulation by the board.

Source: South Carolina Code of Laws [Unannotated], 2009, §40-67-110.

Duties of Health Professionals to the Public under State and Federal Law Licensure law is one method by which the state protects the health, safety, and welfare of its citizens. Another method is to adjudicate malpractice litigation, guided by the common law of torts (see discussion that follows).

Numerous federal statutes also apply to speech-language pathologists and audiologists; a select list of applicable federal law is summarized in Table 6–3. These include the Medicare and Medicaid statutes (the Social Security Act) and related statutes to prevent fraud and abuse: the False Claims Act of 1863 (as amended), and the Anti-Kickback Act of 1943 (as amended). The False Claims Act imposes severe penalties for improper billing, billing for services not rendered, and inadequate documentation. The Anti-Kickback Act prohibits both bribes and kickbacks when referring patients or accepting patient referrals or dispensing products. The Ethics in Patient Referrals Act of 1989 (known as "Stark I" and "Stark II") prohibits health professionals from referring patients to entities in which they have a financial interest. In addition, many providers are subject to the Health Insurance Portability and Accountability Act (HIPAA)'s Privacy Rule pertaining to medical information, and severe penalties attach to individual and institutional providers who breach medical confidentiality (see Horner & Wheeler, 2005a, 2005b; U.S. Department of Health and Human Services, 2003). While perhaps less familiar to some readers, federal antitrust laws prohibiting anticompetitive business practices are also very important (refer to examples in Table 6–3).

Aside from federal agency oversight of the *provision of health care*, the U.S. Equal Employment Opportunity Commission governs the equitable practices of *employers* in the health care workplace. The "civil rights" laws of the United States apply to most employers in the health care industry. Title VI of the Civil Rights Act of 1964 (Public Law 102-166, as amended) prohibits discrimination on the basis of race, color, or national origin, as well as disability, sex, or age, in all programs or activities that receive federal financial assistance (see http://www2.ed.gov/ for policies). Title VII of the Civil Rights Act of 1964 (42 U.S.C. 2000e et seq.; see http://www.eeoc.gov for guidance) prohibits harassment in the workplace—defined by the U.S. Equal Employment Opportunity Commission (EEOC) as "unwelcome conduct that is based on race, color, religion, sex (including pregnancy), national original

TABLE 6–3 Duties of Health Professionals to the Public under State and Federal Laws

Topic	Legal Duties	Source of Law
Licensure of professionals	To adhere to the scope of practice and all governing regulations	State licensure statutes
Participation in public health care programs	To adhere to federal conditions of participation (COPs)	State and federal statutory entitlement programs (e.g., Social Security Act of 1965, as amended; Title XVIII, Medicare, and Title XIX, Medicaid)
Safeguarding medical privacy	To adhere to medical privacy and security rules of HIPAA	Health Insurance Portability and Accountability Act of 1996 (HIPAA, as amended); state statutes
False claims	To submit truthful claims for reimbursement of Medicare or Medicaid services; illegal to submit a false claim with specific intent to defraud or to knowingly or deliberately ignore or recklessly disregard the truth or falsity of the claim	False Claims Act of 1863, as amended

(*Continues*)

(*Continued*)

Kickbacks	To refrain from giving or receiving money or any other thing of value to induce someone to refer a patient or to purchase a good or service that is reimbursable under Medicare or Medicaid	Anti-Kickback Act of 1943, as amended
Self-referral	To refrain from referring patients to facilities in which the health professional has an ownership interest	Ethics in Patient Referrals Act of 1989, as amended (Stark I and II)
Antitrust law (restraint of trade; anticompetitive practices)	To avoid restraining trade or engaging in anticompetitive practices, because a free market is competitive, reduces price, and increases choice and quality Price fixing: Unlawful for competitors to agree on a price (fee schedule) Boycotting: Unlawful for competitors to boycott a third competitor Monopoly: Unlawful for competitors to allocate services to particular geographic regions, thereby creating monopolies	Sherman Anti-Trust Act of 1890, as amended: Section 1: conspiracy; effect on interstate commerce; restraint of trade Section 2: possession of monopoly power; willful acquisition or maintenance of that monopoly power Clayton Antitrust Act (1914, as amended): Prohibits mergers and acquisitions that may reduce the level of competition. Enforced by the U.S. Department of Justice in cooperation with other executive agencies such as the U.S. Office of Civil Rights, the U.S. Department of Health and Human Services, and the U.S. Federal Trade Commission
Civil rights of patients and employees	Prohibits discrimination against individuals accessing public services and those employed by entities receiving federal assistance on the basis of race, color, national origin, disability, sex, or age	Civil Rights Act of 1964. Oversight by the U.S. Equal Employment Opportunity Commission and U.S. Department of Justice
Use, advertising, or promotion of drugs, devices, and biologics without approval	Liability to individuals, manufacturers, and other entities that manufacture, distribute, or advertise unapproved products or advertise and promote off-label uses of approved products	Federal Food, Drug and Cosmetic Act of 1938, as amended; overseen by the U.S. Food and Drug Administration
Product liability	"The accountability of a manufacturer, seller, or supplier of [goods] to a buyer or other third party for injuries sustained because of a defect in a product" (Pozgar, 2012, p. 53)	See Model Uniform Product Liability Act (U.S. Department of Commerce, 1979); state laws vary

(age 40 or older), disability or genetic information" (http://www.eeoc.gov/). (The EEOC website provides laws and best practices regarding harassment and sexual harassment; see also U.S. Department of Justice, 2005, for a compilation of disability rights laws.)

The Food and Drug Administration (FDA) also touches upon speech-language pathologists and audiologists because the FDA is responsible for approving the safety and efficacy of all drugs, biologics, and medical devices; overseeing good manufacturing practices of these products; accurately labeling products as to their intended benefits and potential risks; policing truthful advertising of products governed by the FDA; and ensuring that "off-label" uses of approved products are promoted/advertised appropriately. The governing law is the Federal Food, Drug and Cosmetic Act (FD&C Act, 21 U.S.C. 301 et seq., as amended). When scientific or medical information is promoted, it should follow the FDA's recommendations for "Good Reprint Practices." Similarly, advertisements should follow the FDA's recommendations for "Consumer-Directed Broadcast Advertisements" (see http://www.fda for regulatory information).

Another area of liability for health professionals is "products liability," defined by Pozgar (2012) as "the accountability of a manufacturer, seller, or supplier of [goods] to a buyer or other third party for injuries sustained because of a defect in a product" (p. 53). Liability may attach to negligence, breach of warranty, or strict liability. This is a complex area of the law and is beyond the scope of this chapter (see Pozgar, 2012, pp. 53–56 for an introduction).

The Law of Negligence

The tort of negligence as applied to health professionals is referred to as *malpractice.* This section defines these terms, explains the legal meaning of *standard of care,* and uses hypothetical clinical cases to illustrate how speech-language pathologists and audiologists can be held liable for failing to administer appropriate tests, administering tests in a substandard manner, failing to interpret the tests accurately, and/or failing to recommend or implement appropriate interventions.

Tort A *tort* is a "wrong" experienced by one individual by the actions of another individual (Harris, 2003) whereby the latter person has acted unlawfully (malfeasance) or has failed to act (nonfeasance) when he or she had a legal duty to act. The legal duty arises from the nature of the relationship between the parties as defined by common law or statute. The obligations arising from the law of torts are separate and distinct from obligations arising between parties by voluntary contracts (involving mutual promises between parties). The law of torts as applied to professional malpractice arises after the patient and professional relationship has been established. This is a "special relationship" in the eyes of the law that triggers a legal *duty of care.*

The Tort of Negligence One category of the law of torts is negligence (Glannon, 1995). *Black's Law Dictionary* (1990, p. 1032) defines negligence as "... failure to use such care as a reasonably prudent and careful person would use under similar circumstances." Liability for negligence rests on the bedrock of the *duty of care.*

There are gradations in the types of negligence. *Ordinary negligence* refers to "failure to exercise care of an ordinarily prudent person in same situation" (Black, 1990, p. 1034); *gross negligence* is "the intentional failure to perform a manifest duty in reckless disregard of the consequences as affecting the life or property of another" (Black, 1990, p. 1033); and *per se negligence* is "the unexcused violation of a statute which is applicable" (Black, 1990, p. 1034). Finally, *malpractice* is a subcategory of the law governing negligence and is defined as:

> Professional misconduct or unreasonable lack of skill ... Failure of one rendering professional services to exercise that degree of skill and learning commonly applied under all the circumstances in the community by the average prudent reputable member of the profession with the result of injury, loss or damage to the recipient of those services or to those entitled to rely upon them. It is any professional misconduct, unreasonable lack of skill or fidelity in professional or fiduciary duties, evil practice, or illegal or immoral conduct." (Black, 1990, p. 959)

PROFESSIONAL NEGLIGENCE (MALPRACTICE)

For speech-language pathologists and audiologists, the duty of care arises from the patient-professional relationship itself; it is the formation of this "special relationship" that creates a heightened legal duty of care (i.e., a duty of care above and beyond what ordinary citizens engaged in ordinary activities owe one another). The tort of negligence applies to health professionals when behavior is careless and substandard. In the typical case, negligence is *unintentional.* A health professional may be held liable for harming a patient if the duty of care is breached; an *intent* to harm is *not* required for liability to attach. Furthermore, liability can attach regardless of whether the professional was poorly trained, unprepared, distracted, rushed, fatigued, or ill. When credentialed professionals hold themselves out to the public as "prepared to do the job," they can be held liable for negligence that causes harm.

In 1881, Chief Justice Oliver Wendell Holmes wrote:

> The rule that the law does, in general, determine liability by blameworthiness, is subject to the limitation that minute differences of character are not allowed for. The law considers, in other words, what would be blameworthy in the average man, the man of ordinary intelligence and prudence, and determines liability by that. If we fall below the level in those gifts, it is our misfortune; so much as that we must have at our peril, for the reasons just given. But he who is intelligent and prudent does not act at his peril, in theory of law. On the contrary, it is only when he fails to exercise the foresight of which he is capable, or exercises it with evil intent, that he is answerable for the consequences. (pp. 108–109)

By way of background, consider an example of everyday behavior. The general rule is that ordinary citizens have a duty to act reasonably, particularly when harm is foreseeable. Their behavior is governed by the common law of (ordinary) negligence. If a neighbor plays softball in a backyard with no fence, and a pedestrian on the sidewalk is harmed by a fly ball, the neighbor will probably be responsible to compensate the pedestrian for the injury. The reason for this is that the neighbor has a common law duty to act in a reasonable manner (to build a fence or to refrain from playing baseball in his backyard) in order to avoid foreseeable injuries to his neighbors. When such a case is heard by a jury, the jury must decide whether a "reasonable person," using an average degree of judgment and foresight, would have played softball in a fenceless yard adjacent to a busy sidewalk, or would have taken reasonable and prudent measures to prevent the risk of probable injury to pedestrians.

Health professionals are held to a higher duty of care than ordinary citizens. This higher duty stems from the fact that health professionals have specialized education, hold licenses to practice, and hold out their credentials to the public as skilled and qualified service providers. Health professionals are ethically and legally bound to exercise the level of care that similarly educated and skilled practitioners would provide in similar circumstances while exercising good judgment and acting prudently. Usually, the standard of care is established by the profession itself (and presented at a trial by an expert witness). However, in a court of law, it is the jury that decides the facts and the credibility of witnesses, and the judge who applies the legal standards. Together, the judge and jury will determine whether the *customary* clinical standard of care is adequate to satisfy the *legal* standard of care (duty of care).

Two older cases illustrate that the court has ultimate discretion in appraising whether the prevailing or customary standard of care is adequate as a matter of law (i.e., satisfies a *legal duty of care*). In 1932, Judge Learned Hand of the Second Circuit Court of Appeals opined that the captain of a tugboat named *The T.J. Hooper* was negligent by failing to equip his boat with a radio and thereby causing damage. Judge Hand wrote: "Courts must in the end say what is required; there are precautions so imperative that even their universal disregard will not excuse their omission" (*The T.J. Hooper,* 1932). In a controversial 1974 case, *Helling v. Carey,* the court (citing *The T.J. Hooper*) held an ophthalmologist liable for failing to diagnose a young woman's glaucoma, despite her persistent complaints of deteriorating vision over nine years. At the time, it was not common practice for ophthalmologists to test for glaucoma in individuals younger than age 40. Nevertheless, the court held that reasonable prudence was absent and that customary practice was insufficient as a matter of law.

Duty, Breach, Causation, and Damages

The common law of negligence as applied to health professionals engaged in their professional duties is known as the tort of malpractice. To hold the professional liable, the plaintiff (the person alleging harm who has brought the lawsuit) must prove four elements. If the patient (the plaintiff) presents sufficient evidence, the professional (the defendant) will be held liable for the patient's injuries and be required to pay the patient money in damages.

Duty: The duty required of the professional is the standard of care—the obligation shared by all similarly educated and skilled practitioners in similar circumstances exercising good judgment and prudence.

Breach: The duty was breached (e.g., the practitioner failed to administer an intervention that was indicated or administered a customary intervention in a substandard manner).

Causation: The harm experienced by the patient (plaintiff) was caused by the breach of the legal duty of care.

Damages: The patient experienced harm (e.g., misdiagnosis, physical injury, comorbidity).

Causation is the most difficult element of a malpractice claim for plaintiffs to prove. According to Glannon (1995), different jurisdictions embrace different methods of proving causation. For example, to attach liability, the defendant's conduct must be the *direct cause* of the injury, a *substantial factor* in causing the plaintiff's injury, the *natural and probable consequences* of the defendant's conduct, or a *foreseeable consequence of the defendant's conduct.* In the final analysis, to attach liability to the defendant, the jury must determine that conduct was the *proximate* cause of the injury—in essence, "but for" the defendant's conduct, the plaintiff would not have been harmed.

> Proximate cause means that cause which, in a natural and continuous sequence, unbroken by an effective intervening cause, produces an event, and without which cause such event would not have occurred. (Glannon, 1995, p. 157)

Speech-Language Pathology Imagine a middle-aged individual who experienced bilateral strokes and now presents with a swallowing disorder. A speech-language pathologist, experienced and trained in the use of instrumental procedures, follows the established protocol for pharyngeal examination of swallowing function and consults with specialists in neurology, gastroenterology, and radiology. Following the examination, the speech-language pathologist recommends a nonoral nutritional method. The attending physician places the patient on NPO status (nothing by mouth) and orders insertion of a nasogastric tube. One week later, the patient experiences pneumonia with significant discomfort, a protracted hospital stay, and thousands of additional dollars in medical expenses. The family sues the speech-language pathologist (and all other attending health professionals).

In this hypothetical case, the plaintiff's lawyer will argue, "My client had dysphagia, the speech-language pathologist evaluated him, and her recommendations caused him to get pneumonia." To escape liability, the speech-language pathologist as a defendant will, first and foremost, try to prove to the court and jury that she adhered to the standard of care—that is, she did not breach her legal duty of care. The court might, or might not, allow ASHA practice guidelines to be introduced into evidence but probably will allow an expert witness—another speech-language pathologist with credentials in swallowing disorders—to testify as to the appropriate clinical standard of care. The defendant's lawyer will argue that the patient's underlying bilateral cerebral disease was the superseding (and legal) cause of the patient's pneumonia. In the end, the defendant speech-language pathologist will prevail if she adhered to the legal standard of care (duty of care) for this straightforward reason: If the plaintiff cannot prove that the defendant breached the duty of care, then the plaintiff cannot, as a matter of law, prove that the defendant's conduct *caused* the patient's medical condition. In other words, if no *breach* of a legal duty is found, the plaintiff is precluded from presenting evidence that the defendant's conduct *caused* the harm.

Now imagine a slightly different scenario. The underlying facts are the same, *except* that the speech-language pathologist did not read the medical record thoroughly and missed the fact that the patient had a history of gastroesophageal reflux disease (GERD). Furthermore, the record shows that she did not consult with neurology or gastroenterology, nor did she advise the attending physician to place the patient on reflux precautions. When these facts come to light, the plaintiff's lawyer will be in a stronger position to argue that "but for" the defendant's conduct (actions or inactions), the patient would have avoided the pneumonia and the protracted hospital stay.

Audiology A young adult presents to an audiology clinic with progressive hearing loss. The audiologist's evaluation included an otoscopic examination, a pure-tone audiometric evaluation, and auditory brainstem evoked response (ABER) testing. The audiologist diagnosed a conductive hearing loss and referred the patient to an otolaryngologist for cerumen removal. Two years later, the audiologist is summoned to civil court by her former patient. Her patient alleges that he has been irreparably harmed by the audiologist's failure to diagnose his retrocochlear lesion (an acoustic neuroma). The patient has undergone surgery and now has a permanent hearing loss in one ear, in addition to paralysis of facial muscles on the same side. In this hypothetical case, the plaintiff's lawyer will argue, "My client had a progressive hearing loss, the audiologist evaluated him, and her diagnosis was wrong. As a result of the delayed diagnosis, my patient has undergone surgery and suffers permanent hearing loss and facial disfigurement."

The audiologist (defendant) will, first and foremost, try to prove to the court that she adhered to the standard of care (i.e., recorded a thorough history, administered the appropriate diagnostic tests, and rendered an accurate diagnosis consistent with what a reasonable and prudent clinician in her circumstances would have provided). The court might, or might not, allow ASHA or other practice guidelines and technical reports into evidence but will probably allow an expert—another audiologist with credentials in differential diagnosis of hearing disorders—to testify as to the appropriate clinical standard of care. The plaintiff's lawyer will try to prove that the patient's hearing loss was only partly explained by cerumen and that the audiologist failed to interpret the ABER accurately. In the end, the plaintiff will win his civil malpractice lawsuit if the plaintiff convinces a jury that "but for" the audiologist's failure to correctly interpret the ABER, he would have received a timely diagnosis.

Now imagine a slightly different scenario. The underlying facts are the same, except that the audiologist performed *and interpreted* the audiometric tests appropriately and found no abnormality. Consistent with the audiologic evaluation, she referred the patient to an otolaryngologist, the cerumen was removed, and the patient experienced an immediate improvement in hearing acuity. Nevertheless, one year later, the patient experienced a decline in his hearing, and an acoustic neuroma was diagnosed. The plaintiff's lawyer will once again argue that the audiologist failed to diagnose the retrocochlear lesion. In turn, the defendant's lawyer will attempt to prove that the audiologist's evaluation was consistent with the prevailing standard of care and that the acoustic neuroma manifested itself *after the evaluation*. If the jury agrees, it will find that the acoustic neuroma was the superseding (and legal) cause of the patient's subsequent hearing loss, not substandard care rendered one year before the tumor was manifest. In the end, the defendant audiologist will prevail if she proves she adhered to the standard of care and there was no evidence of a retrocochlear lesion at the time of the evaluation.

Again, the first two elements of a malpractice lawsuit are *duty* and *breach*. In a court of law, the duty of care must be established, typically by expert testimony, and then a breach of this duty of care must be proved (again, by expert testimony). If there is no breach of a legal duty of care, then any harm the patient experienced cannot be causally linked to the malfeasance (or nonfeasance) of the defendant clinician. In the absence of a breach of a legal duty, the patient has no remedy in a civil malpractice lawsuit. On the other hand, if the professional failed to administer the appropriate tests, administered the tests in a substandard manner, failed to interpret the tests accurately, and/or failed to recommend or implement appropriate interventions—*and the breach is causally linked to the patient's harm*—the professional will be held civilly liable to the patient and will be expected to compensate the patient by paying monetary damages.

In summary, this section has contrasted professional negligence (malpractice) in the conduct of clinical care with negligence in everyday affairs to illustrate that professionals have a heightened legal duty to conduct their clinical practices competently and prudently, commensurate with the knowledge and skills they hold out to the public. This section identified duty, breach, causation, and damages as the four elements that must be proved in a court of law to sustain a finding of liability for malpractice. Issues relating to malpractice reform in the twenty-first century are complex, contentious, and beyond the scope of this chapter. Readers are referred to Studdert, Mello, and Brennan (2004), who discuss the prevalence of adverse events and negligence, the rise in health care costs, patient safety issues, and tort reform. These weighty policy issues aside, the best defense to any allegation of malpractice is diligent adherence to the standard of care.

Liability of Health Care Institutions

When health professionals incur legal liabilities, their supervisors or employers are also subject to legal liabilities. Misconduct by health professionals, whether intentional or not, may give rise to "vicarious liability" of health care institutions because the health professionals (1) are "agents" of the institutions; (2) are selected, credentialed, supervised, and/or controlled by the institutions; and/or (3) are acting within the scope of their employment on behalf of the institutions.

TABLE 6–4 Theories of Vicarious Liability and Direct Corporate Liability

Theory of Liability	Description
"Captain of the ship" (traditional label applied to the person in authority)	An individual who exercises supervisory control and authority over health professionals may be liable for their misconduct.
Apparent agency (ostensible agency)	A modern-day application of the captain of the ship doctrine, whereby a health care entity (the principal) may be held liable for the misconduct of health professionals (agents) who act on its behalf; a professional may be deemed "ostensibly" an agent of the health care entity even if not employed by the entity.
Respondeat superior (Latin, "let the master respond")	When health professionals perform functions that are inherent to the operation of the health care entity, and the misconduct occurred within the scope of their employment, the entity may be held liable for their misconduct.
Direct corporate liability	The health care entity has legal duties independent of its employees, such as providing adequate facilities and equipment; having sound hiring, credentialing, and retention practices; and maintaining safety standards. These are nondelegable duties for which the entity can be held directly liable.
Negligence per se	A health care entity may be per se liable for harm resulting from its failure to adhere to a statute or regulation or for negligent implementation of the statute or regulation.
Strict liability (products liability)	Some jurisdictions have held that service providers (individual practitioners or institutions) who regularly sell or dispense products may be held liable (along with manufacturers) for harm that results from defective products.

A fourth theory of corporate liability involves the idea that there are some duties an institution cannot delegate ("nondelegable duties"). These include, for example, providing adequate facilities and equipment; having sound hiring, credentialing, and retention practices; and maintaining safety standards. According to Glannon (1995), the institution "may delegate the *work* but cannot delegate away the *liability* for tortuous acts in the course of the work" (p. 380). The different legal theories of liability are identified in Table 6–4. Readers should note that the application of these theories of legal liability varies not only in relation to the facts of particular cases but also depending on the statutes or case law in the governing jurisdiction—typically in state court (Furrow, Greany, Johnson, Jost, & Schwartz, 1997; Glannon, 1995; Harris, 2003).

MANAGING RISK

The key to preparing for the possibility of a malpractice lawsuit is *prevention.* ASHA's 1994 Technical Report on risk management provides a useful, comprehensive summary of strategies for audiologists, speech-language pathologists, and their employers. The strategies fall into three overlapping categories of activities: quality improvement, risk management, and insurance.

Professionals manage risks (and prevent errors) by embracing practice guidelines promulgated by ASHA, AAA, and other authoritative professional organizations; by engaging in continuing education; and by establishing quality improvement projects for high-risk, high-volume, and problem-prone types of cases. Quality improvement concentrates on maintaining optimal levels of client care; risk management focuses on meeting acceptable levels of care from a legal perspective (ASHA, 1994, p. 243).

Finally, professionals should be sure they have adequate insurance. In many instances, state law will place caps on the tort liability exposure of duly licensed practitioners in the state. Typically, employers will provide insurance for health care providers who could be sued for mistakes that occur during the course of employment. In addition, professionals may purchase professional liability insurance either from their employer, through ASHA, or from independent insurance companies (ASHA, 1994, p. 244).

Standard of Care and Professional Liability Insurance

Imagine a hypothetical case involving "Mary," a clinician holding the Certificate of Clinical Competence in Speech-Language Pathology (CCC-SLP). Mary was employed full time by a hospital to work in the Speech Clinic 8 A.M. to 5 P.M. Monday through Friday. In addition, she worked with patients at home after hours on a private-pay basis. For her work at the hospital, Mary was covered under her employer's blanket professional liability (malpractice) insurance policy, but she did not carry her own professional liability insurance.

Mary was sued by the parents of a child whom she had been treating for a motor speech disorder (spastic dysarthria). The 12-year-old boy had survived a closed head injury from a bicycle accident and began speech therapy one month after his injury. As reflected in Mary's documentation, the stated goal was to improve muscle strength and agility as a basis for improving the effectiveness, efficiency, and intelligibility of speech (Duffy, 2005; Yorkston, Beukelman, Strand, & Hakel, 2010). Therapy consisted primarily of nonspeech oral-motor exercises (NSOME), including repetitive activities such as blowing, sucking, tongue protrusion, lateralization and elevation, cheek puffing, and nonspeech movements against resistance (Lof, 2008; Lof & Watson, 2010). After one year of treatment (three times weekly), the child's speech did not improve.

The case proceeded in several steps. First, the parents filed a civil complaint alleging that their child had made no progress in the effectiveness, efficiency, and intelligibility of his speech, and that NSOME had not been proved to be effective to remediate motor speech disorders. They claimed recovery of treatment costs ($15,000), personal costs (transportation plus hours lost from work, $5,000), and noneconomic damages ($50,000) due to the lost opportunity for their son to benefit from future speech therapy (during his chronic phase of recovery). In short, the parents complained that Mary rendered *unnecessary, unproven, and ineffective intervention*, that is, that there was no support in motor learning theory, logic, or extant evidence that NSOME will improve the ability of speech-impaired individuals to speak more effectively, efficiently, or intelligibly (see also Clark, 2003; Duffy, 2005; Lof, 2008; Lof & Watson, 2010).

Second, Mary's lawyer petitioned the court for "summary judgment," asserting that there were no issues of material fact in dispute and, furthermore, that this was a simple matter of contract and not a case of negligence. The judge ruled that the action at hand was a claim for professional negligence (malpractice) because it pertained to the *standard of care.*

Third, Mary's lawyer asked the court to join Mary's hospital-employer as a plaintiff in the lawsuit because, he asserted, the employer-hospital's liability insurance should cover Mary's potential liability (i.e., that Mary should not be held personally liable). The court rejected this motion, finding that Mary's interaction with the child was on a private basis and not within the scope of her "8-5" responsibilities to the hospital's Speech Clinic. In short, the judge released the hospital from liability.

Fourth, Mary's attorney also asserted at the pretrial hearing that NSOME was widely accepted as the standard of care and that Mary could not be found negligent merely because the intervention she offered did not have the desired outcome. Finally, the attorney asserted that the severity of the child's speech disorder "caused" the lack of treatment effectiveness, not the treatment itself.

The judge ruled that there were numerous material facts in dispute (i.e., he rejected the summary judgment motion) and set a trial date for *Parents v. Mary*. His ruling meant that, at trial, the jury (known in legal circles as "the triers-of-fact") would determine (1) Mary's legal *duty* by hearing testimony from experts in the discipline about the applicable standard of care; (2) whether Mary *breached* that duty; (3) whether the child had been *damaged* by the breach due to ineffective treatment, including economic damages and future noneconomic damages under a "lost opportunity" theory; and, finally, (4) whether Mary's alleged breach *caused* the economic and noneconomic damages alleged by the parents. (Duty, breach, causation, and damages are the essential elements of a negligence lawsuit; all must be assessed by the jury.) As stated earlier, the tort of negligence applies to health professionals when behavior is careless and substandard. A health professional may be held liable for harming a patient if the duty of care is breached; an *intent* to harm is *not* required for liability to attach.

The purpose of this hypothetical case is not to debate the theory, logic, or evidence supporting or refuting NSOME. The reasons for offering this hypothetical case are to stimulate the reader to consider the question of *liability for negligence* through the lens of the law and to consider the question of *liability insurance*. According to Pozgar (2012), "The purpose of liability insurance is to spread the risk of economic loss among members of a group who share common risk" (p. 463). When the professional (the insured) purchases professional liability insurance, he or she pays a premium to an insurance company (the insurer). In turn, the typical professional liability contract obligates the insurer to defend the insured against legal liability risk, namely "the possibility that the insured may become legally liable to pay money damages to another" (p. 464). Typical benefits include the insurer's time to settle cases out of court, payment of attorneys' fees, and/or payment of money damages to the successful plaintiff. In contrast, many insurance carriers do *not* cover punitive damages that might arise in a malpractice case, either as a matter of policy within a specific state, or within the terms of the insurer-insured contract.

Without speculating about the possible outcome of the *Parents v. Mary* trial, the main point is to illustrate why Mary, in her role as a private practitioner, should have carried individual professional liability insurance. If the parents win their lawsuit, and the court awards them $65,000, Mary will be responsible for paying these monetary damages and attorneys' fees. If the court had added Mary's hospital as a defendant, and if Mary had been found negligent, her liability concerns would not necessarily be alleviated. As Pozgar (2012) explains, if the employer has adequate legal grounds—such as the fact that Mary was functioning as an *independent contractor* when she treated the 12-year-old boy after regular office hours—the employer would pay the original damages *and then sue Mary to recover all of its costs* related to her negligent professional conduct (p. 464). Mary's best defense against future lawsuits will be to stay abreast of the standard of care for motor speech disorders—and to purchase individual professional liability insurance.

Research Practices, Research Responsibilities, and Professional Liability Insurance The "responsible conduct of research" (RCR) encompasses many ethical norms that pertain to conducting, reporting, or reviewing of research in nine major domains: data acquisition, management, sharing, and ownership; conflict of interest and commitment; human subjects protection; animal welfare; research misconduct; publication practices and responsible authorship; mentor/trainee responsibilities; peer review; and collaborative science (Horner & Minifie, 2011a, 2011b, 2011c; Macrina, 2005; Office of Research Integrity, 2000; Steiner, 2006; U.S. Public Health Service, 2005). Readers particularly interested in preventing harm to research participants should read the report *Moral Science: Protecting Participants in Human Subjects Research,* produced in December 2011 by the Presidential Commission for the Study of Bioethical Issues.

Horner and Minifie (2011c) reviewed several historical and high-profile cases in which research participants were harmed, resulting in institutional investigations, suspension of research by federal agencies, and legal settlements and/or lawsuits. Agati (2006) cataloged a range of legal cases involving researchers, based in civil rights violations, lack of informed consent, violation of federal regulations, and breach of contract. Recently, the case of Poehlman (*U.S. v. Poehlman*, 2005a, 2005b) illustrates how research misconduct (defined as fabrication, falsification, or plagiarism) may lead to personal and professional liability. Poehlman not only falsified research data in publications and research grants, he also misused millions of federal grant dollars over many years and failed to cooperate with investigators. Poehlman was penalized by debarment from receiving federal grants, financial penalties, and 12 months of incarceration.

Inappropriate research practices may be more prevalent than is commonly thought (Martinson, Anderson, & deVries, 2005). Speech, language, and hearing scientists are advised that liability may attach to inappropriate research practices; mistakes resulting in harm to research participants; or study designs that expose participants to unreasonable physical, psychological, privacy, reputational, or legal risks. To minimize legal risks (liability) associated with their work as scientists/researchers, readers are advised to familiarize themselves with the U.S. Office of Research Integrity's website, which offers many educational materials pertaining to RCR; institutional compliance reports, policies regarding reporting and investigating research misconduct, and links to empirical RCR research.

Readers are referred to a 2011 *Journal of Speech, Language, and Hearing Research* supplement that reports the findings of a project funded by an Office of Research Integrity/National Institutes of Health grant (awarded to S. Moss of the American Speech-Language-Hearing Association) that investigated how RCR is taught and learned in communication sciences and disorders (Minifie et al., 2011) and conducted an empirical survey of publication practices (Ingham et al., 2011). As a precaution, scientists/researchers should consult with their insurance carriers to ensure that their professional liability insurance coverage (held individually or by an employer) is of sufficient scope to cover risks associated with the conduct of research. As explained previously in the *Parents v. Mary* hypothetical, scientists/researchers may find it advantageous to purchase supplemental professional liability insurance for their research activities.

SUMMARY

This chapter explained that the U.S. Constitution and laws written by both state legislatures and Congress have a major role in defining the professional responsibilities of speech-language pathologists and audiologists. The chapter identified numerous sources for professionals' legal obligations—to individual patients, to the state in which a license to practice is held, to public agencies that purchase health care services, and to the public at large. The chapter also outlined the law of negligence (malpractice); explained how health care institutions can also be held vicariously liable for the misconduct of their employees, or can be held directly liable for failures to maintain requisite institutional standards of practice; and illustrated the importance of maintaining professional liability insurance, either through an employer or individually (preferably both).

Although speech-language pathologists and audiologists have a daunting array of obligations, the bases of their legal liabilities lie ultimately in their moral responsibilities to their patients. Pellegrino (1983) articulated why health professionals should be held accountable for the promises they made when they entered the professions.

> To be a professional is to make a promise to help, to keep that promise, and to do so in the best interests of the patient. It is to accept the trust the patient must place in us as a moral imperative…
>
> The nature of the relationships we have described is grounded in the human condition. They impose moral obligations that must transcend standards of moral behavior in society at large. A true professional is, in sum, an ordinary person called to extraordinary duties by the nature of the activities in which he or she has chosen to engage. (pp. 174–175)

CRITICAL THINKING

1. If a patient entered a speech-language pathology or audiology clinic and declared on the intake form that she was HIV positive, would the clinician be permitted, under the law, to refuse to treat this individual? If yes, why? If not, why not?
2. If a child in the public school system was designated as needing speech-language pathology or audiology services, what issues would a clinician need to consider before deciding to treat the child on a one-to-one basis (rather than treating the child while engaged in classroom activities)?
3. If an employer demanded that the speech-language pathologist or audiologist change a billing code to maximize reimbursement, what law(s) would be implicated?
4. If a speech-language pathologist or audiologist had an ownership interest in a clinic, would it be appropriate to refer patients to this clinic? If yes, why? If not, why not?
5. If a speech-language pathologist or audiologist was sued for professional malpractice due to allegedly providing substandard care to a patient, what would be the clinician's best legal defense?
6. If a speech-language pathologist or audiologist was found by the American Speech-Language-Hearing Association's Board of Ethics to have violated a provision of ASHA's Code of Ethics (2010), could the clinician avoid repercussions simply by changing employment or moving to another state? If yes, why? If not, why not?
7. If speech-language pathologists or audiologists wish to engage in telepractice diagnosis or treatment, may the clinicians rely on their license to practice in their home state, or will they be required to seek licensure in other states?
8. Even though various health professionals strive to establish their own standards of care through technical reports and practice guidelines, and even though the disciplines of speech-language pathology and audiology consider themselves to be relatively autonomous, why should the professions be concerned about the *legal standard of care*?
9. Write a hypothetical case involving legal liability of a speech-language pathologist or audiologist in the realm of your choosing (common law duties of care, licensure law, federal law). Explain (with hypothetical facts) what the professional did, and why the professional's conduct came under scrutiny by either an ethics board or a court.
10. Respond to your hypothetical case in two parts. Based on your knowledge of professional liability, (a) defend the professional's conduct on the basis that it was responsible and appropriate under the factual circumstances, and (b) offer counterarguments as to why the professional's conduct might be described inappropriate (and possibly unethical or illegal) as viewed by a licensure board and ethics board, a patient's personal attorney, or a government agency.

REFERENCES

Academy of Neurologic Communication Disorders and Sciences. (2005). Mission statement of the ANCDS. Available from http://www.ancds.org

Agati, A. (2006). Clinical research trials in the courtroom. In J. E. Steiner Jr. (Ed.), *Clinical research law and compliance handbook* (pp. 411–437). Sudbury, MA: Jones & Bartlett.

Age Discrimination in Employment Act of 1967, Public Law 90-202.

American Academy of Audiology. (2005). Code of ethics of the American Academy of Audiology. Available from http://www.audiology.org/

American Speech-Language-Hearing Association. (1994, March). Professional liability and risk management for the audiology and speech-language pathology professions. *ASHA, 36* (Suppl. 12), 25–38.

American Speech-Language-Hearing Association. (2001, Spring). Practices and procedures for appeals of Board of Ethics decisions (p. 193). *ASHA Supplement.* Available from http://www.asha.org/

American Speech-Language-Hearing Association. (2002). Ethical practice inquiries: ASHA jurisdictions. *ASHA Supplement, 22,* 231–232.

American Speech-Language-Hearing Association. (2003). Code of ethics. *ASHA Supplement, 23,* 13–15. Available from http://www.asha.org/

American Speech-Language-Hearing Association. (2004). Statement of practices and procedures of the Board of Ethics (pp. 189–192). Available from http://www.asha.org/

American Speech-Language-Hearing Association. (2005a). Background information and standards and implementation for the Certificate of Clinical Competence in Speech-Language Pathology. Available from http://www.asha.org/

American Speech-Language-Hearing Association. (2005b). Speech-language pathologists providing clinical services via telepractice: Technical report. *ASHA Supplement, 25,* in press. Available from http://www.asha.org/

Americans with Disabilities Act of 1990, 42 U.S.C. §§12101 *et seq.*

Anti-Kickback Act of 1943, 42 U.S.C. §1320a-7b (b)(1)-(2).

Black H. C., Nolan, J. R., & Nolan-Haley, J. M. (1990). *Black's law dictionary.* St. Paul, MN: West Publishing.

Brown v. Board of Education, 347 U.S. 483 (1954).

Canterbury v. Spence, 464 F. 2d 772 (D.C. Cir., 1972).

Civil Rights Act of 1964, 42 U.S.C. §§2000 *et seq.*

Clark, H. (2003). Neuromuscular treatments for speech and swallowing: A tutorial. *American Journal of Speech-Language Pathology, 12,* 400–415.

Clayton Antitrust Act of 1914, (as amended) 15 U.S.C. §§12-27, 52-53.

Council on Ethical and Judicial Affairs. (2002). *Code of medical ethics: Current opinions.* Chicago, IL: American Medical Association.

Cruzan v. Director, Missouri Department of Health, 497 U.S. 261 (1990).

Denton, D. R. (2003, November). Ethical and legal issues related to telepractice. *Seminars in Speech and Language, 24*(4), 313–322.

Dickson, D. T. (1995). *Law in the health and human services: A guide for social workers, psychologists, psychiatrists, and related professionals.* New York, NY: The Free Press.

Duffy, J. R. (2005). *Motor speech disorders: Substrates, differential diagnosis, and management* (2nd ed.). St. Louis, MO: Mosby.

Emergency Medical Treatment and Active Labor Act of 1986 (EMTALA), 42 U.S.C. §1395dd.

Employee Retirement Income Security Act of 1974 (ERISA), 29 U.S.C. §§1001 *et seq.*

Ethics in Patient Referrals Act of 1989 (Stark I and II), 42 USC §1395nn.

False Claims Act of 1863, 31 U.S.C. §§3729 *et seq.*

Federal Food, Drug and Cosmetic Act of 1938, as amended, 21 USC 301 *et seq.*

Federal Patient Self-Determination Act 1990, 42 U.S.C. §1395 cc(a).

Frattali, C. M. (2001). Professional autonomy and collaboration. In R. Lubinski & C. M. Frattali (Eds.), *Professional issues in speech-language pathology and audiology* (2nd ed., pp. 173–182). Clifton Park, NY: Delmar Cengage Learning.

Furrow, B. R., Greaney, T. L., Johnson, S. H., Jost, T. S., & Schwartz, R. L. (1997). *Health law: Cases, materials and problems* (3rd ed.). St. Paul, MN: West Publishing.

Glannon, J. W. (1995). *The law of torts: Examples and explanations.* Boston, MA: Little, Brown.

Griswold v. Connecticut, 381 U.S. 479 (1965).

Harris, D. M. (2003). *Contemporary issues in healthcare law and ethics* (2nd ed., pp. 45–66). Chicago, IL: Health Administration Press.

Health Insurance Portability and Accountability Act of 1996, Public Law 104-191 (August 21, 1995); Standards for Privacy of Individually Identifiable Health Information, 45 C.F.R. Parts 160 and 164 (December 28, 2000, as amended May 31, 2002 and August 14, 2002).

Helling v. Carey, 519 P.2d 981 (Wash. 1974).

Holmes, O. W. (1881). *The common law.* Available from Historic Law Books, Louisiana State University Law Center, Medical and Public Health Law Site, http://biotech.law.lsu.edu/

Horner, J. (2004). Legal implications of clinical documentation. *Perspectives on Swallowing and Swallowing Disorders, 13*(1), 10–16.

Horner, J., & Minifie, F. D. (2011a). Research ethics I: Responsible conduct of research (RCR)—Historical and contemporary issues pertaining to human and animal experimentation. *Journal of Speech, Language, and Hearing Research, 54*, S303–S329.

Horner, J., & Minifie, F. D. (2011b). Research ethics II: Mentoring, collaboration, peer review, and data management and ownership. *Journal of Speech, Language, and Hearing Research, 54*, S330–S345.

Horner, J., & Minifie, F. D. (2011c). Research ethics III: Publication practices and authorship, conflicts of interest, and research misconduct. *Journal of Speech, Language, and Hearing Research, 54*, S346–S362.

Horner, J., & Wheeler, M. (2005a, September 6). HIPAA: Impact on clinical practices. *ASHA Leader,* 10–11, 22–23.

Horner, J., & Wheeler, M. (2005b, November 8). HIPAA: Impact on research practices. *The ASHA Leader,* 8–9, 26–27.

Individuals with Disabilities Education Improvement Act of 2004, Public Law 108-446, 118 Stat. 2647, 20 U.S.C. §§14000 *et seq.*

Ingham, J. C., Minifie, F. D., Horner, J., Robey, R. R., Lansing, C., McCartney, J. H., et al. (2011). Ethical principles associated with the publication of research in ASHA's scholarly journals: Importance and adequacy of coverage. *Journal of Speech, Language, and Hearing Research, 54*, S394–S416.

Keeton, W. P., Dobbs, D. B., Keeton, R. E., & Owen, D. G. (1984). *Prosser and Keeton on torts* (5th ed.). St. Paul, MN: West Publishing.

Lof, G. L. (Ed.). (2008, November). Controversies about the use of nonspeech oral motor exercises for childhood speech disorders [Special issue]. *Seminars in Speech and Language, 29*(4).

Lof, G. L., & Watson, M. (2010). Five reasons why nonspeech oral-motor exercises do not work. *Perspectives on School-Based Issues, 11,* 109–117.

Macrina, F. L. (Ed.). (2005). *Scientific integrity* (3rd. ed.). Washington, DC: ASM Press.

Martinson, B. C., Anderson, M. S., & deVries, R. (2005). Scientists behaving badly. *Nature, 435,* 737–738.

Meador, D. J. (1991). *American courts.* St. Paul, MN: West Publishing.

Miller, T. D. (2001). Professional liability in audiology and speech-language pathology: Ethical and legal considerations. In R. Lubinski & C. M. Frattali (Eds.), *Professional issues in speech-language pathology and audiology* (2nd ed., pp. 63–76). Clifton Park, NY: Delmar Cengage Learning.

Minifie, F. D., Robey, R. R., Horner, J., Ingham, J. C., Lansing, C., McCartney, J. H., et al. (2011). Responsible conduct of research in communication sciences and disorders: Faculty and student perceptions. *Journal of Speech, Language, and Hearing Research, 54*, S363–S393.

Office of Research Integrity. (2000). Final PHS policy for instruction in the responsible conduct of research [Announcement]. *Federal Register, 65*(236), 76647. Available from http://www.ori.dhhs.gov/policies/RCR_Policy.shtml

Paul-Brown, D. (1994). Clinical record keeping in audiology and speech-language pathology. *ASHA, 36*, 40–43.

Pellegrino, E. (1983). What is a profession? *Journal of Allied Health, 12,* 168–175.

Pozgar, G. D. (2012). *Legal aspects of health care administration* (11th ed.). Sudbury, MA: Jones & Bartlett.

Presidential Commission for the Study of Bioethical Issues. (2011, December). *Moral science: Protecting participants in human subjects research.* Washington, DC. Available from http://www.bioethics.gov

Rehabilitation Act of 1973, Section 504, 29 U.S.C. §794.

Scheutzow, S. O. Patient care. In B. M. Broccolo, D. H. Caldwell, A. R. Daniels, et al. (2004). *Fundamentals of health law* (3rd ed., pp. 37–56). Chicago, IL: American Health Lawyers Association.

Schloendorff v. Society of New York Hospitals, 105 N.E. 92, 93 (N.Y., 1914).

Sherman Anti-Trust Act, 15 U.S.C. §§1, 2 (2002). Available from http://www.usdoj.gov/atr/foia/divisionmanual/ch2.htm

Social Security Act of 1965, Medicaid, Title XIX, 42 U.S.C. §§1396-1396v.

Social Security Act of 1965, Medicare, Title XVIII, 42 U.S.C. §§1395-1395ccc.

South Carolina Code of Laws (Unannotated). Speech-Language Pathologists and Audiologists, §§40-67-5 *et seq.* and §§40-1-110 to 40-1-150. Available from http://www.lawsource.com/also/

Steiner, J. E. Jr. (Ed.). (2006). *Clinical research law and compliance handbook.* Sudbury, MA: Jones & Bartlett.

Studdert, D. M., Mello, M. M., & Brennan, T. A. (2004). Medical malpractice. *The New England Journal of Medicine, 350*(3), 283–292.

Tanner, D. C. (2007). Dysphagia malpractice: Litigation and the expert witness. *Journal of Medical Speech-Language Pathology, 15*(1), 1–6.

Tanner, D. C. (2010). Lessons from nursing dysphagia malpractice litigation. *Journal of Gerontological Nursing, 36*(3), 41–46.

Tarasoff v. Regents of University of California, 551 P.2d 334 (Cal. 1976).

The T. J. Hooper, 60 F. 2nd 737 (2d Cir. 1932).

Truman v. Thomas, 611 P.2d 902 (Cal., 1980).

U.S. Constitution. (1787). Available from http://www.house.gov/house/Constitution/Constitution.html

U.S. Department of Commerce. Available from http://www.commerce.gov/

U.S. Department of Commerce (1979, October 31). Model Uniform Product Liability Act. *Federal Register, 44*(212), 62714–62750.

U.S. Department of Health and Human Services. Available from http://www.hhs.gov

U.S. Department of Health and Human Services, Office of Civil Rights. (2003, May). *Summary of the HIPAA privacy rule* [OCR privacy brief]. Washington, DC: Author.

U.S. Department of Justice. Available from http://www.usdoj.gov

U.S. Department of Justice. (2009, July). *A guide to disability rights laws.* Washington, DC: Author, Civil Rights Division, Disability Rights Section. Available from http://www.ada.gov/cguide.htm

U.S. Department of Justice. (2011, March 16). *ADA update: A primer for small businesses.* Washington, DC: Author, Civil Rights Division, Disability Rights Section. Retrived from http://www.ada.gov/regs2010/smallbusiness/smallbusprimer2010.htm

U.S. Equal Employment Opportunity Commission. Available from http://www.eeoc.gov/

U.S. Federal Trade Commission. Available from http://www.ftc.gov/

U.S. Food and Drug Administration. Available from http://www.fda.gov/

U.S. Public Health Service (2005). Public Health Service policies on research misconduct (final rule). *Federal Register, 70,* 28370–28400.

U.S. v. Eric T. Poehlman, Criminal No. 2:05-cc-38-1 [Criminal information] (D. Vt. March 21, 2005a).

U.S. v. Eric T. Poehlman, No. 2:05-cv-66 [Settlement agreement and stipulation for entry of judgment] (D. Vt. March 21, 2005b).

Yorkston, K., Beukelman, D., Strand, E., & Hakel, M. (2010). *Management of motor speech disorders in children and adults.* Austin, TX: Pro-Ed.

7

International Alliances

Linda Worrall, PhD; Louise Hickson, PhD; and Anna O'Callaghan, PhD

SCOPE OF CHAPTER

International alliances in speech-language pathology and audiology involve forming connections among and between nations. These connections or networks, formed either directly through personal contact or indirectly through web-based searches, are increasingly becoming part of clinicians' work and social life (Harasim, 1993). The term *global village* was coined to promote discussion about the possibility of an interconnected world. The concept of a global village is now a reality as we work within a new information age. According to Cheng (1998), a global communicator is someone who is prepared "to learn and embrace cultural and individual diversity" (p. 283). Speech-language pathologists and audiologists have been swept up in the global communication revolution within both their social and professional lives. This global village has had an impact on the professional practice of speech-language pathologists and audiologists. International conferences are only a few hours' travel away, and relevant clinical information is accessible in seconds from the World Wide Web. You might even converse with international colleagues via e-mail, Skype, instant messaging, and telephone.

This chapter has two aims. The first is to outline the benefits of creating and nurturing international alliances—benefits that include broadening one's knowledge base; developing skills; learning new procedures; and pooling resources to develop tests, resources, and/or standards that can be applied in a number of countries. Some of the barriers to developing international alliances (e.g., language barriers, ethnocentrism) are also discussed. The second aim is to examine the two main forms of transnational communication in the professions. Internet use is espoused as a means of forming international alliances, and practice in other countries is also encouraged.

Substantial information and resources necessary for speech-language pathologists and audiologists to practice in other countries are provided as an introduction to how to find jobs in other countries. The main emphasis in this chapter is on the practice requirements for Australia, Canada, New Zealand, South Africa, Ireland, and the United Kingdom. These countries were chosen because they are English speaking and represent the major destinations for English-speaking speech-language pathologists and audiologists. Since 2005, there has also been an agreement of mutual recognition of certification in speech-language pathology among the countries of Australia, Canada, the United Kingdom, and the United States. In 2008, this agreement was extended, and New Zealand and Ireland were included. The implications of this international agreement are discussed later in this chapter. A summary of information about working in developing countries is also included as well as a brief description of the international associations for speech-language pathologists and audiologists.

BENEFITS OF INTERNATIONAL ALLIANCES

Globalization has many advantages, and the benefits are beginning to influence the professions of speech-language pathology and audiology. Many clinicians and researchers are traveling to other countries and are able to learn new perspectives and skills for when they return to their home countries. They may also provide perspectives, skills, and services to the host country. The professions in many developing countries have been assisted by speech-language pathologists and audiologists from countries with longer-established professional bases, such as the United States and the United Kingdom.

Although a summary of information about opportunities for assisting developing countries is contained in this chapter, we focus on the less tangible benefits that international alliances can bring to those who want to interact with fellow professionals from other predominantly English-speaking countries. The benefits include learning new skills, procedures, and perspectives; gaining a greater understanding of cultural diversity; and pooling new and existing resources.

The Benefit of Learning New Skills, Procedures, and Perspectives

Speech-language pathologists and audiologists in various countries frequently use distinct theoretical frameworks and diverse practical techniques and work in very different policy environments. Gaining knowledge about these areas can enrich both the individual clinician and the professions as a whole. New ways are not always better, but it is possible to select particular aspects that will improve practice in another setting. An example is the innovative and exciting use of the social model of disability in aphasia rehabilitation in North York, Ontario, Canada (Kagan & Gailey, 1993) and the City University, London, England (Byng, Pound, & Parr, 2000). These approaches have founded many similar aphasia centers throughout the world, each a little different but reflecting the same principles.

The Benefit of Gaining New Perspectives of Cultural Diversity

As a preface to the introduction of the "World View" section of the *American Journal of Speech-Language Pathology*, Fey (1996) highlights the importance of evaluating trends in professional practice in the United States from the standpoint of the state of the art elsewhere. This is a welcome recognition of the benefits that a leading professional nation such as the United States can obtain from a flow of information into the country. Fey also states that "we cannot develop adequate theories of speech and language disorders or speech and language intervention unless we embrace an international perspective that takes into careful consideration the similarities and differences among cultures and languages across the world" (p. 2).

Cultural diversity within a nation is a feature of everyday life in many countries. Hence, in addition to the influence of global communication networks, population mobility is shaping our future. Nations like Australia, Canada, New Zealand, South Africa, Ireland, the United Kingdom, and the United States have a diversity of cultures within their own borders.

The speech-language pathology and audiology professions are striving to provide relevant services to these populations and need to develop sensitivity to other cultures so they can best service their clients. A benefit of international alliances is greater sensitivity to cultural and linguistic diversity.

The Benefit of Pooling Resources

There are many resources produced in one country that would be useful in other countries; however, only a few of these are distributed internationally, as they may have little commercial value within the local publishing industry. Such resources may nonetheless be extremely useful in other cultural settings. For example, the speech pathology department of a hospital in Australia produced an outcome scale, the Royal Brisbane Hospital Outcome Measure for Swallowing (1998), that has been widely accepted by speech pathologists across Australia. However, as the national market for the scale is relatively small and there is no specific speech-language pathology and audiology publishing company in Australia, this scale is unlikely to be distributed internationally. This occurs despite the scale being one of the only dysphagia outcome rating scales known to have substantial psychometric data (Sonies, 2000; Ward & Conroy, 1999).

An example of pooling of international resources in speech-language pathology is seen in a project related to the American Speech-Language-Hearing Association's *Functional Assessment of Communication Skills for Adults* (ASHA FACS) (Frattali, Thompson, Holland, Wohl, & Ferketic, 1995), which has become a leading functional communication assessment around the world as well as in the United States. The ASHA FACS has gained greater recognition internationally because of the involvement of international contributors in the review process. Items that were not appropriate to other English-speaking countries were identified and discussed. The successful international alliance developed during the original ASHA FACS project has taken on an expanded role for the next phase of the project. The project has evolved into developing a measure of quality of communicative life, the ASHA Quality of Communication Life Scale (Paul, Frattali, Holland, Thompson, Caperton, & Slater, 2005). The international advisory group has been able to offer theoretical perspectives on quality of life issues in their own country, field test the new measure in English-speaking countries outside the United States, and offer suggestions on how the tool might be accepted in countries outside the United States. Hence, a two-way information flow has developed. The end product resulted in wider application and a new appreciation of international perspectives on functional communication and quality of life.

Another example of the benefits of pooling resources is evident in the development of *The International Guide to Speech Acquisition* (McLeod, 2007). This guide was created to assist speech-language pathologists who work with children from a variety of language backgrounds. It provides a general overview of 12 English-speaking dialects and 24 languages other than English. This overview covers speech acquisition (including articulation, phonology, and phonetics) as well as assessment and intervention tools commonly used for each language and dialect. The authors who contributed to this resource include speech-language pathologists from the Middle East, Europe, Canada, the United States, South America, Australia, the United Kingdom, and Asia. Websites by Judith Kuster and Liz Herring also provide a wealth of clinical resources for speech-language pathologists.

In audiology, a group of researchers and practitioners in the International Collegium of Rehabilitative Audiology (ICRA) has worked on a number of projects from a global perspective. For example, it has developed the ICRA noise CD, which is a collection of noise signals that can be used as background noise in clinical tests of hearing aids and possibly for measuring characteristics of nonlinear instruments. It is hoped that these signals might become an international de facto standard. As another example, members of the collegium have developed and promoted the use of the International Outcome Inventory (Cox, Stephens, & Kramer, 2002) for measuring the outcomes of rehabilitation for adults with hearing impairment. The tool is available from the ICRA website in a number of different languages, and recent publications suggest that it is being used worldwide (e.g., Heuermann, Kinkel, & Tchorz, 2005; Hickson, Clutterbuck, & Khan, 2010; Oberg, Lunner, & Andersson, 2007).

Aside from pooling international resources, speech-language pathologists and audiologists may wish to join international associations such as the International Association of Logopedics and Phoniatrics (IALP), the International Society of Augmentative and Alternative Communication, the International Society of Audiology, and the International Association of

Laryngectomees. Membership within these organizations provides opportunities for professionals and students to network, engage in professional development, and present research in annual meetings or conferences with speech-language pathologists and audiologists from around the word (Lubinski, 2011). While the benefits of international alliances are clearly evident, the barriers to international collaboration should be acknowledged, including language barriers, inconsistent professional terminology, and ethnocentrism.

BARRIERS TO INTERNATIONAL COLLABORATION

Language

There are many similarities in professional practice in English-speaking countries; however, there are also many differences, and these can be barriers to cross-cultural communication in the professions. A good example of the differences among these countries is the use of the English language itself. Although English is the global language for international communication, and more than 80 percent of the world's research is published first in English, the language is diverse.

Just as Africaans became a separate language from Dutch within a relatively short period of time, Stevenson (1994) concurs with the editor of the *Oxford English Dictionary* who predicts that American English and British English will drift into two distinct languages. Although American English is the language of the largest nation of speech-language pathologists and audiologists—the United States—other forms of English comprise the language of the professions in Australia, Canada, New Zealand, South Africa, and the United Kingdom. Some of these nations, such as Australia, Canada, New Zealand, and South Africa, use a mix of both American English and British English in their professional language.

Within speech-language pathology and audiology, differences are most noticeable in examples of written language emanating from each country. *Dysphasia* is still the term used most often in the United Kingdom, whereas *aphasia* is used in the United States. In audiology, *immittance audiometry* is the preferred term in the United States, whereas *impedance audiometry* is more commonly used in Australia and the United Kingdom. The profession of speech-language pathology in the United States and Canada is called *speech pathology* in Australia, and *speech and language therapy* in New Zealand and the United Kingdom. In South Africa, *speech and hearing therapists* has been the term for the combined professions of speech-language pathology and audiology (Bortz, Jardine, & Tshule, 1996; Tuomi, 1994). Overall, however, *audiology* is the most commonly used term for the profession worldwide.

Australian speech-language pathologists changed the name of their profession to speech pathology in 1973. British therapists also voted at this time to change their name, but it took until 1990 for them to reach consensus and change their name from speech therapy to speech-language therapy. Terms considered at this time included communication, language, speech and therapist/pathologist/specialist as well as remedial linguistics, communication specialist, communicologist, ortholinguist, logopaedist, and clinical speech pathologist (Patterson, 2005). During the debate to change their name, Professor David Crystal (1973) wrote in the *College of Speech Therapists Bulletin* that speech-language pathologists would never find one term that was comprehensively accurate and immediately intelligible. Nevertheless, he stated that the profession should aim for the least misleading and hope to find a name that reflects the professions' priorities of action. The mutual recognition agreement of certification between the United States, Canada, Australia, the United Kingdom, New Zealand, and Ireland confirms that while speech-language pathologists use different names as a profession they are virtually the same (Patterson, 2005).

Nevertheless, variations in cross-cultural communication affecting terminology in the professions are evident and often cause confusion. An example in speech-language pathology is found in the use of the terms *articulation disorders* and *phonological disorders*. Clinicians in the United States often interpret these terms differently than clinicians in Australia and the United Kingdom. The prevailing meanings in the United States are exemplified by Stone and Stoel-Gammon (1994), who use *phonological disorders* as the generic term that often includes articulation disorders due to structural characteristics or the control mechanism of the speech system (albeit having an impact on the phonological system). In the United Kingdom and Australia, these terms are used to describe two discrete disorders, with phonological disorders implying an underlying cognitive-linguistic deficit and articulation disorders implying an underlying phonetic production deficit. Although connotative meanings of terms such as these may vary even within one country's profession, cross-cultural communication between professions in different countries may encounter difficulties caused by differences in the connotative meaning of professional terms.

Variations in terminology can be traced to variations in educational tradition. For example, in the 1950s in central Europe, the education in speech-language pathology was shaped by phoniatricians. The speech-language pathologists were considered the doctors' assistants, and the professional paradigm was a paramedical one. In Denmark and Norway, the education was a postgraduate education based on teacher training; therefore, the paradigm within which they worked was a pedagogical one (Kjaer, 2005).

The International Classification of Functioning, Disability and Health (ICF) (World Health Organization [WHO], 2001) may provide a solution to the barrier of inconsistent professional terminology. The ICF classifies impairments in terms of body structures and functions, activities, participations, and environmental factors and gives an alphanumeric code to all terms used. Since the classification is international, the whole world agrees that by listing the code b310, we are referring to "voice function," defined as the "functions of the production of various sounds by the passage of air through the larynx" (WHO, 2001). Two purposes are obtained through the use of the ICF: (1) different professions may refer to the same code to mean the same thing, even if they use a different clinical label, and (2) two regions of the world may use the same alphanumeric code as a translation system, despite language, cultural, and clinical label differences (Schindler, 2005). In audiology, there is a World Health Organization-supported project currently working to define the core sets of codes that are relevant to hearing loss. The project is based in Sweden but is led by an international team of researchers who work in the field of audiology (Danermark et al., 2010).

Ethnocentrism

Ethnocentric attitudes are another barrier, and the citation of local references is common to all disciplines, not just speech-language pathology and audiology. An increasing and contentious barrier is the American dominance of the two professions, which has the potential to marginalize the professions in other countries.

The American Speech-Language-Hearing Association has the largest number of speech-language pathology and audiology members in the world. It represents 145,000 members and affiliates who are speech-language pathologists; audiologists; and speech, language, and hearing scientists in the United States and internationally (American Speech-Language-Hearing Association, 2010). Being the largest nation of speech-language pathologists and audiologists, the United States certainly exerts a large influence on the professions of speech-language pathology and audiology in other nations.

There may be some advantages to this, such as the development of common professional terms; however, Americans need to be sensitive to this powerful influence. There are many benefits to be gained from international alliances if the cultural and communication barriers can be identified and overcome.

STRATEGIES FOR INTERNATIONAL ALLIANCES

We encourage professionals to begin appreciating the diversity of the profession across the world by becoming speech-language pathologists or audiologists of the world, rather than professionals of their own specific country. There are two main types of professional transnational interaction. One is via mass communication system contacts such as those of the World Wide Web, and the other is person-to-person international contact, which often involves practicing professionally in another country (Mowlana, 1997). This section contains details about practice in other countries and about other strategies for transnational interaction that do not involve international travel.

Kuster and Poburka (1998) detail the advantages that the Internet provides for bridging research and practice in speech-language pathology and audiology. In addition, these Internet functions, such as chat groups, e-journals, online bibliographies and journal services, websites that describe research and report findings, and simple e-mail can also be useful for bridging the gap between communication disorders professionals throughout the world. For example, in audiology, Balatsouras, Korres, Kandiloros, Ferekidis, and Economou (2003) detail newborn hearing screening resources available on the Internet. These include websites about hearing screening program guidelines and position statements, research laboratories, publications, related organizations and societies, equipment, and data management software, as well as online mailing lists and discussion groups. Addresses for 150 sites are listed. In addition to more specific websites, services such as Audiology Online and Speech Pathology Online are an excellent starting point for surfing the web. Kuster and Poburka (1998) offer many suggestions for learning about research on the Internet. This highlights the need for leadership by the international research community to spearhead cross-cultural communication in both professions. Individuals need to join discussion lists, post their own professional insights on websites, seek information about the profession in other countries of the world via the Internet, request the tables of contents of international journals from publishers' websites, go to specific websites of speech-language pathologists or audiologists in other countries, and correspond if possible through e-mail. The Internet is fast and has already become the most extensive communication and information system worldwide. Thus, speech-language pathologists and audiologists should be keen to embrace it to develop international alliances.

Citing a U.S. commission on international studies by U.S. citizens, Mowlana (1997) concludes that study-abroad programs can have a lifelong impact on values and on understanding of other cultures. "Cross-cultural contact enables persons to understand the complexities of another society and empathize with persons of another culture" (Mowlana, 1997, p. 157). The personal benefits of studying abroad as cited in Speech Pathology Australia's *Speak Out* (2011) include increased self-confidence, improved maturity, greater global networks, better preparedness to face future challenges, and improved creativity while becoming more familiar with individual strengths and weaknesses. Experiences of students studying abroad may range from exchanges (students spend one or two semesters of study in another country while gaining credit for the subjects they study), short-term programs (students complete their clinical practicum hours at a clinic in another country), external volunteer programs (e.g., projects abroad), summer school, or GAP programs. Learning a second or third language during your study abroad may have positive results when you seek employment. Each individual university will provide unique opportunities for international study.

It is recommended that undergraduate and postgraduate students interested in studying abroad contact the departments dealing with international studies at their universities. Experiencing the professions in another country provides a unique understanding of how cultural differences affect the practice of speech-language pathology or audiology. Sensitivity to cultural effects on clinical practice is a prized value of not only individuals but also organizations. One example of international opportunities for speech-language pathology students at the master's level is that designed by Teachers College Columbia University in Bolivia, Cambodia, and Ghana.

International research is also possible. University professors frequently collaborate with researchers in other countries and may encourage students to be part of these studies. Zajdo (2007) discusses how her initial collaborative work in Hungary led to other research in Holland. The Center for International Rehabilitation Research Information and Exchange (CIRRIE) also has funds to help support international components of NIDRR grants. Be sure to follow the requirements for the safeguarding of human subjects in any country in which you do research. Faculty may also be invited to give international presentations and serve on a variety of panels with researchers from around the world.

PRACTICE IN OTHER COUNTRIES

The Internet has facilitated finding a job as a speech-language pathologist or audiologist in another country. Many of the larger professional associations now have websites and often provide information for professionals qualified outside their country. Some also have job vacancies listed on the site. Appendix 7–A contains a summary of the speech-language pathology and audiology entry qualifications, practice requirements, and relevant professional associations in Australia, Canada, New Zealand, Ireland, South Africa, and the United Kingdom. Each country has different arrangements for the admission of people trained overseas to practice, and some reciprocity agreements are in place. The best way to obtain information is to contact the country's professional association. The website addresses included in the appendix are the most convenient way of accessing relevant up-to-date information.

Links to speech-language pathology and audiology professional associations and individual practitioners can be made through large profession-specific websites such those listed in the Resources section of this chapter. In addition, the American Speech-Language-Hearing Association has a list of international resources on its website such as cleft palate and craniofacial treatment programs as well as links to many other useful sites such as an international directory of communication disorders. If your destination country does not have a website, then contact information should be available through your own professional association.

As noted earlier, an agreement of mutual recognition of credentials among the six speech-language pathology professional associations of Australia, Canada, the United Kingdom, Ireland, New Zealand, and the United States came into effect at the beginning of 2009. Boswell (2004) states that benefits of the agreement include identifying common standards of clinical competence, facilitating ongoing exchange of knowledge, promoting greater international understanding of the role of speech-language pathologists, reducing trade barriers, improving mobility for employment abroad, and providing a process for countries interested in mutual recognition of qualifications and credentials. For speech-language pathologists wishing to work in countries covered by the agreement, this agreement does not mean automatic entry into the other countries' professional associations. Each professional association may still require additional certification; however, the agreement means that applicants do not have to have their academic coursework and clinical practicum evaluated as part of the application process. Further details about the specific requirements of each professional association under the agreement are contained on their websites. Note, too, that in the United States, practitioners in both audiology and speech-language pathology may also need to meet teacher certification and/or licensure requirements of individual states to practice. Again, it is best to check with both national organizations and individual states or provinces for practice requirements.

Australia

Speech Pathology Australia (SPA) is the professional association that represents more than 4,200 speech pathologists. SPA is recognized as the national professional standards organization in Australia. It provides services in representation, data collection and collation, public relations, publication, continuing education, member services, and government submissions.

SPA has established educational and clinical standards that applicants are required to meet for admission to membership. For Practicing Membership, applicants are required to have an appropriate degree in speech pathology and meet the Australian standards of practice, including being competent in the use of English within the Australian clinical context. For applicants who graduated more than five years ago, evidence is required of at least 1,000 hours of speech pathology practice within the past five years. The eligibility for membership requirements has changed to a competency-based approach as contained in the Competency-Based Occupational Standards for Entry-Level Speech Pathologists (Speech Pathology Australia, 2001). There is also a requirement for applicants to demonstrate their competence in the area of dysphagia. SPA looks for evidence that graduates have attained the level of competence that would enable students to work independently with dysphagic clients of any age.

The practice or licensing requirements for speech pathologists in Australia vary for the different states and territories. Queensland is the only state in Australia that requires mandatory registration through the Speech Pathologists Board of Queensland before practicing as a speech pathologist. Membership in SPA is not mandatory across Australia; however, employers usually require applicants for speech pathology positions to demonstrate eligibility for current practicing membership in SPA. Some employers state that association membership is obligatory.

The Audiological Society of Australia is the professional association that maintains standards for audiology in Australia and represents more than 1,600 audiologists. To practice, an individual should be eligible for full membership in the society, that is, be a university graduate with tertiary qualifications in audiology and have passed the core knowledge and competencies assessment. To obtain the society's Certificate of Clinical Practice, it is then necessary to complete a graduate clinical internship, which is 12 months of supervised clinical practice. There are currently no official registration or licensing agreements for the practice of audiology in Australia. Although membership in the Audiological Society of Australia is not mandatory, most employers require applicants to have or be eligible for society membership, and membership is required for audiologists to provide services to clients through the Australian Government's Office of Hearing Services funding scheme.

Canada

With more than 5,400 members, the Canadian Association of Speech-Language Pathologists and Audiologists (CASLPA) represents the interests of both professions of speech-language pathology and audiology in Canada. In addition to the national association, there are provincial/territorial associations for speech-language pathologists and audiologists.

These associations have varying practice requirements. CASLPA grants certification to speech-language pathologists and audiologists. To be considered full members of CASLPA, speech-language pathologists and audiologists must meet clinical certification practicum requirements and pass the CASLPA clinical certification examination. Clinical certification with CASLPA is a voluntary process and not a license to practice; however, the association encourages all members to undertake and maintain certification.

Continuing education is a necessary part of maintaining certification; to maintain clinical certification status, members must report a minimum of 45 continuing education equivalents over a three-year cycle. Certification is recognized internationally and facilitates movement not only within Canada but also within the United States.

CASLPA requires that foreign-trained speech-language pathologists and audiologists hold the minimum academic requirement of a graduate university degree. The usual qualification is a master's degree in audiology and/or speech-language pathology or equivalent and proof of having completed 300 clinical practicum hours. All applicants must provide evidence of passing the CASLPA clinical certification exam, have documented evidence of clinical practicum hours and university transcripts indicating the date of conferred degree, and have evidence of education and supervised practicum experience in assessment and treatment in audiology and speech-language pathology according to current CASLPA standards. For speech-language pathology, the total minimum number of clinical practicum hours is specified according to distribution across disorders: developmental language disorders (40 hours), acquired language disorders (30 hours), fluency (10 hours), voice and resonance disorders (10 hours), articulation/phonology disorders (20 hours), dysphagia (10 hours), motor speech (10 hours), and minor audiology (20 hours). A minimum of 50 clinical hours must be with adults and 50 hours with children. A minimum of 100 hours must be spent in diagnostic activities and 100 hours in therapeutic activities.

For membership in the association as an audiologist, applicants must have obtained a master's degree in audiology and have completed 300 hours of clinical practice. These hours must be distributed according to basic audiometric measurement (50 hours), amplification (65 hours), aural rehabilitation and education (25 hours), electrophysiological measurement (10 hours), and minor speech-language pathology (20 hours). Fifty hours must be spent with children, and likewise for adults. A minimum of 100 hours must be spent in assessment and 100 hours in treatment activities. Some provincial associations have different clinical hour requirements than the national association, and these are listed separately on the association's website.

Practice requirements for registration and licensure differ from province to province, and these details can be obtained from the CASLPA website. Information is available for British Columbia, Yukon, Alberta, Northwest Territories, Saskatchewan, Manitoba, Ontario, Quebec, New Brunswick, Nova Scotia, Prince Edward Island, Newfoundland, and Labrador.

Ireland

The Irish Association of Speech and Language Therapists (IASLT) is the national body for speech and language therapy in the republic of Ireland. To become a member of IASLT, speech-language therapists need to hold a bachelor's or master's degree equivalent recognized by the republic of Ireland. Overseas graduates wishing to work in Ireland require evidence of recency of practice, defined as 1,000 hours of clinical practice, and/or conducting research or college/university teaching within the previous five years.

Two organizations represent audiology in Ireland. The professional society representing audiologists is the Irish Society of Audiology (ISA). The Irish Society of Hearing Aid Audiologists (ISHAA) represents audiologists who are in private practice.

New Zealand

The New Zealand Speech-Language Therapists' Association (NZSTA) is the national professional body of speech-language therapy in New Zealand. To be a member of NZSTA, speech and language therapists need to hold a bachelor's or master's degree equivalent, have a minimum of 1,000 hours of clinical experience in the past five years, and have evidence of a record of continuous professional development. The NZSTA association asks that overseas graduates applying for membership under the mutual recognition agreement hold membership with either ASHA, CASLPA, SPA, or the Royal College of Speech & Language Therapists (RCSLT).

When applying to work in New Zealand, NZSTA asks applicants to request a letter of good standing from their home association. ASHA members must also provide certified evidence of 1,000 hours of speech-language pathology practice within the past five years, whereas SPA and CASLPA members are required to provide documented evidence of having completed a year of supervised speech-language therapy practice in the country of certification. Clinical practice is defined as no less than 36 weeks of full-time clinical practice of at least 30 hours per week paid employment.

The entry-level qualification for the practice of audiology in New Zealand is a master's degree. The professional society representing audiologists is the New Zealand Audiological Society (NZAS). Requirements for entry to the society are a master's degree in audiology and a Certificate of Clinical Competence, which involves a year of supervised clinical practice. Although membership in the society is encouraged, it is not a prerequisite for working as an audiologist in New Zealand.

South Africa

The national body for speech-language pathologists, audiologists, and community speech and hearing workers in South Africa is the South African Speech-Language-Hearing Association (SASLHA). The aim of SASLHA is to promote members' best interests in all spheres of professional activity; enhance members' professional competence by providing coordinated learning activities; and lobby and advocate for recognition of the profession by government and private and international bodies. To be a member of SASLHA, speech-language pathologists and audiologists must register with the Health Professionals Council of South Africa. The requirements for registration are a degree from an accepted institution verified by academic transcripts. Speech-language pathology and audiology is a combined four-year undergraduate degree in South Africa, and although postgraduate qualifications can be obtained, they are not necessary for practice.

United Kingdom

The Royal College of Speech & Language Therapists (RCSLT) is the regulating body for overseas speech and language therapists wanting to work in Great Britain and Northern Ireland. To work in the United Kingdom, applicants need to be registered with the Health Professions Council. Under the Mutual Recognition of Credentials Agreement, applicants from Canada and Australia must have completed 12 months of post-qualification work experience to work in the UK. The national association of the applicant's country must also send a letter of good standing, confirming current certification. Evidence of satisfactory completion of the initial year of monitored practice in the UK is required for ongoing certification.

Speech and language therapists must complete a recognized three- or four-year degree course that combines academic study and clinical placements and register with the Health Professions Council to practice in the UK. The practical components of the courses in the UK are very important. These may take place in schools, National Health Service (NHS) hospitals, and community health clinics. The aim of these placements is to help students develop their skills in the assessment and treatment of people with communication disorders.

Audiology in the UK is primarily focused within the NHS. The professional body representing audiologists in the United Kingdom is the British Academy of Audiology (BAA). It replaced the British Association of Audiological Scientists (BAAS), the British Association of Audiologists (BAAT), and the British Society of Hearing Therapists (BSHT) nearly a decade ago. During this time, major changes in education and training, as well as a program of modernization of audiology services within the NHS, culminated in three different ways to qualify as an audiologist. Currently, there are undergraduate programs (a four-year Bachelor of Science in Audiology), master's programs (Master of Science in Audiology), and some fast-track postgraduate diploma conversion programs for those with a Bachelor of Science in another relevant area of science. Membership in the professional body (BAA) is voluntary. Audiologists with a postgraduate qualification (called Clinical Scientists Audiology), however, must register with the Health Professions Council to practice, but audiologists with an undergraduate qualification can register with the Registration Council for Clinical Physiologists (RCCP), although this is currently voluntary. These statutory registration bodies are responsible for setting and maintaining standards of professional behavior, education and training, and maintaining and publishing a register of health professionals who meet these standards.

Further changes in the education and training of audiologists are in progress. As of 2011, audiologists will become part of a professional group called Healthcare Scientists. The education and training route will be through a three-year Bachelor of Science in Healthcare Science (Audiology) for Healthcare Science Practitioners and a three-year Master of Science in Healthcare Science (Audiology). There are higher specialist education and training programs that include doctoral levels of education and training.

Audiologists working in the private sector in the UK are called hearing aid audiologists. The professional body representing this sector is the British Society of Hearing Aid Audiologists (BSHA), and members are required to be registered with the Health Professions Council. To qualify as a hearing aid audiologist requires successful completion of a Foundation Degree (approximately equivalent to the first two years of a Bachelor of Science) as well as experience working within the private sector.

INTERNATIONAL PROFESSIONAL ASSOCIATIONS

Membership in international associations for speech-language pathologists and audiologists can provide valuable opportunities for interaction with fellow professionals worldwide. Although there are many international associations in specialist areas of speech-language pathology and audiology, the major international association for speech-language pathology is the International Association of Logopedics and Phoniatrics (IALP), and the major international association for audiology is the International Society of Audiology (ISA).

International Association of Logopedics and Phoniatrics (IALP)

The IALP is a nonprofit, nonpolitical, and nongovernmental organization whose purpose is to work for the benefit of people with a range of communication disorders (speech, language, voice, swallowing, and hearing). Founded in Vienna in 1924, the association now has more than 300 individual members from 57 countries and is affiliated with 58 national societies from 38 countries (including Australia, Canada, New Zealand, South Africa, the United Kingdom, and the United States). The IALP has informative and consultative status with several United Nations offices, including UNESCO, UNICEF, and WHO. The association also publishes a journal, *Folia Phoniatrica et Logopaedica*, which publishes six issues annually.

International Society of Audiology (ISA)

The statutory purpose of the ISA is to facilitate knowledge, protection, and rehabilitation of human hearing. It also serves as an advocate for the profession and for people with hearing impairment throughout the world. The major activities of the ISA are publications of the *International Journal of Audiology*, a newsletter (*Audinews*), organization of biannual congresses and other events, promotion of international standards in audiology, participation in the organization of affiliated societies, and representation of the multidisciplinary field of audiology in international organizations. Full Membership requires a university degree in audiology or any related field, and Associated Membership includes anyone working in the field of audiology without a university degree or having a professional interest in audiology. Two current members of the ISA must support a membership application.

Other International Professional Associations

Many countries across the world have professional organizations devoted to the study of speech and hearing. ASHA lists these on its website in a section titled "Audiology and Speech-Language Pathology Associations Outside of the United States" (see Resources). Another good source is the International Directory of Communication Disorders, which also lists a wide variety of international groups such as the International Fluency Association, the International Clinical Phonetics and Linguistics Association, the World Federation of the Deaf, and many others.

DEVELOPING AND OTHER NATIONS

In the first edition of this volume on professional issues, Wilson (1994) points out that appropriate speech-language pathology and audiology services are available in developed nations but not in many developing countries. This is particularly the case for speech and language disorders, as hearing impairment has received somewhat more attention internationally. For example, in 1991, the World Health Organization established a Division for the Prevention of Hearing Impairment, which aims to support the formation of organizations and committees in countries worldwide to address prevention issues in hearing impairment. Wilson suggests a number of possible roles for individual professionals who want to get involved with the evolution of the professions in developing countries. These roles include assisting with the development of training programs and services in other countries, acting as advocates for improved services for individuals with communication disorders around the world, joining an international professional association, building a local network of people with international interests, hosting international students, and being an advocate for the professions of speech-language pathology and audiology when traveling in developing countries. There is a danger, however, that these practices promulgate Western imperialism in developing countries. It is suggested, therefore, that those who are interested in working abroad in developing countries are directed to specific agencies and programs such as World Vision International, the Peace Corps, or Volunteer Services Overseas, which have bases in the home country.

One example of Australian speech-language pathologists' work in a developing country is the Trinh Foundation's speech-language therapy for Vietnam program (Trinh Foundation Australia, 2011). The Trinh Foundation is an independent, voluntary, nonprofit organization established in Australia for the following purposes:

- To improve the quality of life of Vietnamese children and adults who suffer from communication and swallowing disorders
- To address this problem by continuing to raise the awareness in Vietnam of speech-language therapy as a profession
- To provide the knowledge, clinical skills, and finances to establish formalized educational courses in speech-language therapy in Vietnam

Vietnam, like many developing countries, has a history of speech-language pathologists visiting the country in volunteer placements for a few weeks to a couple of years, working with locals to provide specialist services and training (Clarke, Roberts, White, & McAllister, 2002; McAllister, Whiteford, Hill, & Thomas, 2006; McAllister & Whiteford, 2008; Whiteford & McAllister, 2006). Increasing survival rates from stroke and degenerative diseases, rapidly increasing head injury rates, and a growing middle class have created demand for formal, ongoing government and privately funded speech pathology services for people in Vietnam with disabilities and rehabilitation needs. Given this demand, the Ear, Nose and Throat Hospital of Ho Chi Minh City requested that the Trinh Foundation Australia organize and deliver a six-week course in key topics in speech-language pathology (voice, swallowing, and speech) to 19 doctors, nurses, audiologists, and physiotherapists from the major hospitals in Vietnam. These practitioners were already working with people with communication and swallowing impairments. Eight Australian speech pathology lecturers and clinical educators volunteered their time to lecture and provide clinical teaching (McAllister et al., 2010). Given the growing number of partially and fully qualified speech-language pathologists in Vietnam, together with the increasing demand for speech-language pathology services, Australian and Vietnamese speech pathologists are working together in their respective hospitals, universities, and governments to create a sustainable university-based degree in speech-language pathology in Vietnam. As of September 2010, the first-ever speech-language pathology course started at Pham Ngoc Thach University of Medicine, Ho Chi Minh City. This course, in the form of a full-time, two-year postgraduate traineeship, has been instigated and financially supported by Trinh Foundation Australia.

Audiologists have a long history of working in developing countries, and a summary of these endeavors is provided in the excellent text *Audiology in Developing Countries* (McPherson & Brouillette, 2008). The book gives a clear overview of the specific challenges involved in hearing health care in developing nations and the ways in which these challenges can be met. It also provides numerous examples of services in developing countries and agencies that support such endeavors. For example, Miles and McCracken (2008) describe the development of audiology skills in Namibia that began with a British audiologist recruited to work at the Eluwa School for the Deaf in northern Namibia in 1996. Other than this one audiologist, at the time there were two other audiologists in Namibia, both of whom were working in the capital city of Windhoek, 650 kilometers south of Eluwa. The British audiologist trained four local teachers to take over the school-based service.

Opportunities exist in many other countries, and various resources are available that may assist the prospective traveler. Many of these countries, but not all, also have audiology training programs. In a small number of countries, speech-language pathology and audiology are considered to be the same profession and therefore are taught conjointly (e.g., India, Brazil, and Israel). Information about a range of countries is available in a number of journals such as the *American Journal of Speech-Language Pathology, American Journal of Audiology, International Journal of Audiology,* and *Folia et Phoniatrica Logopaedica.* For example, articles have appeared on speech-language pathology in the Dominican Republic (Meline, Penalo, & Oreste, 1996), Brazil (Lemos & Bazzo, 2010; Ferreira, 2002), the Philippines (Cheng, Olea, & Marzan, 2002; Roseberry-McKibbin, 1997), Malaysia (Ahmad, 2010; Lian & Abdullah, 2001), Taiwan (Tseng & Wen, 2002), Greece (Tsoukala & Tziorvas, 1995), Malta (Grech, 2002; 2006), Sri Lanka (Wickenden, Hartley, Kariyakaranawa, & Kodikara, 2003; Wickenden et al., 2001), India (D'Antonio & Nagarajan, 2003; Karanth, 2002; Konnai, Jayaram, & Scherer, 2010), Iran (Nilipour, 2002), Israel (Korenbrot, Hertzano, & Ben Aroya, 2002), Uganda (Robinson, Afako, Wickenden, & Hartley, 2003), and Zimbabwe (Wolf-Schein, Afako, & Zondo, 1995), and articles on audiology in Trinidad and Tobago (Ali, 1992), Israel (Bergman & Hildesheimer, 1994), Nicaragua (Saunders, Vaz, Greinwald, Lai, Morin, & Mojica, 2007; Polich, 1995), Germany (Neumann, Keilmann, Rosenfeld, Schonweiler, Zaretsky, & Kiese-Himmel, 2009; Lenarz & Ernst, 1995), and Latin America (Madriz, 2001).

SUMMARY

This chapter has used the concept of the global village to illustrate how international alliances in speech-language pathology and audiology can be developed. It has emphasized the use of the Internet as a means for promoting greater international interaction, but it has also described the professions in five other English-speaking countries of the world.

Barriers to professional communication even within English-speaking countries abound; however, the advantages of international alliances are many. The forces that are driving globalization are powerful, and the professions of speech-language pathology and audiology are not exempt from such a global trend. Indeed, it is suggested that if the professions do not take advantage of international alliances, then the professions will not have the potency to serve those for whom we exist.

CRITICAL THINKING

1. What are the benefits of international alliances in the professions of speech-language pathology and audiology?
2. What are some of the barriers to international alliances, even within the English-speaking world?
3. What are the two main ways of professional interaction across countries?
4. Review the membership and credential criteria for a country outside the United States and compare them with those for ASHA or AAA. What are the similarities and differences?
5. Do an Internet search for information about speech-language pathology or audiology in a country of interest to you. How developed is the profession? What credentials are necessary for practice? How would you go about working in that country if you had the opportunity?
6. Suppose a speech-language pathologist or audiologist from a developing nation asked to come to visit you and discuss professional issues. What topics would be of importance to discuss with this professional?
7. Your family originally came from what is considered a developing country that has only a few qualified speech-language pathologists or audiologists. You have a doctoral degree in your profession and also speak your family's first language. You now have a real desire to return to that country and help develop one of these professions. Is this possible? How would you go about this process? What might be the benefits of this process to you, the country and its citizens, and our professions? What problems might you have in achieving your goals?

REFERENCES

Ahmad, K. (2010). Discharging patients: A perspective from speech-language pathologists working in public hospitals in Malaysia [Editorial material]. *International Journal of Speech-Language Pathology, 12*(4), 317–319.

Ali, J. E. (1992). Audiology in Jamaica and Trinidad and Tobago. *American Journal of Speech-Language Pathology, 1*, 8–9.

American Speech-Language-Hearing Association. (2010, April 21). About the American Speech-Language-Hearing Association (ASHA). Retrieved from http://www.asha.org/about.htm

Balatsouras, D., Korres, S., Kandiloros, D., Ferekidis, E., & Economou, C. (2003). Newborn hearing screening resources on the Internet. *International Journal of Pediatric Otorhinolaryngology, 67*, 333–340.

Bergman, M., & Hildesheimer, M. (1994). Forty years of audiology in Israel. *American Journal of Speech-Language Pathology, 3*, 11–15.

Bortz, M. A., Jardine, C. A., & Tshule, M. (1996). Training to meet the needs of the communicatively impaired population of South Africa: A project of the University of Witwatersrand. *European Journal of Disorders of Communication, 31*, 465–476.

Boswell, S. (2004, October 19). International agreement brings mutual recognition of certification. *The ASHA Leader*, pp. 1, 22.

Byng, S., Pound, C., & Parr, S. (2000). Living with aphasia: A framework for therapy interventions. In I. Papathanasiou (Ed.), *Acquired neurological communication disorders: A clinical perspective*. London, England: Whurr Publishers.

Cheng, L-R. L. (1998). Learning from multiple perspectives: Global implications for speech-language and hearing professionals. *Folia Phoniatrica et Logopaedica, 50*(5), 283–290.

Cheng, W. T., Olea, T. C. M., & Marzan, J. C. B. (2002). Speech-language pathology in the Philippines: Reflections on the past and present, perspectives for the future. *Folia Phoniatrica et Logopaedica, 54*(2), 79–82.

Clarke, S., Roberts, A., White, J., & McAllister, L. (2002). *Clinical placements in Vietnam: Students' stories of their experiences of developing intercultural competence.* Paper presented at the annual conference of Speech Pathology Australia, Alice Springs, May 2002.

Cox, R. M., Stephens, D., & Kramer, S. E. (2002). Translations of the International Outcome Inventory for Hearing Aids (IOI-HA). *International Journal of Audiology, 41*(1), 3–26.

Crystal, D. (1973). Letter to editor. *RCSLT Bulletin, April*, 15.

Danermark, B., Cieza, A., Gagné, J-P., Gimigliano, F., Granberg, S., Hickson, L., et al. (2010). International classification of functioning, disability and health core sets for hearing loss: A discussion paper and invitation. *International Journal of Audiology. 49*, 256–262.

D'Antonio, L. L., & Nagarajan, R. (2003). Use of a consensus building approach to plan speech services for children with cleft palate in India. *Folia Phoniatrica et Logopaedica, 55*(6), 306–313.

Ferreira, L. P. (2002). Speech therapy in Brazil: Forty years of existence, two decades of recognition. *Folia Phoniatrica et Logopaedica, 54*(2), 103–105.

Fey, M. (1996). Inside. *American Journal of Speech-Language Pathology, 5*(2), 2.

Frattali, C. M., Thompson, C. K., Holland, A. L., Wohl, C. B., & Ferketic, M. M. (1995). *Functional assessment of communication skills for adults.* Rockville, MD: American Speech-Language-Hearing Association.

Grech, H. (2002). Speech-language pathology in Malta: Meeting local needs in a global perspective. *Folia Phoniatrica et Logopaedica, 54*(2), 91–94.

Grech, H. (2006). Education in logopaedics in the Maltese Islands. *Folia Phoniatrica et Logopaedica, 58*(1), 36–40.

Harasim, L. M. (1993). *Global networks: Computers and international communication.* Cambridge, MA: MIT Press.

Heuermann, H., Kinkel, M., & Tchorz, J. (2005). Comparison of psychometric properties of the International Outcome Inventory for Hearing Aids (IOI-HA) in various studies. *International Journal of Audiology, 44*(2), 102–109.

Hickson, L., Clutterbuck, S., & Khan, A. (2010). Factors associated with hearing aid fitting outcomes on the IOI-HA. *International Journal of Audiology, 49*, 586–595.

International Collegium of Rehabilitative Audiology (2011, April 21). ICRA organization. Available from http://www.icra.nu/

Kagan, A., & Gailey, G. (1993). Functional is not enough: Training conversation partners for aphasic adults. In A. Holland & M. Forbes (Eds.), *Aphasia treatment: World perspectives* (pp. 199–225). Clifton Park, NY: Delmar, Cengage Learning.

Karanth, P. (2002). Four decades of speech-language pathology in India: Changing perspectives and challenges of the future. *Folia Phoniatrica et Logopaedica, 54*(2), 69–71.

Kjaer, B. E. (2005). Terminology and conception of the profession. *Advances in Speech-Language Pathology, 7*(2), 98–100.

Konnai, R. M., Jayaram, M., & Scherer, R. C. (2010). Development and validation of a voice disorder outcome profile for an Indian population. *Journal of Voice, 24*(2), 206–220.

Korenbrot, F., Hertzano, T., & Ben Aroya, A. (2002). Emerging issues in Israel: Commentaries in a global context. *Folia Phoniatrica et Logopaedica, 54*(2), 72–74.

Kuster, J. M., & Poburka, B. J. (1998). The Internet: A bridge between research and practice. *Topics in Language Disorders, 18*(2), 71–87.

Lemos, M., & Bazzo, L. M. F. (2010). Speech-language pathology formation in the city of Salvador and the consolidation of SUS. *Ciencia & Saude Coletiva, 15*(5), 2563–2568.

Lenarz, T., & Ernst, A. (1995). Audiology in Germany: Before and since reunification. *American Journal of Speech-Language Pathology, 4*(1), 9–11.

Lian, C. H. T., & Abdullah, S. (2001). The education and practice of speech-language pathologists in Malaysia. *American Journal of Speech-Language Pathology, 10*(1), 3–9.

Lubinski, R., (2011, April 11). Speech therapy or speech-language pathology. Retrieved from http://cirrie.buffalo.edu/encyclopedia/en/article/333/

Madriz, J. J. (2001). Audiology in Latin America: Hearing impairment, resources and services. *Scandinavian Audiology, 30*(Suppl. 53), 85–92.

McAllister, L., Thi Ngoc Dung, N., Christie, J., Woodward, S., Thi Kim Yen, H., Thi Bich Loan, K., et al. (2010). Speech therapy services in Viet Nam: Past, present and future. *Acquiring Knowledge in Speech, Language and Hearing, 12*(1), 47–51.

McAllister, L., & Whiteford, G. (2008). Facilitating clinical decision making in students in intercultural fieldwork placements. In J. Higgs, M. Jones, S. Loftus, & N. Christensen (Eds.), *Clinical reasoning in the health professions.* (3rd ed., pp. 357–365). Sydney, Australia: Elsevier.

McAllister, L., Whiteford, G., Hill, R., & Thomas, N. (2006). Learning and reflection in professional intercultural experience: Qualitative study. *Journal of Reflective Practice, 7*(3), 367–391.

McLeod, S. (2007). *The international guide to speech acquisition.* Clifton Park, NY: Delmar Cengage Learning.

McPherson, B., & Brouillette, R. (Eds.). (2008). *Audiology in developing countries.* New York, NY: Nova Science Publishers.

Meline, T., Penalo, S., & Oreste, A. (1996). Speech-language pathology in the Dominican Republic. *American Journal of Speech-Language Pathology, 5*(3), 4–6.

Miles, S., & McCracken, W. (2008). Educational audiology in developing countries. In B. McPherson & R. Brouillette (Eds.), *Audiology in developing countries* (pp. 167–179). New York, NY: Nova Science Publishers.

Mowlana, H. (1997). *Global information and world communication: New frontiers in international relations.* London, England: Sage Publications.

Neumann, K., Keilmann, A., Rosenfeld, J., Schonweiler, R., Zaretsky, Y., & Kiese-Himmel, C. (2009). Guidelines of the German society of phoniatrics and pediatric audiology on developmental speech and language disorders of children. *Kindheit Und Entwicklung, 18*(4), 222–231.

Nilipour, R. (2002). Emerging issues in speech therapy in Iran. *Folia Phoniatrica et Logopaedica, 54*(2), 65–68.

Oberg, M., Lunner, T., & Andersson, G. (2007). Psychometric evaluation of hearing specific self-report measures and their associations with psychosocial and demographic variables. *Audiological Medicine, 5*, 188–199.

Patterson, A. M. (2005). What's in a name? Cross cultural, cross linguistic considerations. *Advances in Speech-Language Pathology, 7*(2), 80–83.

Paul, D. R., Frattali, C. M., Holland, A. L., Thompson, C. K., Caperton, C. J., & Slater, S. C. (2005). *Quality of Communication Life Scale* (ASHA QCL). Rockville, MD: American Speech-Language-Hearing Association.

Polich, L. (1995). Audiology in Nicaragua. *American Journal of Speech-Language Pathology, 4*(3), 6–9.

Robinson, H., Afako, R., Wickenden, M., & Hartley, S. (2003). Preliminary planning for training speech and language therapists in Uganda. *Folia Phoniatrica et Logopaedica, 55*(6), 322–328.

Roseberry-McKibbin, C. (1997). Understanding Filipino families: A foundation for effective service delivery. *American Journal of Speech-Language Pathology, 6*(3), 5–14.

Royal Brisbane Hospital Outcome Measure for Swallowing. (1998). (Available from Speech Pathology Department, Royal Brisbane Hospital, Herston, 4029, Queensland, Australia).

Saunders, J. E., Vaz, S., Greinwald, J. H., Lai, J., Morin, L., & Mojica, K. (2007). Prevalence and etiology of hearing loss in rural Nicaraguan children. *Laryngoscope, 117*(3), 387–398.

Schindler, A. (2005). Terminology in speech pathology: Old problem, new solutions. *International Journal of Speech-Language Pathology*, 7 (2), 84–86.

Sonies, B. C. (2000). Assessment and treatment of functional swallowing in dysphagia. In L. Worrall & C. Frattali (Eds.), *Neurogenic communication disorders: A functional approach.* New York, NY: Thieme Publishers.

Speech Pathology Australia. (2001). *Competency-based standards for entry level speech pathologists.* Melbourne, Australia: Author.

Stevenson, R. L. (1994). *Global communication in the twenty-first century.* New York, NY: Longman Publishing Group.

Stone, J. R., & Stoel-Gammon, C. (1994). Phonological development and disorders in children. In F. D. Minifie (Ed.), *Introduction to communication sciences and disorders* (pp. 149–187). Clifton Park, NY: Delmar Cengage Learning.

Trinh Foundation Australia. (2011). *Speech-language therapy for Vietnam.* Retrieved from http://www.trinhfoundation.org

Tseng, C., & Wen, Y. (2002). Treatment program planning by speech therapists in Taiwan. *Folia Phoniatrica et Logopaedica, 54*(2), 83–86.

Tsoukala, M., & Tziorvas, R. (1995). The development of a new era of speech language pathology in Greece. *American Journal of Speech-Language Pathology, 4*(1), 5–7.

Tuomi, S. K. (1994). Speech-language pathology in South Africa: A profession in transition. *American Journal of Speech-Language Pathology, 3*, 5–8.

Ward, E. C., & Conroy, A-L. (1999) Validity, reliability and responsivity of the Royal Brisbane Hospital Outcome Measure for Swallowing. *Asia Pacific Journal of Speech, Language and Hearing, 4*, 109–129.

Whiteford, G., & McAllister, L. (2006). Politics and complexity in intercultural fieldwork: The Vietnam experience. *Australian Occupational Therapy Journal, 54*(Suppl. 1), S74–83.

Wickenden, M., Hartley, S., Kariyakaranawa, S., & Kodikara, S. (2003). Teaching speech and language therapists in Sri Lanka: Issues in curriculum, culture and language. *Folia Phoniatrica et Logopaedica, 55*(6), 314–321.

Wickenden, M., Hartley, S., Kodikara, S., Mars, M., Sell, D., Sirimana, T., et al. (2001). Collaborative development of a new course and service in Sri Lanka. *International Journal of Language & Communication, 36*(Suppl. 2), 315–320.

Wilson, M. (1994). International perspectives. In R. Lubinski & C. Frattali (Eds.), *Professional issues in speech-language pathology and audiology* (pp. 75–88). Clifton Park, NY: Delmar Cengage Learning.

Wolf-Schein, E. G., Afako, R., & Zondo, J. (1995). Sounds of Zimbabwe. *American Journal of Speech-Language Pathology, 4*(3), 5–14.

World Health Organization. (2001). *International classification of functioning, disability and health (ICF).* Geneva, Switzerland: Author. Retrieved from http://www.who.int/classification/icf/en

Zajdo, K. (2007). International cooperative projects. *The ASHA Leader.* Retreived from http://www.asha.org/Publications/leader/2007/071226/071226c2/

RESOURCES

Internet Sources on International Audiology and Speech-Language Pathology

American Speech-Language-Hearing Association international resources
http://www.asha.org/members/international/ontlassoc/.

Audiology Online
http://www.audiologyonline.com

Caroline Bowen's website
http://speech-language-therapy.com/index.php?option=com_content&view=article&id=3&Itemid=108

Centre for International Rehabilitation Research Information and Exchange (CIRRIE)
http://cirrie.buffalo.edu/

Communication Therapy International
http://icommunicatetherapy.com/resources/web-resources/web-links

Hear 2 Speak Organization
http://hear2speak.org/index.html

Humanitarian Audiology
http://www.isa-audiology.org/humanitarian.asp

International Association of Logopedics and Phoniatrics
http://www.ialp.info/

International Collegium of Rehabilitative Audiology
http://www.icra.nu

International Directory of Communication Disorders
http://www.comdisinternational.com/intl_associations.html

International Society of Audiology
http://www.isa-audiology.org/

Judith Kuster's website
http://www.mnsu.edu/comdis/kuster2/welcome.html

Liz Herring's website
http://herring.org/speech.html/html

Rehab World
http://www.rehabworld.com

SLPGURU
http://www.speechpathologyguru.com/conferences-d5

Speech Pathology Online
http://www.speechpathology.com

INTERNATIONAL VOLUNTEER AGENCIES

Peace Corps
http://www.peacecorps.gov/

Volunteer Services Overseas
http://www.vso.org.uk/

World Vision International
http://www.wvi.org/wvi/wviweb.nsf

APPENDIX 7-A

Professional Practice in Australia, Canada, New Zealand, South Africa, and The United Kingdom

Speech-Language Pathology Entry-Level Country Professional Association Qualifications Practice Requirements

Australia

Speech Pathology Australia
2nd Floor 11-19 Bank Place
Melbourne VIC 3000 Australia
Telephone: +61 3-9642-4899
Facsimile: +61 3-9642-4922
E-mail: office@speechpathologyaustralia.org.au
Website: http://www.speechpathologyaustralia.org.au

Four-year undergraduate bachelor's degree or two-year postgraduate master's degree and meet Australian standards of practice. Competency assessed on the Competency-Based Occupational Standards for Speech Pathologists: Entry Level (Speech Pathology Australia, 2001).

Registration is compulsory in Queensland. Contact details are:
Speech Pathologists Board of Queensland
GPO Box 2438
Brisbane, QLD 4001 Australia
Telephone: +61 7-3225-2509
Facsimile: +61 7-3225-2527
E-mail: speechpathology@healthregboards.qld.gov.au
Website: www.speechpathboard.qld.gov.au

Eligibility for membership in Speech Pathology Australia is often a requirement of employers in other states and territories.

Canada

Canadian Association of Speech-Language Pathologists and Audiologists (CASLPA)
1 Nicholas St, Suite 1000
Ottawa, Ontario, Canada K1N 7B7
Telephone: +1 613-567-9968
Facsimile: +1 613-567-2859
E-mail: caslpa@caslpa.ca
Website: http://www.caslpa.ca/english/index.asp (information is also available on the web in French: http://www.caslpa.ca/francais/index.asp)

Master's degree in speech-language pathology including 300 clinical hours.

Some provinces require between 200 and 300 clinical hours.

Registration/licensure in each of the provinces and territories (see the CASLPA website for specific requirements for each province and territory, as follows: http://www.caslpa.ca/english/index.asp).

Ireland

Irish Association of Speech & Language Therapists
P.O. Box 541
Ballinlough, Co. Cork, Ireland
Telephone: +353-(0)85-7068707
E-mail: info@iaslt.ie
Website: http://www.iaslt.ie

Bachelor's or master's degree equivalent in speech and language therapy.

Documented evidence of having completed one year of clinical practice as a speech and language therapist. Evidence of recency of practice.

New Zealand

New Zealand Speech-Language Therapists' Association (NZSTA)

P.O. Box 38 070
Parklands, Christchurch, New Zealand 8842
Telephone: +64-3-383-1518
E-mail: nzsta@speechtherapy.org.nz
Website: http://www.speechtherapy.org.nz

Four-year undergraduate degree or two-year master's degree in speech and language therapy. Documented evidence of having completed a year of supervised clinical speech-language pathology practice in country of certification. Evidence of recency of practice.

South Africa

South African Speech-Language-Hearing Association

Telephone: +27-86-111-3297
Facsimile: +27-41-379-5388
E-mail: admin@saslha.co.za
Website: http://www.saslha.co.za

Four-year professional bachelor's degree in speech pathology and audiology.

Registration is compulsory. Contact details are: The Registrar, Health Professions Council of South Africa,

Professional Board for Speech, Language, and Hearing Professions
P.O. Box 205 Pretoria 0001 South Africa
Telephone: +27-12-338-9301
Facsimile: +27-12-328-5120
E-mail: info@hpcsa.co.za

United Kingdom

Royal College of Speech & Language Therapists (RCSLT)

2 White Hart Yard
London SE1 1NX England UK
Telephone: +44-20-7378-1200
Facsimile: +44-20-7403-7254
E-mail: info@rcslt.org
Website: http://www.rcslt.org/

Three- or four-year undergraduate degree in speech and language therapy, or professional master's degree, or graduate entry two-year bachelor's degree. One year of supervised membership before eligible for full membership. Evidence of recency of practice. Evidence of satisfactory completion of initial year of monitored practice in the UK is required for ongoing certification. Registration with the RCSLT is not compulsory; however, registration with the Health Professions Council (HPC) is now compulsory. Contact details are:
The Health Professions Council Park House
184 Kennington Park Road
London SE11 4BU England UK
Telephone: +44-20-7840-9802
Facsimile: +44-20-7840-9801
E-mail: registration@hpc-uk.org
Website: www.hpc-uk.org

Audiology Entry-Level Country Professional Association Qualifications Practice Requirements

Audiology

Australia

Audiological Society of Australia

Suite 7 476 Canterbury Road
Forest Hill VIC 3131 Australia
Telephone: +61-3-9416-4606
Facsimile: +61-3-9416-4607
E-mail: info@audiology.asn.au
Website: http://www.audiology.asn.au

Two-year postgraduate master's degree and 200 hours of clinical contact.

Eligibility for membership in the association.

Canada

Canadian Association of Speech-Language Pathologists and Audiologists (CASLPA)

1 Nicholas St, Suite 1000
Ottawa, Ontario, Canada K1N 7B7
Telephone: +1 613-567-9968
Facsimile: +1 613-567-2859
E-mail: caslpa@caslpa.ca
Website: http://www.caslpa.ca/english/index.asp

Master's degree in audiology including 300 clinical hours.

Registration and licensure differ according to province (see the CASLPA website for specific requirements for each province and territory, as follows: http://www.caslpa.ca/english/index.asp).

New Zealand

New Zealand Audiological Society
P.O. Box 9724
Newmarket Auckland 1149 New Zealand
Telephone/facsimile: +64-9-625-1664
E-mail: nzas@xtra.co.nz
Website: http://www.audiology.org.nz

Master's degree in audiology.

South Africa

South African Speech-Language-Hearing Association
Telephone: +27-86-111-3297
Facsimile: +27-41-379-5388
Email: admin@saslha.co.za
Website: http://www.saslha.co.za

Four-year professional bachelor's degree in speech pathology and audiology.

Registration is compulsory. Contact details are:
The Registrar, Health Professions Council of South Africa,
Professional Board for Speech, Language, and Hearing Professions
P.O. Box 205
Pretoria 0001 South Africa
Telephone: +27-12-338-9300
Facsimile: +27-12-328-5120
E-mail: hpcsa@hpcsa.co.za

United Kingdom

British Academy of Audiology (BAA)
Kingston Smith Association Management, Chester House
68 Chestergate, Macclesfield, Cheshire SK116DY
Telephone: +44-(0)1625-664545
Fax: +44-(0)1625-664510
E-mail: admin@baaudiology.org
Website: http://www.baaudiology.org

Master's degree in audiology.

Membership in the association is not mandatory but recommended. Registration with the Health Professions Council (HPC) is compulsory.
Contact details are:
The Health Professions Council Park House
184 Kennington Park Road
London SE11 4BU England UK
Telephone: +44-20-7840-9802
Facsimile: +44-20-7840-9801
E-mail: registration@hpc-uk.org
Website: http://www.hpc-uk.org.

SECTION II

Employment Issues

8

Workforce Issues in Communication Sciences and Disorders

Gail P. Brook, MA

SCOPE OF CHAPTER

This chapter describes the present and future status of the supply of and demand for audiologists, speech-language pathologists, and communication sciences and disorders (CSD) faculty-scholars and researchers in the United States. It begins with a description of the current demographics and employment characteristics of individuals in the professions and discipline. Next, first-year enrollment and graduation data for CSD graduate programs are presented. The chapter concludes with a discussion of factors affecting the future employment of audiologists, speech-language pathologists, and CSD faculty-scholars and researchers. Influential factors include the changing demographics of the U.S. population, medical and technological advances, federal policy, reimbursement, overlapping scopes of practice, and personnel shortages. Data from the American Speech-Language-Hearing Association (ASHA), the Council of Academic Programs in Communication Sciences and Disorders (CAPCSD), the U.S. Bureau of Labor Statistics (BLS), and other relevant sources are presented.

THE CURRENT WORKFORCE

The audiology and speech-language pathology professions comprise individuals who affiliate—and do not affiliate—with ASHA through membership and/or certification. This chapter mainly presents data on the individuals who affiliate with ASHA. Data on the broader population are offered when possible.

ASHA is the professional, scientific, and credentialing association for more than 150,000 members and affiliates who are audiologists; speech-language pathologists; and speech, language, and hearing scientists. The ASHA Certificate of Clinical Competence (CCC) is the internationally recognized professional credential for audiologists and speech-language pathologists. The CCC allows holders to independently provide clinical services and mentor or supervise student clinicians, externs, and clinical fellows. The certificate can be obtained by individuals who have completed a rigorous academic program and a supervised clinical experience and have passed a national exam. Certificate holders are expected to abide by ASHA's Code of Ethics and demonstrate a commitment to remain current in the field.

Licensure, unlike ASHA certification, is mandatory for those states that regulate the practice of audiology and/or speech-language pathology. In many states, regulatory requirements parallel those of ASHA certification, so certificate holders will likely meet the regulatory requirements of their state. As of December 2010, 50 states and the District of Columbia regulated the practice of audiology (American Speech-Language-Hearing Association [ASHA], 2009b). All states and the District of Columbia also regulate the practice of speech-language pathology.

ASHA MEMBERSHIP AND AFFILIATION DATA

As of year-end 2011, ASHA represented 150,079 audiologists; speech-language pathologists; and speech, language, and hearing scientists (ASHA, 2012). Compared with year-end 2010, this number has increased by 4,598—a 3.2 percent increase (ASHA, 2011a). Figure 8–1 illustrates the growth of the ASHA membership and affiliation over the past 10 years. In 2001, 12,511 individuals held certification in audiology; this number grew to 12,844 in 2011, a change of 2.7 percent over 10 years (ASHA, 2002, 2012). The percentage change for the number of ASHA-certified speech-language pathologists over the same time period was 49.5 percent—from 89,364 in 2001 to 133,621 in 2011.

A total of 1,172 individuals held certification in both audiology and speech-language pathology in 2011, compared with 1,392 individuals in 2001, a change of 15.8 percent (ASHA, 2002, 2012). The lack of growth in the number of individuals who hold dual certification may be due in part to the increasing specialization of the professions. It may be more challenging and time intensive to develop the broadening skills and knowledge base that each profession requires to work with individuals across the age, severity, and disorders spectrum.

Demographics

As of year-end 2011, males made up 17.4 percent of audiologists, 4.0 percent of speech-language pathologists, and 26.2 percent of those with dual certification (ASHA, 2012). These percentages have declined from 19.7 percent, 4.9 percent, and 31.7 percent, respectively, over the past 10 years (ASHA, 2002).

With regard to ethnicity, in 2011, 3.1 percent of audiologists, 4.5 percent of speech-language pathologists, and 4.0 percent of those with dual certification indicated they were of Hispanic or Latino origin (ASHA, 2012). The majority of audiologists, speech-language pathologists, and those with dual certification indicated they were white (92.4 percent, 92.8 percent, and 90.8 percent, respectively). These percentages have remained relatively constant over the years and differ significantly from their distribution within the general population. Specifically, individuals of Hispanic origin accounted for 14.8 percent of the total civilian labor force in 2010; this figure is expected to increase to 18.6 percent by 2020 (U.S. Department of Labor, 2012). Individuals who are white accounted for 81.3 percent of the total civilian labor force in 2010; this figure is expected to decline to 79.4 percent by 2020.

A primary objective of ASHA's strategic plan is to increase the diversity and cultural competence of the membership (ASHA, 2011d). This objective includes focusing on males, underrepresented ethnic and racial populations, and bilingual service providers. It also includes providing members with information and

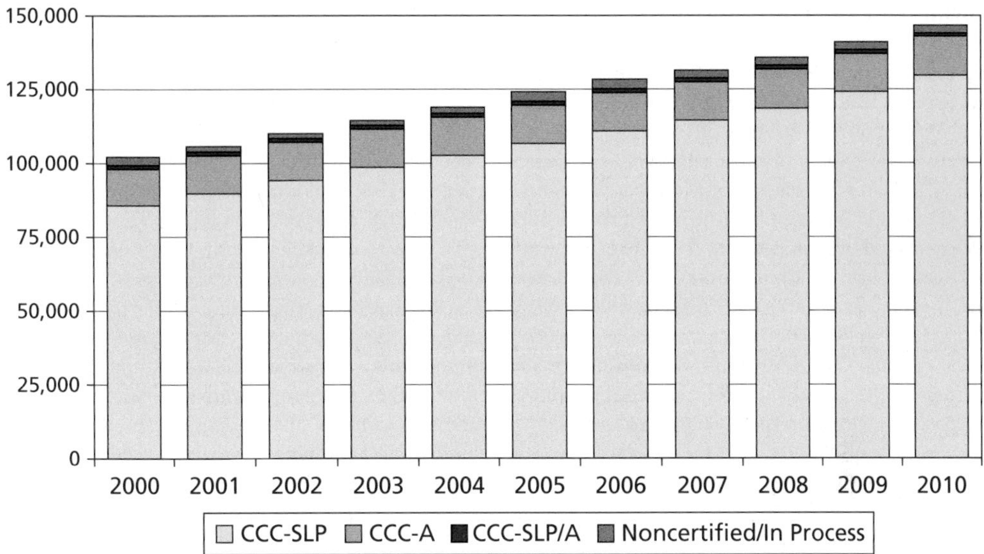

FIGURE 8-1 American Speech-Language-Hearing Association Summary Membership and Affiliation Counts, 2000 to 2011

Adapted with permission from American Speech-Language-Hearing Association summary membership and affiliation counts, 2000 to 2010. Available from www.asha.org.

resources that are available internationally to support the ongoing development of cultural competence. The intended outcome of these efforts is a more culturally and linguistically diverse ASHA membership that is equipped to prepare professionals and provide services to individuals from all backgrounds.

A final demographic to consider is age. In 2011, the median age of audiologists was 47 years, up from 43 years in 2001; the median age of speech-language pathologists was 43 years, down slightly from 44 years in 2001; and the median age of individuals with dual certification was 60 years, up from 54 years in 2001 (ASHA, 2002, 2012).

Employment Characteristics

As of year-end 2011, 71.6 percent of ASHA's membership and affiliation were employed on a full-time basis; 20.4 percent were employed on a part-time basis (ASHA, 2012). Only 1.1 percent were unemployed and seeking employment, well below the January 2012 national unemployment rate of 8.3 percent reported by the U.S. Bureau of Labor Statistics (U.S. Bureau of Labor Statistics [BLS], 2012a).

In 2011, nearly three-quarters of audiologists (72.5 percent) were employed in health care settings, including 47.1 percent in nonresidential health care facilities such as private physicians' or audiologists' offices, 24.3 percent in hospitals, and 1.1 percent in residential health care facilities such as skilled nursing facilities (ASHA, 2012). About 16.2 percent were employed in educational settings, including 8.6 percent in schools and 7.6 percent in colleges and universities. More than one-quarter (27.5 percent) were employed full or part time in private practice, a rate somewhat higher than the rates of the past few years.

As for speech-language pathologists, more than half (57.1 percent) were employed in educational settings, including 54.0 percent in schools and 3.1 percent in colleges and universities. An additional 37.9 percent were employed in health care settings, including 15.6 percent in nonresidential health care facilities, 12.5 percent in hospitals, and 9.8 percent in residential health care facilities. Nearly one-fifth (17.7 percent) were employed full or part time in private practice, a rate somewhat higher than the rates of the past few years.

In 2011, most audiologists (77.9 percent) reported their primary work role as clinical service provider

(ASHA, 2012). Less than one-tenth (8.9 percent) held an administrative position (e.g., executive officer, department chair, or supervisor). A very small percentage (5.2 percent) held a teaching position (0.6 percent were special education teachers and 4.6 percent were college or university professors), 2.6 percent were consultants, and 1.7 percent were researchers. Most speech-language pathologists (78.7 percent) reported their primary work role as clinical service provider. Less than one-tenth (9.3 percent) held a teaching position (7.3 percent were special education teachers and 2.0 percent were college or university professors); 7.3 percent held an administrative position. Only 1.7 percent were consultants and less than 1.0 percent were researchers. These percentages are consistent with those of previous years.

Job and Career Satisfaction

ASHA conducted the 2011 Membership Survey in part to gather information about members' career and job satisfaction and their long-term career plans. The survey shows that audiologists and speech-language pathologists overall have high levels of career and job satisfaction (ASHA, 2011e, 2011f). The majority (86.7 percent of audiologists and 90.8 percent of speech-language pathologists) reported that they are satisfied or very satisfied with their choice of career so far. Respondents also indicated that the most important factors for accepting or staying in a job were the compensation/pay, flexibility to balance life and work, and meaningfulness of the job. As for their long-term career plans, 52.2 percent of audiologists and 50.2 percent of speech-language pathologists reported that they plan to continue working in their career as long as they are able; 32.0 percent of audiologists and 33.1 percent of speech-language pathologists reported that they plan to continue working in their career until they are eligible for retirement.

Salaries of Audiologists In 2010, most audiologists (74.6 percent) were paid an annual salary; the remainder were paid an hourly wage (ASHA, 2010c). The majority (84.6 percent) earned their salary over an 11- or 12-month period (i.e., a calendar year). The remainder earned their salary over a 9- or 10-month period (i.e., an academic year). In 2010, audiologists earned a median calendar year salary of $70,000, excluding bonuses and commissions. They earned a median academic year salary of $65,000, excluding bonuses and commissions. Of those who received a bonus, the median amount was $1,500. Of those who received a commission, the median amount was $14,000. About one-quarter of audiologists (25.4 percent) worked for an hourly wage. Their median hourly wage was $33.04, excluding bonuses and commissions. Of those who received a bonus, the median amount was $600. Of those who received a commission, the median amount was $10,000. More than half (63.0 percent) of the audiologists who earned an hourly wage worked part time (ASHA, 2010b).

Numerous variables, including primary work setting and role, highest academic degree, years of experience in the profession, geographic region, and type of community (i.e., metropolitan/urban, suburban, or rural), affected earnings. For example, audiologists from industry had the highest median calendar year salary in 2010 ($81,121); those from nonresidential health care facilities had the lowest ($65,000; ASHA, 2010a). Administrators earned a median calendar year salary of $92,531 compared with $68,000 for clinical service providers. The median calendar year salary of audiologists who hold the PhD was $96,097, compared with $70,000 for those who hold the AuD and $69,000 for those with a master's degree.

Salaries of Speech-Language Pathologists in Health Care Settings In 2009, more than half (56.1 percent) of speech-language pathologists in health care settings were paid an hourly wage (ASHA, 2009e). Over half of them (52.0 percent) worked full time (ASHA, 2009c). About one-third (34.9 percent) were paid an annual salary (ASHA, 2009e). A small percentage (9.0 percent) were paid per home health visit. In 2009, the median hourly wage of speech-language pathologists in health care settings was $39.50 (ASHA, 2009c). The median annual salary was $70,000 (ASHA, 2009e). The median wage per home health visit was $65.00.

Numerous factors affected earnings. For example, speech-language pathologists from home health settings reported a higher median hourly wage ($60.00) than those from other practice settings (ASHA, 2009a). (See Table 8–1 for data on the annual salaries and hourly wages of speech-language pathologists by type of health care setting.) Administrators, supervisors, and directors earned a median hourly wage of $41.24, compared with $40.00 for clinical service providers. The median hourly wage of speech-language pathologists was highest in the Northeast region of the

TABLE 8–1 2009 Median Annual Salary and Hourly Wage of Speech-Language Pathologists by Their Type of Health Care Setting

Health Care Setting	Annual	Hourly Wage (30 or Fewer Hours per Week)	Hourly Wage (More Than 30 Hours per Week)
Overall	$70,000	$45.00	$36.00
General medical hospital	$73,000	$40.00	$35.00
Rehabilitation hospital	$73,400	$39.00	$35.85
Pediatric hospital	$66,250	$n < 25$	$n < 25$
Skilled nursing facility	$80,000	$45.00	$34.64
Home health/client's home	$66,000	$65.00	$n < 25$
Outpatient clinic or office	$65,000	$55.00	$35.47

Note: ASHA does not report salaries and wages for groups of less than 25.

From "SLP Health Care Survey 2009: Survey Summary Report." Available from the website of the American Speech-Language-Hearing Association: http://www.asha.org/. Adapted with permission.

United States ($47.50); it was lowest in the Midwest ($36.00).

Salaries of Speech-Language Pathologists in School Settings In 2010, most speech-language pathologists in school settings (88.0 percent) were paid an annual salary; the remainder were paid an hourly wage (ASHA, 2010g). The majority (91.1 percent) worked 9 or 10 months per year; the remainder worked 11 or 12 months per year. In 2010, the median academic year salary of speech-language pathologists in school settings was $58,000. The median calendar year salary was $65,000. A small percentage (12.0 percent) worked for an hourly wage (ASHA, 2010e). The median hourly wage was $50.00.

Numerous variables affected earnings. For example, speech-language pathologists in secondary schools had a somewhat higher median academic year salary ($61,786) than those in other school settings (ASHA, 2010d). The most seasoned speech-language pathologists (those with 28 or more years of experience) had a higher median academic year salary than those just starting out ($70,000 and $45,200, respectively). Speech-language pathologists in suburban and metropolitan/urban areas had a higher median academic year salary than those in rural communities ($62,000, $61,000, and $51,000, respectively).

Salaries of Academic and Clinical Faculty in Colleges and Universities A recent salary study by the Council of Academic Programs in Communication Sciences and Disorders (Messick, Currie, Hardin-Jones, & Lof, 2009) reported that the nine-month adjusted base salary for audiology and hearing sciences *academic* faculty was $74,245 (mean) and $67,983 (median). It was substantially lower for audiology and hearing sciences *clinical* faculty: $51,008 (mean) and $49,419 (median). The nine-month adjusted base salary for speech-language pathology and speech-language sciences *academic* faculty was $71,496 (mean) and $66,150 (median). It was substantially lower for speech-language pathology and speech-language sciences *clinical* faculty: $49,335 (mean) and $47,688 (median). Factors other than professional area of focus that influenced salaries included highest academic or clinical degree earned, rank, tenure status, type of institution (i.e., public or private), Basic Carnegie classification of institution, and geographic region of institution (as defined by the Federal Reserve Classification).

U.S. Department of Education Data

Public school employment data are collected by the U.S. Department of Education (ED) and disseminated through the *Annual Reports to Congress on the Implementation of the Individuals with Disabilities*

Education Act (IDEA). According to the *Twenty-Ninth Annual Report to Congress* (U.S. Department of Education, 2010), 1,182 "fully certified" audiologists were employed to provide special education and related services to children and youth ages 3 to 21 with disabilities in the 50 states and the District of Columbia in fall 2004. An additional 253 "not fully certified" audiologists were employed as well. A total of 45,499 "fully certified" and 2,287 "not fully certified" speech-language pathologists were reported for the same time period. Note that ED's definition of *certified* differs from the ASHA definition.

FIRST–YEAR ENROLLMENT AND GRADUATION DATA

ASHA has conducted the Higher Education Data System (HES) Graduate Guide Survey since 2007. This annual survey gathers data on graduate education in CSD, including information on first-year enrollments and degrees granted. It was intended that data collected from the survey would be used to populate EdFind, ASHA's online search engine featuring individualized profiles of graduate programs in CSD; provide state-by-state data on graduate education in CSD; and be used to address important issues in the discipline.

In 2010, a total of 257 academic institutions received the survey, and 229 academic institutions completed and submitted data, representing an 89.1 percent response rate (ASHA, 2011c). Among the 229 institutions completing the survey, data were provided by 97.2 percent of audiology entry-level programs (70 of 72 institutions); 89.1 percent of institutions with master's speech-language pathology programs (220 of 247 institutions); and 91.5 percent of institutions with research doctoral degree (PhD) programs (65 of 71 institutions). The data collected reflect the fall 2009 through summer 2010 academic year.

Regarding first-year enrollments, in 2010, academic institutions reported 787 audiology clinical doctoral (entry-level) students; 7,791 speech-language pathology master's students; and 11 speech-language pathology clinical doctoral (post-entry) students. No speech and hearing sciences master's students were reported. Institutions further reported 21 audiology research doctoral students; 64 speech-language pathology research doctoral students; and 88 speech, language, and hearing sciences research doctoral students.

Regarding graduate degrees granted, in 2010, academic institutions reported granting 548 audiology clinical doctoral (entry-level) degrees; 6,009 speech-language pathology master's degrees; and 14 speech-language pathology clinical doctoral (post-entry) degrees. Institutions also reported granting 19 PhDs in audiology; 33 PhDs in speech-language pathology; and 68 PhDs in speech, language, and hearing sciences.

Trend data on first-year enrollments and graduations are not available, as the data collected through the HES Graduate Guide Survey are not extrapolated to 100 percent of degree-granting institutions.

The National Opinion Research Center conducts the Survey of Earned Doctorates (SED) every year. According to the SED data, from 1999 to 2009, the number of annual doctorate recipients in "speech-language pathology and audiology" in the United States ranged from 86 to 121 recipients (National Science Foundation, Division of Science Resources Statistics, 2010). For the most recent three-year period (2007–2009), the number ranged from 112 to 121 recipients.

Shortage of PhD Students and Faculty in CSD

Data presented by CAPCSD in 1999 suggested that the number of doctoral graduates in audiology and speech-language pathology would not meet the anticipated needs for doctoral-level academic positions in the coming years. In response to these data, ASHA and CAPCSD established a Joint Ad Hoc Committee on the Shortage of PhD Students and Faculty in CSD in 2002. The report of the Joint Ad Hoc Committee included an initial plan to address the shortage (2002–2007). The *Report of the 2008 Joint Ad Hoc Committee on PhD Shortages in Communication Sciences and Disorders* includes information about activities completed to date and a strategic plan (2008–2011) to continue addressing the shortage (McCrea et al., 2008).

In addition to these efforts, a primary objective of ASHA's strategic plan is to improve the science base of the discipline (ASHA, 2011d). This objective includes collaborating with CSD faculty, academic programs, and CAPCSD to (1) address the PhD shortage to increase the quantity and quality of researchers and faculty-scholars and (2) facilitate an increase in the quantity and quality of the discipline's science base, especially with respect to research that advances clinical practice and improves patient/client outcomes. The intended result of these efforts is a science base, supported by a sufficient pipeline of scientists, and the advancement of the professions based on a comprehensive foundation of scientific evidence.

Ensuring a solid foundation of faculty-scholars and researchers is a particular area of concern as the science of the discipline continues to play an increasingly important role in the education and day-to-day practice of audiologists; speech-language pathologists; and speech, language, and hearing scientists. A focus on evidence-based practice, research integrity, and other emerging areas is integral to the future role that the CSD professions and discipline play in service delivery and scientific research and publication. Faculty prepared at the doctoral level are key in delivering this message to future practitioners and applying it to their teaching, research, and publication practices.

A LOOK FORWARD: FACTORS AFFECTING EMPLOYMENT IN FUTURE YEARS

As a student or professional, you may be wondering what the employment forecast is for the coming years. This section discusses employment availability and factors affecting it.

BLS Projections

Based on its research, the BLS projects that from 2010 to 2020, total employment will increase by 20.5 million jobs (BLS, 2012b). About 28.0 percent of the newly created jobs will be in the health care and social assistance industry, which includes public and private hospitals, residential health care facilities, and individual and family services. This industry is expected to grow by 33.0 percent, or 5.7 million new jobs—more than that projected for any other industry. Employment growth will be propelled mainly by an aging population, longer life expectancies, and modern treatments and technologies.

Audiologists and speech-language pathologists fall under the BLS category "healthcare practitioners and technical occupations." The BLS projects that the employment of audiologists will increase from 13,000 in 2010 to 17,800 in 2020 (a 37.0 percent increase)—much faster than average for all occupations. It further projects that the employment of speech-language pathologists will increase from 123,200 in 2010 to 152,000 in 2020 (a 23.0 percent increase)—faster than average for all occupations.

An Older and More Diverse Population

The changing demographics of the U.S. population are a key influential factor in the workforce of CSD professionals. Americans age 65 to 84 are the fastest growing segment of the population (U.S. Census Bureau, 2004). This segment is expected to increase by 38.8 percent from 2010 to 2020 and 30.6 percent from 2020 to 2030. Americans age 85 and older are the second fastest growing segment of the population. This segment is expected to increase by 18.7 percent from 2010 to 2020, 32.1 percent from 2020 to 2030, and 60.5 percent from 2030 to 2040.

The rapid growth of the elderly population is expected to result in a striking increase in the number of people with hearing and balance impairments (BLS, 2012b). The possibility of neurological disorders and associated speech, language, and swallowing impairments is also expected to increase.

Earlier in the chapter, it was noted that the percentage of individuals in the professions from underrepresented ethnic and racial groups is far below that for the general population. According to the U.S. Census Bureau (2004), the non-Hispanic white population is expected to increase by only 2.4 percent from 2010 to 2020 and 1.6 percent from 2020 to 2030. These percentage increases are below those for all other ethnic and racial categories. Hispanics (of any race) are expected to increase by 25.1 percent from 2010 to 2020 and 22.3 percent from 2020 to 2030; that translates to an increase of at least 12 million individuals over each decade.

The percentage of white Americans in the U.S. population is expected to increase by only 6.4 percent from 2010 to 2020 and 5.8 percent from 2020 to 2030 (U.S. Census Bureau, 2004). The percentage of African Americans in the population is expected to grow by 12.1 percent and 11.2 percent, respectively, during the same time periods. The percentage of Asian Americans in the population is expected to increase by 26.3 percent from 2010 to 2020 and 25.5 percent from 2020 to 2030. The percentage of "all other races" (i.e., American Indian or Alaska Native, Native Hawaiian and Other Pacific Islander, and multiracial individuals) is expected to grow by 27.9 percent and 25.5 percent, respectively, during the same time periods.

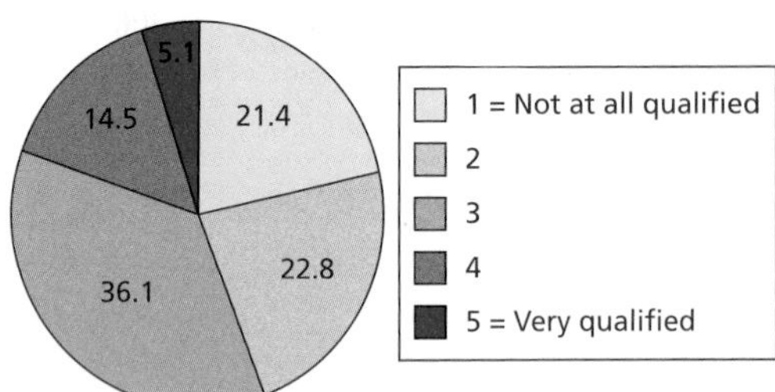

FIGURE 8-2 Audiologists' Self-Perception of Qualifications to Address Cultural and Linguistic Influences on Service Delivery and Outcomes
Adapted with permission from 2010 Audiology Survey Summary Report: Number and type of responses. Available from the website of the American Speech-Language-Hearing Association: www.asha.org.

The ability to work with and provide services to individuals from diverse ethnic and racial backgrounds is of major importance. For a 2010 survey, audiologists were asked to use a 5-point scale (from *not at all qualified* to *very qualified*) to rate how qualified they believe they are to address cultural and linguistic influences on service delivery and outcomes (ASHA, 2010c). As displayed in Figure 8–2, overall, only 5.1 percent rated themselves as 5 (*very qualified*). Ratings ranged from 3.2 percent in nonresidential health care facilities to 9.2 percent in colleges and universities. Nearly one-quarter (21.4 percent) rated themselves as 1 (*not at all qualified*). Ratings ranged from 8.6 percent in colleges and universities to 29.9 percent in industry.

For a 2009 survey, health care–based speech-language pathologists were asked to use a 5-point scale (from *not at all qualified* to *very qualified*) to rate how qualified they believe they are to provide services to multicultural populations (ASHA, 2009e). Overall, only 5.8 percent rated themselves as 5 (*very qualified*). Ratings ranged from 3.2 percent in skilled nursing facilities to 13.2 percent in pediatric hospitals. More than one-tenth (12.1 percent) rated themselves as 1 (*not at all qualified*). Ratings ranged from 4.4 percent in pediatric hospitals to 19.6 percent in skilled nursing facilities.

Health care–based speech-language pathologists were also asked in 2009 to identify the clinical approaches they had used in service delivery to address cultural and linguistic influences on communication in the past 12 months (ASHA, 2009e). Nearly half (44.0 percent) used interpreters/cultural brokers; 33.4 percent modified their assessment strategies or procedures; 24.7 percent acquired translated materials; 18.2 percent referred clients to bilingual service providers; 15.1 percent translated therapy tools; and 14.5 percent translated written materials, including consumer information. More than one-third (36.2 percent) had not used any of the above-mentioned approaches in the past 12 months.

For a 2010 survey, school-based speech-language pathologists were asked to use a 5-point scale (from *not at all qualified* to *very qualified*) to rate how qualified they believe they are to provide services to multicultural populations (ASHA, 2010g). Overall, only 7.6 percent rated themselves as 5 (*very qualified*). About 2.5 percent of those working in special day and residential schools and 16.0 percent in administrative offices rated themselves as very qualified. Less than one-tenth (8.0 percent) rated themselves as 1 (*not at all qualified*). Four percent of those in administrative positions and 12.5 percent in special day and residential schools rated themselves as not at all qualified.

In 2010, school-based speech-language pathologists were also asked to indicate who provided services to children with speech-language disorders who are English language learners (ELLs) (ASHA, 2010g). Almost half (49.5 percent) provided services to them in English; 8.2 percent indicated trained interpreters were used; 6.2 percent provided services to them in the learner's native language; 5.2 percent indicated a bilingual speech-language pathologist was contracted; 3.7 percent indicated reliance on untrained interpreters (e.g., family members); and 2.0 percent indicated bilingual speech-language pathology assistants. More than one-third (40.4 percent) had no ELL students. Of those who did, the median number of students in their typical monthly caseload was three in 2010, up from two in 2008 (ASHA, 2008b, 2010g).

These data suggest a need for education—both preparatory and continuing—for all audiologists and speech-language pathologists in working with individuals from diverse cultural, ethnic, and racial backgrounds. See Chapter 24 for more discussion of cultural diversity.

Medical and Technological Advances

Medical and technological innovations continue to have an impact on the supply of and demand for audiologists and speech-language pathologists. As an example, medical advances have improved the survival rate of premature infants and trauma and stroke patients, who may then need assessment and treatment for communication-related disorders (BLS, 2012b). Technological advances in hearing aids may increase the demand for audiologists. Digital hearing aids have become smaller in size and more effective in reducing feedback. Demand for them may be driven by those who change from analog to digital hearing aids, those who want new hearing aids, or those for whom the now less-visible devices are of interest. The development and application of augmentative and alternative communication (AAC) devices and systems also have served to expand the client and patient base.

Telepractice

Telepractice provides another example of how technological advances may affect the supply of and demand for audiologists and speech-language pathologists. However, it is emerging as a factor in and of itself and its impact remains unknown. Telepractice involves "the application of telecommunications technology to the delivery of professional services at a distance by linking clinician to client, or clinician to clinician, for assessment, intervention and/or consultation" (ASHA, 2011e, 2011f). It may allow clinicians to provide services more efficiently, more quickly, and to more patients. Individuals in geographically rural and remote areas, as well as those who are homebound, also may benefit through greater access to audiology and speech-language pathology services.

The use of telepractice by audiologists and speech-language pathologists may affect either end of the supply-demand spectrum. On one side, telepractice may result in decreased demand as fewer clinicians are needed to provide services. Conversely, an increased demand may result as individuals who previously did not have access to services seek the assistance of audiologists and speech-language pathologists through technology. Issues related to technology and telepractice are discussed in Chapter 26.

Federal Policy

The passage of federal laws and regulations addressing the needs of individuals with disabilities has resulted in a continued and growing demand for audiologists and speech-language pathologists. Federal law guarantees special education and related services to all eligible children with disabilities through the Individuals with Disabilities Education Improvement Act of 2004. This act addresses numerous key issues surrounding the provision of services related to audiology and speech-language pathology, including personnel qualifications, early intervention, ELLs, assistive technology, learning disabilities, Individualized Education Programs (IEPs), and funding.

The U.S. Department of Education reported that the number of children with disabilities, ages 6 to 21, served in the public schools in the 50 states and the District of Columbia under IDEA Part B in fall 2005 was 6,021,462 (U.S. Department of Education, 2010). Of these children, 1,143,195 (19.0 percent) received services for speech or language impairments; 71,484 (1.2 percent) received services for hearing impairments. These figures do not include children who have speech, language, or hearing problems secondary to other conditions.

Trend data suggest a continued emphasis on early intervention. The number of children with disabilities, ages 3 to 5, served in the public schools in the 50 states and the District of Columbia under IDEA Part B in fall 2005 was 698,938 (U.S. Department of Education, 2010). Of these children, 325,895 (46.6 percent) received services for speech or language impairments; 7,777 (1.1 percent) received services for hearing impairments. Again, these figures do not include children who have speech, language, or hearing problems secondary to other conditions. Note that of all the disabilities for which children ages 3 to 5 were served, "speech or language impairments" were the most prevalent. It is anticipated that early intervention services will continue to grow as the nation places a higher priority on prevention and early intervention.

The early identification and diagnosis of hearing disorders in infants and toddlers is part of the national public health agenda. As of December 2010, all 50 states and the District of Columbia had Early Hearing Detection and Intervention (EHDI) laws or voluntary compliance programs that screen hearing (ASHA, 2011b). As this issue continues to be brought before state legislatures, states may enhance existing EHDI programs or enact mandates, thereby continuing to increase the demand for audiologists to oversee and perform hearing screenings.

The No Child Left Behind (NCLB) Act was signed into law in January 2002. This act is designed to improve student achievement through greater accountability, personnel standards, and assessments. Title I of the act focuses on improving the academic achievement of disadvantaged students. Title III focuses on language instruction for limited English proficient (LEP) and immigrant students. The act may positively impact the demand for special education teachers, including audiologists and speech-language pathologists.

The Rehabilitation Act Amendments of 1998 assist Americans with disabilities in pursuing careers through vocational training and rehabilitation. This act continues to serve as one of the most important laws for adult consumers of audiology and speech-language pathology services.

The Assistive Technology (AT) Act of 2004 eliminated a sunset provision that threatened many assistive technology programs (ASHA, 2004). The AT Act funds state programs that provide assistive technology devices and services to individuals with disabilities, such as those provided by audiologists and speech-language pathologists. With ongoing federal funding, programs will have the ability to continue offering assistive technology devices and services to individuals who seek them. See Chapter 13, Health Care Legislation, Regulation, and Financing, and Chapter 15, Education Policy and Service Delivery, for more discussion of these issues.

Reimbursement

The BLS cautions that growth in the employment of audiologists will be restrained by limitations on reimbursements made by third-party payers (i.e., health insurance companies, health plans, or publicly funded programs) for the tests and services they provide (BLS, 2011). The BLS further cautions that growth in the employment of speech-language pathologists in health care settings may be limited in the short-term by restrictions on reimbursement for therapy services. Still, the long-term demand for speech-language pathologists should continue to increase as more individuals with disabilities or limited function seek therapy services. The BLS also projects that the number of speech-language pathologists in private practice will increase as hospitals, skilled nursing facilities, and schools strive to contain costs by increasingly contracting out therapy services.

Overlapping Scopes of Practice

Individuals from other professions may be perceived as competitors for the audiology and speech-language pathology market share. Overlapping scopes of practice may allow other professionals to provide speech, language, hearing, and swallowing assessments and treatment. According to a 2009 survey (ASHA, 2009e), 10.3 percent of health care–based speech-language pathologists reported that professionals other than speech-language pathologists were providing primary swallowing services (e.g., assessment, treatment, instrumental studies) in their facility. This figure is fairly consistent with those of previous years (12.4 percent for 2007 and 12.9 percent for 2005; ASHA, 2005, 2007). The figure for 2009 ranged from 2.9 percent of speech-language pathologists in skilled nursing facilities to 47.0 percent of those in pediatric hospitals.

ASHA recently surveyed audiologists, speech-language pathologists, and National Student Speech Language Hearing Association (NSSLHA) members about what they thought were the most important or "hottest" professional topics in the discipline (ASHA, 2011g). Scope of practice made the top 10 list for all three groups. In open-ended comments, some audiologists expressed concern about encroachment by technicians and hearing instrument specialists. Cerumen management was identified as another scope of practice issue. Quite a few speech-language pathologists commented on the blurred boundaries between themselves and other professionals in schools (e.g., early childhood special education teachers, general education teachers, ELL teachers, and reading specialists). A number of students touched on the use of speech-language pathology assistants or aides and how it impacts the role of speech-language pathologists in the workplace.

American Association for Employment in Education Data

The 2008 *Educator Supply and Demand* research report by the American Association for Employment in Education presents job market data on 62 education fields including audiology and speech pathology. The report indicates that the audiology field is one of 23 fields with "some shortage." The speech pathology field is one of 14 fields with "considerable shortage" (American Association for Employment in Education, 2008). These data are another indicator that the job market for school-based audiologists and speech-language pathologists will be strong in future years.

ASHA Job Market Data

In recent years, a survey item has been included on several major ASHA data collection initiatives to assess the job market for audiologists and speech-language pathologists. The question and response categories were patterned after definitions used by the BLS. The question reads as follows:

> Based on your own observations and experiences, rate the current job market for your profession in your type of employment facility and in your geographic area.
>
> 1. Job openings more numerous than job seekers
> 2. Job openings in balance with job seekers
> 3. Job openings fewer than job seekers

As shown in Figure 8–3, speech-language pathologists perceived far greater shortages of personnel in both health care and school settings compared with audiologists. Only 15.7 percent of audiologists responding to a 2010 survey (ASHA, 2010c) reported that job openings were more numerous than job seekers. Note that this is a substantial decline from 2008, when 30.0 percent of audiologists reported that job openings exceeded job seekers (ASHA, 2008a). Responses to the 2010 survey varied by the type of facility in which the respondent was employed. The greatest disparity between job openings and job seekers appeared to be in industry, where 23.9 percent of audiologists reported that job openings were more numerous than job seekers.

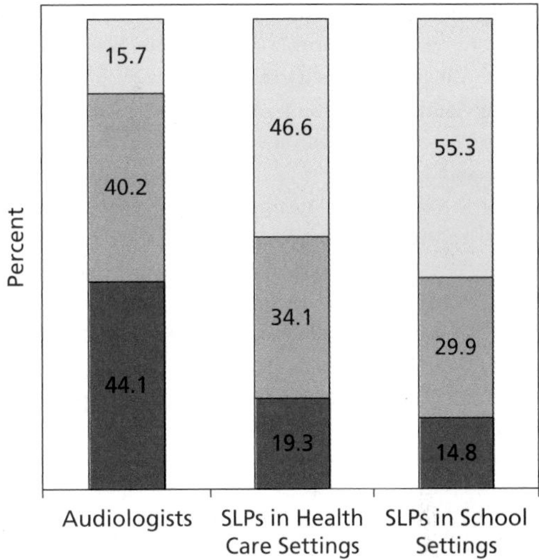

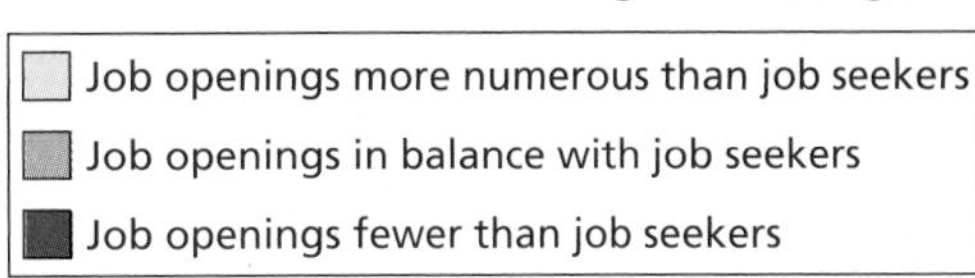

FIGURE 8-3 Reponses to ASHA Workforce-Related Questions by Profession/Setting, 2009–2010

Adapted with permission from 2011 SLP Health Care Summary Report: Number and type of responses and 2010 Audiology Survey Report: Number and type of responses. Available from www.asha.org, the website of the American Speech-Language-Hearing Association.

Almost half (46.6 percent) of speech-language pathologists in health care settings reported that job openings were more numerous than job seekers (ASHA, 2009e). Note that this is a decline from 2007, when 59.1 percent of respondents reported that job openings exceeded job seekers (ASHA, 2007). In 2009, the largest gap between job openings and job seekers appeared to be in home health/client home settings and skilled nursing facilities, where 61.0 percent and 56.2 percent of respondents, respectively, reported that job openings were more numerous than job seekers.

Across all health care settings, more job openings were reported by speech-language pathologists in the Pacific states (Alaska, California, Hawaii, Oregon, and Washington; 57.4 percent) than in other states (ASHA, 2009d). More openings were also reported by speech-language pathologists in rural areas (52.0 percent) compared with those in suburban and metropolitan/urban areas (48.0 percent and 44.0 percent, respectively). More than one-quarter of respondents (25.0 percent) further indicated that there were funded, unfilled positions for speech-language pathologists at their facility (ASHA, 2009e). Note that this is a decline from 2007, when 36.8 percent of respondents indicated that there were funded, unfilled positions for speech-language pathologists at their facility (ASHA, 2007). In 2009, the percentage ranged from 20.2 percent in general medical facilities to 35.4 percent in home health/client home settings.

In response to a 2010 survey (ASHA, 2010g), 55.3 percent of school-based speech-language pathologists reported that job openings were more numerous than job seekers. Note that this is a decline from 2008, when 71.9 percent of respondents reported that job openings exceeded job seekers (ASHA, 2008b). In 2010, respondents who worked in multiple school settings and administrative offices reported the largest gap between job openings and job seekers. Nearly two-thirds (63.7 percent) of those in multiple school settings and 61.5 percent of those in administrative offices reported that job openings were more numerous than job seekers.

Across all school settings, more job openings were reported by speech-language pathologists in the Pacific states (78.9 percent) than in other states (ASHA, 2010f). More openings were also reported by speech-language pathologists in metropolitan/urban areas (59.0 percent) compared with those in rural and suburban areas (57.0 percent and 52.0 percent, respectively).

Respondents who reported there was a shortage of speech-language pathologists in their type of school setting and geographic area were asked to indicate the impact of the shortage. Most (81.1 percent) indicated "increased caseload or workload" (ASHA, 2010g). More than half (51.6 percent) indicated "decreased opportunities for appropriate service delivery."

A primary objective of ASHA's strategic plan is to advance efforts that safeguard the discipline and professions (ASHA, 2011d). This objective includes addressing clinical personnel shortages. The intended outcome of this effort is a decline in the number of reported openings for audiologists and speech-language pathologists in health care and educational settings.

SUMMARY

This chapter provided a description of the demographics and employment characteristics of individuals in the professions and discipline. It also presented salary and job and career satisfaction data and information on first-year enrollments and graduations in CSD graduate programs. Steps taken to address the PhD shortage were also summarized. The chapter closed with employment projections and a discussion of factors that may affect future employment. These factors included the changing demographics of the U.S. population, medical and technological innovations, federal laws, reimbursement for services, overlapping scopes of practice, and personnel shortages. Data from ASHA and other organizations and agencies were used to evaluate the impact of these factors on the future supply of and demand for audiology and speech-language pathology professionals.

CRITICAL THINKING

1. How has the number of ASHA-certified audiologists, speech-language pathologists, and individuals with dual certification changed over the past decade? What are the advantages and disadvantages of having dual certification?
2. How does the ethnicity and race of ASHA-certified audiologists and speech-language pathologists compare with that of the U.S. population as a whole? What strategies would you suggest to encourage more individuals from underrepresented ethnic and racial groups to enter the professions of audiology and speech-language pathology?
3. Suppose you are a human resources administrator in a health care or school setting. What would you do to recruit and retain qualified audiologists and speech-language pathologists in your setting?
4. What variables affect the earnings of audiologists, speech-language pathologists, and CSD faculty?
5. How might the forthcoming changes in the general workforce (using information from the BLS) affect the future number of audiologists and speech-language pathologists?
6. How might changes in the demographics of the U.S. population affect the supply of and demand for audiologists and speech-language pathologists in future years? How would you use demographic information to help you in deciding where you might like to work?
7. Which federal laws or regulations might have an impact on the audiology and/or speech-language pathology workforce and in what way?

8. What is meant by overlapping scopes of practice? Give some examples of this. How does this concept affect the availability of employment for you?

9. Why is the shortage of doctoral students in our professions so important? How does it affect our educational institutions? What could the schools of higher education do to make doctoral study more accessible and affordable for potential students?

REFERENCES

American Association for Employment in Education. (2008). *Educator supply and demand in the United States*. Available from http://www.aaee.org

American Speech-Language-Hearing Association. (2002). *American Speech-Language-Hearing Association summary membership and affiliation counts for the period January 1, 2001, through December 31, 2001*. Available from http://www.asha.org/

American Speech-Language-Hearing Association. (2004, November 16). Assistive technology bill signed into law. *The ASHA Leader*. Available from http://www.asha.org/

American Speech-Language-Hearing Association. (2005). *2005 SLP Health Care Survey frequency report*. Available from http://www.asha.org/

American Speech-Language-Hearing Association. (2007). *2007 SLP Health Care Survey frequency report*. Available from http://www.asha.org/

American Speech-Language-Hearing Association. (2008a). *2008 Audiology Survey summary report: Number and type of responses*. Available from http://www.asha.org/

American Speech-Language-Hearing Association. (2008b). *2008 Schools Survey summary report: Number and type of responses*. Available from http://www.asha.org/

American Speech-Language-Hearing Association. (2009a). *SLP Health Care Survey report: Hourly wage trends, 2005–2009*. Available from http://www.asha.org/

American Speech-Language-Hearing Association. (2009b). *State licensure trends: States regulating audiology and speech-language pathology*. Available from http://www.asha.org/

American Speech-Language-Hearing Association. (2009c). *2009 SLP Health Care Survey report: Hourly and per visit wages*. Available from http://www.asha.org/

American Speech-Language-Hearing Association. (2009d). *2009 SLP Health Care Survey report: Workforce and work conditions*. Available from http://www.asha.org/

American Speech-Language-Hearing Association. (2009e). *2009 SLP Health Care Survey summary report: Number and type of responses*. Available from http://www.asha.org/

American Speech-Language-Hearing Association. (2010a). *2010 Audiology Survey report: Annual salaries*. Available from http://www.asha.org/

American Speech-Language-Hearing Association. (2010b). *2010 Audiology Survey report: Hourly wages*. Available from http://www.asha.org/

American Speech-Language-Hearing Association. (2010c). *2010 Audiology Survey summary report: Number and type of responses*. Available from http://www.asha.org/

American Speech-Language-Hearing Association. (2010d). *Schools Survey report: SLP salary trends, 2004–2010*. Available from http://www.asha.org/

American Speech-Language-Hearing Association. (2010e). *2010 Schools Survey report: SLP annual salaries and hourly wages*. Available from http://www.asha.org/

American Speech-Language-Hearing Association. (2010f). *2010 Schools Survey report: SLP workforce/work conditions*. Available from http://www.asha.org/

American Speech-Language-Hearing Association. (2010g). *2010 Schools Survey summary report: Number and type of responses, SLPs*. Available from http://www.asha.org/

American Speech-Language-Hearing Association. (2011a). *American Speech-Language-Hearing Association summary membership and affiliation counts for the period January 1, 2010, through December 31, 2010*. Available from http://www.asha.org/

American Speech-Language-Hearing Association. (2011b). *Early hearing detection and intervention action center.* Available from http://www.asha.org/

American Speech-Language-Hearing Association. (2011c). *State-by-state data on graduate education in communication sciences and disorders for academic year 2009–2010.* Available from http://www.asha.org/

American Speech-Language-Hearing Association. (2011d). *Strategic pathway to excellence: ASHA's strategic plan.* Available from http://www.asha.org/

American Speech-Language-Hearing Association. (2011e). *2011 Membership Survey CCC-A summary report: Number and type of responses.* Available from http://www.asha.org/

American Speech-Language-Hearing Association (2011f). *2011 Membership Survey CCC-SLP summary report: Number and type of responses.* Available from http://www.asha.org/

American Speech-Language-Hearing Association. (2011g, March 10). The top ten hottest topics in communication sciences and disorders. *The ASHA Leader.* Available from http://www.asha.org/

American Speech-Language-Hearing Association. (2012). *American Speech-Language-Hearing Association summary membership and affiliation counts for the period January 1, 2011, through December 31, 2011.* Available from http://www.asha.org/

McCrea, E., Creaghead, N., Goldstein, H., O'Rourke, C., Ryals, B., & Small, L. (2008). *Report of the 2008 Joint Ad Hoc Committee on PhD Shortages in Communication Sciences and Disorders.* Available from http://www.asha.org/

Messick, C., Currie, P., Hardin-Jones, M., & Lof, G. (2009). *2008–2009 Salary Survey of Graduate Programs: Preliminary report.* Available from http://www.capcsd.org

National Science Foundation, Division of Science Resources Statistics. (2010). *Doctorate recipients from U.S. universities: 2009* [Special report NSF 11-306]. Retrieved from http://www.nsf.gov/statistics/nsf11306

U.S. Bureau of Labor Statistics. (2011). *Occupational outlook handbook, 2010–11 edition.* Retrieved from http://www.bls.gov/oco/

U.S. Bureau of Labor Statistics. (2012a). *Labor force statistics from the current population survey.* Retrieved from http://data.bls.gov/timeseries/LNS14000000

U.S. Bureau of Labor Statistics. (2012b). *Occupational outlook handbook, 2012–13 edition.* Retrieved from http://www.bls.gov/ooh

U.S. Census Bureau. (2004). *U.S. interim projections by age, sex, race, and Hispanic origin: 2000–2050.* Retrieved from http://www.census.gov/population/www/projections/usinterimproj/

U.S. Department of Education, Office of Special Education and Rehabilitative Services, Office of Special Education Programs. (2010). *29th annual report to Congress on the implementation of the Individuals with Disabilities Education Act, 2007: Vol. 2.* Washington, DC: Author.

U.S. Department of Labor. (2012). *Civilian labor force, by age, sex, race, and ethnicity, 1990, 2000, 2010, and projected 2020.* Retrieved from http://data.bls.gov/cgi-bin/print.pl/news.release/ecopro.t01.htm

RESOURCES

American Speech-Language-Hearing Association. (2011). *Explore the professions.* Available from http://www.asha.org/

American Speech-Language-Hearing Association. (2011). *Start a career: Job search tips.* Available from http://www.asha.org/

American Speech-Language-Hearing Association. (2012, May 15). ASHA members: 150,000 strong and growing. *The ASHA Leader.* Available from http://www.asha.org/

Council of Academic Programs in Communication Sciences and Disorders
Website: http://www.capcsd.org

U.S. Department of Labor, Bureau of Labor Statistics
Website: http://www.bls.gov

9

Finding Employment

Rosemary Lubinski, EdD

SCOPE OF CHAPTER

This chapter focuses on the process of and strategies for obtaining employment in speech-language pathology or audiology. It is followed by a new chapter that discusses how to build your career in the professions once you have gained employment. Professional employment is the natural and hoped-for culmination of academic coursework and clinical practicum in your area of specialty. This chapter begins with a discussion of the paths a career in speech-language pathology or audiology may take. Discussion then focuses on how you can create a dynamic and individualized "game plan" for obtaining a clinical position. Major steps in this plan of action include creating a self-inventory, researching potential work settings, preparing a cover letter and resumé, and practicing interviewing techniques. Specific suggestions for accomplishing each stage are highlighted. The chapter concludes with a discussion of how to accept a job offer and how to approach a desired or imposed change in employment settings. New to the chapter is information related to Internet applications and resumé style, career fairs, telephone and meal interviews, and using social media in employment searches.

CAREER DEVELOPMENT

You are entering professions with good employment potential. Your search for professional employment as an audiologist or speech-language pathologist is actually the beginning of a career development ladder. An exciting and challenging aspect of becoming a communication disorders professional is that there are many settings in which to work, a variety of types of clients across the age span, and numerous opportunities for branching upward and outward within the professions. Although many of you will remain in your first professional position, it is likely that for a variety of reasons you will move vertically within your profession into supervisory positions; change jobs within your field and move to a different setting or client population; become self-employed; or continue your education and move into academia, research, or management. A small percentage of you will switch to a related field such as education or medical/rehabilitation administration or take off time for family care.

It has also become more common for professionals to bridge two or more workplace settings. Increasing numbers of professionals work in educational settings and "moonlight" in home health care, early intervention, or private practices during evenings, weekends, holidays, or summers. These professionals need to be prepared to meet the assessment and intervention needs of children and adults with a wide variety of disorders. Funding difficulties in health care in recent times precipitated some decrease in the availability of positions in health care and clinical settings and a move by some professionals to educational and private practice settings. It remains to be seen if this trend will continue and what long-term impact it may have on speech-language pathology and audiology services in health care settings.

EMPLOYMENT SETTINGS

Speech-language pathologists and audiologists work in a wide variety of employment settings. About 54 percent of ASHA-certified speech-language pathologists are employed in educational settings, including public and private schools, developmental learning centers, specialized schools such as schools for the deaf, language development programs, state schools for those with developmental disabilities, and colleges or universities (ASHA, 2010). About 40 percent of ASHA speech-language pathologists and about 75 percent of audiologists are employed in health care facilities including hospitals, residential health care facilities, and nonresidential health care facilities (ASHA, 2009a). Forty-two percent of audiologists are employed in private practice settings as are about one-quarter of speech-language pathologists (ASHA, 2008; ASHA 2009b). Table 9–1 delineates the variety of settings that employ professionals in our disciplines. (See Chapter 8 for more specific demographics of workforce characteristics of speech-language pathologists and audiologists.)

The majority (76 percent) of professionals in speech-language pathology and audiology are employed as clinical service providers (ASHA, 2009c). Such professionals are

TABLE 9–1 Primary Employment Settings for Speech-Language Pathologists and Audiologists

Educational Facilities

- Public and private schools
- Preschools and day care programs
- Speech-language development programs
- Developmental centers
- Head Start programs
- Day care and treatment centers
- State schools and intermediate facilities for children with developmental disabilities
- Special schools

Health Care Facilities

- Acute care hospitals
- Subacute care facilities
- Psychiatric hospitals

(Continues)

(*Continued*)

- Pediatric hospitals
- University hospitals
- Veterans Administration Medical Centers
- Inpatient rehabilitation centers
- Outpatient rehabilitation programs
- Hospital and clinic outpatient speech and hearing centers
- Residential health care facilities: nursing homes, adult care facilities, group homes, assisted living care
- Adult day care programs
- Nonresidential care facilities: home health, community speech and hearing centers, physicians' offices
- Public health departments

Colleges and Universities

- Academic teaching programs
- Administration
- Clinical service delivery
- Research
- Supervision

Private Practice

Corporate Speech-Language Pathology

Industry

The Uniformed Services

Research Agencies

Other

employed on a full-time basis, typically 35 to 40 hours per week, for either the 12-month calendar or the 9- to 10-month school year, on a part-time basis, or by contract (PRN). PRN means that the professional is paid on an hourly or per-service rate, generally with no fringe benefits and no guaranteed number of hours per week of employment. The compensation rate may appear high for these positions, but it may not include federal, state, or local deductions and may include only limited benefits or none at all. In a time of budget cutbacks, a number of settings have turned to PRN employment, whereby the facility pays either a private contractor or an agency on an as-needed basis. School districts with large vacancy rates may also contract with private practice consultants to augment their workforce.

JOB SEARCH

Some of you will be fortunate to obtain a job through your practicum, externship, or internship. Most, however, will need to actively search for employment. Finding and securing the best job involves a strategic plan. This process begins with self-assessment and job analysis, preparing a cover letter and resumé, and getting ready for and participating in an interview. Hopefully, these steps will lead to a job offer for you.

Self-Assessment and Job Analysis

The first step begins with objective self-assessment of skills, motivations, and constraints. This is your opportunity to view yourself through the eyes of an employer. This step is followed by an analysis of potential employment settings. Knowing yourself makes you better able to market yourself to an employer.

Self-Analysis The search for employment is affected by personal, economic, and job availability factors. You may be restricted geographically in the job search because of family circumstances, personal preference to remain in a particular area, or limited finances to support relocation. You may live in areas that have few available employment settings and lack opportunities to complete a Clinical Fellowship (CF) or a fourth-year externship experience. Appropriate positions may not be available just when you are ready for employment. Such factors may necessitate a geographic move. Some new graduates may have a commitment to a financial sponsor of their graduate education to work in a particular setting or area. Others may desire and have the resources to relocate to what they perceive as a highly desirable area at this stage in their lives.

The search for first employment begins with answering several critical questions about yourself:

1. What is my career goal at this time? What do I see myself doing in the profession of audiology or speech-language pathology in 3, 5, and 10 years?
2. What type of job tasks do I like to do? Of these tasks, in which ones do I have special expertise?
3. What type of setting(s) and clientele attracts me at this time?
4. Do I like to work independently or on a team?
5. How does my immediate career goal affect my long-range career aspirations?
6. What special skills, knowledge, and paid and unpaid experiences do I have that will make me attractive to employers of desired settings?
7. What special skills and experiences would I like to acquire?
8. What geographic areas are attractive to me as sites of employment?
9. What employment settings in those areas match my career goals?
10. What personal, economic, and job availability factors limit my search for employment either in my home area or in a relocation area?
11. What personal, economic, and job availability factors enhance my opportunities to seek employment away from my home area?
12. What factors will contribute to a feeling of job satisfaction?
13. What are my personal and professional weaknesses? How would I accommodate to these in an interview or job?
14. Who might help me in preparing to seek employment?

Answering these questions in an honest way is essential. List specific actions that describe your personal, clinical, and technical capabilities gained from academic, paid, and unpaid employment experiences. For example, what tests and procedures have you *administered*? What programs have you *designed, managed,* or *supervised*? Employers will also be interested in skills and experiences you have had other than those related to speech and hearing. For example, do you speak and understand a foreign language? Do you have particular computer skills, business management or leadership skills, or specialized knowledge of areas such as geriatrics or pediatrics? Have you had research experiences that would be useful in the employment setting? All employers will be interested in your ability to work as a productive member of an educational or health care team. Finally, ask yourself what aspects of a job are likely to give you the greatest satisfaction. Are you interested in direct client care or more interested in program development and supervision? Are you interested in working with a variety of disorders, or would you prefer to specialize? Are you more comfortable with children or older adults?

Never forget that you may have gained valuable skills outside the workplace. For example, consider the skills you gained from other types of activities such as those related to organization and implementation of programs with special populations. Individuals who have changed careers or who have managed their homes and families often have valuable skills that will be attractive to employers.

During serious consideration of these questions that arise during this pre-job analysis stage, some geographic areas and settings will be eliminated. You may feel that options to relocate are limited until your spouse completes school or because of the need to support elderly parents. Some of you may lack the finances needed to support a move to another area, to meet the costs of housing in that particular area, or simultaneously to repay outstanding loans while incurring the costs of relocation. Note that it is appropriate to ask potential employers if they are able to assist with these costs. Some of you may be willing to incur financial debt to pursue an especially challenging and professionally fulfilling position in a desired setting, with a special population, and/or in a geographically ideal area. Hopefully, you will literally be in the "right place at the right time."

Targeting a Position As this pre-job self-analysis reveals your employment options, certain settings and geographical areas will emerge as best suited for you at this point in your professional development. The next step is to learn more about the reality of meeting individual personal employment goals in those settings and areas.

Begin by making contacts through your own academic and clinical faculty. Be prepared to discuss career goals and personal assets and limitations. Faculty are likely to be aware of the scope of positions that match your academic and clinical preparation. In addition, through their participation in local, state, and national organizations and committees, faculty may know of positions available beyond the immediate area of the college or university setting.

A similar discussion with off-campus graduate practicum supervisors may reveal current or potential employment opportunities. Sometimes these individuals will not know of specific positions available in other areas, but they may know professionals in those areas who could be of assistance to you. This is called networking, an invaluable means of entry into the professional world. Networking is building alliances that may lead to information about prospective jobs. Such discussions with faculty and supervisors serve as preinterview practice and will also be helpful to these individuals in writing recommendations for you.

You may also meet potential employers or those who know of an upcoming job by attending professional association meetings and conferences at the local, state, or national levels. Introduce yourself to colleagues and tell them about your professional employment interests. It is good to have a business card handy with your contact information to give to the individual. This is one of those "You never know situations." Opportunity may be sitting right next to you at the program. If networking leads to employment, be sure to thank the original contact person.

Most academic programs will have some means of transmitting information to students about potential employment. Departments frequently receive announcements about jobs that they will post online, on a bulletin board, in a department job binder, or in areas where students congregate. Some student associations take responsibility for disseminating this information to their members. All of these sources are updated frequently. Contacting alumni from your department may also lead to employment opportunities.

Another source of employment opportunities includes employment listings in journals, bulletins, and publications such as *The ASHA Leader,* the monthly journal of the American Speech-Language-Hearing Association; *Advance for Speech-Language Pathologists and Audiologists,* a biweekly publication for speech-language pathologists and audiologists in health care settings; listings offered by local and state professional organizations; special employment bulletins posted in an academic department; national newspapers such as the *New York Times* (Sunday edition); and community newspapers. Some newspapers publish a special section devoted to employment on a weekday in addition to weekends. The annual conventions of the American Speech-Language-Hearing Association and the American Academy of Audiology offer special opportunities to peruse employment listings, list one's name under "Employment Wanted," and meet with potential employers on-site. Similar employment opportunities occur at conventions of state speech-language-hearing associations and meetings of other related professional organizations. Positions are posted online at the ASHA Career Center.

The American Academy of Audiology has a number of networking opportunities available on its website including its annual convention, listservs, social media, and online directories. HearCareers is its online resource for posting and finding positions in audiology.

Be sure to review the employment section of professional journals in related areas such as education, physical therapy, occupational therapy, and hospital administration. Job seekers interested and prepared for a position in academia might review possible listings in the *Chronicle of Higher Education.* Listings of governmental job positions are available through individual city and state departments of labor and the United States Civil Service Commission.

Career fairs may be offered by colleges, school districts, or other agencies where potential employers are available to offer information about their settings and possibly interview job candidates. Always have paper resumés available to distribute, and be prepared for a possible interview. Dress professionally and consider every interaction as a means to another interview or job offer.

The newest and frequently used source for jobs is the Internet, which provides copious information about job search strategies and access to information about all types of domestic and worldwide professional settings. Some sites may have nationwide announcements while others are geographically specific. For example, school districts frequently combine to create one website to advertise positions available in their specific geographic area. Check these sites frequently as information change is rapid. New Internet sources include social media such as Linkedin, Facebook, and Twitter.

If you apply through any websites, be sure to keep a copy of all your correspondence, e-mail addresses, and passwords. Internet applications should be filled out as completely, accurately, and error free as possible. See the Resources section at the end of this chapter for samples of sources of employment.

Remember that employers and human resource personnel now check the Internet to research who you are. The Internet is the twenty-first-century portal to information about you. You should do a number of thorough searches using Google, MSN, Yahoo, and any other available search engines to determine what information is on the Internet about you. Do not forget to check blogs, microblogs, location-based social networks, social networks, social photo and video sharing networks, and wikis for your name. Also check people search engines including PeekYou, Pipl, Wink, and Dogpile. Be sure to identify and sanitize if possible any personal information that may be considered objectionable to a potential employer.

Tory Johnson (2006) of ABC News states that employers will check for your digital dirt or all the "hobbies, photos, rants, and raves available on the Internet through websites, profiles on social networking, and comments on blogs." What is considered acceptable or the "norm" in college may be considered inappropriate to employers. Either delete comments about you or deactivate the features on social networking sites that are negative or may be perceived as inappropriate. Never complain about your current practicum or employment on social media sites. Be prepared to explain any such material that cannot be eliminated from the Internet. You want to carefully control your personal and professional images on the Internet prior to and after employment.

Yet another option for identifying employment in a target geographic area is to do some pre-employment research on settings that match your goals and skills. For example, if you are interested in working in an acute care hospital in Chicago, (1) obtain a list of hospitals accredited by the Joint Commission or the Commission on Accreditation of Rehabilitation Facilities (CARF); (2) review the directory of hospitals published by the American Hospital Association or your state health department; (3) contact the local professional organization for a listing of hospitals; (4) obtain lists of hospitals from the local Chamber of Commerce; (5) check the Sunday edition of major metropolitan newspapers for position announcements; (6) review the listings of hospitals in the phone book; or (7) check the Internet for a listing of hospitals in the target area. You can then research specific hospitals and review the information they present on the web. Yellow Pages on the Internet (http://YP.com) can be used to find specific addresses and phone numbers of hospitals.

A final option for seeking potential employers is to sign with a search firm. Not common in the field of communication disorders, particularly at the entry level, this is a more likely avenue for professionals seeking high-level clinical or academic administration positions and those willing to change geographic areas. Two types of search firms are available: those that work specifically for you and those that are retained by client hospitals or agencies to fill specific vacancies. If you choose to work with a search firm, it is prudent to have all details regarding expectations and results in writing before making any payment for this service. It is also wise to consult with an attorney or the Better Business Bureau before signing a contract with a search firm.

Pre-Employment Research Doing some pre-employment research on potential employers will be invaluable in clarifying career goals, in preparing a resumé, and in asking for references to tailor recommendations to a potential employment setting. The primary goal of this research is to optimize a match between your skills, experiences, and career objectives and the particular institutional and departmental objectives, programs, and needs. Answer the following questions by reviewing employers' websites and brochures and by talking to those familiar with the setting. To make a careful analysis of options, begin by making a list of standard questions to be answered about each setting. Following are some areas to include on an analysis sheet:

- Name of setting
- Address
- Phone number of setting, personnel department, and communication disorders department
- E-mail address of setting, personnel department, and communication disorders department
- Full name of person(s) heading the communication disorders department (include degree, if possible)

- Number of positions currently filled within the communication disorders department and number of openings
- Description of the communication disorders program (e.g., pediatric head trauma, adult neurogenic disorders, central auditory processing disorders)
- Gaps in the program that you could fill, such as assessment of patients with autism, phonological disorders, dementia, dysphagia assessment and treatment, instrumental procedures to assess respiratory and laryngeal functioning, hearing aid assessments, balance system assessment, augmentative communication system selection and training
- Availability of a CF position or fourth-year experience with the necessary mentoring to meet ASHA licensure/certification requirements

Although it will not be possible to visit all potential employers for a preapplication visit, inspection of the analysis sheet should reveal several settings that match your goals, skills, and experiences and that potentially have positions available. You may be able to arrange an informal site visit of these settings, thus providing more opportunities to know how to tailor an eventual cover letter and resumé to that particular institution (Baker, 1989). The site visit may also help eliminate the setting as a potential place of employment.

These site visits have a dual objective: You discover more about the program, and the program representative begins to know more about you as an employee. Even in times of economic constraints on communication disorders programs, there are potential employment opportunities. It is essential to call ahead and make an appointment with the director/codirector of the communication disorders program, the director of rehabilitation, or the director of the specific division in which the communication disorders program is located. In educational settings, the coordinator of speech-language pathology or the director of pupil personnel services is the likely professional to conduct interviews. In some large settings, communication disorders may be located in more than one branch of the facility. For example, in some hospitals speech-language pathology may be located in outpatient rehabilitation, neurology, and/or ENT. In some educational facilities, it may be a separate program or subsumed under special education, special services, or some other department. Audiology may be associated with speech-language pathology, ENT, or rehabilitation, or it may be its own department. You should never arrive unexpectedly, and after the visit, you should send a typed thank-you letter or e-mail to the host.

Continued Self-Analysis After selecting a list of potential employers, you need to continue your pre-employment self-analysis. This will involve objective consideration of assets and deficits versus the skills needed to work successfully in the target setting(s). For example, if visitation to a large metropolitan hospital reveals that 50 percent of the current caseload involves diagnosis and treatment of dysphagia and you have no academic or clinical experience in that area, this setting should be eliminated as a potential place of employment until continuing education and further experience in that area can be fulfilled. Although potential employers generally realize that few applicants, particularly those entering first professional employment, can be prepared in all areas, they will want to hire someone who can best fulfill the job requirements with minimal immediate on-the-job training. At this point, you have identified a number of possible employment settings and it is time to prepare a cover letter and resumé.

Cover letters and resumés may be sent either through traditional paper copies or via e-mail. Regardless of the style you use, it is critical that these documents be *letter perfect*. The following section includes general suggestions that can be applied to both paper copies and e-mail versions. More specific suggestions for Internet delivery appear later in the chapter.

COVER LETTER

Your cover letter is equally important as the resumé in marketing yourself to a potential employer. This is usually the *first* impression an employer has of you as a job applicant. The cover letter is a powerful tool in sparking interest in the resumé. A well-prepared cover letter and resumé are essential in obtaining an interview, the situation in which you actually "sell" yourself. Beatty (1989) maintains that the cover letter reflects an applicant's motivation, organization, and knowledge about the agency. Employers use the cover letter as a critical screening device even before reviewing a resumé. Considerable time should be spent in the preparation of each letter. Target the letter to the specific agency to which you are applying. Do not use a "one size fits all" cover letter. In *The Perfect Cover Letter,* Beatty (1989) suggests that applicants have between 20 and 40 seconds to attract the employer's attention and stimulate interest in the resumé. Detailed suggestions for preparing the cover letter can be found in numerous publications obtainable in a library or bookstore, in materials available through a college or university's career planning and placement office, or on websites. Many colleges have extensive materials, resources, and online examples to help you prepare your cover letter and resumé. These suggestions can be divided into those focusing on style and those focusing on content. Remember that this is a business letter and should incorporate business style. See Appendix 9–A at the end of this chapter for a sample cover letter.

Cover Letter Style Suggestions

1. Confine the letter to one page. Avoid a long letter. If you are applying for college-level teaching, administration, and research positions, you may need more pages.
2. Professionally type the letter or use a word processor to guarantee that the layout and design are stylistically appropriate for a business letter.
3. Use a 10- to 12-point font size that is clearly readable.
4. If sending a paper copy, use good-quality, 20-pound, 8.5-by-11-inch bond paper in a neutral color with matching envelopes. A white background is better than colored when sending copies via e-mail.
5. All letters should be originals, never copies.
6. Use appropriate business letter style, such as full or modified block style, including return address, date, agency address, salutation, body of letter, closing, signature, and typed name. Do not right justify or center align the cover letter.
7. Each letter should be personalized to the person who is responsible for making hiring decisions in your target department. Be sure to have the correct full name, spelling, title, and address.
8. Address the person by the appropriate title: Dr., Mr., Mrs., Ms. Never send a letter addressed "To Whom It May Concern" or "Dear Sirs." If you are unsure whether a person has a doctorate, it is best to research the individual so that you correctly address the individual.
9. Use complete, well-constructed sentences in an active voice. Avoid overly lengthy or complex sentences.
10. Check grammar and spelling. Do not rely solely on the spelling or grammar checker included in computer programs.
11. Put the cover letter aside for a few days and then recheck a printed version of the letter.
12. Be sure to sign the letter legibly.
13. Keep and file appropriately a copy of all letters.
14. Check that you have the appropriate letter with its matching envelope.

Cover Letter Content Suggestions

The cover letter should focus on your major strengths and accomplishments that meet the employer's needs. Do not repeat every item on your resumé. Generally, the letter contains three major paragraphs that complement the resumé:

Paragraph 1 introduces you, states the target position by name, mentions how you learned of the position, and excites the reader about you as a potential employee. You need a hook that draws the reader to want to know more about you. If appropriate, include the name of a person who has suggested that you apply for the position or the name of the agency employee who met you at a screening interview. Specify why you are a desirable candidate for the position.

Paragraph 2 focuses on your experiences and assets and how these might meet or enhance the needs of the target department or agency. Review your self-analysis and that of the agency to highlight how you can enhance the organization. Review your list of action verbs (see Table 9–2) that describe your skills and experiences and choose those that might provoke interest in your resumé. Include another paragraph if you must elaborate on some skills or experiences that are of special importance to this job setting. Impart a confident tone without bragging.

Paragraph 3 is the "action" section in which you request an interview, tell the employer to expect a call to arrange an appointment for an interview at a convenient time, and state a willingness to provide additional

TABLE 9–2 Sample Action Verbs

administered	edited	organized
aided	enhanced	performed
analyzed	established	programmed
appraised	evaluated	provided
assessed	examined	recommended
assisted	facilitated	rehabilitated
communicated	formed	researched
counseled	generated	stimulated
created	implemented	submitted
demonstrated	interpreted	supervised
designed	lectured	taught
developed	managed	tested
diagnosed	measured	trained
directed	monitored	undertook
documented	observed	utilized

information. State if you are enclosing additional information such as a resumé. Mention when you are available for an interview and how you can be reached. If you are going to be in the geographic area, mention the date. This paragraph usually ends with an expression of appreciation to the employer for considering the letter and resumé.

RESUMÉ

The resumé or curriculum vitae (CV) is the second important tool for marketing yourself to a potential employer. The purpose of the resumé is to secure an interview for a specific position. For job seekers entering their first professional employment, this document will be an initial presentation of their academic and clinical background. Remember that preparation of a resumé provides organized data to use in completing online Internet applications as well. Experienced professionals will need to review and update their resumés regularly to ensure that career developments such as additional clinical or administrative responsibilities, teaching, continuing education, and supervision are included. The major hallmarks of a quality resumé are that it is well organized, concise, prioritized, readable, truthful, and polished (Eubanks, 1991). Keep in mind that your resumé shows an employer how well you can prioritize and organize information (Nazareth College of Rochester, 2011).

You will have to decide what type of resumé fits your objectives and skills. Resumés can be classified as chronological, functional, targeted, or combination. Chronological resumés list your education, experiences and skills, and extracurricular achievements typically in reverse chronological order (most recent first). Most employers expect this type of resumé. Functional resumés separate your skills and accomplishments into categories that reflect your job objective. This type of resumé highlights what you have done rather than when and where you gained the skills. Targeted resumés emphasize your skills and achievements that meet the specific needs of the agency to which you are applying. Combination resumés combine chronological and functional styles.

Again, as in the cover letter, the suggestions for preparing a resumé can be divided into style suggestions and content suggestions. Many bibliographic resources provide more in-depth suggestions, and some are presented at the end of this chapter. Finally, the resumé should reflect you as an individual and not be a sterile, dull document. Avoid packaged resumés with "fill in the blank" formats. Several drafts will be necessary until one emerges that is clear, concise, creative, and reflective of you, the job seeker. Some suggestions for style and content standards are given next. See Appendix 9–B for a resumé sample.

Resumé Style Suggestions

1. Some job applicants may want to work with a commercial resumé preparation expert to enhance resumé style. Be sure to investigate the quality and reputation of the resumé preparation service. The work done by someone else reflects you, the job applicant, not the preparer. Some colleges also provide such resumé preparation or review services in their career placement offices.
2. The resumé should be limited to one or two pages, particularly for individuals entering the field. Those with extensive experience *may* require more space.
3. Preparation of an outline helps to organize the major information to be presented. The major words of the outline become the bold headings of the resumé. These headings easily alert the reader to important information.
4. A consistent chronological format should be used to present the history of education and employment. The advantage of listing the most recent data first (reverse chronological order) is that the reader knows immediately your most recent experiences and skills.
5. A resumé must be "readable" (Eubanks, 1991). This means that the font is an appropriate size, usually 12 to 14 points for headings and 10 to 12 for text; margins are 1 inch on all sides; headings are in bold or in all-capital type to focus the reader; and indentions are used to separate information and are consistent in style across the resumé. Bullets may be helpful in setting off information. Avoid a "busy" look to your resumé.
6. If sending a paper copy, use high-quality, 20-pound, 8.5-by-11-inch paper in a neutral color (usually white), as in your cover letter. Unusual colors or border designs should be avoided as a means of attracting attention.
7. Avoid artwork and backgrounds as they tend to be distracting.
8. Prudent use of varying typefaces is crucial. Headings should stand out but not distract the reader. Bullets may be helpful in setting off information.
9. Avoid centering or right aligning your resumé. Left-aligned text with clear and consistent headings, bolding, or italicizing tends to be clear and professional.
10. A resumé that is dense with information prevents the reader from quickly scanning the document and finding information.
11. Brief, jargon-free phrases are the best choice, and avoid the use of "I."
12. Pictures are generally inappropriate. You want your resumé to be reviewed with an objective attitude, which may be compromised if a picture is included.
13. The resumé must be checked several times on separate days for typographical, grammatical, spelling, or content errors. The resumé should not contain any erasures or corrections.
14. Someone else should proofread the resumé for both style and content. Qualified people to do this include faculty and supervisory staff, a college or university's career planning and placement office, previous employers, and colleagues. Check a grammar book or dictionary for additional help.
15. All copies prepared by commercial duplicating should be checked carefully. Ink smudges, shadows, jagged staples, and torn or missing pages reflect negatively on the job applicant.

Resumé Content Suggestions

1. **Identification section:** The first section of the resumé should feature identifying information, including name; current and permanent addresses; phone number for the applicant to be reached

during business hours of the job search; and business address and phone number, if it is appropriate to be contacted at that setting. Brenner (2005) recommends including a straightforward e-mail address, not something "cutesy" such as honeybunny@xyzmail.com. Also be sure that your voice mail has a professional greeting. Do not enter salary information.

2. **Job/career objective:** Resources differ in advising whether a career objective should be included in the resumé or cover letter. Some suggest it is too restrictive, whereas others argue that it focuses the employer on your goals. If an objective is included, it should be brief but comprehensively describe the type of position you wish to obtain. You may need to customize your objective if you are applying to different types of settings. Limit your objective to one or two sentences.
3. **Education:** List in chronological or reverse order your earned degrees, full name of college or university where they were obtained, city and state, and dates. Education is listed first by recent graduates or those applying for college/university positions. Recent graduates may include their GPAs if they are especially outstanding—at least 3.5 on a 4-point scale.
4. **Certification and licensure:** Briefly list any special certifications or licensures you hold or for which you have completed all requirements to date. This is important as employers will know immediately if you are qualified for the position or what supervision you might need to complete these qualifications.
5. **Experience or work history:** This section lists relevant paid professional positions, or in the case of new entrants to the workforce, practicum positions. The purpose of this section is to describe the quantitative and qualitative results of each accomplishment. For example, employers are interested in programs developed, skills learned, revenues generated, and individuals served. Information can be presented in chronological or reverse order: dates of employment/participation, setting name and address, and job title. You should list job duties, highlighting special components of the program (e.g., developed a kindergarten language screening program in an inner-city public school, implemented an in-service program on hearing problems of elderly residents for nursing staff). Use your list of active verbs in this section.
6. **Publications:** Any published books, monographs, chapters, or articles should be included here with full bibliographic referencing as seen in professional journals, or what is commonly referred to as American Psychological Association (APA) format. This is the place to include the title of your dissertation or thesis.
7. **Honors:** Include here any professional or academic awards or scholarships/traineeships.
8. **Presentations:** This section focuses on presentations to professional associations, including title, copresenter(s) (if any), name of conference, date, location, and whether invited or competitive.
9. **Professional affiliations:** This segment lists the name(s) of any professional local, state, national, or international associations to which the applicant belongs. Included also are special roles within such organizations, including committee chair or conference organizer.
10. **Continuing education:** This section is reserved for professionals who have participated in postgraduate training or education. It is usually listed after Employment History.
11. **References:** If references are included, they should be listed on a separate page from your resumé. Only the names of people who have given explicit approval to serve in this capacity can be listed. Recommendations for obtaining references will be discussed later in this chapter.
12. **Personal data:** Resources differ on whether to include personal information such as age, ethnic background, marital status, and number of children. On the positive side, this information reflects the job applicant more personally and often is the icebreaker during an eventual interview for the employer. Conversely, such information may be used to discriminate in subtle ways. This is a good topic to discuss with a faculty adviser or supervisor before you complete your resumé. If in doubt, do not include this information.

E-Mail Style Issues

E-mail applications, letters, and resumés are becoming common. First, remember that e-mail correspondence represents you just as much as hard-copy materials. You want the recipient to open, read, and not delete your e-mail (*Riley Guide*, 2010). Check everything carefully before you press the Send button as there is no way to retrieve the mail once it is sent. Check spelling of all words including the recipient's name. Be sure to use complete words and full sentences that reflect standard American writing style. Do not use any e-mail or texting acronyms.

You should have an unambiguous subject line so that the recipient will open your e-mail and any attachments. You do not want the recipient to consider your e-mail as spam. For example, "Application for Speech-Language Position" or "Follow-up on AAA Interview" would attract the recipient's attention. Never leave the subject line blank or say "Read this." Your e-mail address should also include your name and not an inappropriate alias. For example, Jane.Doe@biguniversity.edu would be more acceptable than talksalotgirl@something.com.

Always begin the e-mail with a personal greeting such as "Dear Mr. Smith." The content of the e-mail should state explicitly its purpose. For example, you might say why you are sending the e-mail and the nature of the attachments. Keep the content crisp, focused, and as short as possible. You will need a signature block that closes your e-mail. Give your full name, mailing address, e-mail address, and phone numbers. Do not include any graphics or background in your e-mail.

Be sure to follow the specific directions of an employer who has requested that you send a cover letter and/or resumé via e-mail. Always send your actual cover letter and resumé as attachments. Give the attachments clear names. If you are using Microsoft Word documents, include the appropriate extension such as ".doc." In general, it is best to avoid sending PDF files to employers. Keep a copy of all e-mail letters and attachments you send and the addresses of the recipients. Do not expect a recipient to respond immediately. Some professionals check their mail frequently, some on a daily basis, and some may wait to respond. If you have not heard from an employer to whom you have sent e-mail correspondence in three days, call the person as a follow-up. Finally, remember that e-mails are not secure. If you are sending a job-seeking e-mail from a computer at your current job, your employer may have the right to see your correspondence.

Be sure that your resumé is electronically formatted for e-mail delivery if it is not included as an attachment. If you are not familiar with how to prepare plain text or text-only copy, get advice from a friend or colleague. You should also have a resumé version that is scannable. A one-page resumé is best for e-mail delivery. Keep it focused, crisp, and uncluttered. Check that your resumé looks good on all e-mail systems. If you are posting your resumé on job sites, research the databases and read privacy statements before you submit personal information included in a resumé. Some experts suggest that you remove any personal contact information from resumés posted on large databases and simply use e-mail addresses designed specifically for your job search. Remember to delete your resumés from databases once you have obtained employment. Finally, never link your resumé to personal websites or social media sites. See the Resources section for suggested web resources on Internet correspondence.

Fax Delivery

You may also be asked to fax your cover letter and resumé to an employer. Be sure to have the correct fax details. Do not send fax documents unless requested. Also, call potential employers to notify them that the fax has been sent and confirm that it has been received. This may be an opportunity to talk to the employer about any issues. Fax quality is dependent on using white paper with a clear black font and setting the fax machine to high resolution. Many fax machines will provide a confirmation that the fax has been received. Again, keep a copy of all fax correspondence.

LETTERS OF RECOMMENDATION

Why are recommendations so important for you? Good written or oral recommendations are essential in separating you from other applicants with similar or even superior backgrounds. In choosing references, you should consider what the employer wants to know. Although employers are interested in academic achievements, they are more interested in clinical and personal characteristics. Through these letters or conversations, the employer should see a well-rounded, multidimensional professional. Employers want to know the following types of information:

- Do you have the professional skills to carry out the responsibilities of the position? What professional or student experiences do you have that will support these statements?

- What particular professional skills do you have? How have they been exhibited? How have these skills enhanced your present employment/practicum?
- What will you be like as a professional? Employers want to know about your ability to communicate orally and in writing, your reliability and punctuality in completing tasks, your ability to initiate without direction, your creativity, and your commitment to your position. They want to know if you will easily "fit in" with the existing program and if you are willing to grow professionally as demands change.
- What is your self-initiative growth potential? Do you demonstrate a sense of independent career development, such as voluntary attendance at workshops, creative problem solving, and participation in journal groups?
- How flexible are you? Do you demonstrate adaptability to changes in schedule, cancellations, and client needs?
- How do you communicate verbally with clients and their families? How do you communicate with other professionals?
- Do you have professional writing skills for diagnostic reports, daily notes, and progress reports? How familiar are you with a variety of report writing styles appropriate to the setting? For example, can you complete Medicare reports or Individualized Educational Plans?
- What will you be like as a colleague? Are you appropriately assertive? Do you know how to work on a team? How well do you take direction and criticism?
- What are you like as a person? Some reference to family or personal background helps the potential employer know you better.

Who Is a Best Recommender?

You need to carefully consider both the number and types of individuals who can serve as your personal references. Only ask people who are truly familiar with your work-related skills and qualities. Students entering the employment field for the first time generally rely on academic and clinical faculty as well as outside placement supervisors. It is advantageous to have a balance of academic faculty and clinical supervisors who can reflect on both professional and personal skills. Some first-time applicants may ask current and/or former employers who are familiar with their work ethic and skills. Generally, most applicants have between three and five references. Personal references should never be submitted. Only list people who have agreed to serve as a reference. Remember that employers will generally call some or all of your references even if they have provided a letter of recommendation.

Be prepared when approaching someone to provide a reference. This involves calling ahead and, if necessary, making an appointment to discuss reference needs. You should provide the individual with a copy of your cover letter, your resumé, the name of the target employer and intended individual(s) to whom the reference should be sent, and a brief description of the target position. This information helps individualize the reference letter for a particular employer. Students should generally include a listing of courses completed, grades earned in those courses, and departmental grade point average. Clinical supervisors might like to see copies of semester clinical evaluations. This is the time to highlight your clinical and academic accomplishments. Tell your references where you are applying, and if you know it, the name of the person who will contact them and when. Keep your references current on any changes in your resumé or other activities that may influence your employment.

If you are using a college's or university's career placement reference forms, these should be given to your reference person. These forms usually have a place for the applicant to waive the right to see the reference. It is to your advantage to waive your right to the letter because the employer then perceives that the letter is an honest and frank opinion of you. If you are asking for letters to individual employers, provide typed full names, full addresses, and stamped envelopes. Politely ask your reference writers if they are prepared to offer positive recommendations.

Job applicants who are not currently in a college setting but who want to ask an academic or clinical faculty member for a recommendation may need to "refresh" the individual's memory. This can be done by describing any special experiences you had with the reference writer in class or clinical practicum. Employed professionals seeking new jobs may find it difficult to obtain references for several reasons. First, the applicant may not want supervisors or colleagues to know about the potential change of jobs. Second, colleagues may not be in a position to comment on all of your skills. Other sources of recommendations include former employers and other supervisory staff with the proviso that the current job search be kept confidential. If at all possible, references should be sought from your current supervisor, or you should be prepared to discuss in an interview why this information is not available.

Students frequently ask reference writers to give them the letters of recommendation to distribute to potential employers as they go for interviews. These may be "generic" letters addressed "To Whom It May Concern." Not all writers will agree to this request. Some writers may prefer to send the letters individually as the need arises, and others may prefer to submit the letter to an on-file service in Career Services. Some will give you the letter in an envelope that has been signed across the sealed flap. Do not be discouraged if reference writers prefer to send individual letters, as they may perceive that this is more professional and to your advantage.

You should create a reference page and attach it to your resumé. Be sure all information is correct and current about your references. Include full name, title, organization, address, phone number, and e-mail address. Check all spelling and information. Some resumé resources suggest that you should not give your reference page until asked by a prospective employer.

If you are leaving a position, do not assume that a place of employment will give you a letter of recommendation. Some workplaces will document only that you have worked for them and dates of employment. Some professionals in your workplace may offer informal references for you that are off the record. Know the policy of your workplace regarding letters of recommendation, and if you are able to obtain recommendations, ask before you list anyone on the attachment to your resumé.

Be sure to send a written thank-you note or e-mail to each person who has written a letter of recommendation for you as soon as the letters are sent or you have an interview. These persons have done you a professional courtesy, and you may need them to follow up with a phone call or a form to complete. It is also polite to let your recommenders know what job you have accepted.

INTERVIEW

If you have been called for an interview, it means you are likely one of several individuals whose cover letter and resumé have sparked an interest in the employer. Consider the interview a series of phases: the preinterview, the interview, and the follow-up. Discussion of how to handle phone interviews is given at the end of this section.

Preinterview

Preparation for the interview is critical because this is when you really have the opportunity to sell yourself to a potential employer. Review of your preapplication analysis is essential, combined with information about the setting gathered from professors, supervisors, colleagues, or friends. This information base provides you with confidence to make knowledgeable and constructive comments about the position. Your preparation should lead you to answer both directly and indirectly the major question employers want answered during the interview: "Why should we hire you?" You should critically review your clinical assets and deficits with a mind to the target position, leading to a clear concept of what you can or cannot do. Be prepared to answer questions about these areas in a pressure situation. Edis (1989b) states that overestimation of abilities is likely to hinder you, although "openness about your faults may also suggest that you are a self-aware and honest person" (p. 55). You must be prepared to articulate how your skills and experiences can match or enhance the target position and setting. Although you do not want to present yourself as a false master of all skills, this is not the time to assume that the employer knows your special skills and assets. Use strong, confident language without being aggressive, and highlight achievements without being arrogant (King, 1993).

Practice and Role-Play Practice or rehearsal is the most important strategy of the preinterview phase. This step involves writing out potential questions and answers and rehearsing them by yourself or, even better, with another person who has some knowledge of the potential position. Role-playing with a fellow student or colleague is an excellent preparation and desensitizing strategy (Davis, 1989). Role-playing gives you an opportunity to "think on your feet" and answer questions that you might not have considered otherwise.

It also provides an opportunity for you to prepare questions to ask during the interview. Role-playing the employer gives you an opportunity to predict questions that might be asked. Your questions reveal a great deal about your preparation, interest in the position, and insight into the employer's programs. Video- or audio-taping the simulated interview provides opportunities to review and refine problem areas, particularly in nonverbal communication. On the other hand, you do not want to be so "programmed" for the interview that you appear robot-like and cannot easily adjust to unexpected questions. The interviewer is trying to get a sense of how quickly, logically, and insightfully you think, solve problems, and relate to people.

Types of Interview Questions Some interviewers will ask general open-ended questions that give you freedom to respond, such as "Tell us about yourself." When responding to this question, focus on what qualifies you for this position, including academic and clinical experiences. Another interviewer might ask specific questions about particular skills such as "How much clinical experience do you have in doing swallowing studies?" A third interviewer might present a case for you to analyze, for example, "We recently had a patient with a ______ diagnosis. How would you go about evaluating this individual?" One common interviewing technique is to ask applicants to provide examples of how they managed a situation similar to the job requirements. For example, you might be asked to describe a time when you worked on a team to develop a new program. Try to respond with specific information that reflects positively on your skills and accomplishments whenever possible.

Be prepared to ask a few questions during the course of the interview or at its conclusion. Avoid questions that are obvious or purely self-centered, such as vacation and benefits. Employers cannot discriminate against any group (age, gender, disability, etc.) in their hiring practices, but it is hard to prove why someone is or is not hired for a given position. If you ask questions during the interview that are limited to vacation, maternity leave policies, health and disability benefits, and sick leave, the employer may surmise that you will be taking time off during employment. This may make you appear to be a less reliable worker than another candidate. Asking a few insightful questions demonstrates that you are interested in the position and have been thinking critically during the interview.

The questions listed in the next section can be used as sample questions for role-playing. This list is not exhaustive, but the act of role-playing both the employer and interviewee is likely to generate more questions. Remember that the interviewer will not ask all of these questions but is likely to sample questions about your background, interests, specific abilities, and motivations. The Internet also offers sites that include possible types of interview questions; see the Resources section at the end of the chapter for some examples.

Possible Questions from Employer

1. Tell me about yourself.
2. How did you become interested in speech-language pathology? Audiology?
3. What are your primary professional interests? What clinical populations are you interested in? How did you develop these interests?
4. What are your long-term career goals? Where do you see yourself in 5 years? 10 years?
5. Why are you interested in the position of _____?
6. What types of clinical skills do you have that will fulfill this position?
7. How would you plan an assessment for _____?
8. What intervention methods do you find appropriate for a _____ case?
9. How much experience have you had with _____?
10. How would you handle a patient or family member who cried?
11. What experience do you have in completing reports for _____? (e.g., Medicare, insurance)
12. What computer experience do you have?
13. What would you do if...? Have you ever...?
14. In what ways might you make a contribution to our program?
15. What do you see as your strengths? Weaknesses?
16. How would you describe your interpersonal skills?
17. How do you handle criticism?
18. Tell me about your most recent clinical placement/job?
19. What did you like most about that placement? The least?

20. What problems did you have to deal with in that placement/position? How did you handle the problem?
21. What were your greatest accomplishments during that placement/position?
22. Do you see yourself in a supervisory position?
23. What is your salary requirement?
24. What questions do you have for me?

Polished Professionalism of Attire and Style

It is critical to project an image of polished professionalism during the interview. This involves tasteful, well-fitting, clean, and pressed classic clothing; polished, comfortable shoes; conservative accessories; and immaculate personal grooming. It is best to dress conservatively in a suit and to avoid conspicuous, trendy colors and patterns, ornate jewelry, heavy makeup, extremely high-heeled shoes or sandals, bare midriffs or legs, short skirts, and strong fragrances. Men should wear a tie and two-piece matching suit or dress pants and a sport coat. Check your appearance standing and sitting. It is prudent to wear your interview outfit during one of your rehearsals to check its fit and to solicit a review from a professional colleague regarding its appropriateness. Remember to check seams, buttons, tags, hanging threads, lint, and other tailoring before wearing the outfit to the interview itself. Turn off all electronic devices such as cell phones and pagers before you enter the agency and never take or make a phone call once you have arrived.

Before the interview, gather several extra sets of your resumé, pen and paper, and reference letters if not already sent to the interviewer. Carry these in a small briefcase or portfolio. Women should avoid carrying both a purse and a briefcase if possible. A frequent question regarding style of attire is "What if the professionals in the setting wear casual clothes? Won't I look inappropriate in a suit or professional dress?" The answer is no. You are participating in an interview and should dress for that role. Many organizations have dress codes that prohibit visible tattoos and body piercings, acrylic nails, denim, capri pants, sandals, T-shirts, sweatshirts, and so forth. If conforming to such a dress code would be personally difficult for you, then that is not the organization where you would want to work. Increasingly, hospital and clinic-based programs are allowing clinicians to wear scrubs, particularly if there is any risk of exposure of their clothing to body fluids. There are few professional settings in speech-language pathology or audiology where anything less than business attire would be allowable.

Location of Interview

Before the interview, you should check the location of the facility, parking availability and cost, and needed travel and time arrangements. Be sure you know the name of the individual who will be interviewing you. If the interview is not at the clinical facility, be sure it is in a public place and check the identity of the individual. Interviews at professional conventions are common, and you should consider this a formal interview although it may appear casual. Interviews in restaurants are also common and are discussed later in the chapter.

Never be late or super early for an interview. A 10- to 15-minute early arrival gives you time to refresh, introduce yourself to the receptionist and thank him or her for assistance, find the restroom, review materials about the facility, or complete further application forms provided at that time. Dispose of any cigarettes, chewing gum, candy, or breath mints before entering the building. Turn off all electronic equipment. All of these preparations for the interview will give you a sense of confidence to participate in the interview in a meaningful and positive manner.

Paying for Interview Expenses

If you are invited to an out-of-town interview, you may or may not have your travel, lodging, and food expenses covered. The person who invites you will discuss this with you at the time of the invitation. If you are unsure if the potential employer will pay for your expenses, ask but never assume that there will be reimbursement unless specifically stated. A few employers pay for the visit, but it is not a general practice for entry positions, and you may be expected to pay your own way. If your expenses are covered, the employer may or may not make travel and lodging reservations for you. You should in all cases keep a detailed account of your expenses and be prepared to submit the receipts at the time you seek reimbursement. If you make your own arrangements, be sure to keep your expenses moderate, avoiding what may be perceived as inappropriate expenses such as alcohol and in-room movies. Again, if you are unsure of what the employer will reimburse, check ahead of time.

Interview

The interview should be perceived as a conversation or information exchange between you and the interviewer. Consideration has already been given to your cover letter, resumé, and letters of reference, so this is your opportunity to convince the employer that you are the best person for the job and will "fit in" to the culture of the program. Krannich and Krannich (2003) state that impressions that the applicant makes during the first five minutes of the interview are critical in obtaining the position. Remember that this is your opportunity to make a good impression and give yourself an "edge" over other applicants.

The interview itself will progress through stages. The first part of the interview, the greeting or introduction, is when the first impression of you is formed. It begins with a firm handshake, eye contact between the interviewer and you, a smile, and a few preliminary remarks or "chitchat." These social comments usually focus on the weather, travel to the interview, common personal interests, and so on. Be sure to address the interviewer by his or her name, for example, Miss Smith or Dr. Jones. If you are unsure of the pronunciation of the interviewer's name, ask. Do not sit until offered a chair and take the one offered by the interviewer or the one closest to that person. Sit upright, comfortably, but not casually. The interviewer will lead with opening questions such as "Tell me why you are interested in this position." Another direction an interviewer may take is to encourage you to talk about why you are interested in speech-language pathology or audiology in general. You may be asked to describe your relevant clinical experiences.

Some interviews may begin with the most open of comments: "Tell me about yourself." The underlying agenda of this question focuses on answering: What kind of person are you? What kind of employee will you be? Edis (1989a) states that interviewees should be aware of the style of questions being presented and the focus of the interview. Do the questions tend to be open and allow you a great deal of freedom to answer? Are the questions closed, requiring yes or no responses with little room for elaboration or explanation? There may be some "leading questions" that suggest the expected response such as "How would you deal with a confrontational mother during an interview?"

Applicants should be aware that employers are not allowed by federal law to ask personal questions such as age, race, citizenship, health, credit history, disabilities, marital status, children, child care needs, and religion. "To be legally acceptable a question has to be related to the job and asked of all candidates, irrespective of sex" (Edis, 1989a, p. 47). You should be prepared to deal with such questions, however, because they may occur in both direct and indirect ways. For example, during the preliminary informal remarks, questions about personal life may appear in innocuous ways. You should tailor your answer to your advantage by discussing the job-related quality the interviewer is seeking. Unfortunately, not answering such a question may be subtly held against you. Another tricky question centers on length of time between jobs. Do not say that you have missed out on other jobs, only that you are looking for the right position where you can contribute your skills. Refocus the question by returning to your qualifications. Keep all information truthful, open, and succinct without being terse.

During the interview, you should be sensitive to your own and the interviewer's nonverbal behavior. Interviewers will be aware of eye contact, body posture, gestures, tone of voice, and rate of speech. Active, careful listening skills during the interview are essential. You need to pay attention to both the overt question and what may be underlying the message. The interviewer expects appropriate feedback through nods and smiles and relevant responses and questions. This is not the time to let your mind wander from the topic or situation or allow yourself to be distracted by anything in the environment.

Questions You Might Ask During the Interview

Interviewers will expect you to have some questions and will ask you for them usually toward the end of the interview. If the interviewer does not solicit them, ask them at this time. Be sure to carefully review information about the position and the facility prior to the interview and write down questions that emerge from that review. Do not ask obvious questions just to ask a question. Typical questions include, but are not limited to, the following:

- What assistance will I have for completing licensure and certification requirements and applications?
- Who will mentor my first year of employment?

- Where will I work? (if more than one clinical site)
- What materials, tests, and equipment will be available to me?
- What opportunities are there for continuing education?
- What assistance is there for relocation?

Be sure to write down the answer to the questions and thank the interviewer for providing responses.

What Is the Interviewer Evaluating?

The interviewer is assessing simultaneously your professional and interpersonal qualities, including intelligence; motivational characteristics; interpersonal skills and personality strengths and weaknesses; competence, knowledge, and experience; and interest in the job (Krannich & Krannich, 2003). In addition to assessing your professional competence and problem-solving skills, employers are evaluating your appearance of honesty, responsibility, stability, confidence, enthusiasm, and ability to communicate ideas clearly, precisely, and sensitively. You are being evaluated as much on personal skills as on professional knowledge and experience. Employers are looking to see if you can do the job and are a good fit for the position (Golper & Brown, 2004).

Employers are likely to have several equally qualified applicants for a position. Thus, in addition to strong clinical skills, the interviewer will be searching for the best fit: an employee who will match with existing staff and capably implement the agency's goals. At a time when many agencies are focusing on team care, the interviewer will be looking for your ability to share ideas, to act in a leadership role without being dominant, and to generate new ideas. The employer wants to hire an individual who will enhance the organization and will search for the individual who comes as close to the ideal as possible. The employer is seeking to determine not only professional interests and skills but also longevity as an employee and desire for promotion. Having reasonable career aspirations increases an applicant's value as an employee. Your goal is to project these qualities.

It is not unusual for employers to involve a number of people in an interview, especially if the position is one that involves working on a team. This approach allows the group you will be working with to get a sense of how well you will fit with the team and permits you to ask questions of individuals with whom you could ultimately work. This is a great time to ask clinician-to-clinician questions (e.g., How are caseloads assigned? Is weekend coverage required? What kind of documentation system does the facility use? Are staff members happy with that?) Even if you are given the opportunity to meet with clinicians or individuals other than the hiring manager, you will most likely end the visit with a brief meeting with the interviewer you met with initially.

There are a number of issues that you should not bring up during the interview, including the fact that you may feel desperate for a job, the job is desirable because of its geographical location, or salary expectations.

End of Interview

You will sense when the interview is coming to a close. The interviewer may have given you a timed agenda if you will be meeting with others. The interviewer will also send nonverbal signals that the interview is concluding, for example, by looking at a watch or asking if you have questions. Keep in mind throughout the interview that its purpose is to be offered a position. Thus, during the closing of the interview you should clearly articulate your interest in the position. The closing of the interview also gives you an opportunity to express appreciation for the interview and briefly summarize your strengths as they relate to the target position. This is when you tell the interviewer where and when you can be reached for further discussion about the position. A student's permanent address may be more useful than a college address. Currently employed applicants must tell the employer the best methods for correspondence. For example, if you are currently employed, give a home phone number for a message to be left on a telephone answering machine, a cell phone number, or an e-mail address. These methods allow you to reply to the interviewer at a convenient location and time.

If you sense that the interview did not go well, or you feel the setting is not a good match for you at this time, it is still important to end the interview with a positive attitude. Never let your discouragement or lack of enthusiasm show. The interviewer may be a source for future positions or may know of opportunities in other settings that better fit your skills and needs. A polite and sincere exit is important.

Telephone Interviews

You may be asked to participate in a telephone interview. This may be a screening interview or a first interview before you are asked to come into the agency and meet with supervisors or staff. Phone interviews may be with one interviewer or a panel of people in a conference call. Prepare as diligently for this interview as for an in-person one. Practice a phone interview with a friend before the real experience. In addition, simulate the ambience of an interview by dressing professionally, arranging for child or pet care to eliminate interruptions, and eliminating all background distractions. Never smoke, chew gum, or eat during the interview. It is acceptable to have a drink of water available. Use a landline or be sure your cell phone is well charged and in a strong cell-receiving area. Talk clearly and a little slower while using full, well-formed sentences. Keep a pen and paper handy to note information or questions you might have. Have your resumé in front of you and a list of prepared questions but avoid sounding as though you are reading answers to questions. Call the interviewer by his or her title throughout the interview. Finally, consider your nonverbal communication during the interview. Are you projecting a positive and confident image through the phone? Always thank the interviewer for his or her time. The interviewer will tell you the next step following the phone interview. If you are asked to do an interview using Skype or another Internet visual program, keep the previous suggestions in mind, dress professionally, and monitor background disruptions.

Meal Interviews

Interviews may include breakfast, lunch, or dinner with your primary interviewer and possibly a panel of other employees. Use your best general American dining etiquette during the meal. If you are unsure what constitutes appropriate meal etiquette, check the Internet or a variety of print etiquette books available in the library or bookstores. Remember that the interviewer is evaluating you in this context. You will need to converse and eat while demonstrating good table manners. In choosing your meal, follow the lead of the interviewer, though it is best to choose simple, easy-to-eat food that is not messy or has unpleasant odors. Most resources state it is best to avoid alcohol, even if your host is drinking. Avoid criticizing the food or being rude if the service is inadequate. Do not offer to pay for the meal, but be sure to thank your host. If you go to the home of the interviewer, be sure to mingle among the guests and, again, thank the host and hostess for their hospitality.

Postinterview Follow-up

Within two days after the interview, you should send a typed thank-you letter or an e-mail thank-you to your interviewer. Again, if you are sending a paper letter, appropriate business letter style should be used on 8.5-by-11-inch, good-quality bond paper. This letter gives you a chance to express your appreciation for the interview, renew interest in the position, briefly restate major qualifications, and explain any unresolved issues raised during the interview. Be sure to proofread carefully the hard-copy letter or e-mail. Follow all e-mail etiquette and style issues discussed previously and keep a copy of the correspondence.

Allen (1992) suggests that if an applicant has not heard from the employer within one week of sending a follow-up letter, a phone call to the interviewer is appropriate. This is actually a courtesy to the interviewer or hiring manager. The interviewer may simply not have had time to contact you and can now let you know the status of the hiring process. You should prepare for this phone call as carefully as you did for the interview through practice and role-playing. This phone call shows that you are sincerely interested in the position and are willing to go a step further to obtain the job. Monday is not a good time to make such a call as it tends to be the busiest day of the week. The interviewer may tell you the employer has selected another candidate. If the interviewer states that the position has been given to someone else, express appreciation for the interview and ask the interviewer to keep your resumé on file for future consideration.

Second Interview

In some agencies, a second interview (or third) will be offered to those candidates who appear most qualified for the position, sometimes called the short list. It is likely the applicant will be called to schedule this appointment. This interview may be with the program director or another individual in an administrative capacity within the organization. For example, when applying to an educational setting, the applicant now may be interviewed by the director of pupil personnel services, the principal of the school, or the director of special education; in a hospital, the meeting may be with the director of rehabilitation or the head of otolaryngology. In some cases, the second interview will also include an opportunity to meet either formally or informally with a select group of current employees. You may be asked to have lunch with one or more staff members. Be sure to have enough money with you to pay for your lunch if it is not covered by the institution. In some settings such as academia, there may be a reception at a faculty home for you to meet other faculty and their families in a more informal context. Try to circulate during the event to meet as many faculty members as you can.

Is This Where I Want to Work?

Although it may seem that an interview is one-sided and the interviewee is the only person being judged, an interview ought to allow an applicant to judge the qualities of the organization that will influence his or her determination of *is this where I want to work*? (Golper & Brown, 2004). When making that determination, consider factors such as the following:

- What is the reputation of this program? Will I be proud to say I work here?
- What is the financial stability of the program?
- What are the program's vision, mission, and values?
- Is the facility clean and well maintained?
- Are there sufficient supplies and materials?
- Will I have my own computer?
- Will I have sufficient privacy to do my desk work?
- Do people seem happy?
- What is the staff turnover?
- Are the support and clinical staff friendly, respectful, and welcoming?
- Do people appear to behave and dress in a professional manner?
- Are there others in the program who are a part of my ethnic or cultural group?
- Does the staff work as a team or independently?
- Can I see myself making friends here?
- Is there someone who could be a good mentor for me?
- Is the supervisor someone I can trust? Does he or she demonstrate good leadership?

Red Flags

While you are interviewing, you may get a "feeling" that this job has problems. Common red flags may include issues such as the following:

- The interviewer is rude, abrupt, or ignores staff as you visit the agency.
- The interviewer challenges you rather than inviting your responses.
- The interviewer takes numerous calls or accesses media during your interview without apologizing.
- You need to find your own CF or fourth-year experience mentor.
- The salary is comparatively higher than you would expect for your experience and the position.
- The person who previously worked in the position left after a very short time.
- You are not invited to speak with current employees or given other access to them.

FORMAL OFFER

Once the decision to hire you has been made, a formal offer will be made. Although many offers will be made by phone, a written offer is essential. Tammelleo (1989) states, "To avoid misconceptions, disappointments or possibly even a lawsuit, get the job offer in writing" (p. 74). The written offer should explicitly state the title of the position, period of employment, duties expected, salary, steps for salary increments, beginning date of employment, benefits package, and any other conditions of employment. Such conditions include appropriate supervision of the CF or fourth-year clinical experience, necessary certifications or licensure, pre-employment physical, employee evaluation procedures, continuing education opportunities, and expectations. Some of this information will be presented in an employee manual or handbook. Details presented in this document serve as an agreement between the newly hired individual and the agency (Allen, 1992). The more you know about the conditions of employment, the easier it will be to make an informed decision regarding acceptance or rejection of that position. Remember that the "cemetery of broken job dreams... is full of verbal hiring miscommunications" (Kennedy, 1998, p. A-14).

Whenever possible, consider the offer for a few days (not too long) before accepting. An offer should be accepted with a sense of confidence that this is the best position and that all aspects of the position are clear. You might discuss the offer with respected colleagues or individuals who wrote your letters of recommendation. Issues to consider at this time include salary, cost of relocation and living expenses in a new area, quality of life in the environment in which you will live and work, challenges inherent within the position, and opportunities for advancement and continuing education. These factors become even more important when an applicant has more than one offer at a time. If you have more than one desirable job offer, you may decide to negotiate with both to obtain the best working conditions and salary.

SALARY

Two frequent questions job seekers ask are: "Should I bring up the topic of salary during the interview?" and "What is a reasonable salary?" You should be prepared to discuss salary expectations and benefits, although interviewers differ on whether they will introduce this line of discussion during a first interview. It is best to secure the position before you bring up the topic. Challenger (1997) states that "bringing up money too early in the interviewing process is one of the main reasons prospective jobs are lost. (It) sends a negative message to the employer that you are more interested in yourself than the job" (p. I-1). Although graduating students are often not in a position to negotiate salaries, you should be prepared to discuss what you consider is a fair salary for you.

To gauge a fair salary, you should do some research in the area in which you are applying. Other professionals in the target geographical area may provide data on beginning or range of salaries. New employees are not likely to get salaries above the average for that position and geographical area. There can be a vast difference between geographical locations, usually related to the cost of living. Individuals with more professional experience need to factor in their experience and expectations.

Do not try to secure a job by naming a salary that is lower than what is considered fair for your educational level and experience in the particular setting and geographical area. This sends a negative message to the employer that you lack confidence in yourself. Similarly, naming a salary that is far higher than your background warrants will price you out of the market. If you do ask for a salary higher than average or have another offer that exceeds the one presented, be prepared to make a case for your qualifications or provide evidence of another better offer. It is more important to impress the employer with your value and potential contributions to the facility before you enter into salary negotiations. It is also best to refrain from asking questions about vacations, bonuses, and other benefits until a job offer has been made.

PART-TIME AND FLEXTIME POSITIONS

Some of you may prefer a part-time position so you can devote time to your families or other professional or personal interests. New graduates must know the requirements for part-time work to meet ASHA guidelines for successful CF completion as well as the mandates of certification and/or licensure. Part-time positions have become popular in many settings, and they usually pay only for direct clinical service and provide few or no benefits. Such positions may appear to have higher hourly salaries than full-time positions. In fact, these positions are usually paid on a strict per-hour or per-session basis and may not include paid time for traveling to and from client homes, report writing, or conferencing with caregivers or others. There may be a different, usually lower, pay schedule for team or staff meetings. Travel may be reimbursed at a specified rate per mile if you are providing home care.

It is important to know the salary schedule for services offered, reimbursement in the case of client cancellations, requirements for makeup sessions, travel compensation, and tax deductions from your paycheck. It is wise to consult with an accountant if you are doing part-time work to ensure that you are following federal and state tax guidelines. Part-time employers may require that you do a specific number of hours of continuing education per year. This may be provided through the facility, or it may be considered your own obligation to fulfill and document. Finally, clinical testing and therapy materials may or may not be available from part-time employers. This is an important question to pose during an interview so that you are prepared to provide comprehensive services requested. Again, discussion with an accountant is important so you have appropriate documentation for any deductions you might be entitled to in contractual work.

Flextime

Some employers may offer you alternative work schedules such as "flextime employment." Flextime allows you to work your full- or part-time job at variable times to meet your personal needs. Flextime includes flexible hours, workdays, holidays, or other arrangements as long as the job duties are accomplished to meet the mission and staffing of the agency. Some agencies have staggered start and ending times to the day. For example, in some hospitals, staff may work 12- to 14-hour days three days per week including some weekends per month. Flextime arrangements may be particularly attractive to clinicians who are also caregivers. Such options, when available, may reduce your stress and help you manage other areas of your life while maintaining your job. If this is not an alternative in your facility, you could propose it. Be sure to check your employer's requirement for full- versus part-time employment as this also affects your benefits package.

LOCUM POSITIONS

If you accept a fill-in position for a defined length of time, for example, for a maternity leave or for a CF year, be sure to discuss options with your supervisor for when the position ends. You should not assume that the position will continue. The position may end, or you may need to reapply for another position within the organization. Some employers may also have different salaries for the locum position versus the full-time regular position. If you need to move on to another position, be sure to seek a positive recommendation from this employer and leave your work in an appropriate manner for the returning professional.

BENEFITS

You likely will receive a variety of benefits while employed. The number and array of these depend on the setting, the position, your length of employment, and full- or part-time status. Some settings offer a hiring or sign-on bonus, ranging from a few hundred to several thousand dollars, as a means to entice you to accept a position. Find out when the bonus will be paid and if you must maintain employment for a specified length of time to receive it (Messmer, 1999). When evaluating salary, be sure to consider the entire benefits package, including retirement (401(k)) and defined pension plans, the number of paid holidays, fringe benefits, continuing education benefits, paid professional development days, parking costs, reimbursement for licensure and certification fees, reimbursement for professional association dues and memberships, uniform allowances, flexible hours, opportunities for overtime, and so on. In areas where housing is expensive, some agencies may offer corporate housing, a housing bonus, and/or a moving allowance. Some agencies have what are called "noncompete" clauses in their contracts, forbidding you from working for a competitor for a specified amount of time after leaving the agency. An assortment of typical benefits is given in Table 9–3. Remember that some of these benefits are for you alone, and some may cover family. Increasingly, both employer and employee contribute to cover the cost of these benefits. Your benefits package may be valued at 20 to 40 percent of your salary, and some options may not be taxable. Check your employee handbook or the personnel office for specifics.

RETIREMENT

While discussion of retirement may appear incongruous in a chapter devoted to finding employment, both young and mature professionals need to be aware of the retirement plans available through their employers. Retirement plans may or may not be available for part-time employees. Check your employee handbook or raise this question after you have been offered a position so that you know the retirement program to which you are entitled. Retirement planning is a serious and lifelong process and involves new financial tools,

TABLE 9–3 Possible Benefits Offered to Employee

Medical/health insurance	CF supervision
Vision/dental plans	Resource library
Retirement/pension plans	24-hour support from consultants
401(k) plans	Licensure assistance
Paid vacation/holidays	Direct deposit
Paid sick leave	Second language learning opportunities
Paid personal/educational leave	Tuition reimbursement
State/national dues	Opportunities for bonuses
Certification/licensure fees	Opportunities for research
Moving allowance/expenses	Travel reimbursement
Housing/housing allowance	Mobile phone plans or reimbursement
Uniform allowance	Child care allowance/dependent care
Malpractice insurance	Parking
Life insurance	Business travel insurance
Disability insurance	Commuting cost reimbursement
Health club membership	Cell phone for business use
Employee assistance programs	Profit sharing or stock options

including individual retirement accounts. While some settings offer traditional, defined pension plans sponsored and managed by the employer, more are offering "self-directed" programs in which you will both contribute to and direct the investment (Kiplinger Washington Editors, 2005). Good questions to ask your employer include the amount of employer versus employee contributions, time to investiture, transferability, and opportunities for extra contributions and profit sharing. Again, discussion with an accountant or financial planner may be helpful in understanding your retirement options.

SUMMARY

The focus of this chapter has been on how to secure employment. Key concepts can be summarized in single words: self-knowledge, research, networking, preparation, practice, style, and follow-up. Securing fulfilling employment is a deliberate process that begins with self-evaluation and research into employment settings. These analyses help you to tailor and prepare your cover letter and resumé—marketing tools that hopefully will solicit an interview. Careful preparation for the interview gives you confidence and helps you to project a winning image. Contacts made during interviews can serve as networks for future career moves. Securing employment may be a challenging experience but will result in the fulfillment of your career aspirations. Chapter 10 continues with how to build your career once you have secured employment.

CRITICAL THINKING

1. What characteristics of a cover letter and resumé attract the attention of an employer? What characteristics detract?
2. What skills and experiences do you have that will be attractive to an employer?
3. What are the key ingredients in a successful interview?
4. Why and how should you follow up after an interview?
5. What are the differences in the job search process for someone seeking first employment versus an experienced professional?
6. What are some differences between sending a hard-copy versus an e-mail cover letter and resumé to a prospective employer? Create a rubric or checklist for what your hard-copy and e-mail documents should contain and look like.
7. What are some important facts part-time employees should know about their positions?
8. What types of benefits are valuable to you at this stage of your life? What benefits might you want or need in 10 years?
9. A frequent question posed by graduate students is, "I'd like to work for a few years in a hospital and then when I have a family, switch to the schools. Is this realistic?" How would you answer this question?
10. After an interview, you felt that you really "blew it." How would you know this? What would you do now?
11. Prepare a hard copy of your resumé and have a peer and a professional colleague critique it. What needed improvement?

REFERENCES

Allen, J. (1992). *The perfect follow-up method to get the job.* New York, NY: John Wiley.

American Speech-Language-Hearing Association. (2008). *2008 Audiology Survey summary report: Number and type of responses.* Rockville, MD: Author.

American Speech-Language-Hearing Association. (2009a). *SLP Health Care Survey 2009. Workforce and work conditions.* Rockville, MD: Author.

American Speech-Language-Hearing Association. (2009b). *2009 Membership Survey summary report: Number and type of responses.* Rockville, MD: Author.

American Speech-Language-Hearing Association. (2009c). *2009 SLP Health Care Survey summary report: Number and type of responses.* Rockville, MD: Author.

American Speech-Language-Hearing Association. (2010). *2010 Schools Survey summary report: Number and type of responses, SLPs.* Rockville, MD: Author.

Baker, J. (1989). Preparing a curriculum vitae. *Nursing Times, 85,* 56–58.

Beatty, R. (1989). *The perfect cover letter.* New York, NY: John Wiley.

Brenner, L. (2005, June 12). How to land your first job. *Parade Magazine,* 18.

Challenger, J. (1997, September 14). How to negotiate salary: Don't settle for less than you have to. *Buffalo News,* I–1.

Davis, W. (1989). Simulated job interviews as learning devices. *Academic Medicine, 64,* 438–439.

Edis, M. (1989a). The interview: 2. Games people play. *Nursing Times, 85,* 45–47.

Edis, M. (1989b). The interview: 1. Rules of the game. *Nursing Times, 85,* 54–55.

Eubanks, P. (1991). Experts: Making your resumé an asset. *Hospitals, 65,* 74.

Golper, L., & Brown, J. (Eds.). (2004). *Business matters: A guide to business practices for speech-language pathologists.* Rockville, MD: ASHA Publications.

Johnson, T. (2006). *Dusting your digital dirt.* Retrieved from http://abcnews.go.com/GMA/TakeControlOfYourLife/story?id=1729525&page=1

Kennedy, J. L. (1998, September 12). When it's time to resign, do it with savvy. *Buffalo News,* A–14.

King, J. (1993). *The smart woman's guide to interviewing and salary negotiation.* Hawthorne, NJ: Career Press.

Kiplinger Washington Editors. (2005). *Retire worry-free* (5th ed.). Chicago, IL: Dearborn Trade Publishing.

Krannich, C., & Krannich, R. (2003). *Interview for success* (8th ed.). Woodbridge, VA: Impact Publications.

Messmer, M. (1999). *Job hunting for dummies* (2nd ed.). New York, NY: Wiley.

Nazareth College of Rochester. (2011). *Resumes and cover letters.* Retrieved from http://www.naz.edu/career-services/career-services

Riley Guide. (2010). Retrieved from www.rileyguide.com

Tammelleo, A. D. (1989). Ways to pin down an employer's promise. *Registered Nurse,* 52, 74–78.

RESOURCES

Securing Employment

ADVANCE. This free weekly publication of Merion Publications lists available employment positions by geographic area. For information, write to 2900 Horizon Drive, Box 61556, King of Prussia, PA 19406-0956. Website: http://www.ADVANCE-forSPandA.com.

American Academy of Audiology. In addition to job listings and opportunities for interviews at the annual convention, check for current job listings at http://www.audiology.org. For information, write to 11730 Plaza America Drive, Suite 300, Reston, VA 20190, or call 800-AAA-2336.

ASHA Publications and Website. The monthly publication *The ASHA Leader* has a section on employment opportunities. The ASHA website (http://www.asha.org/about/career) has numerous resources for job tips, finding jobs, resumé writing, interviewing, and salary negotiations. You may also post a job resumé and search available jobs online.

College Department Listings. Most college or university departments receive notices of job vacancies. These may be posted or available in a department administrator's office or in student areas. Check your local communication disorders department for such information.

Local Library and Bookstores. Check your local library or bookstore for the section on employment or business. There are dozens of texts on topics such as interviewing, resumé preparation, and follow-up methods.

Professional Conventions. There is a Placement Center at the annual ASHA convention held each November. State conventions may also have the same service.

State and School District Websites. Individual states may have listings of jobs. For example, in New York State, search the term "NYS Teaching Jobs" and you will be directed to job listings in educational settings in that state. Many school districts list their available positions online.

Federal Government Uniformed Services Positions

Air Force (civilian)
Civilian Personnel Headquarters
U.S. Air Force, The Pentagon
Washington, DC 20331
Phone: 703-697-3127

Air Force (military position)
U.S. Air Force Health Professions
4815 Fredericksburg Road
San Antonio, TX 78229-3627
Phone: 210-341-6802

Dependent Schools on Military Bases
Department of Defense
Office of Dependent Schools
4040 N. Fairfax
Arlington, VA 22203
Phone: 703-696-3033

Navy
U.S. Navy Recruiting District Washington
Presidential Building, Room 285, 6525 Belcrest Road
Hyattsville, MD 20782-2082
Phone: 301-394-0500

U.S. Public Health Service Recruitment
500 Fishers Lane 4A-18
Rockville, MD 20857
Phone: 800-279-1605
Website: http://www.usphs.gov

Internet Sources

Note: The following sources are fluid and should be checked periodically for their availability and current Internet addresses.

Advance Publications
http://www.ADVANCEforSPandA.com

Allied Healthcare Professionals
http://www.AlliedVIP.com

American Hearing Aid Associates
http://www.ahaanet.com/

America's Health Care Source
http://www.healthcaresource.com

America's Job Bank
http://www.jobsearch.org

ASHA
http://www.asha.org/careers/

Audiology Jobs
http://www.audiologyJobs.net

Audiology Job Web
http://www.audiologyinfo.com/websites/jobweb

Audiologyonline.com
http://www.audiologyonline.com

Career Builder.com
http://www.careerbuilder.com

Career Path
http://www.careerpath.com

craigslist
http://craigslist.org

HireTherapy.com
http://www.ihiretherapy.com

MedHunters
http://www.medhunters.com

MedSearch
http://www.medsearchcorp.com

MiracleWorkers
http://www.miracleworkers.com

Monster.com
http://www.monster.com

Rehab.Career.com
http://www.rehabcareer.com

Rehab Quest
http://www.rehabquest.com

Rehabworld.com
http://rehabworld.com

SLPJOB.com
http://www.slpjob.com

Speech Pathology.com
http://www.speechpathology.com

Therapy Jobs
http://www.therapyjobs.com

Sample Interview Questions

http://www.best-interview-strategies.com/questions.html

http://www.espan.com/docs/intprac.html

http://www.studentcenter.com/brief/virtual/virtual/htm

Internet Resumé Preparation Sources Examples

CollegeGrad.com
http://www.collegegrad.com/jobsearch/Best-College-Resumes

The Damn Good Resume
http://www.damngood.com

Riley Guide
http://www.rileyguide.com

Susan Ireland's Resume Site
http://susanireland.com/resume

State and Local Association Resources

Contact your state or local professional association to determine if it has a job listing or matching service. For state association contact information, visit ASHA's website, http://www.asha.org.

Appendix 9-A

Sample Cover Letter

123 Prescott Avenue
Rochester, New York 14226
March 29, 2012

Rochelle Peteers, PhD
Director Audiology Program
Fairwell Rehabilitation Hospital
5342 Burroughs Way
Toronto, ON M3B 2R2
Canada

Dear Dr. Peteers:

I am very interested in the position of clinical audiologist at Fairwell Rehabilitation Hospital. I was informed of this position by my recent fourth-year clinical experience supervisor, Dr. Bernard Trippe, who is in private audiology practice in Rochester, New York. I will receive my AuD from the University of Buffalo on June 1, 2012, by which time I will have met all requirements for CASLPA registration and New York State Licensure.

Given the cultural and linguistic diversity of your clientele, I understand your clinic's growing need for foreign language expertise. As a clinician proficient in six languages, including English, Spanish, Italian, French, Mandarin, and Cantonese, I am uniquely suited to helping the Fairwell Rehabilitation Hospital Audiology Program reach a higher level of client service—one that truly meets the needs of the multiethnic Greater Toronto area.

During my doctoral program at the University of Buffalo, I provided more than 3,000 hours of diagnostic and counseling services to children and adults in clinic, hospital, education, and private practice settings. I earned more than 300 hours in fitting digital hearing aids. My culminating project focused on follow-up audiology services for children who have received a cochlear implant. I presented the results of my study at a recent convention of the American Academy of Audiology in Baltimore, Maryland. I was also recipient of the Jack Katz Scholarship for my work with school-age children with central auditory processing disorders.

I believe that my skills and experience would enable me to make a valuable contribution to the Fairwell Rehabilitation Hospital, and I would greatly appreciate an opportunity to discuss my qualifications with you in person. I will call within the coming week to arrange an appointment as your schedule allows. I can be reached by telephone at 716-839-5555 at any time, or by e-mail at lincsmith21@abcd.edu.

Sincerely,

Linda Chau-Smith

Appendix 9-B

Sample Resumé

Johanna B. Smith
jbsmith@abcd.edu

25 Devon Lake Lane
Buffalo, NY 14226
(716) 555-6629

EDUCATION

University at Buffalo, Buffalo, NY
MA in Speech-Language Pathology, May 2012
Member of National Student Speech-Language-Hearing Association
Research in Literacy Scholarship
Who's Who Among Students in American Universities and Colleges

Cornell University, Ithaca, NY
BA in Spanish and Linguistics, May 2009
Graduated Summa Cum Laude, Phi Beta Kappa

PRACTICUM EXPERIENCES

Graduate Clinician Speech-Language Pathology

Waterville Elementary School, Buffalo, NY January–May 2012

- Provided assessment and intervention services for severely impaired bilingual children in individual and group settings
- Presented a six-week communication enhancement education program for Spanish-speaking parents
- Conducted hearing screenings for preschool program
- Developed Individual Education Programs for school-age children

Hardwick Neurological Hospital, Buffalo, NY September–December 2011

- Provided assessment and intervention clinical services for outpatient adult aphasia program
- Conducted weekly adult aphasia group program
- Provided assistive communication assessments for children with severe neurological impairments
- Assisted with bedside and videofluoroscopic swallowing evaluations

University at Buffalo Speech-Language and Hearing Clinic January–August 2011

- Provided comprehensive diagnostic assessments and therapy for adults and children with aphasia, motor speech disorders, phonological disorders, voice disorders, and stuttering in individual and group settings
- Conducted intensive six-week group language program for high school students

- Performed hearing screenings for elders at Amherst Senior Center
- Conducted weekly speech and language screenings at Bright Beginnings Head Start Program

VOLUNTEER

Literacy Volunteers of America Buffalo Branch September 2010–present

PRESENTATION

Smith, J., and Duncan, J. (April 2011). *Techniques for Enhancing Language and Literacy of Older Students.* Paper presented at the Annual Convention of New York State Speech-Language-Hearing Association, Saratoga Springs, New York.

SPECIAL ABILITIES

Fluent in Spanish and American Sign Language

Program variety of assistive and augmentative devices

REFERENCES WILL BE SENT UPON REQUEST

10

Building Your Career

Marva Mount, MA
Melanie W. Hudson, MA

SCOPE OF CHAPTER

This chapter is written by two professionals who have more than 60 years of combined professional experience in a variety of settings in addition to volunteer service to professional associations. Professional experience reveals particular issues that are as important to building your career as your technical expertise and knowledge. We begin with your first year of professional practice and the issues you will face. We then move to what it is like to be a mentor/preceptor, work ethics and professional codes of ethics, organization, time management, productivity, teamwork, politics in the workplace, networking, performance evaluations, advancement, and factors to consider when changing employment. We examine how each of these issues plays a distinct part in professional growth and success.

YOUR FIRST YEAR OF CLINICAL PRACTICE

You should be very pleased that you have obtained employment in your first professional clinical position. It is now your responsibility to know what licensure and teacher or other professional certifications you will need to obtain, the details of the process, the requirements, the forms to complete, and the deadlines that must be met. Keep in mind that you may not stay in this position forever, and thus, it is best to consider all your options regarding licensure and certification. This is also the time to sit down with your mentor and discuss your schedule, specific responsibilities, materials, equipment, and anything else that will help you get started. Review your department's policies and procedures manual, and take a look at sample diagnostic protocols and reports; observe others working; and get a real feel for what the job entails. Meet the other professionals with whom you will be working and administrative/support staff so that you know who can help you when you have questions. You are no longer a student, and you will be expected to be "ready to go" with less direct supervision.

THE CLINICAL FELLOWSHIP EXPERIENCE AND THE AuD CLINICAL PRACTICUM

Although some employers and work settings do not require ASHA certification, you should make every attempt to complete the certification process as you begin your career. As part of the interview process, you should have determined that your employer will provide a proper Clinical Fellowship (CF) experience for you, including a designated mentor and any additional support you will need to complete your CF experience in accordance with ASHA (1997) requirements. Therefore, both you and your mentor need to learn the requirements for certification completion.

The Speech-Language Pathology Clinical Fellowship (SLPCF) leading to ASHA (1997) certification consists of a minimum of 36 weeks of full-time (minimum 35 hours per week) clinical practice, or no less than 1,260 hours accumulated within 48 months of the beginning date of the CF experience. Professional experience of less than five hours per week may not be counted toward the SLPCF, nor can experience of more than 35 hours per week be used to shorten the length of the experience. At least 80 percent of the total hours must be in direct clinical contact, including assessment, diagnosis, evaluation, screening, treatment, family/client consultation, and/or counseling related to the management of the disorders that fit within the scope of practice. Therefore, *the length of the CF experience may vary according to the productivity level in the various types of work settings.*

Mentors of clinical fellows must engage in no fewer than 36 supervisory activities during the CF experience, including six hours of on-site observations during each third, or *segment*, of the experience, for a total of 18 hours of on-site observation. Use of real-time, interactive video and audio conferencing technology is permitted as a form of on-site observation. The other 18 monitoring activities may be through correspondence, telephone, and the like and may include evaluation of written reports, discussions with professional colleagues of the CF, and so on. Clinical fellows should maintain a log of all on-site visits and, when possible, other monitoring activities. It is also *the responsibility of clinical fellows* to ensure that their mentors are fulfilling the necessary monitoring requirements throughout the experience.

Assessment of the clinical fellow's performance may be both informal and formal, but one formal means of assessment must be the Clinical Fellowship Skills Report and Rating Form. The rating form portion is the Clinical Fellowship Skills Inventory (CFSI), a scale designed along a five-point continuum that is completed at three intervals (segments) during the CF experience. Clinical fellows should complete this rating form with their mentors. A minimum score of 3 on the core skills in the final segment of the experience is required to complete the CF experience. When all requirements for completion of the CF experience have been met, the SLPCF Report and Rating Form is completed jointly by the clinical fellow and the mentor and submitted to ASHA. Individual states may also require submission of the SLPCF Report and Rating Form to their respective licensure boards. Again, it is the responsibility of CFs to know what the requirements may be for the state in which they are practicing, understanding that ASHA will defer to a state's licensure or certification requirements that are more stringent than those of ASHA. The summative assessment used for ASHA certification is the Praxis series examination in speech-language pathology administered by the Educational Testing Service. Applicants for certification need to score a minimum of 600 to obtain the CCC in speech-language pathology within two years of graduation.

To meet ASHA certification requirements in audiology, all academic coursework and clinical practicum must have been initiated and completed in a program that holds accreditation by the Council on Academic Accreditation in Audiology and Speech-Language Pathology (CAA). Effective January 1, 2012, all applicants for audiology certification are required to have an earned doctoral degree. Although many accredited clinical doctoral programs in audiology offer the Doctor of Audiology (AuD) degree, the Council for Clinical Certification's (CFCC) requirement for an earned doctoral degree does not exclude any specific designator (PhD, EdD, or ScD) to meet this standard. The graduate degree may be in any area as long as completed coursework and clinical practicum are sufficient to successfully meet the knowledge and skill requirements mandated by the audiology certification standards.

Applicants for ASHA certification in audiology must complete 1,820 hours of supervised clinical practicum at the graduate level. Hours may be counted for direct patient/client contact, consultation, record keeping, and administrative duties relevant to audiology service delivery. Supervision must be provided by individuals who hold the ASHA Certificate of Clinical Competence (CCC) in audiology and must be sufficient to ensure the welfare of the patient and the student in accordance with the ASHA Code of Ethics. The amount of supervision must also be appropriate to the student's level of training, education, experience, and competence.

Supervision must include direct observations, guidance, and feedback to permit the student to monitor, evaluate, improve performance, and develop clinical competence. ASHA policy allows students to receive pay for services they provide within the clinical practicum setting. However, some academic programs or state licensure laws may have policies that prohibit students from being paid for their practicum work. In such cases, ASHA defers to the university's or state's decision about such payment.

Upon completion of the required coursework and supervised clinical practicum, the Application for Certificate of Clinical Competence in Audiology is submitted to ASHA, including the verification of receipt of graduate degree. The summative assessment used for ASHA certification is the Praxis series examination in audiology administered by the Educational Testing Service, and applicants need to score a minimum of 600 to obtain the CCC in audiology.

Once the CCC has been awarded in either speech-language pathology or audiology, ASHA Certification Maintenance Standards require that all certificate holders (CCC-A and CCC-SLP) must accumulate 30 Certification Maintenance Hours (CMHs) of professional development during each three-year certification maintenance interval to maintain their ASHA Certificates of Clinical Competence.

The American Board of Audiology (ABA) (2011) offers provisional certification for those doctoral students who have completed their required coursework in an AuD program in addition to 375 contact hours of patient care. These are the same hours that are accrued as practicum experience while taking the first two or three years of audiology coursework in an AuD program. These hours may be obtained on or off campus and not necessarily in any particular sequence, as long as they are directly supervised by a licensed audiologist. All hours should be documented, typically on a form provided by the individual university program. These hours do not count toward the 2,000 hours of mentored professional practice required for ABA board certification.

For the student in an AuD program, the required 2,000 hours of mentored professional practice is equivalent to the residency, or 12 months of mentored work in audiology. The supervisor (preceptor) must hold a state license and/or be a certified ABA audiologist. The individual seeking ABA Board certification has two years in which to accrue the required 2,000 contact hours. Upon completion of the mentored professional practice, and when a minimum score of 600 has been achieved on the national exam in audiology, the Professional Practice Summary and Verification Form is submitted to the ABA, along with academic transcripts. Once ABA Board certification has been earned, it is valid for three years during which time 60 hours of approved continuing education must be acquired. Note that requirements for certification from ASHA and AAA may change, and it is your responsibility to monitor these changes as they apply to you. Do not depend on your employer to monitor any changes in certification or licensure.

MENTORING

"Mentoring works best when it focuses on the entire person versus focusing on skill development alone." (Harvard Business Review)

As you begin your career in the field of speech-language pathology or audiology, you will require the support and guidance of a mentor or preceptor as you work toward establishing yourself as an accomplished professional. Your mentor or preceptor serves as a coach or guide, employing less of a "hands-on" but more of an indirect style of supervision than you experienced as a student clinician.

In its *Gathering Place Mentoring Manual*, ASHA explains that mentors provide a support system during critical stages of career development. This helpful tool describes a mentor as a good listener, knowledgeable, nonjudgmental, candid, and honest. It explains that a mentor is one who provides constructive feedback and networks to find and provide resources to assist the mentee with gaining personal success. Finally, a mentor is one who is willing and able to devote the time required to develop skills in others while being eager to learn themselves.

A mentor/preceptor may be assigned to you within your work setting, or you may be required to identify one. The ASHA website has information on how to find a mentor, if necessary. A mentor or preceptor is typically a more senior, respected professional in your field who will take a personal interest in your career development. It is important that you establish a good working relationship with your mentor or preceptor to gain the maximum benefit from this worthwhile relationship, which is collaborative in nature (ASHA, 2008a).

You and your mentor/preceptor should discuss how often you will be communicating and what modes of communication work best for each of you. Frequent contact, at least initially, is important to build trust and establish a mutual respect. This contact will gradually allow for each person to respect the experiences and views of the other, even when not in agreement. It will also serve to establish the relationship as a two-way street to promote flexibility and enjoyment.

At the first meeting, you and your mentor/preceptor will work together to establish goals that offer you a challenge as you grow professionally. As you tackle these goals together, ASHA (2008b) recommends that you describe and measure your own progress and achievement to promote independence and confidence in your work. You may need to develop a tool for self-assessment to serve this purpose, or there may be a ready-made tool available from your employer or professional organization. See Chapter 25 for more information about setting goals and assessment.

The focus of the relationship with your mentor/preceptor will be on sharing information that requires critical thinking while maintaining an open line of communication. You may be discussing how you can take better data, what strategies you could utilize to improve client outcomes, or how you and your mentor/preceptor can improve your communication with one another. Both you and your mentor/preceptor must possess good interpersonal communication skills and be able to openly share ideas, suggestions, and concerns as part of this process.

Effective communication is such an important component of the relationship with your mentor/preceptor, and it is important to remember the role that both verbal and nonverbal communication plays in all of our relationships. Because much of our communication with another person is through tone of voice, appearance, and interpersonal and/or written interactions, we must be ever mindful of the message we send to others. Open communication will assist with navigating through problem areas when they arise and in the negotiation of resolutions to potential areas of conflict.

At times, you and your mentor/preceptor may be required to have a *difficult conversation*. For instance, you may need to tell your preceptor that he is interfering during your diagnostic sessions, causing you to feel inadequate in front of your patients. Or your mentor may be of the opinion that an area of your clinical treatment is inadequate. These types of situations require a dialogue that is based upon a predetermined plan. Maintaining open lines of communication is supported by deciding ahead of time in what manner this type of conversation will take place.

During these conversations, each party must invite joint problem solving and be willing to consider and understand both points of view. Good communication skills require the separation of the problem from the person. Effective communicators will listen first and talk second, to assist with establishing facts necessary to explore all options in a nonjudgmental way. The goal in this collaborative relationship is to work together to find solutions to all situations that arise and to utilize conflict as an additional way to promote both personal and professional growth.

Both you and your mentor/preceptor must recognize that the relationship will evolve over time as you become more proficient and move from a novice to a proficient speech-language pathologist or audiologist. This relationship is an excellent opportunity for you to examine your response to constructive feedback and for you to learn how to not only listen to and accept guidance but to offer your suggestions to others in a positive way. Your relationship with your mentor/preceptor sets the stage for your professional growth as a clinician and as a leader in your chosen profession.

WORK ETHIC AND PROFESSIONAL CODE OF ETHICS

In the professions of speech-language pathology and audiology, the landscape is ever changing, and top jobs can be difficult to find and to keep. To remain competitive in this type of work environment, you must instill in yourself a good work ethic where you are committed to being the best employee you can possibly be. Terms that are often synonymous with work ethic include diligence, dedication, enthusiasm, energy, focus, initiative, reliability, honesty, and steadfastness, to name a few. You want to become "indispensable." So how does one begin to develop these characteristics within the work setting?

Work Ethic

Instilling a good work ethic is a process that develops during your growth as a professional. Learning about employer expectations is the first step in this process. Within your work setting, you will have an employee policies and procedures manual, which contains information regarding a variety of topics specific to your facility (see Chapter 19 for details on the Policies and Procedures Manual). Work topics that may be covered in a facility policies and procedures manual include attendance and punctuality, discrimination, sexual harassment, confidentiality, disability accommodations, conflicts of interest, substance abuse, misconduct regarding technology (e-mail specifically), and federal and state laws and regulations such as FERPA, IDEA, HIPAA, and Medicaid, to name a few. In addition, you will need to familiarize yourself with all state licensure and/or certification rules and requirements regarding scope of practice, delegation of work, and ethical conduct. You should learn about these policies and procedures early on in order to be educated and fully informed and to prevent problems that could arise from your lack of knowledge.

The Council of Academic Programs in Communication Sciences and Disorders (CAPCSD) (Schwartz, Horner, Jackson, Johnstone, & Mulligan, 2007) document *Eligibility Requirements and Essential Functions* describes a set of knowledge and skills requisite to the practice of speech-language pathology to function in a broad variety of clinical situations. Although written for students in graduate programs, it established guidelines that may be applied to working professionals, including both speech-language pathologists and audiologists. The document identified five areas of focus necessary to be effective as a professional: communication, motor, intellectual-cognitive, sensory-observational, and behavioral-social.

The behavioral/social area plays an important role in any discussion of work ethic, as it addresses the display of mature professional relationships. The requirements and essential functions included in this section of the CAPCSD document are displaying respect for others; conducting oneself in an ethical and legal manner, to include upholding the ASHA Code of Ethics as well as all federal privacy policies; maintaining general good physical and mental health and self-care; the ability to adapt to changing and demanding environments; managing time effectively; the acceptance of suggestions and constructive criticism; and appropriate professional dress. Each of the areas described and discussed within this document is an essential ingredient in the development of a good work ethic.

Code of Ethics

In addition to developing a solid work ethic, you should be cognizant of the code of ethics of your professions and maintain ethical standards for yourself in every aspect of your job. ASHA (2010) explains that a code of ethics is the fundamental principles and rules considered essential for the preservation of the highest standards. ASHA goes on to state that "ethical principles are vital to the responsible discharge of obligations by the speech-language pathologist and audiologist" (Preamble). Therefore, it is imperative that you are familiar with the ethical standards that govern your practice, including the ASHA Code of Ethics, the AAA Code of Ethics, the ethical code for the state in which you work, and the ethical code of conduct required for your place of employment and any other professional association that you are affiliated with.

If you are faced with an ethical dilemma, what should you do? For instance, your employer has asked you to submit a billing statement to an insurance provider for client hours for which you have no documentation. You should begin by exploring what the possible courses of action are and what the outcomes could be for each of those actions. In your place of employment, it is always a good idea to be familiar with what is permissible (can be done or not done), impermissible (must never be done under any circumstance), obligatory (cannot change and must always be done, regardless of circumstance or personal feeling), or necessary. Having this foundation will assist you in your decision-making process and prevent you from making decisions that are contrary to your workplace.

Let us explore what the potential benefits and burdens are for each action that you investigate. Sue Hale (2006) describes an ethical decision-making process that is as powerful as it is simplistic. She suggests that you follow a four-step decision-making process that requires that you (1) recognize that you may have an ethical issue, (2) gather information on the issue, (3) evaluate the situation, and (4) make a decision and test it using your definition of ethics and your knowledge of ethical practices. You should also familiarize yourself with what the outcomes could possibly be for ethical misconduct, should it occur. Violations such as falsification of documents and/or records or violation of laws associated with professional regulations, or felony or misdemeanor convictions for matters involving moral turpitude, for example, may result in sanction or revocation of your credentials.

Developing and maintaining a solid work ethic and adhering to principles of professional ethical conduct are as important to your success as knowledge of clinical skills. The choices we make in our personal lives can affect our professional lives in ways that we may not have even considered until it is too late to repair the damage. Employee personnel policies and procedures and your professional code of ethics are important tools. They are there to serve as your road map and compass as you navigate your career. See Chapter 5 for more information on professional ethics and Chapter 6 for discussion of professional liability.

BEING ORGANIZED

Did you know the average human being in our society loses an hour per day due to disorganization and poor time management? That is more than two weeks per year! As you develop your career path, you will need to learn how to work efficiently in order to best serve the needs of your clients and to maintain a healthy work-life balance. Employing strategies of organization and time management will also help in the prevention of job burnout.

Many believe being organized is the foundation of success. Being organized typically means keeping things in predictable places or arranging things in an orderly or structured manner. An organized work space is one in which materials can easily be located and where distractions are minimal. It is not as easy as being neat, which may simply mean maintaining cleanliness in a state of disorganization. Knowing where all items are on a consistent basis helps to maintain the flow of your workday and eliminates the need to waste time searching for what you need. We will examine several strategies for organization.

Start by scheduling a specified amount of time for organizing your space and begin by organizing your desk. Look through everything initially and make decisions about what to discard and what to keep. For those items you choose to keep, make a clearly labeled file immediately for those items. As you locate tasks that are in process, make a to-do file to place those items in so you can find them readily and complete them on time. Do not be afraid to throw things away. Find a box to place items in that require shredding, and place those items there for shredding at a later time. Do the same with file cabinets, desk drawers, bookshelves, and any other area where disorder abounds.

You also need to organize the information you are required to obtain and maintain in your work environment. By organizing your information, you will ensure that time lines are kept and compliance is maintained. Organizing your information properly will also help you remember critical information. Information can be organized by utilizing filing systems that make sense to you personally, where you can physically manipulate your information when necessary. In the age of technology, many choose to organize their information on the computer for easy access so they do not have to find a location to store and file information within their limited office space. Organize your computer files for your information there as well so you do not have to spend valuable time searching for information due to disorganization of your computer filing system.

There are two sobering statistics from time management experts Dodd and Sundheim (2005), authors of *The 25 Best Time Management Tools and Techniques*:

1. We use only 20 percent of the papers we file.
2. We spend at least 75 hours per year looking for lost papers, which averages out to about 13 minutes per day.

They suggest three types of files to organize the "paper" in your life. This system may also be applied to your computer filing system. One file should be an Action file. This file is for projects you are currently working on. The Reference file is the second type of file, and this file should include those things you need to keep for future reference. The third and final file type is the Reading file. These files are filled with those things you wish to read. Every paper you choose to keep should fit into one of these file types. If it does not, you should consider discarding it.

According to Silber (2004), author of *Organizing from the Right Side of the Brain*, we all have different styles that guide how we organize ourselves. Understanding your individual style can assist you as you employ strategies for organization. The manner in which you organize your information will be dependent on many factors, including if you are a "right brainer" or a "left brainer."

"Right brainers" are creative and visually oriented, with a need to see things in order to make sense of them. They usually get totally caught up in the moment and completely lose track of time. Filing papers and clearing desk space can make them feel as if they are being suffocated and as if their creativity is stifled. For "right brainers," many organizational strategies typically suggested will not be effective tools for them. They will need to try a wide variety of strategies to see what is most effective.

"Left brainers," on the other hand, like to feel in control of everything, particularly the environment around them. They are linear and structured and must compartmentalize to feel organized. They must finish things at regular intervals and put things away in order to feel that sense of accomplishment. Work environments tend to try to force individuals into a "left brain" way of doing business because, in the work environment, neatness and punctuality are highly valued. For "left brainers," many organizational strategies typically suggested will be effective tools for them.

Having an organized work space with easy access to information and materials will save you time, energy, and frustration. It is a good idea to have specific places where items are always kept, and therefore easily accessible to you. Once you have initiated an organizational system that meets your needs and works for you, make an effort to maintain that system, even if it requires a few extra minutes of your day. You will reap the benefits of working smarter, not harder.

TIME MANAGEMENT

Many events in our day rob us of our time. Most often, our time is lost due to the three major factors of *disorganization*, *procrastination*, or *interruptions*. As we have already discussed, disorganized work spaces and disorganized information systems rob of us valuable time. Follow the guidelines for organization explored earlier in this chapter to avoid having disorganization rob you of your valuable time.

We can add *procrastination* to the list of time robbers. Why do we procrastinate? If we can answer that question, we can avoid the pitfalls procrastination will cause. Usually, we procrastinate because we are overwhelmed, because we do not estimate correctly the amount of time a project will take us, because we would much prefer to be doing something else, because we fear failure or the inability to complete a task, or because we strive for perfection that is not required or necessary. If you find that you are procrastinating, examine the possible reasons. Once you find out why you are procrastinating at a particular time and on a particular project, you can follow some simple rules to move forward.

First, have a realistic sense of time, and work within the time frame that you have available. Work from a to-do list, and tackle challenging projects first. Set small deadlines for yourself along the way, and share those deadlines with colleagues in order for them to encourage and support your progress. Find what motivates you (reward, sense of accomplishment) and expect problems along the way so you are not disappointed or frustrated when they occur. Remember, no one is perfect and mistakes are likely. Have reasonable expectations for yourself and for others. Expect the unexpected, and plan accordingly.

In his book *How to Get Control of Your Time and Your Life*, Lakein (1996) recommends using the "Swiss Cheese Method" when you have an overwhelming project to complete. The idea is simple. Get started by "poking holes" in your project or by completing *instant tasks* that take five minutes or less. If you hit a dead end with one task, try another. This series of completing instant tasks will help you feel as though you are getting a handle on what you need to do to finish the project by tackling small tasks one at a time.

Dodd and Sundheim (2005) explain that we live in a world of *urgent*. They say if something demands our attention, it usually gets it, no matter what we are doing. They go on to explain that occasional urgency is not a problem. However, a steady diet of it can become a huge drain on your time and other resources. They suggest making lists of some type, such as a weekly to-do list, a daily to-do list, a master list that has everything you need to do, or some type of checklist for frequently occurring activities. When making lists, they suggest you think strategically, cut out the excess, and focus on main priorities.

They also suggest utilizing the "ABC System" as a way to prioritize. Using this system, you rank each item on your list as *A=high priority, B=medium priority, C=low priority*. This system is designed in order for you to complete all of your "A" activities each day, and fill in with "B" and "C" activities as time permits. This system is designed to assist you with crossing things off your list that really matter in the overall scheme of your day.

The final area for us to explore in terms of good time management is the issue of *interruption*. Most interruptions occur when the priorities of someone else are in conflict with what you have planned. You can minimize interruptions in order to improve time management by having a schedule planned for your daily activities and by sticking to it. Within that schedule, look at all the activities you are required to complete as a part of your current position as a speech-language pathologist or audiologist in your current work setting.

Scheduling suggestions include flex scheduling, where you change your schedule as new duties and responsibilities find their way to you. Utilize ASHA resources by accessing the Workload Time Survey (ASHA, 2002) to fully understand where your time is actually going. Incorporate the use of calendars, day planners, online calendar systems, wall calendars, desk calendars, and to-do lists to adequately schedule, maintain, and plan for all aspects of your day.

Because time with your clients/students/patients is typically the most important part of your day, you should plan your schedule for that first. In addition, schedule time for the planning of your therapy, for consultation and collaboration with family members and with colleagues, for the completion of diagnostics, for completion of paperwork and compliance issues, and for time to review and answer e-mail and voice mail.

When reviewing your e-mails, decide if the e-mail is something you can delete, if it is something you need to act on, or if you need to file it. If you do not need to delete it or act on it, then you should file it. When setting up electronic files, remember it is better to have fewer large files than it is to have many small ones. Finally, make an appointment with yourself to clean out your e-mail and voice mail at least once a month.

Plan for designated "office hours" and make conscious decisions regarding when you will be available to colleagues. Try not to encourage interruptions by always making yourself available to others. Understand that lack of planning on the part of someone else should not constitute an emergency for you. Suggest to colleagues that you schedule a designated time with them rather than have a conversation with them when you are unable to provide them with your undivided attention. By doing this, you enable your coworkers to work independently as well.

As a last resort, remove yourself from areas or activities where the interruptions seem to occur most often. Expect that interruptions will occur throughout the workday, and plan accordingly. Above all, do not use interruptions as a way to avoid your work. Sometimes, this will be tempting, particularly if you have an unpleasant or challenging task to complete. You may be tempted to allow interruptions to delay beginning those projects. And try to take advantage of those unexpected bits of time that become available to you to tackle unfinished and/or ongoing tasks.

"Pareto's Principle," or the "80/20 rule" (Dodd & Sundheim, 2005) can also assist us with the management of our time. This principle assumes the notion that 20 percent of our effort will lead to 80 percent of our result. By utilizing this concept as we face our daily tasks, we are better able to set our priorities, prevent overplanning, prevent procrastination, and eliminate interruptions by focusing primarily on the most important tasks we face each day.

When managing your time, it is all about your plan. A plan gives you an overall view of what must be accomplished, and it saves you valuable time in the long run. Making a plan and sticking to it will ensure that your work life has balance and that you are productive in your job.

PRODUCTIVITY

Now that we have explored the importance of organization and time management, we will discuss productivity in the workplace. Productivity is important for both personal and professional growth. When you are productive in your work, you obtain more enjoyment from your job and are less likely to be complacent or unhappy with where you work. Your confidence in your performance typically results in positive work behaviors, positive work relationships, superior work performance, better performance evaluations, and higher compensation. When you are more productive, you are more efficient and more creative and have more energy.

It is important to implement your therapy effectively and efficiently to achieve the highest levels of success with those you serve in the least amount of time possible. In some work settings, specified *productivity standards* are in place that you must meet in order to maintain employment. In those settings, productivity is usually described in percentage amounts, such as 80 percent. That figure translates into the amount of time during your total working hours in which you are expected to be providing direct services, or accruing "billable" hours. You need to know what those standards are in your work setting and comply accordingly.

To begin your road to productivity, you may want to look at a few things to focus your attention as you begin your new job. First, you will want to set target goals for each day, with some "mini" goals built in so that you can identify, more efficiently, time requirements for the tasks that you have to complete. Break those larger tasks into smaller tasks, and then stick with the task until it is completed. You will find that by doing so, you can also group like tasks together in order to complete them in less time.

In addition, it is necessary for you to be able to problem solve and make decisions efficiently in order to remain productive. Time wasted in the decision-making process can erode your productivity. Have a set amount of time for the decision-making process, a plan for how you will make decisions, and then stick with that plan. Force yourself to make important decisions within the time frame that you set. Recognize that your problem is your responsibility until it is solved, and "own" the problem until you resolve it. You may have to solicit the assistance of others to help you solve the problem; however, you are ultimately responsible for the resolution.

At the end of each workday, identify the task that you will begin the next day, and prepare for that task in advance by readying the materials you will need to complete the task (Pavlina, 2007). The next day, you will be able to begin working on that task immediately. If you are interrupted at the beginning of the day with unplanned events, you will be less likely to get "off track" if you have planned ahead and have a clear vision for the new day.

You are paid to do a specific job based on your specific skill set, within a specified time frame. In your job as a speech-language pathologist or audiologist, multitasking is necessary on a daily basis. Steve Pavlina (2007) has a blog with many helpful suggestions regarding productivity. He states that in order to multitask and maintain productivity, we must handle our jobs with flexibility and decreased distraction. Setting deadlines is crucial in order to prioritize tasks and remain highly productive for long periods of time.

Being productive in the workplace improves your performance as you become more self-sufficient in organizing your daily tasks. Productivity goes along with developing a good work ethic, and it goes hand in hand with time management and organization. By organizing your daily tasks, prioritizing your tasks, and keeping track of your progress, you can maintain a very productive schedule and meet employer productivity expectations, if required. Just as with organization and time management, we must utilize such strategies to assist us with being and remaining productive.

Heathfield (2011), a human resource professional who writes extensively for an online human resources website, suggests that you maintain a portfolio that demonstrates your productivity. The portfolio may document assignments, projects, and personal achievements. She also recommends that you keep copies of appraisals and/or evaluations, samples of your work, and written feedback from employers and colleagues, organized in chronological order. This effective strategy will demonstrate your productivity as you take on and complete new tasks and assignments. You should ask team members for letters of recommendation, and add those to your growing portfolio for future career conversations.

The satisfaction derived from a "job well done" fuels us on to do more, be more, accomplish more. When you are productive, you gain more mastery of yourself and your work environment and are more likely to achieve both your professional and personal goals. By achieving these goals, you are more aligned with the goals of your coworkers and employer and therefore better able to obtain success personally and make a significant contribution to the workplace.

TEAMWORK

Teamwork is paramount in the professions of speech-language pathology and audiology. In a team environment, you find shared values, shared vision, inspiration, and energy. Team members must be able to empower, coach, and reward themselves as well as their colleagues. In successful work settings, you find shared credit for accomplishments, ideas, and contributions. In environments where individuals embrace the team concept, you find those capable of rewarding themselves rather than those who have the expectation that others will reward them. True team environments help all parties find their own personal rewards on the way to "greatness."

As you begin your career, you will be assigned a number of tasks commensurate with your job description. Some of those assigned tasks may not be ones you will find appealing. However, it is important to understand that most assignments serve as potential growth opportunities and will require that you engage in them willingly. Be the employee that asks for new assignments that will challenge you, both personally and professionally, and allow others to see the extent of your diversity as a team member.

When taking on a new assignment, particularly one that is more challenging, try to create a vision of how you will accomplish it, and share that vision with your fellow team members. Through this vision, and a sense of shared values, you and your team members can establish goals that will benefit all parties while you energize and inspire one another. In this kind of collegial environment, you assist each other with achieving those goals as you coach and reward one another.

As your confidence and skills continue to grow, request more challenging work, ask for assignments that require increased responsibility, and exhibit over time that you deserve them. Contribute to the workplace by offering your unique qualifications in order to enhance the work setting and contribute to the effectiveness of the team as a whole. To perform well, be certain you understand the project you are undertaking, as well as all deadlines associated with it. Meet deadlines without fail, and ask for assistance if you require it. It is imperative that you check and recheck your work before providing it to your supervisor, mentor, or fellow team member. Ask for constructive feedback from colleagues as you complete tasks together, and keep a positive attitude when that feedback is provided.

Heathfield (2011) discusses building relationships with your coworkers. Being friendly and supportive of coworkers contributes to your success and visibility. Show your creative talents, mediate conflicts, demonstrate your willingness to experiment, and take advantage of opportunities to participate in seminars, training events, and classes. As you learn new things, *share* them. Forget the "them versus me" attitude. Your ability to work well with other team members is the key to your success. The goals of your workplace become your goals, and you need to fully understand how your work complements the work of others, and vice versa.

In today's workplace, jobs are demanding and much is required of you as a professional. Remember that success is attributable to a pattern of mutually beneficial interpersonal relationships, and this includes being part of a team. Being part of a true team environment allows you to celebrate shared victories while examining defeats in an environment rich with trust and respect for one another.

POLITICS IN THE WORKPLACE

Before you step inside the building where you will begin your new job, you need to do some homework. Do some research and find out everything you can about your new employer, including the employer's philosophy or mission statement, goals and strategic plans, and corporate structure or staff roster. Make an attempt to meet someone who works there before you start, as it is nice to see a familiar, friendly face on your first day. Learning as much as possible before that first day will keep you from feeling overwhelmed and possibly unwelcome.

During the first few weeks, do your best to make a positive, lasting impression. When it comes to interacting with your coworkers, spend more time observing rather than offering opinions, and planning rather than acting. There will be plenty of opportunities for you to demonstrate your talents, skills, and personality attributes. Show how eager you are to learn and not how eager you are to instruct.

Keep in mind that you are the "new kid in town" and that relationships among your new coworkers were formed before your arrival. It will not go unrecognized that you have the power to destabilize some of those relationships before you have even found out where the restrooms are located. So tread carefully as you begin to form working and, certainly, personal relationships with your coworkers.

Rosenberg McKay (2010) shares four rules that will help you grasp the importance of understanding the politics within your new setting. First, she stresses the importance of listening and observing before suggesting any changes. You may have some great ideas and see a better way to do things, but until you are able to appreciate the dynamics of your surroundings, your suggestions may be met with negative reactions. Suppose a clinical fellow (CF) working in an elementary school observes what appears to be unused office space in a much more desirable location than the room to which she has been assigned. She approaches the principal in the hallway as he is speaking with a parent and mentions the "unused, wasted office space" that would be better utilized if she were permitted to relocate. As it turns out, the parent to whom the principal is speaking is the PTA president and the "unused, wasted office" is the PTA office. The CF has not only offended the PTA president but has made a negative impression on the principal.

Second, she suggests that you be aware of the "office troublemaker," adding that every office has one. This is the individual who will try to warn you about other employees and stirs up trouble only to later pretend to have nothing to do with it. Listen to what this person tells you but refrain from making a comment. For example, the AuD extern has just met a coworker who proceeds to warn him about the mean-spirited clinic director. He tells him that the clinic director, among other negative things, always assigns the most difficult patients to the newest person hired. Mr. Talkative adds that this is how the director is able to make an early determination as to the competence of the new employee. The extern now faces with dread the first patient encounter, assuming that it will be a very difficult case and that the director is prepared to give him a poor evaluation. Be aware that even though there may be some truth in what he says, it may be greatly exaggerated, or only based upon his personal experiences. In time, you will be able to form your own opinions based upon your own experiences, and you will not need Mr. Talkative to help you in this process.

The third rule is to mind your manners, as people may not remember your politeness but they are sure to remember rude behavior. The CF who heard a funny but off-color story on the radio while driving to work cannot resist the temptation to share it with his coworkers during the lunch break at the skilled nursing facility. What made it even funnier to the CF was that it had to do with an elderly individual, with striking similarity to one of the patients in the facility. When he told the joke, no one laughed and one individual even left the room to finish her lunch elsewhere. Such stories have no place in the workplace, especially if you are the new employee and do not know how your coworkers would react.

The last rule is to keep your ear to the grapevine but do not contribute to it. Although you can gain valuable insight into office dynamics by paying attention to what is being said, you may also damage your reputation by making statements that have no substance. Suppose a new employee heard the news that a coworker was leaving. This news came soon after she overheard a patient complaining loudly about the poor manner in which the coworker had fitted a hearing aid. The new employee concluded that this was the reason for the coworker's departure, and added to the story by saying that the coworker was probably fired. The coworker was in fact not fired but was moving to another city to take care of an ailing family member. Furthermore, the angry patient was known to be unreasonably difficult and had always expressed his displeasure with any audiologist who fitted his hearing aids. Contributing to the grapevine is never good practice, particularly when you are new.

Every work setting has its own culture, its own set of unwritten rules, and its own climate for developing professional and personal relationships. It is important to take time to understand and appreciate how these factors may influence and contribute to your own professional growth and development. Remember that it is a small world and your reputation can follow you for years. Your willingness to listen, observe, discourage unproductive interactions, avoid gossip, and show consideration for others will go far in helping you achieve success in the workplace.

NETWORKING

"*The true measure of a man is how he treats someone who can do him absolutely no good.*" - Samuel Johnson

You have probably heard people say "It's not what you know, it's who you know." That may be especially true in today's culture of being connected to one another in so many ways. Your friends, acquaintances, and professional colleagues are a vast resource for you as you navigate the professional world. Having the knowledge and skills to perform your job well is your primary focus, but having the ability to demonstrate your knowledge and skills to your professional colleagues is also a very important part of building your career.

There are many benefits that come with professional networking, including sharing knowledge, finding new approaches to the way you do your job, and creating new opportunities that contribute to your professional growth and development. Networking allows you to meet with other speech-language pathologists and audiologists who might have had similar challenges in the past that you are facing today. By sharing knowledge, they are able to help you demonstrate possible solutions to these challenges while also learning to appreciate your individual talents and skills.

Many audiologists and speech-language pathologists have used networking to supplement their ability to do things well and to expand their careers in directions that go beyond the clinical setting. They have, in essence, developed networking into an art form and would offer the following tips:

1. When starting a new job, try to get to know as many people as possible, particularly the "key players." Do not isolate yourself, and be sure to take advantage of non-work-related activities to be with your colleagues, such as lunch, after-hours activities, and so on.
2. Join your professional associations and become active by signing up for a committee, helping out at a conference or meeting, editing a publication, etc.
3. Make yourself noticeable by volunteering for responsibilities at your worksite and in your professional organizations, particularly the ones that may be the most unpopular, and follow through with them.
4. Approach someone who appears to be "well connected" and ask how you can help them with their projects, etc., thereby having them serve as an informal mentor.
5. Establish specific networking goals, such as making important contacts, establishing and advancing professional relationships, and widening your professional contact base.
6. Do not exhibit blatant self-promotion by trying to be the star of the show. Make a genuine effort to include others in your activities, be a true team player by learning how to share responsibility, and adopt a "share the wealth" philosophy. (These are also key elements in developing leadership skills.)
7. Show a genuine and sincere interest in those individuals within your network by focusing on building a relationship with them that relates to goals you share in common.

Your place of employment and your professional associations offer the best opportunities for you to develop your professional networking skills. Attending staff meetings and informal faculty get-togethers, eating lunch in the employees' break room, and volunteering at professional conferences are just a few of the ways your knowledge, interests, skills, and talents will be recognized by your colleagues. There are also opportunities for networking within your university alumnae associations, religious groups, civic associations, political organizations, and special interest/hobby clubs, to name a few. These can serve as excellent opportunities for you to meet and establish relationships with individuals with whom you share common interests that extend beyond the worksite, while enabling you to practice your networking skills.

Another way to network is through the use of social networking sites on the Internet such as Facebook and LinkedIn. These sites are an effective way to stay in touch with people you already know and want to get to know better. Keep in mind that when you take advantage of these sites for the purpose of networking, your communication exchanges should only reveal information about you that is appropriate for all readers.

Therefore, you must pay careful attention to choice of topics, language style, and photos in order to project a professional image.

Networking plays a significant role in the growth and development of the new professional. Opportunities for establishing networking relationships exist both in and out of the workplace. Successful networking results in the establishment and maintenance of long-term relationships that are mutually beneficial. These relationships are built on confidence and trust, and require planning, time, effort, nurturing, diplomacy, integrity, and good judgment. Professional networking becomes an integral component of building a career that is both productive and meaningful over the course of time.

PERFORMANCE EVALUATIONS

Evaluations of employee performance are a component of any job. The purposes of performance evaluations are typically to provide a system of accountability, promote quality assurance, support professional growth and development, and promote performance improvement. They should also provide an opportunity for feedback and serve to rejuvenate and renew the employees' approach to their work. Most employers have an evaluation system in place for employees at all levels. Some frequently used types of performance evaluations include top-down, peer-to-peer, 360-degree, and self-assessment performance reviews.

The top-down evaluation involves the assessment of the employee by the direct supervisor. The supervisor is typically someone who works closely enough with the employee to be familiar with the employee's specific strengths and weaknesses. This form of assessment often includes a rating scale or a narrative, or a combination of both. Most graduate student clinicians would have experienced being evaluated with an assessment tool of this type. An offshoot of this type of performance evaluation is referred to as a "matrix" evaluation. This is used when an employee works for multiple supervisors or managers, perhaps in several facilities, and is thereby evaluated by several of these individuals.

The peer-to-peer evaluation requires employees at the same level to review each other. The rationale for this type of evaluation is that no one is in a better position to observe performance than a coworker. There are some obvious problems with this type of evaluation, including level of experience and qualifications for assessing performance, personality issues, and the possibility of negative reviews getting back to fellow workers. This can be an effective format in certain situations, for example, a team of clinicians co-treating a patient where specific content knowledge is required.

The 360-degree performance assessment (U.S. Office of Personnel Management, 1997) incorporates input from different types of individuals, including coworkers, customers/clients, supervisors, and individuals who may be working "under" the individual, such as a supervisee. There are some obvious benefits to having multiple sources of input for the purpose of performance assessment, but employees may be reluctant to give candid feedback about their manager or supervisor out of fear that the manager finds out. In addition, outside contacts may feel unqualified or simply too busy to provide meaningful feedback. If this type of assessment is used, a human resources manager should coordinate the process to ensure confidentiality of subordinate reviewers.

Self-assessment performance reviews are effective when combined with other types of performance assessments, including the previous three presented. With this type of assessment, employees are asked to rate their performance, often using the same form that a supervisor uses to review them. Having employees complete the assessment performance prior to the supervisor's review can set a positive tone for the evaluation session. An example of this type of performance review is used for ASHA certification for speech-language pathologists during their clinical fellowship experience, as described in the following section. Because the mentoring relationship is a collaborative one, the CF and the CF mentor complete this rating scale together, and they discuss further action for improvement as part of the process.

Your employer will most likely have an established performance appraisal process in place upon your arrival. As part of your orientation to the job, it is important that you become acquainted with the manner in which your performance will be evaluated. The types of performance appraisals are varied and your employer may use one or any combination of appraisals, depending on your setting, responsibilities, pay grade or level, or even the culture of your individual working environment. Your participation in the performance appraisal process provides you with an opportunity to help you improve your skills and promote your own professional growth and development.

CONTINUING EDUCATION

Once employed, you will be expected to keep abreast of advances and changes within your profession. Your employer will want you to have the latest assessment and intervention skills and use evidence-based practice. Maintenance of certification and licensure will also require documentation of continuing education (CE). Be sure to know these requirements for the credentials you hold. You do not want to jeopardize your credentials because you did not fulfill continuing education mandates or to feel pressured to find an appropriate program to meet your goals. Your employer may offer on-site educational programs or you may participate in local, state, or national conferences that provide continuing education programs. There is a growing number of online CE programs, too. It is critical to keep a log of these activities and proof of attendance. Your employer may contribute to the cost of attendance, and in all cases, you should keep receipts for reimbursement or tax purposes.

PROMOTION AND ADVANCEMENT

Once employed, you may find that opportunities are possible for advancement within the current program, within the larger organization, or even within other settings. Individuals become aware of available positions through professional publications, networking, or direct solicitation to apply for a position. Advancement can take the form of moving upward to positions of more direct program responsibility such as supervisory roles, or it can take place laterally with the individual remaining in a similar position but assuming new responsibilities or a new type of caseload. For example, in some programs, individuals may become team leaders or have special duties such as coordinator of quality improvement or continuing education. Increasingly, programs have "career ladders" intended to promote staff development and leadership and provide opportunities for new challenges, without employees having to be "promoted" to a supervisory position. Advancement both vertically and laterally can be challenging and contribute to a more fulfilling career.

Before advancement, some basic questions arise. What duties does the new position entail? What are prerequisite technical and personal skills and credentials for fulfilling the position? Will the new responsibilities be challenging or constitute a professional or personal burden? Will the prestige or financial reward be adequate to compensate for new responsibilities? For example, if promotion entails increased travel, is this possible within your current lifestyle? What personal accommodations, such as the need for child care, would be required? Should an advanced position be attractive, the application process will be similar to that already described in Chapter 9: preapplication analysis, preinterview preparation, interview(s), and final offer. A major difference in seeking an advanced position within a present organization is that the interview will be with familiar individuals. Careful preparation is no less important for a longtime employee. In some cases, a current employee may be competing with individuals from both within and outside the organization whose credentials and experiences are equal or superior to your own.

If you decide to apply for advancement within your present organization, you need to be prepared psychologically for a rejection. Some individuals may perceive this as an overwhelming personal rebuff by colleagues, and it may affect their ability to work productively in that setting. This is an important concept to consider as you apply for promotions within your setting. Having a positive support network is vital to helping you cope if such a rejection occurs. While rejection does not usually mean that your current position is in jeopardy, this may be a good time to reevaluate your goals and have a frank discussion with trusted colleagues about your options at this time.

CHANGING EMPLOYMENT

An employee may change employment settings for any number of reasons. These reasons include job loss, relocation, unreasonable demands in the current position, lack of opportunities for professional growth, infrequent raises, boredom or burnout, lack of employer appreciation, or readiness to assume new or increased responsibilities associated with a different position (Raudsepp, 1990). Recent changes in Medicare reimbursement for long-term care and outpatient rehabilitation services have seriously affected employment in medical settings. Thus, some professionals may make a job change by choice, whereas others will find this an unwelcome event in their lives.

The new job search may begin while you are currently employed, or the process may begin after resignation or termination from a position. Securing a new position while currently employed presents some challenges. If you are currently employed, you may not want your employer to know that you have begun a job search. If the job search becomes public, how will this knowledge affect your current position? How available can you be for interviews? If you feel that you do not want your current employer to know about a potential move, you will need to change options for references. You also must be prepared to take time off from work to attend interviews, either on the phone or in person.

In the case of relocation or a mutually agreeable job change, your current employer will be the best possible reference in securing new employment. In the situation in which a position has ended before beginning a job search, you again have to evaluate the helpfulness of a former employer. Targeted employers will want to know the circumstances of why you left the last position and generally will want some reference from that employer. It is important to consider that a current employer is the most important reference for the future; therefore, conditions under which the applicant leaves should be positive—"a graceful exit" (Kroner, 1989). When an employee leaves, employers are sometimes asked to indicate on the termination documentation if they "would" or "would not" rehire this individual. That is a question often asked by future employers when calling for references on a terminated employee. An ungraceful exit, such as leaving without sufficient notice for your employer to find a replacement, or leaving without completing required paperwork, is not likely to get a "would rehire" response.

Before you resign from a current position, be sure to have the new offer in writing. Check your current employer's policies and procedures manual for contractual information on what time period constitutes sufficient notice of termination. Your present employer must then receive notification of your intended departure. Include in this letter your exit date, the title of your new position and employer, and the last date of work. It is also dignified to inform your boss before telling coworkers and meet with this person in a formal exit interview. Exit interviews should be positively focused on making an orderly and courteous transition between you and your replacement (Kennedy, 1998). Before leaving a current position, all work should be summarized for a successor, and all required paperwork must be updated, completed, and filed. Some employers will require you to help train a replacement, so an overlap time may be necessary. How a departure is handled can positively or negatively affect the tone of future references from the employer.

Many speech-language pathologists and audiologists have felt the impact of changes in Medicare and other insurance reimbursement in medical settings. Some have lost their jobs while others have had positions changed or hours reduced. Although this is likely to be a time of anger, despair, and frustration, it is also an important time to know what your options are financially and vocationally. Be sure to consider psychological support during this time of unwelcome transition. Some human resources departments will have such support available to assist you.

Financial Considerations

If you are faced with an impending loss of a job, it is critical to plan for the time when you may be without a regular income. To be prepared, (1) know your financial assets and monthly expenses and make a realistic financial plan, (2) reduce all unnecessary expenses, (3) build a three- to six-month cash reserve, (4) reduce debt, (5) know the rules regarding any 401(k) or retirement plans to which you have contributed, (6) discuss mortgage and insurance coverage with qualified professionals, (7) investigate your agency's severance package options and negotiate the best one, (8) plan for health insurance while unemployed (e.g., COBRA option), and (9) claim your unemployment benefits.

The Interval between Jobs

It may take you more time than you had anticipated finding new employment. This is an important time to review your skills and update them as this demonstrates a commitment to learning and self-improvement. For applicants who have been unemployed for an extended time, the prospective employer will want to know if and how you have kept your clinical skills up to date.

Applicants need to provide clear, concise, and honest answers to these questions. All attempts should be made to redirect the interviewer to the applicant's interest in and qualifications for the present position. It is prudent to maintain your professional certification, licensure, and continuing education requirements during any extended periods from active work. You should also use this opportunity to maintain contact with other professionals. This is an excellent example of the value of professional networking that you have hopefully established prior to this time.

Changing jobs is never an easy prospect, whether or not by choice. Careful planning must be a part of any job change. The conscientious professional will ensure a smooth transition for the successor, leaving the former job site in "turnkey" condition. Financial considerations are also part of this planning and should always play an important role in your career choices. Particularly if the job change is related to stress or burnout, you may want to consider psychological support and/or career counseling during this time of transition. Networking relationships should continue to be developed and maintained both during the transition period and upon entering the new employment setting. Finally, once you have entered the new setting, treat it as you would any new job, remembering that first impressions do count and that your reputation, although it may precede you and will certainly follow you, is always a work in progress.

SUMMARY

Your decision to enter the profession of audiology or speech-language pathology requires more than the acquisition of clinical knowledge and skills. Many important issues affect your ability to build your career in a positive direction, leading to job fulfillment and professional success. You must understand the nature of the collaborative relationship you have with your mentor/preceptor and develop effective communication skills as part of that and all relationships in your work setting. In addition to having a solid appreciation for a good work ethic, you will need to adhere to a professional code of ethical conduct established by your professional association. Effective time management and good organizational skills will help you prioritize and keep you motivated as you perform your day-to-day tasks while increasing productivity. Being an effective member of a team, understanding the political culture of your workplace, and maintaining a supportive professional network will also help you as your career develops. Performance evaluations are a required component of any job, and you should play an active role in the assessment process as you make advances in your career path. The CF experience and the audiology clinical practicum serve as launch pads for the beginning professional, and it is important to be familiar with the requirements leading to certification. Finally, when changing employment, either by choice or not, you need to consider many factors as you continue to build your career with confidence, competence, and success.

CRITICAL THINKING

1. What are some of the dynamic differences you should anticipate as you move from working with a clinical supervisor in a university setting to a mentor in your professional workplace? What role do interpersonal communication skills play in this relationship?
2. Your preceptor has made a comment in front of your patient that you perceived as calling into question your competence. You are embarrassed and would like to have a difficult conversation with your preceptor to address the situation. What is the predetermined plan that you and your preceptor have decided upon for such a dialogue? What factors should you keep in mind during the conversation to make it a productive one for both of you?
3. You are preparing to discharge a client from services at a private clinic where you work. The clinic director has asked you to keep a client on your caseload in order to ensure revenue for the practice. What steps should you take to address the situation? Why is ethical behavior important as you build your career?

4. You have been too busy to keep up with the amount of paperwork that seems to be piling up on your desk. How can you tackle this problem immediately, and what strategies can you employ to avoid this situation in the future?
5. Your colleague has told you that he stays in his office during lunch and avoids non-mandatory staff functions because he has "too much work to do." His clinical knowledge and organizational skills appear to be excellent, so he is frustrated that many of his coworkers do not include him when discussing caseload management issues. He is also disappointed that his director recently overlooked him for a promotion for which he thought he was well suited. He has asked you for advice, so what would you tell him?
6. Your employer has informed you that due to budget cuts, your position has been eliminated and you will need to find employment elsewhere. Develop a "game plan" that will ensure some financial stability while you seek new employment. What role will your professional networking play during this time period? What factors should you consider during your search for a new position?
7. What is meant by having a "work ethic"? Why is it important to develop a realistic work ethic as you begin your first professional position? How is work ethic related to time management?
8. You need to take a leave from your job for family reasons. How would you go about this? What should you do to prepare your replacement until you return to your position?
9. As a professional, you will be evaluated each year by a supervisor. What performance criteria will go into this evaluation? Should performance criteria for a first-year professional be the same as those for a seasoned professional? Suppose you do not agree with the evaluation your supervisor has given you. What would you do?
10. You are the director of a large clinical program that has few opportunities for your staff to get promoted. What could you do to encourage and reinforce innovation, dedication, and service among your staff without promoting them?

REFERENCES

American Board of Audiology. (2011). *Board certification in audiology.* Retrieved from http://www.americanboardofaudiology.org/faq/faqs.html

American Speech-Language-Hearing Association. (1997). *ASHA membership and certification handbook.* Rockville, MD: Author.

American Speech-Language-Hearing Association. (2002). *A workload analysis approach for establishing speech-language caseload standards in the schools: Guidelines.* Retrieved from http://www.asha.org/policy

American Speech-Language-Hearing Association. (2008a). *Clinical supervision in speech-language pathology [Technical report].* Retrieved from http://www.asha.org/policy

American Speech-Language-Hearing Association. (2008b). *Knowledge and skills needed by speech-language pathologists providing clinical supervision.* Retrieved from http://www.asha.org/policy

American Speech-Language-Hearing Association. (2010). *Code of ethics.* Retrieved from http://www.asha.org/policy

American Speech-Language-Hearing Association. (n.d.) *Gathering place mentoring manual.* Available from http://www.asha.org/uploadedFiles/students/gatheringplace/MentoringManual.pdf

Dodd, P., & Sundheim, D. (2005). *The 25 best time management tools and techniques: How to get more done without driving yourself crazy.* Orlando, FL: Peak Performance Press.

Hale, S. (2006). *Ethics: It's more than common sense.* Available from http://www.asha.org/uploadedfiles/practice/ethics/NSSLHAEthicspresentation.pdf

Heathfield, S. (2011). *Human resources and career planning.* Retrieved from http://humanresources.about.com/cs/perfmeasurement/a/pdp.htm

Kennedy, J. L. (1998, September 12). When it's time to resign, do it with savvy. *Buffalo News*, A–14.

Kroner, K. (1989). Take the gamble out of changing jobs. *Nursing, 20*, 111–118.

Lakein, A. (1996). *How to get control of your time and your life.* New York, NY: New American Library.

Pavlina, S. (2007). *Personal development for smart people.* Retrieved from http://www.stevepavlina.com/

Raudsepp, E. (1990). Knowing when to look for a new job. *Nursing, 20*, 136–140.

Rosenberg McKay, D. (2010). *Your first job. Making a good impression.* Available from http://careerplanning.about.com/cs/firstjob/a/first_job.htm

Schwartz, I., Horner, J., Jackson, R., Johnstone, P., & Mulligan, M. (2007). *Eligibility requirements and essential functions.* Minneapolis, MN: Council of Academic Programs in Communication Sciences and Disorders.

Silber, L. (2004). *Organizing from the right side of the brain: A creative approach to getting organized.* New York, NY: St. Martin's Press.

U.S. Office of Personnel Management. (1997). *360-degree assessment: An overview.* Available from http://www.opm.gov/perform/wppdf/360asess.pdf

RESOURCES

American Speech-Language-Hearing Association. (2000). *Background information and standards for implementation for the certificate of clinical competence in speech-language pathology.* Rockville, MD: ASHA, Council on Professional Standards in Speech-Language Pathology and Audiology.

American Speech-Language-Hearing Association. (2007). *Responsibilities of individuals who mentor clinical fellows.* Retrieved from http://www.asha.org/policy

American Speech-Language-Hearing Association. (2008). *Clinical supervision in speech-language pathology.* Retrieved from http://www.asha.org/policy

American Speech-Language-Hearing Association. (2010). *Certification.* Retrieved from http://www.asha.org/about/membership-certification/

Covey, S. (1989). *The 7 habits of highly effective people.* New York, NY: Simon & Schuster.

Covey, S. (1995). *The 7 habits of highly successful people.* DVD series available from http://www.enterprisemedia.com/product/00038/habits_highly_successful_people.html

Gibbons, M. *Self-directed learning.* Available from http://www.selfdirectedlearning.com/personal-development/how-can-i-find-my-strengths.html

Hudson, M. W. (2010). Supervision to mentoring: Practical considerations. *Perspectives on Administration and Supervision, 20*, 71–75.

Lowry, C. M. (1989). *Supporting and facilitating self-directed learning.* Retrieved from http://www.ntlf.com

Silber, L. (1998). *Time management for the creative person.* New York, NY: Three Rivers Press.

Internet Sources

Note: The following sources are fluid and should be checked periodically for their availability and current Internet addresses.

About.com: Career Planning
http://careerplanning.about.com/cs/firstjob/a/first_job.htm

About.com: Human Resources (Susan Heathfield)
http://humanresources.about.com/b/
http://humanresources.about.com/od/workrelationships/u/work.success.htm

ASHA Gathering Place Mentoring Manual
http://www.asha.org/students/gatheringplace/explore.htm
http://www.asha.org/students/gatheringplace/benefit.htm

Hubpages.com
http://hubpages.com/hub/10-Things-you-must-know-before-starting-that-New-Job

Milwaukeejobs.com
http://www.milwaukeejobs.com/

Personal Development for Smart People (Steve Pavlina)
http://www.stevepavlina.com/

Planet of Success
http://www.planetofsuccess.com/blog/2010/effective-networking-tips-professional-networking/

Thedigeratilife.com
http://www.thedigeratilife.com/blog/index.php/2008/12/05/got-laid-off-lose-your-job/

Wikihow.com
http://www.wikihow.com/Network

whatithinkabout.com
http://www.whatithinkabout.com/8-starting-a-new-job-tips/

Your-career-change.com
http://www.your-career-change.com/starting-a-new-job.html

11

Professional Autonomy and Collaboration

Janet E. Brown, MA
Jaynee A. Handelsman, PhD

SCOPE OF CHAPTER

Autonomy is the foundation of our professional identity as audiologists and speech-language pathologists (SLPs), while collaboration connects you to the broader clinical community of service providers. Anyone receiving professional services expects to receive them from an individual who meets established standards as a qualified professional and who can provide independent judgment based on knowledge and experience. At the same time, we expect the professional treating us to consult and collaborate with individuals from other disciplines when it is appropriate. External factors such as national and state regulations, facility policies, and payer requirements now place additional constraints on professional decision making. This chapter defines and describes professional autonomy from an official standpoint and discusses some of the challenges of autonomy and collaboration in real-life situations.

DEFINITIONS OF AUTONOMY AND COLLABORATION

Autonomy simply means the ability of an individual or group to make independent decisions regarding behavior. According to Princeton University's WordNet® (2003), it is defined as freedom from the arbitrary exercise of authority, which includes political and personal independence, and is synonymous with liberty and self-direction. Being autonomous, then, means being independent in mind or judgment and being self-directed (American Heritage, 2000). When the word is used to apply to a group, it also refers to self-governance and being free from the control of outside forces.

Speech-language pathology and audiology are recognized to be autonomous professions devoted to clinical service delivery, education, and research in the areas of normal and disordered human communication (American Speech-Language-Hearing Association [ASHA], 1986). ASHA defined an autonomous profession as "one in which the practitioner has the qualifications, responsibility, and authority for the provision of services which fall within its scope of practice" (p. 53). While being autonomous does not mean that an individual or group is free from being monitored or regulated by external bodies such as licensure boards, it does mean that individuals within the professions have the authority to define qualifications for practice, ethical standards, scopes of practice, and preferred practice patterns.

Collaboration refers to working together to accomplish a mutual goal. According to the dictionary, collaboration is particularly relevant to intellectual effort and includes cooperation (Princeton University, 2003). Collaboration, as it relates to the discipline of communication disorders, is important to providing optimal services to people served and can occur between speech-language pathologists and audiologists. This type of collaboration occurs on a regular basis when children who have hearing loss are evaluated and managed by audiologists and speech-language pathologists who serve as members of a cochlear implant team. Collaboration could also occur with other professions. For example, in a medical setting, audiologists typically work with physicians to establish plans of care for individuals with balance system disorders. Similarly, speech-language pathologists may collaborate with physicians to establish plans of care for clients being treated for head and neck cancer. Therefore, while collaboration, by definition, would appear to be at odds with autonomy, we know that both are important to the discipline as a whole and to individuals within the professions of speech-language pathology and audiology. The following sections discuss the application of factors related to autonomy and collaboration in these professions.

Sources of Professional Autonomy

One of the factors related to establishing professional autonomy is the definition of qualifications for practice, which is covered in detail in Chapter 3. Historically, the criteria for obtaining the Certificate of Clinical Competence (CCC) have been used to define the qualifications for entry into the professions. Specifically, the CCC-SLP is awarded to individuals in the profession of speech-language pathology who have met the minimum criteria specified by the Council for Clinical Certification (CFCC), and the CCC-A is awarded to individuals in the profession of audiology meeting the specified criteria (Council for Clinical Certification, 2005, 2011). The current criteria for certification in speech-language pathology and audiology are discussed in detail in Chapter 3 of this text.

Other qualifications for clinical practice are determined by the location and setting in which an individual practices. All states require state licensure. Generally, individuals within the professions are included on licensure boards and in so doing participate in crafting the rules for practice included in licensing bills. Similarly, individuals working in the schools may be required to hold teacher certification, and clinicians employed in hospital settings may be required to obtain specific credentialing. While other stakeholders may be included in determining the specific qualifications for practice in these cases, involvement of individuals within the professions is important to our professional autonomy.

Ethical standards for the professions are specified in the Codes of Ethics of our professional organizations. Specifically, ASHA's Code of Ethics (ASHA, 2010a) sets forth the essential principles and rules necessary to preserve the highest standards of ethical behavior and integrity that are vital to the responsible practice of SLPs; audiologists; and speech, language, and hearing scientists. The ASHA Code of Ethics applies to individuals who are members, certificate holders, and those in the certification process. See Appendix 5–A in Chapter 5 for the current Code of Ethics. Similarly, the Code of Ethics of the American Academy of Audiology (AAA) specifies what that organization considers to be appropriate professional ethical standards for audiologists and student members of AAA in an effort to protect the integrity of the profession (American Academy of Audiology [AAA], 2011). See Appendix 5–B in Chapter 5 for the current AAA Code of Ethics.

The principles and rules specified by the ASHA Code of Ethics outline ethical behavior as it relates to professionals honoring their responsibility to people served by holding their welfare paramount, honoring their responsibility to achieve and maintain the highest level of competence, honoring their responsibility to the public, and honoring their responsibilities to the professions, including relationships with colleagues, students, and members of allied professions.

While certification and licensure requirements specify the minimum qualifications to practice speech-language pathology and audiology, the Code of Ethics holds individuals within the professions to a higher standard. In addition to meeting the requirements of certification, the Code requires that "Individuals shall engage in only those aspects of the professions that are within the scope of their professional practice and competence, considering their level of education, training, and experience" (Principle II, Rule B). Thus, while there may not be a legal constraint to accepting a job in any setting, the Code of Ethics mandates that an individual has adequate training in the specific area of practice and with a given population to provide services competently. For example, a speech-language pathologist may decide to accept a new job at a hospital because of increased professional opportunities and increased salary. While previous hospital experience may satisfy the potential employer in terms of credentials for practice, if the new job includes working in the Neonatal Intensive Care Unit (NICU), competence in the area of feeding disorders in infants would be a necessary prerequisite from an ethical perspective. Similarly, although vestibular assessment and rehabilitation are within the scope of practice of audiology and employers may expect audiologists to conduct vestibular testing and perform particle repositioning maneuvers when indicated, the Code of Ethics compels audiologists and SLPs to refrain from practicing in any area in which adequate knowledge and skills have not been acquired.

The areas of practice within the professions are outlined in scope of practice documents. The ASHA scope of practice document for audiology (ASHA, 2004c) describes the services provided by qualified audiologists serving in various roles, serving as a reference for interested parties about the profession and informing ASHA members, certificate holders, and students of the professional activities for which the CCC-A is required. Similarly, the scope of practice document in speech-language pathology (ASHA, 2007) specifies areas of practice within the profession and defines professional activities for which the CCC-SLP is required.

ASHA's *Preferred Practice Patterns for the Profession of Speech-Language Pathology* (ASHA, 2004b) were created to enhance the quality and consistency of professional services in speech-language pathology by outlining procedural aspects of clinical service delivery across all practice settings. Similarly, the *Preferred Practice Patterns for the Profession of Audiology* (ASHA, 2006) provides a framework for quality patient care delivery across all settings in which audiologists practice. Both documents are organized by procedure as defined by the scopes of practice and other ASHA documents. The audiology document includes 23 individual practice patterns, while the speech-language pathology document includes 47 practice patterns. Each practice pattern in both documents refers to fundamental components and guiding principles as specified.

The scope of practice and preferred practice patterns define the realm of speech-language pathologists' and audiologists' professional activities and the populations and disorders they serve. In combination with certification, licensure, and codes of ethical professional conduct, they serve the purpose of protecting consumers by defining the qualifications for practice and the scope of the professions. Not only do these guidelines provide information about what is within the scopes of the professions, they prevent SLPs and audiologists from performing procedures that fall into the scopes of other professionals. For example, it is clear that SLPs may not interpret magnetic resonance imaging (MRI) studies and audiologists may not place tympanostomy tubes. The documents are dynamic and subject to periodic review. Accordingly, new procedures or areas of practice are added when appropriate, just as dysphagia became part of the scope of practice for speech-language pathologists in the 1980s and audiologists have added cerumen management and intraoperative surgical monitoring to their practice. Ideally, individuals within the professions are responsible for defining the scopes of practice and for articulating the preferred practice patterns. However, as speech-language pathologists and audiologists add areas of practice or when our scopes overlap with those of other professions, other stakeholders are likely to become more involved. See Chapter 3 on competencies and Chapter 5 for more information on ethics.

Legal Autonomy of the Professions

Being a certified and/or licensed professional allows SLPs and audiologists to work in the setting of their choice and to be in private practice as long as they comply with professional ethics and state regulations. As individuals practicing within autonomous professions, SLPs and audiologists may see clients without a physician's prescription or order. This is in direct contrast to physical therapists (PTs) and occupational therapists (OTs), who in many states must have a prescription from a physician in order to provide clinical services. State licensure boards, which exist to regulate practice and protect consumers within the state, have deemed that consumers can consult speech-language pathologists and audiologists without physician prescriptions. While the specific rules within the license may limit the scope of practice of audiologists or SLPs within a given state, or may require physician referral for the completion of certain types of services, audiologists and SLPs are able to practice independently. This means that they can independently determine which tests to administer, interpret results, make a communication diagnosis, and provide intervention without direction from a physician. Autonomy does not mean that clients are best served by having professionals operating in a vacuum without physician consultation, but it allows professionals to use independent judgment. Note that the term *prescription* is used specifically to refer to professions that can only provide services when prescribed by a physician. On the other hand, referrals are often part of the process required by payers to initiate SLP or audiology services.

Referrals

Institutional employment settings that provide clinical services, including hospitals, clinics, schools, and other settings, must have policies and procedures to ensure consistency and accountability for the manner in which the services are provided. Facilities are often accountable to government agencies such as the state department of health or state education agencies to be in compliance with state policies. Facilities may also seek accreditation by voluntary accrediting organizations such as the Joint Commission or CARF International (originally the Commission on Accreditation of Rehabilitation Facilities). Government agencies may audit client records and accounting practices, and accrediting organizations may perform periodic reviews to ensure that facilities are adhering to specified requirements or standards. Standards and procedures that are developed within institutions or facilities to comply with accrediting groups seek to ensure the quality and safety of the services to people served and to establish administrative procedures for the facility's streamlined and efficient operation.

Within health care organizations, it is common for policies and procedures to require that physicians initiate referrals for services from other professions, including speech-language pathology and audiology evaluations or interventions. Typically, the "privilege" of admitting a client to the facility is limited to only members of the medical staff with certain credentials, such as licensed physicians. Essentially, the facility (hospital, rehabilitation inpatient facility, skilled nursing facility) provides a setting for physicians to admit and care for their clients. The admitting physician, therefore, is legally responsible for decisions regarding the nature and extent of services provided and thus is required to "order" all services—from the level of nursing care required to the client's diet. In care settings managed under health maintenance organizations (HMOs), an outpatient referral from a primary care physician (PCP) is typically required for any specialty consultation or service (e.g., otolaryngology, radiology, audiology, speech-language pathology). This serves a dual purpose of ensuring that the primary care physician coordinates and participates in all aspects of the client's care, and it establishes a "gatekeeping" process for ensuring that physicians document their authorization for services for insurance purposes. While SLPs and audiologists have the right to practice independently, communication and collaboration with medical professions are often essential for optimal client care. Policies and procedures regarding how referrals are managed can be used to facilitate that collaboration.

In addition to complying with standards for quality and safety, health care providers are also responsible for meeting the bottom line—namely, generating sufficient revenue to pay for salaries, supplies, and operating costs of the facility. This financial reality means facilities and individual providers must meet requirements set by various payment sources, including Medicare, Medicaid, private health plans, HMOs, preferred provider organizations (PPOs), and private contracts. Inasmuch as the insurance providers and others are free to establish criteria for payment, it may be difficult for SLPs and audiologists to keep up with current standards. In reality, it often seems that professionals are asked to shoot at moving targets to obtain payment for services, and it is typical for physicians and insurance company administrators to be involved in making decisions about covered services. For example, payers for speech, language, and/or swallowing services typically require that a physician serve as a gatekeeper and attest to the need for the services by signing a referral. In some cases, then, SLPs must advocate for authorization of services by persuading the primary care physician that specific services are needed. Similarly, an SLP in private practice may be required to obtain a referral from a physician so that payment can be received from a client's health insurance plan.

Increasingly, schools use medical reimbursement resources such as Medicaid to pay for services provided to eligible children. In addition to the introduction of the "medical model" of requiring a physician referral for the clinician to provide services that will be reimbursed, the involvement of Medicaid creates additional challenges within educational settings because of the definition of who is a "qualified provider." Although Medicaid's guidelines specify that only a certified and/or licensed professional can provide services, individual state regulations regarding the provision of SLP services in the schools may be less stringent and include individuals with a bachelor's degree or a teaching credential (ASHA, 2004a). In this case, Medicaid's definition of *qualified provider* may exceed the requirements of the schools, leaving certified SLPs in the uncomfortable position of having to supervise individuals who are not certified but who are deemed qualified by the state. ASHA has developed policy documents that provide guidance to SLPs in these situations: *Medicaid Guidance for Speech-Language Pathology Services: Addressing the "Under the Direction of" Rule* (2004a).

In summary, while a physician's referral may be required for insurance purposes or to comply with an organization's policies and procedures, speech-language pathologists and audiologists are legally autonomous in terms of their ability to practice and make independent clinical decisions. Furthermore, SLPs and audiologists are bound by their ethical codes to make clinical decisions based upon independent clinical judgment within their scope of practice and professional competence.

Prescription and Threats to Professional Autonomy

As noted previously, health care facilities or educational settings develop policies and procedures that establish a process for delivering services. However, SLPs and audiologists must participate in the development of the policies and procedures affecting their services so they do not conflict with professional and ethical guidelines. For the same reasons that SLPs and audiologists must practice only in the areas in which they have knowledge and skills, ASHA's Code of Ethics also compels individuals to maintain independent clinical judgment (ASHA, 2010a). Specifically, the Code states that "Individuals shall not provide professional services without exercising independent professional judgment, regardless of referral source or prescription" (Principle IV, Rule J). A challenge to both professional autonomy and ethical behavior can occur when working with physicians who provide referrals for services. As autonomous professionals, SLPs and audiologists conduct assessments and develop treatment plans. When a physician's referral includes prescriptive requirements that conflict with a clinician's professional judgment, professional autonomy is compromised. Furthermore, the clinician is faced with an ethical dilemma. For example, despite a physician's referral order for treatment five times a week for four weeks for a client with severe dementia, the speech-language pathologist may determine that this intensity and length of treatment is inappropriate given the client's limited prognosis and functional goals. Similarly, while a physician might refer a client for amplification and may specify a particular amplification arrangement, the audiologist who ultimately fits the amplification must be responsible for determining what system is in the best interests of those served, including consideration of personal and situational variables as well as hearing status.

The Issues in Ethics statement on *Prescription* by the Board of Ethics discusses the challenges to professionals whose professional responsibilities may be restricted by prescription: "...if a certificate holder

[does] ... not challenge prescriptive mandates where the welfare of the person served is at risk, the certificate holder could be held in violation of the Code of Ethics" (ASHA, 2010b). Thus, certified professionals have an ethical obligation *not* to comply with prescriptions or team decisions that fail to serve the client's best interest.

Employer Challenges to Professional Autonomy

Audiologists and speech-language pathologists who are employees may also encounter institutional policies that can infringe on their professional autonomy. For example, many health care settings set productivity targets for staff (e.g., 10 patients per day, 24 billable units). If these targets are presented as absolute requirements, clinicians might feel pressed to treat patients who are inappropriate for services or to treat them for a longer period than is clinically justifiable. They may even feel pressured to shade their clinical documentation to justify reimbursement. Similarly, when productivity guidelines are based on number of patients seen or number of procedures completed, audiologists or SLPs may be pressed to spend an inadequate amount of time with any given patient. For example, many clinical settings allow 30 minutes for completion of a comprehensive audiological evaluation. While that time frame might be appropriate for cooperative adult patients, it might be inappropriate for patients with more complex needs. Any time professionals are asked to engage in practices that contradict their professional judgment or are otherwise unethical or illegal, they have an ethical obligation to refuse to comply. Furthermore, professionals should be involved in the establishment of clinical guidelines within the settings in which they are employed.

Employers who are not audiologists or speech-language pathologists may be unfamiliar with the scopes of practice, preferred practice patterns, and the Code of Ethics for audiologists and SLPs. They may be unaware that professionals who are both licensed and certified must adhere to the highest or most stringent standard of the state licensing law and ASHA. When supervisors are professionals such as otolaryngologists, nurses, or physical therapists, they form expectations about the practice and ethics of audiology and SLP based on their knowledge of their own profession. Some conflicts over professional judgment versus facility policies can be resolved by educating the supervisor about audiology and SLP professional standards and providing relevant policy documents. In other situations, when financial pressures on a facility result in practices that place the client at risk for a poor outcome, professionals should raise the issue of potential liability for malpractice, negative publicity, or client dissatisfaction. Larger institutions appoint corporate compliance officers and risk managers to ensure quality of services and compliance with state and federal regulations.

Being supervised by a member of another profession can also present challenges in terms of how audiologists and SLPs are evaluated on their individual performance. ASHA's policy on *Professional Performance Appraisal by Individuals Outside the Professions of Speech-Language Pathology and Audiology* stipulates that a supervisor from another profession may evaluate the performance of general responsibilities by an audiologist or SLP, but that a member of the same profession should evaluate clinical performance (ASHA, 1993). Where this is not feasible, the policy recommends the use of self-evaluation or peer review.

Autonomy and Liability

Autonomy comes with increased risk. SLPs and audiologists who are engaged in clinical practice, particularly private practice, are vulnerable to liability claims in the event of injury or other unfavorable outcomes. Physicians pay large sums for malpractice insurance because their decisions and actions can result in serious and permanent injury to an individual. While SLPs and audiologists are much less likely to cause such serious harm directly, it is important to remember that individuals can be held liable for their clinical actions and client care decisions. Therefore, clinicians should exercise good judgment in deciding whether to confer with the primary care or other physician before treating a disorder related to a health condition (e.g., stroke, traumatic brain injury, cerebral palsy) as well as the timing of communication and consultation during and following treatment. Although consultation with other health care providers may not be strictly required, clinical judgment would dictate that clinicians be aware of any potentially complicating medical history before initiating treatment. In addition, complications that occur during treatment warrant additional communication. Read more about liability issues in Chapter 6.

MODELS OF COLLABORATION

In its broadest sense, collaboration simply means working with others. Applied to the practice of speech-language pathology and audiology, it could refer to working with a wide range of professionals from health care, education, and community services, as well as with members of the client's individual support network. According to current definitions of evidence-based practice, the people served, including the client and designated family members or caregivers, are an essential part of the treatment team (see Chapter 29), in that their wishes need to be taken into account when making clinical decisions. ASHA's position statement on evidence-based practice emphasizes the role of the client in the following definition: "The term *evidence-based practice* refers to an approach in which current, high-quality research evidence is integrated with practitioner expertise and client preferences and values into the process of making clinical decisions" (ASHA, 2005). Regardless of the professional setting, collaboration in clinical care includes the incorporation of the people served into the diagnostic and treatment team.

Medical Model

In health care, collaboration can assume many forms, depending on a variety of factors, including the medical diagnosis and the health care setting. In some medical settings, formal multidisciplinary or interdisciplinary teams may be established to develop a structure and process to manage clients with complex problems. Payer requirements can either support or work against team evaluations and treatment. Payers seldom pay for two professional services that bill for simultaneous procedures; typically only one provider can charge for a procedure when providers are "co-treating" or they have to split the time being billed. However, collaboration is highly encouraged in certain care areas. For example, a stroke or traumatic brain injury team might include members representing various professions, including neurology, physiatry, nursing, psychology, speech-language pathology, occupational therapy, physical therapy, and social work. Individual team members typically conduct an independent evaluation of each client, after which the team members confer to develop a plan of care that includes some or all of the professions represented. Similarly, cleft palate teams, at minimum, will consist of an otolaryngologist or plastic surgeon, a dentist or orthodontist, a speech-language pathologist, and an audiologist. A neonatal intensive care unit may have a feeding team composed of a pediatric gastroenterologist, pulmonologist, nurse, lactation specialist, speech-language pathologist, dietitian, and occupational therapist. A balance and falls prevention team may consist of an audiologist and a physical therapist or occupational therapist along with one or more physicians (otolaryngologist, geriatrician, neurologist, physiatrist, psychiatrist). Because these multidisciplinary and interdisciplinary teams are formed to address specific client care needs, they are likely to establish procedures for conducting assessments, coordinating the treatment plan, and meeting periodically to review progress and update the plan.

Collaboration in a medical setting may also be less formal and still involve individuals from a variety of professions. For example, a client coming in to the emergency room with complaints of dizziness is likely to be seen initially by an emergency room physician and support personnel, who may consult with other physicians including neurologists, otolaryngologists, and radiologists. Following initial evaluations designed to rule out life-threatening conditions and the initiation of medical management, the client may be referred for additional outpatient testing or admitted into the hospital. Depending upon the initial medical diagnosis and the nature of the client's symptoms, audiologists may be called upon to provide assessment of hearing and vestibular system function and to provide recommendations regarding the need for audiologic and/or vestibular rehabilitation. In this instance, collaboration is essential to providing optimal care for the client, and the audiologist serves as an important member of the health care team and may ultimately direct the treatment decisions.

Educational Model

Participation in interdisciplinary teams is also an important role of SLPs and audiologists working in school settings. In fact, procedures for collaboration among various professional groups to plan and deliver services to identified students are legally mandated under the Individuals with Disabilities Education Act (IDEA) and other state guidelines. For example, students' Individualized Education Program (IEP) teams consist of the parents, teacher(s), special education teacher(s), and professionals from other relevant disciplines who are working with the student. Various models of service delivery for the schools involve collaboration among the SLP, the classroom teacher, and other relevant professionals (ASHA, 2010c). For a detailed description, the reader is referred to Chapter 15.

As is the case in a medical environment, interdisciplinary teams may be formed to address specific disorders or client care needs. Examples of such teams include a dysphagia team and an augmentative and alternative communication (AAC) team. Teams are also appropriate for coordinating the educational services for children with hearing loss. These teams may be based in a single school or consist of specialists who provide evaluation and consultation within an entire school district. This type of collaboration may incorporate both the educational and medical model, as referrals for evaluation and/or treatment may include hospital or clinic-based services as well as school-based services. The role of the SLP or audiologist may be as team leader, team member, or consultant.

Collaboration and Scope of Practice

Collaboration can occur as joint diagnosis or treatment of the client or in the form of consultation to confirm that goals and treatment approaches complement one another. Each professional typically conducts an assessment focusing on those aspects of care that fall within his or her scope of practice. In some cases, the assessment or a portion of it can be conducted jointly so that simultaneous behavioral observations are made by more than one member of the team, which serves to facilitate later discussion among team members and to minimize the burden on the client. One application of this approach is in the completion of a developmental assessment of an infant by an interdisciplinary team. In other instances, it may be more efficient or informative for each professional to administer his or her own test battery separately and subsequently compare results.

Several challenges are associated with the evaluation and management of complex disorders when multiple disciplines are involved. To provide optimal care and to minimize problems with billing and reimbursement for services, professionals with overlapping scopes of practice should collaborate in advance to ensure that they are not duplicating assessments. For example, if both an SLP and an OT evaluate a client who has had a stroke, it is appropriate for the SLP to report on the speech, language, cognitive-communication, and swallowing aspects of the assessment, while the OT may report on the individual's ability to perform activities of daily living, including grooming, dressing, and feeding, with comments on how cognitive skills such as sequencing, problem solving, and safety awareness affect these activities. In this situation, the SLP and OT may discuss their findings and collaborate to reinforce compensatory strategies for the client's cognitive-communication deficits while working on different tasks. On the other hand, if the client demonstrated only problems with swallowing and both professions remain involved in developing treatment plans for addressing swallowing problems, the overlap could result in a denial of payment for one of the services provided. Furthermore, the overlap may result in confusion for the individuals served and for other members of the health care team.

ROLE AMBIGUITY AND SCOPE OF PRACTICE

In the past decade, concerns about budget limitations or personnel shortages have led external decision makers in some situations to delegate core activities of speech-language pathologists and audiologists to other disciplines. Examples come from many practice settings for both professions. In some skilled nursing facilities and other health care settings, swallowing evaluations or treatments have been assigned to occupational therapists, who also include swallowing as part of their scope of practice. In school systems across the country, educators have proposed reducing the credentials for "speech therapists" in their districts or actually created new titles (e.g., "communication specialist") to take on some of the caseload of speech-language pathologists. In some medical practices, hearing testing and vestibular assessments have been delegated to minimally trained support personnel supervised by physicians. In situations in which services are shifted to a less qualified provider, clients may be placed at risk.

Early intervention programs, frequently funded by state Medicaid programs, have also given rise to concerns about overlap in scope of practice. Many programs stipulate that a single provider (from the discipline in which the most intervention is needed or from "developmental interventionists") will deliver services to the child—which can range from motor skills to language stimulation—with input from other professionals. When these services are provided in the child's "natural environment" (e.g., the child's home), the provider delivering services must be keenly aware of the need to consult with other professionals monitoring the child's progress to ensure that the intervention is appropriate and to determine when reevaluation is needed. Such practices have given rise to concerns about the appropriateness of other professionals addressing language development and swallowing and the effectiveness of those services. When hearing loss is involved, concerns are also raised about the adequacy of knowledge and skills of the service provider related to aural habilitation. See Chapter 16 for more in-depth discussion of early intervention.

Escalating concerns about professional boundaries, often referred to as "encroachment," resulted in ASHA forming a committee in 2006 to study the issue. The Coordinating Committee of the Vice President for Speech-Language Pathology Services conducted a survey of speech-language pathologists and examined the issue from multiple perspectives. The committee concluded that the term *role ambiguity* was a less negative view of overlapping scopes of professional practice when the goal is to provide service to the "whole" client using a practice model that is most appropriate to the client's needs—ranging from a parallel model to a highly interdisciplinary and integrative approach (ASHA, 2009).

INTERPROFESSIONAL TRAINING

In a rising trend, the Institute of Medicine (IOM) has emphasized the importance of interdisciplinary teaming as an important component in improving patient care rather than focusing on separating disciplines to protect scopes of practice. In its 2003 report *Health Professions Education: A Bridge to Quality*, the IOM urged greater coordination in the preservice and continuing education of professionals from different disciplines (Institute of Medicine, 2003). The report advocates developing a core set of competencies across disciplines, with coordination of accreditation, certification, and licensure for the professions. While this call seems at present to be a distant vision, there have been some initial responses on the part of related professional organizations (i.e., physicians, nurses, and pharmacists) to collaborate in establishing a national interprofessional clearinghouse for professional education.

This development could be considered a sequel to the concept of a "multiskilled" professional that was the subject of research and exploration in the 1980s and 1990s. In an effort to streamline services and reduce costs, the notion of a "rehabilitation specialist" who could be cross-trained to address multiple areas of professional service was considered and ultimately rejected by ASHA (ASHA, 1997). Reasons for rejecting cross training of clinical skills included the differences in preparation, education, experience, and autonomy of different professional providers. ASHA's *Multiskilled Personnel* document (1997) acknowledged that cross training of basic patient care skills, administrative skills, nonclinical skills, and possibly the activities of support personnel may be feasible and assist in delivering more efficient care.

Adding Basic Client Care Skills

The concept of speech-language pathologists and audiologists becoming cross-trained in basic client care skills has continued to grow since the multiskilled personnel debate was addressed in the 1997 ASHA document.

In trying to achieve the greatest efficiency of services or streamline the use of staff, schools or health care organizations may ask speech-language pathologists and audiologists to perform tasks that they never before had considered to be within their purview as professionals but that are performed by other professional and even nonprofessional staff.

ASHA concluded that SLPs and audiologists may perform basic client care skills if they have been trained and if they demonstrate competence in that skill, in accordance with the Code of Ethics. Examples of basic client care activities include taking blood pressure readings (which is frequently a routine part of home health visits), performing client transfers (such as from a wheelchair to a bed), and performing suctioning (which may be a frequent part of client care in a hospital specializing in tracheotomized and/or ventilator-dependent patients). While audiologists and

SLPs may view the addition of these activities as burdensome, in some settings they may facilitate optimal client care and safety. For example, an audiologist may encounter a patient becoming less responsive during an evaluation, in which case being able to take a blood pressure reading is important. Similarly, when clients arrive for balance function testing in a wheelchair, they may need to be safely transferred to another chair for the evaluation. As is true with the provision of clinical services that are within the scopes of practice of the professions, SLPs and audiologists are compelled by their Code of Ethics to perform only those services for which they have adequate knowledge and skills. If professionals do not feel comfortable performing a task after being trained, they should discuss the matter with their supervisor or consider seeking employment in another setting.

ADDITIONAL THREATS TO AUTONOMY

While many of the challenges to autonomy are common for audiology and speech-language pathology, audiology has faced some that are unique to that profession. Audiologists have struggled to become the point of entry for individuals with hearing and balance disorders and been met with opposition from many fronts. Physicians have argued that they should remain the gatekeepers of services to protect clients from potential harm, and physician groups have lobbied Congress to thwart legislative attempts to enable clients to initiate hearing care through audiologists. In addition, Medicare policies have historically restricted the payment for audiologic testing to those instances in which the testing is determined to be medically necessary. Furthermore, the Medicare Physician Fee Schedule, which includes the procedures that fall within the scope of practice of audiology, and which is frequently used by private insurance companies to determine coverage for services, has not recognized that the professional work of audiologists enables them to be reimbursed for interpretation of test data (ASHA, 2011). While physicians can completely bill and be paid for the professional component for each of the procedures that are performed by audiologists, audiologists remain unable to directly collect for professional fees. Inasmuch as the billing codes that are used belong to the American Medical Association, physicians have been able to maintain fairly tight control over access to reimbursement by audiologists.

INTERDEPENDENCE OF AUDIOLOGY AND SPEECH-LANGUAGE PATHOLOGY

Audiology and speech-language pathology are viewed as separate professions within one discipline. Intuitively, that position makes sense since both professions address aspects of the discipline of human communication sciences and disorders. As the scopes of practice have expanded, each profession has added areas of practice that are more specialized, creating increased separation between the professions and giving rise to tensions. For example, AAA has espoused the position that it is and must be the primary professional home of audiologists and that audiology must separate itself from speech-language pathology to become an autonomous profession. Essentially, AAA asserts that ASHA cannot rightfully represent the interests of audiologists. That position has created conflict within the profession of audiology and the discipline as a whole. See Chapter 4 for further discussion of ASHA and AAA as professional associations.

In reality, while there are clear areas of separation, there is a great deal of overlap in the knowledge that is required for the practice of audiology and the practice of speech-language pathology. For example, both professions require an understanding of normal anatomy and normal communication processes, including hearing, speech, and language. Audiologists must understand normal speech perception to make clinical decisions about the rehabilitation of hearing loss, including the fitting of hearing aids and the programming of cochlear implants. Similarly, speech-language pathologists must appreciate the impact of hearing loss on language perception, including its impact on clients' performance on speech and language assessments. The management of infants and young children with hearing loss must include input from both professions. The overriding purpose of improving hearing is to facilitate better communication (listening, speech, and language). Both professions also have relevance for literacy issues. In addition, the diseases and disorders that cause clients to need SLP and audiology services frequently cross several domains: hearing, balance, speech, language, cognition, and swallowing. Optimal care of clients across the life span requires audiologists and SLPs to collaborate. For all of those reasons, regardless of whether the professions continue to be viewed as members of a single discipline, it is evident that the professions of audiology and speech-language pathology are interdependent.

COLLABORATION AND CONFIDENTIALITY

While collaboration is an important part of coordinating and maximizing treatment, clinicians must be sure they protect the client's privacy and confidentiality by not disclosing information without the client's permission. The Health Information Portability and Accountability Act (HIPAA) of 1996 and state laws establish guidelines about the privacy of protected medical information and impose sanctions against individuals or institutions that do not protect the client's privacy. For example, the client must give written permission to send a report or videotape for a second opinion from a colleague at another hospital. The client also must give consent for his or her case to be discussed with family members. For that reason, the manner in which professionals conduct business may be affected. For example, leaving detailed messages on an answering machine that include protected information is prohibited. Audiologists and SLPs must be vigilant in obtaining necessary consents before discussing any aspect of care with anyone in order to maintain client confidentiality.

SUMMARY

As professions, speech-language pathology and audiology are constantly evolving and the scopes of practice and preferred practice patterns within the discipline of communication sciences and disorders are periodically reviewed and modified. Your professional autonomy depends upon the involvement of the professions in crafting those documents and in determining ethical practice standards and policies regarding reimbursement for services. Both autonomy and collaboration are subject to the influence of evolving practice and reimbursement trends. The complexity of disorders, populations, and service delivery systems can challenge the autonomy of the speech-language pathologist or audiologist in independent decision making. However, collaboration, when conducted with mutual respect and established procedures, can benefit and enhance outcomes for the people served and for other stakeholders. The key to achieving a successful balance between professional autonomy and collaboration is involvement of audiologists and SLPs in self-determination by taking a leadership role in setting their own standards of practice and shaping the policies and procedures within their work settings that will affect their autonomy. Ultimately, professional autonomy and collaboration within and outside of the discipline strikes a balance to benefit both the people served and the professionals themselves.

CRITICAL THINKING

1. What would you do if a physician orders a modified barium swallow but you think the client's dementia will make him unable to cooperate?
2. What referral or authorization (if any) would a licensed SLP need to work on accent modification with an individual in his home if he were paying privately?
3. How do institutional and reimbursement constraints affect the autonomy of SLPs and audiologists?
4. What is the difference between a multiskilled provider and a multidisciplinary team? Consider the settings in which you have done practicum or worked professionally. What teams were in place? How did teamwork facilitate or impede what you do professionally? Why?
5. What unique challenges to autonomy have audiologists faced? What can be done to ameliorate these challenges?
6. In what ways are audiology and speech-language pathology interdependent, and is that relationship helpful or harmful to the discipline and to people served?

REFERENCES

American Academy of Audiology. (2011). *Code of Ethics of the American Academy of Audiology.* Available from http://www.audiology.org/

The American Heritage Dictionary of the English Language (4th ed.). (2000). New York, NY: Houghton Mifflin.

American Speech-Language-Hearing Association. (1986). Autonomy of speech-language pathology and audiology. *ASHA, 28*, 53–57.

American Speech-Language-Hearing Association. (1993). *Professional performance appraisal by individuals outside the professions of speech-language pathology and audiology* [Technical report]. Available from http://www.asha.org/policy

American Speech-Language-Hearing Association. (1997, Spring). Position statement: *Multiskilled personnel. ASHA, 39* (Suppl. 17), 13.

American Speech-Language-Hearing Association. (2004a). *Medicaid guidance for speech-language pathology services: Addressing the "under the direction of" rule.* Available from http://www.asha.org/

American Speech-Language-Hearing Association. (2004b). *Preferred practice patterns for the profession of speech-language pathology.* Available from http://www.asha.org/

American Speech-Language-Hearing Association. (2004c). *Scope of practice in audiology.* Available from http://www.asha.org/policy

American Speech-Language-Hearing Association. (2005). *Evidence-based practice in communication disorders.* Available from http://www.asha.org/

American Speech-Language-Hearing Association. (2006). *Preferred practice patterns for the profession of audiology.* Available from http://www.asha.org/policy

American Speech-Language-Hearing Association. (2007). *Scope of practice in speech-language pathology.* Available from http://www.asha.org/policy

American Speech-Language-Hearing Association. (2009, December 15). Role ambiguity and speech-language pathology. *The ASHA Leader.*

American Speech-Language-Hearing Association. (2010a). *Code of ethics.* Available from http://www.asha.org/policy

American Speech-Language-Hearing Association. (2010b). *Prescription.* Available from http://www.asha.org/policy

American Speech-Language-Hearing Association. (2010c). *Roles and responsibilities of speech-language pathologists in schools.* Available from http://www.asha.org/policy

American Speech-Language-Hearing Association. (2011). *Analysis of 2011 Medicare fee schedule.* Available from http://www.asha.org/Practice/reimbursement/medicare/feeschedule/

Council for Clinical Certification in Audiology and Speech-Language Pathology of the American Speech-Language-Hearing Association. (2005). *2005 Standards and implementation procedures for the certification of clinical competence in speech-language pathology.* Available from http://www.asha.org/

Council for Clinical Certification in Audiology and Speech-Language Pathology of the American Speech-Language-Hearing Association. (2011). *2011 Standards and implementation procedures for the certification of clinical competence in audiology.* Available from http://www.asha.org/

Institute of Medicine. (2003). *Health professions education: A bridge to quality.* Retrieved from http://www.iom.edu/Reports/2003/Health-Professions-Education-A-Bridge-to-Quality.aspx

Princeton University, Cognitive Science Laboratory. (2003). WordNet® 2.0. Available from http://wordnet.princeton.edu/

12

Support Personnel in Communication Sciences and Disorders

Diane R. Paul, PhD
Susan Sparks, MA

SCOPE OF CHAPTER

Many individuals help to support the work of speech-language pathologists and audiologists including families, administrative and secretarial staff, teachers and instructional aides, psychologists and social workers, other therapists and professional staff, interns, and volunteers. This chapter focuses specifically on those individuals who are hired in a professional capacity and have some degree of training and supervision to extend our services. They perform services that are prescribed, directed, and supervised by licensed and/or certified speech-language pathologists or audiologists.

Support personnel have been used in the communication sciences and disorders since the early 1970s. Their use has been a topic of debate, particularly in the field of speech-language pathology, with passionate views on both sides. Those favoring the use of support personnel believe that access to care is improved, frequency and intensity of service are increased, and the skills of professionals are better used. Those opposing argue that the quality of care may be compromised and the services of professionals devalued. Proponents say use of support personnel is in the best interest of consumers; opponents say consumers may be misled (Breakey, 1993; Werven, 1993). The dynamics of the service delivery system, in tandem with cost controls and personnel needs, have led to the development of new and changing state and national policies related to the training, supervision, and use of support personnel in the professions of audiology and speech-language pathology (American Academy of Audiology [AAA], 2010a; American Speech-Language-Hearing Association [ASHA], 1992b, 1998b, 2004g).

In many health care and education settings across the country, speech-language pathologists (SLPs) and audiologists are experiencing escalating caseloads and increasing paperwork in conjunction with shrinking budgets and personnel shortages (particularly for school-based SLPs) (ASHA, 2010c). In response, some facilities and institutions have chosen to employ support personnel to assist their professional staff. Support personnel, known by a variety of terms (e.g., *aides, assistants, OTO techs, paraprofessionals, paratherapists, SLPAs,* and *technicians*), have been employed by professionals in communication sciences and disorders as a way to extend and expand services. They are considered support staff rather than substitutes or replacements for qualified professionals.

The purpose of this chapter is to provide information about the use, training, supervision, responsibilities, and effectiveness of support personnel in the professions of speech-language pathology and audiology. Specifically, the chapter includes information on the rationale, concerns, professional policies, state regulations, current use, training recommendations, supervision requirements, job responsibilities, reimbursement, research, and future directions related to speech-language pathology and audiology support personnel. A glossary of key terms used in this chapter is provided in the appendix.

RATIONALE FOR THE USE OF SUPPORT PERSONNEL

The growing and diverse needs of individuals with communication and related disorders increase the demand for speech-language pathology and audiology services (Bureau of Labor Statistics, 2011a, 2011b). This growing demand for communication services is one of the converging factors leading to the use of support personnel in communication sciences and disorders. Other influences include federal legislation sustaining the education rights of students with disabilities, the Individuals with Disabilities Education Improvement Act of 2004 (IDEA, 2004), including the right of students to be assessed in their native language, and increasing caseloads due to (1) recognition of the value and need for early intervention services (ASHA, 2008; Feldman, 2004; Guralnick, 2005, 2011; Joint Committee on Infant Hearing, 2007); (2) aging of the population with concomitant health needs (Administration on Aging, 2002; Kochkin, 2009); (3) need to care for individuals with hearing loss resulting from occupational noise (AAA, 2003; ASHA, 2004a); and (4) expanding scopes of services in audiology and speech-language pathology (AAA, 1997, 2004; ASHA, 1997, 2001, 2004d, 2004e).

Thus, because of the growing need for services, combined with the rising health care and education costs and personnel shortages, some SLPs and audiologists have identified roles for support personnel in the delivery of service for children and adults with communication disorders. First we will consider the rationale for two of the roles, serving as interpreters/translators in bilingual/bicultural environments and working on collaborative teams in classrooms.

The need to use bilingual/bicultural support personnel in speech-language pathology and audiology has increased as the U.S. population continues to diversify with respect to language and culture (U.S. Census Bureau, 2010). Because only 7.1 percent of ASHA members and certificate holders are nonwhite, 3.8 percent are Hispanics or Latino (ASHA, 2010b), and less than 6 percent are bilingual (ASHA, 2009a), it often is not possible to match a clinician to a client's cultural and linguistic background (ASHA, 2004c). Consequently, the assistance of professional interpreters and cultural brokers is often necessary to provide culturally and linguistically appropriate services (ASHA, 2004e; Lynch & Hanson, 2004). ASHA has a profile of individuals who have self-identified that they are bilingual service providers (ASHA, 2009a).

Executive Order 13166, which reinforces Title VI of the Civil Rights Act (U.S. Department of Justice, 2000), reminds facilities that receive any type of federal funds, including Medicaid/Medicare, that they must develop a plan to provide equal access to services for people with limited English proficiency. IDEA 2004 also requires that assessment be conducted in a child's native language. Support personnel who share the same language and/or culture with a client may fill these roles to help meet the needs of a multilingual population, provided there is ongoing training, planning, and communication (ASHA, 1985a, 2004b; Langdon & Cheng, 2002). In the 2008 and 2010 ASHA Schools Surveys, SLPs were asked how they provided services to English language learners. In both years, 2.0 percent of respondents indicated they use bilingual SLP assistants. In the 2009 ASHA Membership Survey, 12 percent of respondents indicated that they employ support personnel to provide services to users of other languages (ASHA, 2008, 2010c).

IDEA 2004 recognizes the use of paraprofessionals and assistants as adjuncts to the team of service providers in the schools. In accordance with state law, paraprofessionals and assistants who are appropriately trained and supervised may be used to assist in the provision of special education and related services for children with disabilities. In addition, the state must adopt a policy that requires local educational agencies to take measures to recruit, hire, train, and retain highly qualified personnel, including paraprofessionals, to provide special education and related services to children with disabilities. Special education paraprofessionals who provide instructional support in Title I programs (Improving the Academic Achievement of the Disadvantaged) also must meet the requirements of the Elementary and Secondary Education Act (ESEA), reauthorized as the No Child Left Behind Act (NCLB, 2002).

The use of alternative service delivery models for SLPs in the schools also has prompted the use of SLP assistants. Although the prevailing SLP service delivery model in the schools has been and continues to be a "pullout" model (ASHA, 1995a, 2010c), it may not be the best model for fostering natural, contextually based communication interactions. In recent years, the recognition of the need for more functional outcomes has led to an extension of service into the classroom (Cirrin et al., 2010; Paul-Brown & Caperton, 2001). The use of SLP assistants who work directly in the classroom has been a means to integrate speech and language goals into the curriculum, generalize learned concepts, enhance carryover of functional skills, and reinforce SLP goals in the student's natural setting (Gerlach, 2000; Goldberg & Paul-Brown, 1999; Pickett, 1999; Pickett & Gerlach, 1997).

The appropriate use of trained, supervised, and less costly support personnel may be one way to meet the growing service needs of people with communication disorders and still maintain the role of the fully qualified SLP and audiologist (Paul-Brown & Goldberg, 2001). The use of support personnel in various roles (e.g., interpreters/translators, classroom collaborators) may provide a means to supplement services for a diverse population, extend services in natural settings, free professionals to dedicate more time to those individuals with more complex conditions, and fulfill increasing managerial responsibilities (ASHA, 2004b).

CONCERNS ABOUT THE USE OF SUPPORT PERSONNEL

Some audiologists and SLPs have expressed concerns about the impact of using support personnel on service delivery. Some believe that support personnel (1) may be hired in lieu of qualified providers, (2) may be used to increase caseload size, (3) may be asked to provide services for which they are not trained, or (4) may receive inadequate supervision. Audiologists are concerned about otolaryngologists hiring support personnel, specifically otologic technicians (OTO techs), instead of hiring or referring to audiologists.

In many school settings, demand for SLPs outweighs supply. Indeed, 55 percent of SLPs responding to ASHA's 2010 Schools Survey (ASHA, 2010b) indicated that job openings were more numerous than job seekers in their school. Employers may be tempted to hire assistants to fill a persistent vacancy. According to the ASHA Schools Survey (ASHA, 2010b), 23.4 percent of respondents reported that "increased use of support personnel" was one impact of the shortage of SLP clinical service providers in school settings. There is a concern about quality of services when the motivation for using support personnel is to respond to a personnel shortage rather than to extend and enhance service.

Another area of concern is when a bilingual assistant is asked to work with clients without adequate supervision or support. Although using a bilingual assistant may be beneficial, there is the potential for misuse or overuse if the assistant has not been trained appropriately or is asked to go beyond an assistant's job responsibilities (e.g., inappropriately expected to conduct evaluations and create treatment plans for bilingual clients). Furthermore, the ability to speak a second language does not automatically qualify someone to be a translator or interpreter, nor does it mean that the individual has the skills necessary to serve as an SLP assistant or audiology assistant (ASHA, 1985a, 2004c; Langdon & Cheng, 2002).

Clearly, inappropriate use of support personnel could have far-reaching and negative effects on the professions (ASHA, 1992b). One way to ensure that the quality of care is not compromised is for SLPs and audiologists to adhere to national and state laws and follow professional ethic statements and guidelines so that support personnel receive appropriate training and supervision and only provide services within a limited scope of job responsibilities. Even in the absence of mandatory state requirements, SLPs and audiologists should adhere to these professional guidelines. Another way to promote the appropriate use of support personnel is through education and awareness initiatives, such as providing information to administrators, principals, school boards, hospital boards, otolaryngologists, and others responsible for personnel or hiring decisions about the role of supervised support personnel and their job responsibilities in comparison to the scope of practice of the supervising SLPs and audiologists.

Recently, ASHA created a new program as another means to give ASHA and its members a stronger, more credible voice in explaining the proper use of support personnel with defined boundaries for how they are used. ASHA supports the use of support personnel to ensure both accessibility and the highest quality of care while addressing productivity and cost-benefit concerns. The ASHA Board of Directors established an affiliation category for support personnel in speech-language pathology and audiology in 2009. Starting in 2011, ASHA began offering associate status to support personnel who work under the supervision of an ASHA-certified speech-language pathologist or audiologist. Applicants are required to adhere to ASHA's guidelines for SLP assistants or support personnel in audiology, perform only tasks that are appropriate for SLP or audiology assistants, adhere to state laws and state licensure requirements for SLP and audiology assistants, and pay the requisite annual fees (McNeilly, 2010).

Benefits for associate status for support personnel through ASHA are networking opportunities (e.g., joining special interest groups), professional development programs, ASHA online and print resources, and participation on ad hoc committees. They cannot vote or hold elected office within ASHA, and ASHA will not credential support personnel who are affiliates of ASHA.

EVOLVING PROFESSIONAL POLICIES AND PRACTICES

State licensure boards and professional organizations have responded to the concerns about misuse of support personnel by providing regulations, policies, and reports with specific guidance. ASHA (2004b, 2004g, 2011a), the American Academy of Audiology (AAA, 1997, 2006, 2010a), the Council for Exceptional Children (Consortium of Organizations on the Preparation and Use of Speech-Language Paraprofessionals in Early Intervention and Education Settings, 1997), and the National Joint Committee on Learning Disabilities (1998) are among the professional organizations representing SLPs and/or audiologists that have developed documents to provide guidance for the appropriate use and supervision of support personnel in those education and health care settings in which support personnel are employed. All of the professional policies rely on the clinical judgment and ethics of qualified professionals. This includes decisions regarding the delegation of tasks and the amount and type of supervision to provide. Table 12–1 presents a chronology of the policies that professional organizations have developed over the past 43 years to guide the practice and performance of speech-language pathology and audiology support personnel.

Ethical Responsibilities

ASHA's Code of Ethics and Issues in Ethics statements have provided a general framework for the supervision of support personnel in the professions of audiology and speech-language pathology. The first reference in the ASHA Code of Ethics was in the 1979 Code, specifically, Principle of Ethics II, Ethical Proscription 4, which stated that "Individuals must not offer clinical services by supportive personnel for whom they do not provide appropriate supervision and assume full responsibility." The first ASHA Issues in Ethics statements to address support personnel highlighted the professional and ethical responsibilities of the supervising professionals and emphasized the dependent role of the "communication aide" (ASHA, 1979).

TABLE 12–1 Chronology of Ethical and Professional Practice Policies Related to the Use of Support Personnel in Audiology and Speech-Language Pathology

- 1969—ASHA developed guidelines for the use of communication aides.
- 1973—Council for Accreditation in Occupational Hearing Conservation started training and certifying hearing conservationists.
- 1979—ASHA referenced *supportive personnel* in the Code of Ethics and issued an Issues in Ethics statement highlighting the professional and ethical responsibilities of the supervising professionals and emphasizing the dependent role of the *communication aide*.
- 1981—ASHA revised its guidelines for supportive personnel.
- 1988—ASHA developed a technical report about the use of SLP support personnel with underserved populations.
- 1990—ASHA revised the Code of Ethics and included a proscription about service delegation.
- 1992—ASHA developed a technical report on issues and the impact of support personnel in speech-language pathology and audiology. The 1992 and 1994 revised Code of Ethics dealt with the delegation of support services.
- 1994—ASHA approved a position statement supporting the establishment and credentialing of categories of support personnel in speech-language pathology.
- 1995—ASHA approved guidelines for the training, credentialing, use, and supervision of SLP assistants.
- 1996—ASHA convened a consensus panel to develop a strategic plan for approving speech-language pathology assistant programs and credentialing SLP assistants. The plan was used as a framework to develop a training approval process and credentialing process for SLP assistants.
- 1997—Consortium of Organizations on the Preparation and Use of Speech-Language Paraprofessionals in Early Intervention and Education Settings developed guidelines for three levels of paraprofessionals in education settings: aides, assistants, and associates. The assistant category parallels the ASHA SLP assistant guidelines. Consortium organizations included ASHA; Council for Exceptional Children, Division for Children's Communication Development and Division for Early Childhood; Council of Administrators of Special Education; and Council of Language, Speech, and Hearing Consultants in State Education Agencies.
- 1997 and 1998—AAA and ASHA published separate position statements and guidelines for support personnel in audiology.
- 1998—National Joint Committee on Learning Disabilities developed a report on the use of paraprofessionals with students with learning disabilities.
- 2000—Council on Academic Accreditation in Audiology and Speech-Language Pathology developed criteria and procedures for approving technical training programs for SLP assistants, the Council on Professional Standards in Speech-Language Pathology and Audiology developed criteria for registering SLP assistants, and the Council for Clinical Certification in Audiology and Speech-Language Pathology (CFCC) developed the implementation program.
- 2001—ASHA revised its Code of Ethics, added the terms *assistants, technicians, or any nonprofessionals* to the term *support personnel* and mandated informing people served about the credentials of providers.

(*Continues*)

TABLE 12–1 Chronology of Ethical and Professional Practice Policies Related to the Use of Support Personnel in Audiology and Speech-Language Pathology (*Continued*)

- 2002—ASHA developed knowledge and skills statements for supervisors of SLP assistants.
- 2003—ASHA voted to discontinue the registration program for SLP assistants and the approval process for SLP assistant training programs as of December 31, 2003, due primarily to financial concerns.
- 2003—ASHA revised its Code of Ethics and elaborated on delegation and supervision of support personnel.
- 2004—ASHA issued a new Issues in Ethics statement on support personnel.
- 2004—ASHA revised its position statement for support personnel in speech-language pathology and its guidelines for SLP assistants to remove references to SLP assistant credentialing.
- 2006—AAA published a new position statement to define the function of the audiologist's assistant.
- 2010—ASHA revised its Code of Ethics and continues to set forth rules concerning accurate representation of credentials, delegation of tasks, and supervision for assistants, technicians, and support personnel.
- 2010—AAA updated its position statement about the use of an audiology assistant. The rationale is provided in a 2010 task force report.
- 2011—ASHA updated its position statement and guidelines for audiology support personnel. The document addresses preparation, supervision, and ethical considerations for audiology assistants.
- 2012—ASHA is updating the speech-language pathology assistant guidelines and developing new online resources related to support personnel in audiology and speech-language pathology.

The 1990 ASHA Code of Ethics used the same language and also had the first reference to "delegation" with its proscription not to delegate "any service." The 1992 ASHA Code and its revision in 1994 both dealt with the delegation of "support services." The 2001 ASHA Code added the terms *assistants, technicians, or any nonprofessionals* to the term *support personnel* and mandated that members had an affirmative requirement to "not misrepresent the credentials of assistants, technicians, or support personnel and shall inform those they serve professionally of the name and professional credentials of persons providing services."

The 2003 revision of the ASHA Code maintained this requirement pertaining to representation of credentials and added requirements pertaining to delegation of tasks and supervision. The 2010 revision of the ASHA Code continues to set forth rules concerning accurate representation of credentials, delegation of tasks, and supervision (ASHA, 2010a). An ASHA Issues in Ethics statement (ASHA, 2004f) discusses a variety of training options and tasks and indicates that support personnel should be supervised by ASHA-certified audiologists and/or SLPs.

AAA's Code of Ethics also puts forth a rule pertaining to delegation and supervision of support personnel by its audiology members. Specifically, Rule D states, "Individuals shall provide appropriate supervision and assume full responsibility for services delegated to supportive personnel. Individuals shall not delegate any service requiring professional competence to unqualified persons" (AAA, 2011).

Chronology of Professional Practice Policies

In addition to the policies related to ethical use of support personnel, professional organizations also developed documents to guide professional practice. In

1970, ASHA published its first professional practice guidelines on the use of support personnel in audiology and speech-language pathology. These guidelines, revised in 1981, delineated training needs, scope of responsibilities, and amount of supervision for support personnel in audiology and speech-language pathology (ASHA, 1970, 1981). The following two sections address professional practice policies specific to either SLP or audiology support personnel.

SLP Support Personnel

In a 1995 position statement, ASHA endorsed the use of support personnel in speech-language pathology for the first time, rather than only providing guidance for their use (ASHA, 1995b). In 1996, the earlier ASHA guidelines from 1981 were revised to address one category of support personnel, *speech-language pathology assistants,* defined as "support personnel who perform tasks as prescribed, directed, and supervised by certified SLPs, after a program of academic and/or on-the-job training" (ASHA, 1996, p. 22). SLP assistants were differentiated from SLP aides, who usually have a narrower training base and more limited responsibilities relative to the duties of assistants. Like the first two ASHA guideline documents, the 1996 guidelines specified a scope of responsibilities and outlined the type and amount of supervision required. Some of these decisions were influenced, in part, by the less restrictive policies developed by other professions with a longer history using support personnel, such as occupational therapy and physical therapy (ASHA, 1992b). The ASHA guidelines were more prescriptive than those of the other professions to avoid the risk of assistants working outside of their limited scope of responsibilities or being hired in the place of SLPs (ASHA, 1996).

The ASHA guidelines also called for training at the associate degree level rather than just on-the-job training and recommended a credentialing program for assistants and for assistant-level training programs. ASHA's plan to credential SLP assistants and approve training programs started with the 1995 position statement supporting the establishment and credentialing of categories of SLP support personnel (ASHA, 1995b). In 2000, criteria for approving technical training programs and for registering SLP assistants were developed by the Council on Academic Accreditation in Audiology and Speech-Language Pathology (CAA) (ASHA, 2000a) and the Council on Professional Standards in Speech-Language Pathology, respectively (ASHA, 2000b). Recommendations for assistant-level tasks, knowledge required, and where this knowledge could and should be obtained were based in part on a job analysis of SLP assistants conducted by the Educational Testing Service (Rosenfeld & Leung, 1999). ASHA established implementation dates of January 2002 for the approval process for training programs and January 2003 for the SLP assistant registry process. The CAA was responsible for implementation of the technical training approval process and the CFCC was responsible for implementation of the assistant registration program. ASHA's commitment to these programs was linked to the receipt of sufficient fees to cover administrative costs paid by training programs and individuals seeking registration. When those revenues fell well short of what was required, the decision was made to discontinue the approval process for SLP assistant training programs and the registration program for SLP assistants as of December 31, 2003. In 2004, the ASHA position statement for SLP support personnel and guidelines for SLP assistants were revised to remove references to SLP assistant credentialing. Relevant portions of the criteria for SLP assistant technical training programs and assistant registration that related to training, use, and supervision were folded into the revised SLP assistant guidelines (ASHA, 2004b, 2004g).

ASHA has developed other documents and products over the years to assist professionals who choose to employ support personnel in various settings. These include a report on using support personnel with underserved populations (ASHA, 1988), knowledge and skills for supervising SLP assistants (ASHA, 2002a), and practical tools and forms for supervising SLP assistants (ASHA, 2009c) and for using and supervising SLP assistants working in school settings (ASHA, 2000c).

Audiology Support Personnel

Multiple professional organizations are involved in the use of audiology support personnel. In 1997, a Consensus Panel on Support Personnel in Audiology was convened with members of the Academy of Dispensing Audiologists, AAA, Educational Audiology Association, Military Audiology Association, and National Hearing Conservation Association and developed a position statement and guidelines (AAA, 1997). ASHA developed its own audiology support personnel position statement and guidelines (ASHA, 1998b) that differed only in its requirement for supervisors to hold the ASHA Certificate of Clinical Competence in Audiology. The policy documents leave decisions about specific activities and supervision to the discretion of the supervising audiologist: "Support personnel may assist audiologists in the delivery of services where appropriate" (ASHA, 1998b, p. 59). The supervising audiologist is expected to provide competency-based training specific to job needs. According to the ASHA guidelines, supervising audiologists have the full responsibility for determining the specific type of training activities, the assigned tasks, and the nature and amount of supervision provided for support personnel (ASHA, 1998b, 2011a).

The AAA also developed a position statement to guide audiologists on the education and job responsibilities of "audiologist's assistants" in 2006 and updated it in 2010 (AAA, 2006, 2010a). The updated position statement was based on the rationale articulated in an "Audiology Assistant Task Force Report" (AAA, 2010b). The AAA statement indicates that audiology assistants may be assigned duties at the discretion of an audiologist, provided that the assistant has a minimum of a high school diploma and competency-based training (AAA, 2010a).

Support personnel in audiology are trained and used in a variety of employment settings, such as industry, schools, private clinics, and Veterans Administration hospitals and other military hospitals and medical centers. In industrial and military settings, assistants may help with the prevention of hearing loss resulting from noise. Occupational hearing conservationists have been trained and certified by the Council for Accreditation in Occupational Hearing Conservation (CAOHC) since 1973. They may be audiometric technicians, occupational health nurses, engineers, and others who do audiometric testing and help to fit hearing protection devices for employees (Suter, 2002). The CAOHC is an interdisciplinary group that currently includes representatives from nine organizations. Its mission is to provide education about noise in the workplace and to prevent noise-induced hearing loss in industry. A certificate program for otolaryngology personnel (CPOP) has been promoted by the American Academy of Otolaryngology–Head and Neck Surgery (AAO-HNS) and the American Neurotology Society to train otolaryngology office personnel to become OTO techs and conduct hearing testing. The program includes a self-study reading component, a two-and-a-half-day workshop, and six months of supervision by an otolaryngologist. The list of tasks these groups delegate to an OTO Tech closely matches the scope of practice of audiologists. Professional audiology organizations such as AAA and ASHA are concerned about the overlap of responsibilities and the blurring of professional and technical level boundaries, particularly when otolaryngologists hire OTO techs rather than audiologists and bill for the services. Those endorsing the use of OTO techs suggest that their use can free up time for audiologists to perform more complex hearing and balance services.

Some audiologists have argued that the move to the doctoral level for the profession of audiology may lead to increased use of audiology support personnel to have a less costly option for the more technical aspects of the profession (Thornton, 1993). One of the reasons that audiologists decided not to require a higher education degree or credential for support personnel is to have the educational level and scope of responsibilities as distinct as possible between technical-level and professional-level personnel. Rather than have prescriptive policies related to education and tasks, audiologists prefer to determine independently what support personnel should do and how they should be trained.

STATE REGULATION

Thirty-eight states have laws or regulations governing the use of support personnel in speech-language pathology and/or audiology, an increase of four states since 2007. Some states that regulate speech-language pathology and audiology do not permit the use of support personnel. Of the states that regulate the use of support personnel, a wide range of educational requirements is found. A few states have different requirements for different levels of support personnel, ranging from a high school diploma or equivalent to a bachelor's degree in communication disorders with enrollment in a master's degree program. Continuing education for support personnel is required in 20 states. This number has doubled since 2007. A variety of titles are used to designate support personnel in the professions, with *assistant* and *aide* being the most common. State agencies (licensure boards) currently regulating support personnel also have a variety of differing supervision requirements. See ASHA's website for state-specific information.

Supervisory Requirements

To ensure that support personnel do not exceed the boundaries of their education and experience, most states that regulate support personnel have imposed one or more supervision requirements. Some states limit the number of support personnel that one licensed SLP or audiologist may supervise. Some states specifically prescribe the amount of direct and indirect supervision that a supervisor must provide to the support personnel. Some states specifically define what activities may or may not be performed by support personnel, and others simply provide a general statement that support personnel are the responsibility of the licensed SLP or audiologist and should be appropriately supervised given their individual education and experience.

In addition to state regulatory agencies, state education agencies may credential support personnel to work solely in schools to support service delivery provided by qualified professionals. Some school districts hire assistants under the classification of teacher assistants. If a state regulates support personnel (i.e., under the term of *assistant, aide, paraprofessional,* or *apprentice*), then individuals who wish to become employed in that state must meet the state requirements for practice under a licensed professional. ASHA also requires that audiologists and SLPs hold the Certificate of Clinical Competence to supervise support personnel (ASHA, 2005a). Information about the regulation of support personnel in schools in all states and contacts for state licensure boards or departments of education are available from the ASHA website.

State regulations may differ from professional policies. In those states where there is a conflict, ASHA guidelines indicate that professionals should abide by whichever legal mandates or professional policies are more stringent (ASHA, 2004b). ASHA and the National Council of State Boards of Examiners for Speech-Language Pathology and Audiology developed a set of guiding principles addressing state laws/regulations and ASHA standards, guidelines, and requirements to clarify the relationship to help professionals meet both their legal and ethical obligations (ASHA, 1998a).

CURRENT USE OF SUPPORT PERSONNEL

Survey data were reviewed to determine the current use of SLP and audiology support personnel in educational and health care settings. Having more time to work with clients/patients with more complex needs (71 percent of audiologists and 36 percent of SLPs) and having fewer clerical duties (64 percent of audiologists and 33 percent of SLPs) were two of the primary effects reported from the use of support personnel (ASHA, 2009b). Other effects reported from using support personnel by approximately one-quarter of the audiologists and SLPs who currently employ one or more at their facility were to increase frequency or intensity of service and respond to personnel shortages. The main reasons reported for not using support personnel were that they were not budgeted or not needed. Also, some audiologists (25 percent) and SLPs (29 percent) indicated that larger caseloads or workloads were an effect of using support personnel. Changes in the employment rates of support personnel over time also were explored for each profession and are discussed in the following sections.

SLP Support Personnel

Forty-one percent of school-based SLPs and 32 percent of health care-based SLPs reported that there was one or more SLP support personnel employed at their facility (ASHA, 2009b). For those currently using one or more support personnel, the median number reported was three for school-based SLPs and two for SLPs based in health care settings. These SLPs indicated that support personnel assist primarily in the following five ways: (1) assist with clerical duties (56 percent), (2) follow treatment plans or protocols developed by the SLP (48 percent), (3) assist with informal documentation as directed by the SLP (48 percent), (4) document client performance (45 percent), and (5) collect data for monitoring quality improvement (40 percent).

It is difficult to discern clear-cut trends in employment rates of support personnel for SLP assistants. The use of SLP assistants in the schools appears to have remained stable between 1999 and 2006. At least one SLP assistant was reported in their employment facility by 21 percent, 18 percent, and 18 percent of the school-based SLPs according to the 1999 Omnibus Survey, 2003 Omnibus Survey, and 2006 ASHA Schools Survey, respectively. Apparently, an increase in the use of SLP assistants occurred in 2009, based on the ASHA Membership Survey when 41 percent of SLPs in school settings reported using SLP support personnel.

A stable pattern of use also appears between 1999 and 2003 for health care-based SLPs. At least one assistant was reported to be employed by 16 percent and 14 percent of health care-based SLPs according to the 1999 Omnibus Survey and 2003 Omnibus Survey, respectively (ASHA, 1999, 2003a). However, in 2002, only 2 percent of SLPs in health care settings reported that they employ SLP assistants (ASHA, 2002b). Between 8 percent and 13 percent reported that they employ other support personnel, such as rehabilitation technicians (ASHA, 2002b), which may account for the difference in percentages compared to the other years. Similar to school settings, it appears that use of support personnel may be increasing in health care settings, based on the 32 percent in these settings who indicated on the ASHA 2009 Membership Survey that they employ one or more SLP support personnel.

Audiology Support Personnel

A 2001 survey of audiologists showed that 45 percent hired assistants or previously hired assistants in their practices (Hamill & Freeman, 2001). A 2004 survey of AAA members showed that approximately 28.4 percent of audiologists employed assistants (AAA, 2006). A 2005 report from the U.S. Department of Veterans Affairs by Robert Dunlop revealed a 619 percent increase in the number of audiology support personnel in Veterans Administration hospitals from 1996 to 2004 with a decrease in the ratio of audiologists to support personnel from 24:1 in 1996 to 5.26:1 in 2004 (as cited in AAA, 2006).

According to the 2009 ASHA Membership Survey (ASHA, 2009b), 43 percent of audiologists reported that one or more support personnel were employed at their facility. The median number of support personnel reported by audiologists was two. More than half of the audiologists who had one or more support personnel at their facility indicated that support personnel provided three current services: (1) assist with taking histories, record keeping, and scheduling (70 percent); (2) assist with infection control (69 percent); and (3) troubleshoot amplification devices and hearing aids (63 percent).

The use of audiology support personnel appears to be relatively stable over the past 10 years. The 2009 data from audiologists on the ASHA Membership Survey (43 percent employ one or more support personnel) are consistent with the employment of audiology support personnel based on the 2001 survey of audiologists by Hamill and Freeman (45 percent).

TRAINING FOR SUPPORT PERSONNEL

Support personnel should not be permitted to work with individuals unless the supervising SLP or audiology professional is confident that the support person has obtained a reasonable amount of training and possesses appropriate skills.

Training SLP Support Personnel

Training requirements for SLP support personnel vary across the country. ASHA's guidelines are national in scope and were developed to promote greater uniformity in training requirements (ASHA, 2004b). Currently, ASHA recommends completion of an associate degree from a technical training program with a program of study specifically designed to prepare the student to be an SLP assistant. The ASHA guidelines suggest that SLP assistants complete coursework, fieldwork, and on-the-job training. The guidelines also recommend that the assistant demonstrate necessary technical skills to fulfill the SLP assistant job responsibilities. The document includes a sample curriculum, fieldwork recommendations, and a sample technical proficiency form. As of June 2012, ASHA is aware of 23 operational associate degree programs for SLP assistants in 12 states. Some of these programs have training opportunities through distance learning and collaborations between community colleges and universities. The coursework and fieldwork experiences required in the SLP assistant training program typically differ from those at the bachelor's, preprofessional, or master's professional levels. It is a challenge for SLP assistant training programs in community colleges to locate textbooks that are written specifically for SLP assistants. Often the programs must use more advanced textbooks that are written for SLP students and omit the sections that do not apply, such as those related to assessment and diagnosis and detailed theoretical discussions.

Assistant-level training programs are not specifically intended to be the start of a career ladder to professional-level positions; however, some programs lend themselves to such opportunities. Assistant training programs also may be another avenue for students, including bilingual and bicultural students, to seek their bachelor's and master's degrees in communication sciences and disorders. Universities do not always accept coursework from the SLP assistant training program to transfer to the bachelor's degree programs.

Knowledge and skills needed to be an SLP assistant are distinctly different from those needed to be an ASHA-certified SLP. Academic programs/institutions have the discretion to determine which academic coursework completed in technical training programs will be accepted for transfer to a bachelor's degree program. Students interested in pursuing a career as an SLP are encouraged to verify the transferability of credits between assistant training programs and bachelor's programs. Students also are encouraged to investigate the requirements of graduate educational programs to ensure that basic science courses taken at the undergraduate level will be acceptable to the graduate program (ASHA, 2005a).

Training Audiology Support Personnel

Support personnel in audiology are expected to have at least a high school diploma or equivalent and are expected to have competency-based skills needed to perform assigned tasks (AAA, 2010a; ASHA, 1998b). According to the professional policies, training for support personnel in audiology should be planned and implemented by the supervising audiologist. In addition, the training process needs to encompass all assigned tasks; include information on roles and functions; and be (1) well designed, (2) specific to the assigned task, (3) competency based, and (4) provided through a variety of formal and informal instructional methods (AAA, 2010a; ASHA, 1998b). Training programs for audiology support personnel include a structured technician program provided by the military, formal training programs in colleges or universities, occupational hearing conservation technician programs, and on-the-job training programs by audiologists.

An example of training programs for audiology support personnel at colleges or universities is the program of study for audiologist's assistants at Nova Southeastern University. The distance learning program offers self-paced training modules in the areas of diagnostic testing and amplification. Students go to a website for course materials, tests, and tutorials.

The training program offered by CAOHC for occupational hearing conservationists involves successful completion of a practical and written exam after a 20-hour course on a variety of topics such as social and legal ramifications of noise on people and pure-tone audiometric procedures. CAOHC also offers an eight-hour recertification course; recertification is required every five years. CAOHC also certifies course directors, the majority of whom are audiologists (ASHA, 2004a).

SUPERVISION OF SUPPORT PERSONNEL

Audiologists and SLPs may delegate services to support personnel only with appropriate supervision (ASHA, 2003b). It is essential that the supervising professional has the knowledge and skills needed to provide such supervision (ASHA, 2002a). Supervisors who do not speak the same language as the assistant are still responsible for supervising the assistant. Ideally an interpreter would be provided. However, if an interpreter is not available, it is still possible, without specific knowledge of the spoken language, to observe assistant–client interactions and determine responses to cues and modeling. Supervisors should use their knowledge and skills of typical development and interactions for observations and to monitor progress. Management and supervision skills are not synonymous with the skills needed to be a highly qualified SLP or audiologist. Many professionals have not received specific supervisory training during their preservice education programs. To become a competent supervisor and manager, professionals may consider taking continuing education courses that target these areas. The amount and type of supervision provided should be based on the skills and experience of the support person, the needs of patients/clients served, the service delivery setting, the tasks assigned, and other factors such as initiation of a new program, orientation of new staff, and change in patient/client status (ASHA, 1998b, 2004b). The goal for the supervising professional is to ensure that support personnel restrict their clinical activities to prescribed tasks in contrast with the goal of independent clinical practice for supervision of students and clinical fellows (ASHA, 1985b; Paul-Brown & Goldberg, 2001).

The supervising SLP or audiologist is responsible for the actions of support personnel. Specifically, SLP or audiology supervisors would be held responsible and could be subject to sanctions if their assistants performed activities beyond the scope of their job responsibilities. Thus, any alleged violation of the Code(s) of Ethics governing the supervising professionals should be reported to the AAA Ethical Practices Board or the ASHA Board of Ethics for adjudication. According to the revised Issues in Ethics statement on *Support Personnel* (ASHA, 2004f), "It is the responsibility of ASHA members and certificate holders to ensure that support personnel under their supervision behave in an ethical manner. . . ." Thus, although ASHA does not have jurisdiction over support personnel, ASHA members and certificate holders are vicariously liable for the unethical conduct of support personnel they supervise and can sanction them if they are found in violation.

State laws pertaining to supervision vary and may differ from professional policies. This means that SLPs and audiologists need to check specific state regulations to determine amount of supervision required and qualifications for supervisors of assistants in a particular state. ASHA (2004b) provides the following guidance to assist SLPs and audiologists when state laws are more or less stringent than ASHA policies regarding supervision of support personnel:

> Fully qualified professionals and support personnel are legally bound to follow licensure laws and rules that regulate them and their practice in the state in which they work. Use of support personnel is not permitted in every state. ASHA members also are ethically bound to follow ASHA guidelines. (p. 5)

Concerns are ever present about the potential for inappropriate actions by support personnel and the lack of consequences when there are no state regulations to govern the use of SLP or audiology support personnel. Currently, no professional organization has direct oversight of the actions of support personnel in audiology or speech-language pathology. This is of particular concern when an SLP assistant or audiology support personnel is working under the supervision of a professional who is not required to be ASHA-certified and/or is employed in a state where there is no law that addresses the use of SLP or audiology support personnel.

Supervision of SLP Assistants

ASHA provides specific guidance related to the amount and type of supervision for SLP support personnel. For an SLP assistant in training, ASHA recommends no less than 50 percent direct supervision (ASHA, 2004b). The minimum amount of supervision suggested for a trained assistant is 30 percent weekly (at least 20 percent direct) for the first 90 workdays and 20 percent (at least 10 percent direct) after the initial work period. Direct supervision means "onsite, in-view observation and guidance by the SLP while an assigned activity is performed by support personnel," and indirect supervision "may include demonstrations, record review, review and evaluation of audio- or videotaped sessions, and/or interactive television" (ASHA, 2004d, p. 3). The ASHA assistant guidelines recommend that an SLP supervise no more than three SLP assistants at the same time (ASHA, 2004b). According to the 2011 ASHA Membership Survey, speech-language pathologists report that they provide direct supervision for an average of 30.6 percent of the speech-language pathology assistant's time and indirect supervision for 21.8 percent of the speech-language pathology assistant's time (ASHA, 2011c).

The supervising SLP has responsibility for establishing a means of documenting the supervision of the SLP assistant. Even when faced with time and workload pressures, the SLP is expected to adhere to these supervision guidelines. Although national and state guidelines are available to guide decisions about the amount of direct and indirect supervision, it remains the supervising SLP's responsibility to determine the type and exact amount (beyond the minimum) of supervision that each SLP assistant requires. For example, some SLP assistants may require more guidance and oversight to complete the required documentation. Another SLP assistant may need mentoring to ensure adherence to the rules and regulations of the facility. The SLP makes these decisions on the basis of the SLP assistant's individual strengths and technical proficiency.

Supervision of Audiology Support Personnel

Neither ASHA nor AAA has prescribed supervisory requirements for training support personnel in audiology; nor are there professional policies that set a specific amount of supervision after training or that specify a maximum number of support personnel to be employed. The supervising audiologist has the sole responsibility for these decisions (AAA, 2010a; ASHA, 2011a). According to the 2011 ASHA Membership Survey, audiologists report that they provide direct supervision for an average of 36 percent of the audiology assistant's time and indirect supervision for 31 percent of the audiology assistant's time (ASHA, 2011b).

With regard to supervision of OTO techs, an otolaryngologist is responsible for providing supervision during the six-month portion of the training period.

Thereafter, the OTO Tech works loosely under the supervision of the physician. However, this is similar to a physician providing supervision to anyone in the physician's office who provides patient care as governed by the state's medical practices act. Presumably, a credentialed audiologist also may supervise the OTO Tech consistent with the Code(s) of Ethics governing the audiologist and provided the physician accepts this role for the audiologist (American Academy of Otolaryngology–Head and Neck Surgery, 2012).

JOB RESPONSIBILITIES OF SLP ASSISTANTS

According to the ASHA guidelines, the SLP should be involved in the hiring of an assistant (ASHA, 2004b). Because the assistant must be supervised by a licensed and certified SLP, the supervising SLP should make decisions about the specific tasks and activities assigned to the SLP assistant. The SLP should advise the administrator of a facility or school principal that it is the supervising SLP's responsibility to select the clients/patients, assign responsibilities, and determine the amount and type of supervision needed. Viewed collectively across states, support personnel have a broad scope of responsibilities ranging from clerical duties to clinical activities. ASHA has delineated a restricted set of tasks that an SLP may delegate to an SLP assistant and those services that only an SLP can provide (ASHA, 2004b).

It is the responsibility of the supervising SLP to make certain that SLP assistants engage only in those activities that are within their job responsibilities. The SLP assigns students/clients to an SLP assistant on the basis of the student's needs and the SLP assistant's level of experience. The SLP assistant may be assigned to work with clients/students on previously learned, less clinically challenging, or more rote or repetitive skills. For example, the SLP may assign an SLP assistant to work on increasing generalization after the SLP has worked with a student to establish a specific sound. Support personnel also may work as members of a team in health care and education settings (Longhurst, 1997). In schools, IDEA has institutionalized the practice of using teams to determine the most appropriate course of action for each student and to collaborate and develop the Individualized Family Service Plan (IFSP) or the Individualized Education Program (IEP).

JOB RESPONSIBILITIES OF AUDIOLOGY SUPPORT PERSONNEL

The supervising audiologist is responsible for planning and delegating tasks that a support person may perform. Examples of tasks that have been delegated to support personnel by supervising audiologists include daily visual and listening checks on hearing aids and auditory trainers for children in public schools (Johnson, 1999); assisting with hearing screenings, hearing aid monitoring, and use of assistive listening devices in rehabilitation hospitals (Johnson, Clark-Lewis, & Griffin, 1998); learning ways to optimize communication during interactions with people with hearing loss and assisting with hearing conservation programs at worksites (ASHA, 2004a; Suter, 2002).

The audiologist has exclusive responsibility for a variety of clinical activities. Audiology support personnel may not interpret data; determine case selection; transmit clinical information, either verbally or in writing, to anyone without the approval of the supervising audiologist; compose clinical reports; make referrals; sign any formal documents (e.g., treatment plans, reimbursement forms, or reports); discharge a patient/client from services; or communicate with the patient/client, family, or others regarding any aspect of the patient/client status or service without the specific consent of the supervising audiologist (ASHA, 1998b, p. 60).

REIMBURSEMENT OF SERVICES PROVIDED BY SUPPORT PERSONNEL

Medicare policy currently does not recognize SLP or audiology assistants, regardless of the level of supervision. An otolaryngologist, however, can bill for work performed by OTO techs.

Private insurers may cover licensed or registered SLP assistants. One must query each payer to verify coverage. Private insurers may or may not provide a different rate of reimbursement for services provided by an SLP or audiologist as opposed to an SLP or audiology assistant. Services provided by professionals and their assistants are considered skilled services, as the assistants are implementing the treatment devised by the SLP or audiologist. Most private insurers do not cover services that do not require the skills (directly or indirectly) of an SLP or audiologist. There are some clear definitions of what type of activity constitutes a skilled service in the *Medicare Benefit Policy Manual* (ASHA, 2005b): "The services must be of such a level of complexity and sophistication, or the patient's condition must be such that the services required can be safely and effectively performed only by or under the supervision of a qualified speech pathologist." Nonskilled activities include "Non-diagnostic, non-therapeutic, routine, and repetitive and reinforced procedures ... which may effectively be carried out with the patient by any nonprofessional (e.g., family member, restorative nursing aide) after instruction and training is completed."

Each state has considerable latitude in administering its Medicaid program. The federal regulation states that services may be rendered "by or under the direction of" a qualified SLP, but a state may still prescribe the qualifications of the subordinate practitioners. A state would be more likely to assign a Medicaid provider number to SLP assistants if they were registered or licensed in the state.

The federal regulations for Medicaid specifically recognize services provided by audiology support personnel if such services are provided under the direction of a qualified audiologist. According to regulations, the supervising audiologist must have face-to-face contact with the client in the beginning and periodically throughout the treatment. An audiologist must provide adequate supervision of support staff as well as keep documentation of the supervision and ongoing involvement in the case. If an audiologist is employed by a Medicaid agency, clinic, or school, the federal regulations require that the audiologist's employment terms allow for adequate supervision of support personnel. Although specific supervision ratios are not stated, regulations do require that these ratios be "reasonable and ethical and in keeping with professional practice acts" (Preamble to Federal Regulations, 2004).

RESEARCH RELATED TO SUPPORT PERSONNEL

To determine the effectiveness of using support personnel to extend the clinical work of SLPs and audiologists, a systematic literature search of published English language studies was conducted using 22 electronic databases. The studies, which spanned several decades, needed to be relevant to various clinical questions and contain original data or purport to be systematic reviews of the literature. Following is a summary of the studies for four clinical questions.

Have Any Studies Compared SLP or Audiology Assistants with Professionals?

No studies were identified that compared audiology assistants with professional service provision. Some studies compared treatment outcomes by SLP assistants and SLPs, primarily of elementary school children with articulation disorders and adults with aphasia.

Studies with Children A large-scale, blinded, randomized, controlled trial was designed to compare language outcomes following direct versus indirect and individual versus group treatment for 161 children (6 to 11 years) with primary language impairment (Boyle, McCartney, Forbes, & O'Hare, 2007; Boyle, McCartney, O'Hare, & Forbes, 2009). The study also had a control group of children that received "usual levels of community-based speech and language therapy." The authors provided an intervention manual with suggested procedures and activities, which focused primarily on comprehension vocabulary, grammar, and narratives (McCartney et al., 2004). Speech-and-language therapists conducted the direct interventions and speech-and-language therapy assistants conducted the indirect interventions with individuals or small groups of children attending inclusive schools in Scotland, UK. The study found no significant differences in language outcomes between direct and indirect treatment or between individual and group treatment based on post-intervention testing. All groups showed short-term improvements in expressive language outcomes. Receptive language skills proved to be more intractable and did not show improvements regardless of the intervention group (Boyle, McCartney, O'Hare, & Law, 2010). The authors suggested that the assistants acted effectively with these children because of the lack of differences in language outcomes across groups. Language outcomes did not improve for a cohort intervention group when "school staff" rather than SLPs or speech and language assistants conducted indirect, consultative language treatment (McCartney, Boyle, Ellis, Bannatyne, & Turnbull, 2011). A cost analysis of the different modes of treatment revealed that indirect assistant-led group therapy was the least costly option and therapist-led individual therapy was the most costly (Dickson et al, 2009).

Additional studies involving children, most conducted in the mid-1970s, found no significant differences in the articulation outcomes of children with mild-to-moderate speech disorders when comparing treatment by *trained paraprofessionals* (also called *supportive personnel* or *speech therapy aides*) and professional clinicians; children in both groups showed improvements in articulation (Alvord, 1977; Costello & Schoen, 1978; Gray & Barker, 1977). Sounds that were not targeted for treatment showed no change for children in either the aide or clinician group (Gray & Barker, 1977).

One study reported no significant differences between groups of children with learning disabilities with "perceptual deficits" treated by trained "perceptual-aides" and "therapists" (including occupational, physical, recreational, and language); improvements were noted in motor skills, visual and somatosensory perception, language, and educations skills in children from both treatment groups (Gersten et al., 1975). One study reported that four out of five young children made more progress on computer-based language tasks when a parent volunteer provided the training compared with an SLP (Schery & O'Connor, 1997). Small sample size and lack of statistical comparison make these results difficult to interpret.

A mother–child home program administered by paraprofessionals was compared with interventions by professionals that were tailored to the cognitive and language needs of two-year-old children. Children in both groups showed similar improvements; however, the children were still delayed in cognitive and language functioning at age four in both groups (Scarr, McCartney, Miller, Hauenstein, & Ricciuti, 1996).

Studies with Adults Studies comparing nonprofessionals and professionals providing clinical services for adults focused primarily on volunteers working with individuals with aphasia. Patients showed improvement in communication, and no differences were found in the amount of progress made for adults who received services from professionals compared with those receiving services from untrained volunteers (David, Enderby, & Bainton, 1982; Meikle et al., 1979). In a study with trained volunteers, men with aphasia showed improvement in their communication during treatment but not when treatment was discontinued. These results were similar to patients with aphasia who received treatment from SLPs (Marshall et al., 1989). In a study that compared three different treatment approaches and a no-treatment condition, two of the treatments for patients with aphasia were administered by professionals, and one was administered by "trained nonprofessionals" (Shewan & Kertesz, 1984). The two approaches administered by professionals showed significant differences compared with the nontreatment condition; the treatment method used by nonprofessionals approached significance. It is not possible to determine whether the difference in significance level was due to the treatment approaches themselves or to differences between nonprofessionals and professionals. In another study of patients with aphasia, comparisons were made among clinic treatment by an SLP, home treatment by a trained volunteer, and deferred treatment. No significant differences were found among the three groups after the deferred-treatment group received treatment by a professional (Wertz et al., 1986).

Studies Comparing Service by Professionals and Support Personnel Ideally, supervising professionals should only assign tasks to support personnel that can be performed with the same level of quality as professionals. The studies available reveal no differences in treatment outcomes for children or adults when the services provided by assistants are compared with those provided by professionals. The consistency between outcomes for professionals and support personnel is encouraging for those who employ or wish to employ assistants. Clearly, more research, with a large enough sample for adequate statistical power and sound methodology, is needed.

Do Any Studies Show the Effectiveness of SLP or Audiology Assistants?

The studies described for the first clinical question (i.e., comparing clinical service by assistants with professionals) also address the second question of the effectiveness of SLP or audiology assistants. All of the previously cited studies showed that children and adults made improvements when SLP assistants were used. Other studies have been conducted that show the effectiveness of SLP or audiology assistants but did not have a comparison group of professionals.

Effectiveness of Support Personnel in SLP The few studies conducted on the effectiveness of SLP support personnel focus primarily on their use with children with articulation and expressive language disorders and adults with aphasia or dementia.

Studies with Children SLP support personnel have been used to conduct speech and language screening programs for children. In a pilot program, existing school personnel serving as "aides" were trained to screen the speech and language skills of elementary-age children. The aides were reported to administer the screening tests accurately to make appropriate referrals for those children with a high probability of having speech and language problems (Pickering & Dopheide, 1976). In another pilot screening program, "paraprofessionals" screened young children between 19 and 21 months during home visits for language delay. Screening data from the administration of a standardized screening test were found to be reliable, valid, and sensitive in identifying children for further assessment (Pickstone, 2003).

Children with speech sound disorders showed improvement when they received speech services from SLP support personnel. A study of articulation treatment for elementary-age children by trained paraprofessionals reported that 83.5 percent of the treated sounds were used correctly in a conversational sample (Galloway & Blue, 1975). Improvements in speech production were reported for children treated by students (Hall & Knutson, 1978), "communication aides" (Van Hattum et al., 1974), and paid aides and volunteers (Scalero & Eskenazi, 1976).

Studies focused on improving language skills in children also demonstrated improvements when services were provided by SLP support personnel. A single-participant study reported increases in communication (e.g., percentage of correct information and words per minute) when a "nonprofessional" provided a structured maintenance program for an individual with epilepsy and language and cognitive impairments (Wright, Shisler, & Rau, 2003). Teachers in another study reported that 41 percent of their 22 kindergarten students showed improvement after receiving computer-aided language enrichment by volunteers, although the outcomes were not quantified (Schetz, 1989). "Nonprofessional tutors" were used to help first-grade children develop phonological and early reading skills (Vadasy, Jenkins, & Pool, 2000). Tutors provided one-to-one instruction for 30 minutes, four days a week, for one school year in phonological skills, letter-sound correspondence, decoding, rhyming, writing, spelling, and reading. Tutored children received significantly better reading, spelling, and decoding scores than students who did not receive tutoring. The tutored children continued to do better than nontutored children in decoding and spelling after second grade. An exploratory study used "specialist teaching assistants" to conduct speech and/or language intervention for 35 children (four to six years old) for four one-hour sessions over 10 weeks. The children, from an inclusive school in the UK, showed improvement in targeted language outcomes and on a standardized language test. Differences also were noted on a questionnaire comparing speech and language performance at school and at home before and after intervention (Mecrow, Beckwith, & Klee, 2010).

Positive outcomes in speech and language also were shown when children with severe disabilities received services from SLP support personnel. In one study, two psychiatric aides who served as "paraprofessional teachers" were trained to use a structured language training program with children with severe disabilities. In this study, matched pairs of children were randomly assigned to an experimental or control condition. Results showed that the children in the experimental group who received language training by the aides for two months showed improvement in language (e.g., identifying and labeling objects) and social skills (Phillips, Liebert, & Poulos, 1973). Another study trained undergraduate students to use behavioral principles to develop the verbal behavior of young children with severe disabilities with limited verbal repertoires (Guralnick, 1972). Five of the eight children showed progress in their development of communication skills (e.g., imitation of sounds, sustaining eye contact, using gestures). Another article reported on the use of blind and partially sighted high school students who were trained and paid to serve as "speech assistants" in a residential school to provide extra class practice for younger children with visual impairments who had speech problems (Briggs, 1974). Although data were not collected on the speech outcomes of the students receiving services, the author reported that most appeared to benefit from the additional practice provided by the assistants.

Studies with Adults Adults with aphasia showed communication improvements when treatment was provided by support personnel, including relatives (Lesser, Bryan, Anderson, & Hilton, 1986), untrained volunteers (Griffith, 1975; Griffith & Miller, 1980; Lesser & Watt, 1978), and "community volunteers" (Lyon et al., 1997). Similarly, adults with "communication handicaps" showed increased responsiveness, verbalizations, and social interactions when trained volunteers were used as an adjunct to professional treatment (Mueller, 1990). Trained volunteers were judged to be better conversational partners for adults with aphasia than were untrained volunteers (Kagan, Black, Duchan,

Simmons-Mackie, & Square, 2001). The individuals with aphasia showed significant improvements in social skills and message exchange skills when interacting with volunteers who received supported conversation training. These changes were not seen in the adults with aphasia who interacted with the untrained volunteers.

Support personnel also have been used successfully with adults with dementia. One article described a "partnered volunteering" language and memory stimulation program for adults with Alzheimer's disease. The study reported positive changes in language and memory on pre- and posttests after two semesters of service by student volunteers from speech-language pathology or psychology (Arkin, 1996). Another study used nursing assistants to enhance discourse skills of nursing home residents with dementia. In this study, one group of nursing assistants was trained and supervised using communication techniques and memory books with the residents. A control group paired nursing assistants with residents with dementia but did not use specific communication or memory tools. The conversational skills of residents in the treatment group were more coherent and had fewer vague "empty phrases" compared with the no-treatment control group. The nursing assistants in the treatment group also used more "facilitative discourse strategies" (e.g., encouragement, cuing) than assistants in the control group (Dijkstra, Bourgeois, Burgio, & Allen, 2002).

Effectiveness of Support Personnel in Audiology

Only one study was identified that addressed the use of support personnel for individuals with hearing loss. A Canadian consumer organization trained seniors with hearing loss to serve as peer models and provide support for other seniors with hearing loss in long-term health care facilities or in the community (Dahl, 1997). The volunteers were trained to assist with hearing aid care, use of assistive listening devices, and strategies for coping with hearing loss. Within a five-month period, the volunteers totaled 288 weekly half-day visits. The seniors receiving support found the visitor program to be helpful. An informal follow-up evaluation one year after the project showed continued visits by some of the volunteers and the addition of new trained volunteers.

Four studies were identified that addressed whether audiometric technicians could determine which patients could be fitted with a hearing aid without the need for a medical referral. One study was conducted to determine if "physiological measurement technicians" could safely prescribe hearing aids without medical supervision. The technicians reportedly failed to mention the presence of active inflammatory ear disease in the referral letter for three of eight cases where middle ear disease was present. The authors concluded that review by ear, nose, and throat (ENT) medical staff was needed before prescription of a hearing aid (Bellini, Beesley, Perrett, & Pickles, 1989). In the other studies, the authors concluded that the audiology technicians made accurate assessments of patients to determine if they required a hearing aid referral to an ENT (Koay & Sutton, 1996; Swan & Browning, 1994; Zeitoun, Lesshafft, Begg, & East, 1995). For example, a "senior audiology technician or higher grade" working in a general practitioner's office determined that 23 percent of the 135 patients required medical referral before being fitted for a hearing aid. The ENT review of the same patients showed 100 percent agreement with the audiology technicians (Koay & Sutton, 1996).

Effectiveness of SLP and Audiology Support Personnel

The effectiveness of SLP and audiology support personnel remains an open question. Only a few studies are available and most studies were conducted in the 1970s and 1980s. The methodological quality of many of the studies was poor (e.g., no control group, few participants, no randomized groups, few statistical comparisons) or not accessible, with the exception of a more recent 2007 study (Boyle et al., 2007). The available studies appeared to show that the use of SLP assistants could be effective in improving speech production for children with articulation disorders or conversational skills for adults with aphasia or dementia. Audiometric technicians appear capable of determining which patients need a medical referral before being fitted for a hearing aid.

Do Any Studies Show the Effectiveness of Training Programs for SLP or Audiology Assistants?

No articles were found through the literature search that provided data on the effectiveness of SLP or audiology assistant training programs. None were found that compared different types of training modules. A few articles described training programs to prepare SLP assistants. For example, two articles described statewide public school programs for support personnel working with children with articulation disorders (Blodgett & Miller, 1997; Scalero & Eskenazi, 1976). One article described four model preservice training programs for communication assistants working in the schools with students with language and hearing problems (Shinn-Strieker, 1984). Another article presented a university program for preprofessional undergraduate students working as communication aides in schools (Hall & Knutson, 1978), and one described a program based in a rehabilitation center to train support personnel in speech-language pathology to work with individuals with traumatic brain injury (Werven, 1992).

Future Research Issues

In 1977, Gray and Barker wrote that "there is little substantive information about whether or not [aides] can reliably and effectively provide services" (p. 534). Almost 35 years later, this same statement can still be made. There is a paucity of high-quality efficacy research on the use of support personnel in audiology or speech-language pathology. Among the few studies conducted, there is some evidence of comparable outcomes between supervised SLP assistants and professionals, particularly when services are limited to more repetitive treatment activities. Although some studies demonstrate that SLP assistants and audiology support personnel can carry out assigned tasks, most are descriptive rather than empirical. Except for a controlled trial in the UK (Boyle et al., 2007), few research designs go beyond a low level of evidence using case studies with no randomization or control group. Research also is needed pertaining to the optimal amount or type of supervision necessary for assistants with various amounts of experience and to determine the effectiveness of different types of training programs for support personnel. The use of appropriately trained and supervised support personnel may be a viable option in some settings as a means to enhance the frequency and intensity of service delivery in the professions of audiology and speech-language pathology. However, more evidence, and better-quality evidence, is needed before the value of support personnel in communication sciences and disorders can be ascertained.

SUMMARY

The intended use of support personnel is to supplement and not supplant the work of the qualified professional. The SLP and audiology assistant may be hired to increase the frequency, intensity, efficiency, and availability of services by following a specific set of job responsibilities. However, the licensed and certified professional ultimately remains responsible for the training, selection, management, and supervision of the assistant. It is also the professional's obligation to inform the consumer of the level of training and expertise of the assistant so that at no time is the assistant represented as an SLP or audiologist. The professional retains the legal and ethical responsibility for all services provided or omitted. The professional and the assistant need to work as a team to support the communication needs of the individuals they serve. Although ASHA currently does not credential assistants, a number of states regulate their use. In these states, the use of assistants can be monitored, ensuring that the assistants are used in a legal manner in terms of education and supervision. Adherence to professional guidelines also serves as a means of monitoring ethical clinical practice. The limited research available suggests that services provided by assistants are effective, although much more quality research is needed to determine the degree of effectiveness and optimal amount of supervision and to make comparisons with a professional level of service.

CRITICAL THINKING

1. What are some of the factors that have led to the use of SLP and audiology assistants?
2. What specific job responsibilities are appropriate for SLP and audiology assistants? What are some activities/tasks that are not appropriate for assistants?
3. How have our state laws and national associations addressed the issue of assistants? Consider issues such as training, regulating, certifying, supervising, and ensuring that standards and ethics are not being compromised.
4. How might the inclusion of SLP and audiology assistants in our professions help to address the needs of our linguistically diverse community? When using assistants as interpreters or translators, how should training and supervision issues be addressed?

5. According to the available research, does the use of assistants diminish or enhance the effectiveness of treatment? What additional information do we need to make a more objective analysis of the effectiveness of assistants and ensure comparability with professional-level service?
6. As the supervisor of an assistant, list and describe your responsibilities and necessary knowledge and skills.
7. Consider the following: As an SLP, you work in a school district with a large number of students whose primary language is Spanish. Your administrator hires and assigns an assistant to you. The assistant has a bachelor's degree in communication sciences and disorders and is fluent in Spanish. The administrator states that the assistant will be doing all of the Spanish language testing as well as writing and managing the IEPs and working with the families of all students on your caseload whose primary language is Spanish. What are the ethical and legal implications? How might you address them in this scenario?

REFERENCES

Administration on Aging. (2002). *Statistics: A profile of older Americans: 2002. Future growth.* Retrieved from http://www.aoa.gov/aoaroot/aging_statistics/profile/2002/2002profile.pdf

Alvord, D. J. (1977). Innovation in speech therapy: A cost-effective program. *Exceptional Children, 43,* 520–525.

American Academy of Audiology. (1997, May/June). Position statement and guidelines of the consensus panel on support personnel in audiology. *Audiology Today, 9*(3), 27–28.

American Academy of Audiology. (2003, October). *Preventing noise-induced occupational hearing loss.* Available from http://www.audiology.org/

American Academy of Audiology. (2004, January). *Audiology: Scope of practice.* Available from http://www.audiology.org/

American Academy of Audiology. (2006). Position statement on audiologist's assistants. *Audiology Today, 18*(2), 27–28.

American Academy of Audiology. (2010a, September). *Position statement: Audiology assistants.* Available from http://www.audiology.org/

American Academy of Audiology. (2010b). Audiology assistant task force report. *Audiology Today, 22*(3), 68-73.

American Academy of Audiology. (2011). *Code of ethics.* Available from http://www.audiology.org/

American Academy of Otolaryngology–Head and Neck Surgery. (2012). *Certificate program for otolaryngology personnel (CPOP).* Retrieved from http://www.entnet.org/conferencesandevents/cpop.cfm

American Speech-Language-Hearing Association. (1979). *ASHA policy regarding support personnel.* Rockville, MD: Author.

American Speech-Language-Hearing Association. (1981, March). Guidelines for the employment and utilization of support personnel. *ASHA, 23,* 165–169.

American Speech-Language-Hearing Association. (1985a, June). Clinical management of communicatively handicapped minority language populations. *ASHA, 27*(6), 3–7.

American Speech-Language-Hearing Association. (1985b, June). Clinical supervision in speech-language pathology and audiology. *ASHA, 27*(6), 57–60.

American Speech-Language-Hearing Association. (1988, November). Utilization and employment of speech-language pathology supportive personnel with underserved populations. *ASHA, 30,* 55–56.

American Speech-Language-Hearing Association. (1992). *Technical report: Support personnel: Issues and impact on the professions of speech-language pathology and audiology.* Rockville, MD: Author.

American Speech-Language-Hearing Association. (1995a). *ASHA 1995 Omnibus Survey.* Rockville, MD: Author.

American Speech-Language-Hearing Association. (1995b, March). Position statement for the training, credentialing, use, and supervision of support personnel in speech-language pathology. *ASHA, 37* (Suppl. 14), 21.

American Speech-Language-Hearing Association. (1996, Spring). Guidelines for the training, credentialing, use, and supervision of speech-language pathology assistants. *ASHA, 38* (Suppl. 16), 21–34.

American Speech-Language-Hearing Association. (1997). *Preferred practice patterns for the profession of audiology.* Available from http://www.asha.org/policy

American Speech-Language-Hearing Association. (1998a, June). *Guidance principles addressing state law/regulations and ASHA standards/guidelines/requirements.* Rockville, MD: Author.

American Speech-Language-Hearing Association. (1998b). Position statement and guidelines on support personnel in audiology. *ASHA, 40* (Suppl. 18), 59–61.

American Speech-Language-Hearing Association. (1999). *ASHA 1999 Omnibus Survey.* Rockville, MD: Author.

American Speech-Language-Hearing Association. (2000a). *Council on Academic Accreditation in Audiology and Speech-Language Pathology: Criteria for approval of associate degree technical training programs for speech-language pathology assistants.* Rockville, MD: Author.

American Speech-Language-Hearing Association. (2000b). *Council on Professional Standards in Speech-Language Pathology and Audiology: Background information and criteria for registration of speech-language pathology assistants.* Rockville, MD: Author.

American Speech-Language-Hearing Association. (2000c). *Working with speech-language pathology assistants in school settings.* Rockville, MD: Author.

American Speech-Language-Hearing Association. (2001). *Scope of practice in speech-language pathology.* Rockville, MD: Author.

American Speech-Language-Hearing Association. (2002a). *Knowledge and skills for supervisors of speech-language pathology assistants.* Available from http://www.asha.org/policy

American Speech-Language-Hearing Association. (2002b). *Speech-language pathology health care survey.* Available from http://www.asha.org/

American Speech-Language-Hearing Association. (2003a). *ASHA Omnibus Survey.* Available from http://www.asha.org/

American Speech-Language-Hearing Association. (2003b). *Code of ethics.* Rockville, MD: Author.

American Speech-Language-Hearing Association. (2004a). *The audiologist's role in occupational hearing conservation and hearing loss prevention programs: Technical report.* Available from http://www.asha.org/policy

American Speech-Language-Hearing Association. (2004b). *Guidelines for the training, use, and supervision of speech-language pathology assistants.* Available from http://www.asha.org/policy

American Speech-Language-Hearing Association. (2004c). *Knowledge and skills needed by speech-language pathologists and audiologists to provide culturally and linguistically appropriate services.* Available from http://www.asha.org/policy

American Speech-Language-Hearing Association. (2004d, November). *Preferred practice patterns for the profession of speech-language pathology.* Available from http://www.asha.org/policy

American Speech-Language-Hearing Association. (2004e). *Scope of practice in audiology.* Available from http://www.asha.org/policy

American Speech-Language-Hearing Association. (2004f). *Support personnel.* Available from http://www.asha.org/policy

American Speech-Language-Hearing Association. (2004g). *Training, use, and supervision of support personnel in speech-language pathology.* Available from http://www.asha.org/policy

American Speech-Language-Hearing Association. (2005a). *Frequently asked questions: Speech-language pathology assistants.* Available from http://www.asha.org/

American Speech-Language-Hearing Association. (2005b). *Medicare benefit policy manual.* Available from http://www.asha.org/

American Speech-Language-Hearing Association. (2008). *Roles and responsibilities of speech-language pathologists in early intervention: Technical report.* Available from http://www.asha.org/policy

American Speech-Language-Hearing Association. (2009a). *Demographic profile of ASHA members providing bilingual and Spanish-language services.* Retrieved from http://www.asha.org/uploadedFiles/Demographic-Profile-Bilingual-Spanish-Service-Members.pdf

American Speech-Language-Hearing Association. (2009b). *2009 Membership Survey summary report: Number and type of responses.* Retrieved from http://www.asha.org/uploadedFiles/2009MembershipSurveySummary.pdf

American Speech-Language-Hearing Association. (2009c). *Practical tools and forms for supervising speech-language pathology assistants.* Rockville, MD: Author.

American Speech-Language-Hearing Association. (2010a). *Code of ethics.* Available from http://www.asha.org/policy

American Speech-Language-Hearing Association. (2010b). *Highlights and trends: ASHA counts for year end 2010.* Retrieved from http://www.asha.org/uploadedFiles/2010-Member-Counts.pdf

American Speech-Language-Hearing Association. (2010c). *2010 Schools Survey summary report: Number and type of responses, SLPs.* Retrieved from http://www.asha.org/uploadedFiles/Schools10Frequencies.pdf

American Speech-Language-Hearing Association. (2011a). *Audiology support personnel: Preparation, supervision, and ethical considerations* [Guidelines, Position statement]. Available from http://www.asha.org/policy

American Speech-Language-Hearing Association. (2011b). *2011 Membership Survey. CCC-A survey summary report: Number and type of responses.* Available from www.asha.org

American Speech-Language-Hearing Association. (2011c). *2011 Membership Survey. CCC-SLP survey summary report: Number and type of responses.* Available from http://www.asha.org

American Speech-Language-Hearing Association, Committee on Supportive Personnel. (1970). Guidelines on the role, training, and supervision of the communication aide. *ASHA, 12,* 78–80.

Arkin, S. (1996). Volunteers in partnership: An Alzheimer's rehabilitation program delivered by students. *American Journal of Alzheimer's Disease, 11,* 12–22.

Bellini, M. J., Beesley, P., Perrett, C., & Pickles, J. M. (1989). Hearing-aids: Can they be safely prescribed without medical supervision? An analysis of patients referred for hearing-aids. *Clinical Otolaryngology and Allied Sciences, 14,* 415–418.

Blodgett, E. G., &. Miller, J. M. (1997). Speech-language paraprofessionals working in Kentucky schools. *Journal of Children's Communication Development, 18,* 65–79.

Boyle, J., McCartney, E., Forbes, J., & O'Hare, A. (2007). A randomized controlled trial and economic evaluation of direct versus indirect and individual versus group modes of speech and language therapy for children with primary language impairment. *Health Technology Assessment, 11*(25), iii–iv, xi–xii, 1–158.

Boyle, J. M., McCartney, E., O'Hare, A., & Forbes, J. (2009). Direct versus indirect and individual versus group modes of language therapy for children with primary language impairment: Principal outcomes from a randomized controlled trial and economic evaluation. *International Journal of Language and Communication Disorders, 44*(6), 826–846.

Boyle, J., McCartney, E., O'Hare, A., & Law, J. (2010). Intervention for mixed receptive-expressive language impairment: A review. *Developmental Medicine & Child Neurology, 52*(11), 994–999.

Breakey, L. K. (1993, May). Support personnel: Times change. *American Journal of Speech-Language Pathology, 2*(2), 13–16.

Briggs, B. M. (1974). High school speech assistants in a residential school for the blind. *Education of the Visually Handicapped, 6*(4), 119–124.

Bureau of Labor Statistics, U.S. Department of Labor. (2011a). *Occupational outlook handbook* (2010–11 ed.). Audiologists. Available from http://www.bls.gov/oco/ocos085.htm

Bureau of Labor Statistics, U.S. Department of Labor. (2011b). *Occupational outlook handbook* (2010–11 ed.). Speech-language pathologists. Available from http://www.bls.gov/oco/ocos099.htm

Cirrin, F. M., Schooling, T. L., Nelson, N. W., Diehl, S. F., Flynn, P. F., Staskowski, M., et al. (2010, July). Evidence-based systematic review: Effects of different service delivery models on communication outcomes for elementary school–age children. *Language, Speech, and Hearing Services in Schools, 41,* 233–264.

Consortium of Organizations on the Preparation and Use of Speech-Language Paraprofessionals in Early Intervention and Education Settings. (1997, January). *Report of the Consortium of Organizations on the Preparation and Use of Speech-Language Paraprofessionals in Early Intervention and Education Settings.* Reston, VA: Author.

Costello, J., & Schoen, J. (1978). The effectiveness of paraprofessionals and a speech clinician as agents of articulation intervention using programmed instruction. *Language, Speech, and Hearing Services in Schools, 9,* 118–128.

Dahl, M. O. (1997). To hear again: A volunteer program in hearing health care for hard-of-hearing seniors. *Journal of Speech-Language Pathology and Audiology, 21,* 153–159.

David, R., Enderby, P., & Bainton, D. (1982). Treatment of acquired aphasia: Speech therapists and volunteers compared. *Journal of Neurology, Neurosurgery, and Psychiatry, 45,* 957–961.

Dickson, K., Marshall, M., Boyle, J., McCartney, E., O'Hare, A., & Forbes, J. (2009). Cost analysis of direct versus indirect and individual versus group modes of manual-based speech-and-language therapy for primary school-age children with primary language impairment. *International Journal of Language and Communication Disorders, 44*(3), 369–381.

Dijkstra, K., Bourgeois, M., Burgio, L., & Allen, R. (2002). Effects of a communication intervention on the discourse of nursing home residents with dementia and their nursing assistants. *Journal of Medical Speech-Language Pathology, 10*(2), 143–157.

Feldman, M. A. (Ed). (2004). *Early intervention: The essential readings.* Malden, MA: Blackwell.

Galloway, H. F., & Blue, C. M. (1975). Paraprofessional personnel in articulation therapy. *Language, Speech, and Hearing Services in Schools, 6,* 125–130.

Gerlach, K. (2000). *The paraeducator and teacher team: Strategies for success.* Seattle, WA: Pacific Training Associates.

Gersten, J. W., Gersten, J. W., Foppe, K. B., Gersten, R., Maxwell, S., Mirrett, P., et al. (1975). Effectiveness of aides in a perceptual motor training program for children with learning disabilities. *Archives of Physical Medicine & Rehabilitation, 56,* 104–110.

Goldberg, L., & Paul-Brown, D. (1999). *Strategies for the effective use of speech-language pathology assistants in the classroom.* Proceedings of the Seventh Annual Comprehensive System of Personnel Development Conference, National Association of State Directors of Special Education, Alexandria, VA.

Gray, B. B., & Barker, K. (1977). Use of aides in an articulation therapy program. *Exceptional Children, 43,* 534–536.

Griffith, V. E. (1975). Volunteer scheme for dysphasic and allied problems in stroke patients. *British Medical Journal, iii,* 633–635.

Griffith, V. E., & Miller, C. L. (1980). Volunteer stroke scheme for dysphasic patients with stroke. *British Medical Journal, 281,* 1605–1607.

Guralnick, M. J. (1972). A language development program for severely handicapped children. *Exceptional Children, 39,* 45–49.

Guralnick, M. J. (Ed.). (2005). *The developmental systems approach to early intervention.* Baltimore, MD: Paul H. Brookes.

Guralnick, M. J. (2011). Why early intervention works: A systems perspective. *Infants and Young Children, 24*(1), 6–28.

Hall, P. K., & Knutson, C. L. (1978). The use of preprofessional students as communication aides in the schools. *Language, Speech, and Hearing Services in Schools, 9,* 162–168.

Hamill, T., & Freeman, B. (2001). Scope of practice for audiologists' assistants: Survey results. *Audiology Today, 13*(6), 34–35.

Individuals with Disabilities Education Improvement Act of 2004, Pub. L. No. 108-446, 20 U.S.C. § 1400 *et seq.* (2004).

Johnson, C. E. (1999). Dimensions of multiskilling: Considerations for educational audiology. *Language, Speech, and Hearing Services in Schools, 30,* 4–10.

Johnson, C. E., Clark-Lewis, S., & Griffin, D. (1998). Experience, attitudes, and competencies of audiologic support personnel in a rehabilitation hospital. *American Journal of Audiology, 7,* 1–6.

Joint Committee on Infant Hearing. (2007). *Year 2007 position statement: Principles and guidelines for early hearing detection and intervention.* Available from http://www.asha.org/policy

Kagan, A., Black, S. E., Duchan, J. F., Simmons-Mackie, N., & Square, P. (2001). Training volunteers as conversation partners using "supported conversation for adults with aphasia" (SCA): A controlled trial. *Journal of Speech, Language, and Hearing Research, 44,* 624–638.

Koay, C. B., & Sutton, G. J. (1996). Direct hearing aid referrals: A prospective study. *Clinical Otolaryngology and Allied Science, 21,* 142–146.

Kochkin, S. (2009, October). MarkeTrak VIII: 25-year trends in the hearing health market. Retrieved from http://www.betterhearing.org/pdfs/M8_hearing_loss_trends_2009.pdf

Langdon, H. W., & Cheng, L. L. (2002). *Collaborating with interpreters and translators.* Eau Claire, WI: Thinking Publications.

Lesser, R., Bryan, K., Anderson, J., & Hilton, R. (1986). Involving relatives in aphasia therapy: An application of language enrichment therapy. *International Journal of Rehabilitation Research, 9,* 259–267.

Lesser, R., & Watt, M. (1978). Untrained community help in the rehabilitation of stroke sufferers with language disorder. *British Medical Journal, ii,* 1045–1048.

Longhurst, T. (1997). Team roles in therapy services. In A. L. Pickett & K. Gerlach (Eds.), *Supervising paraeducators in school settings: A team approach* (pp. 55–89). Austin, TX: Pro-Ed.

Lynch, E. W., & Hanson, M. J. (Eds.). (2004). Developing cross-cultural competence: A guide for working with children and their families (3rd ed.). Baltimore, MD: Paul H. Brookes.

Lyon, J. G., Cariski, D., Keisler, L., Rosenbek, J., Levine, R., Kumpula, J., et al. (1997). Communication partners: Enhancing participation in life and communication for adults with aphasia in natural settings. *Aphasiology, 11,* 693–708.

Marshall, R. C., Wertz, R. T., Weiss, D. G., Aten, J. L., Brookshire, R. H., Garcia-Bunuel, L., et al. (1989). Home treatment for aphasic patients by trained nonprofessionals. *Journal of Speech and Hearing Disorders, 54,* 462–470.

McCartney, E., Boyle, J., Bannatyne, S., Jessiman, E., Campbell, C., Kelsey, C., et al. (2004). Becoming a manual occupation? The construction of a therapy manual for use with language impaired children in mainstream primary schools. *International Journal of Language and Communication Disorders, 39*(1), 135–148.

McCartney, E., Boyle, J., Ellis, S., Bannatyne, S., & Turnbull, M. (2011). Indirect language therapy for children with persistent language impairment in mainstream primary schools: Outcomes from a cohort intervention. *International Journal of Language and Communication Disorders, 46*(1), 74–82.

McNeilly, L. (2010, November 23). ASHA will roll out associates program in 2011. *The ASHA Leader.* Retrieved from http://www.asha.org/Publications/leader/2010/101123/ASHA-Will-Roll-Out-Associates-Program-in-2011.htm

Mecrow, C., Beckwith, J., & Klee, T. (2010). An exploratory trial of the effectiveness of an enhanced consultative approach to delivering speech and language intervention in schools. *International Journal of Language and Communication Disorders, 45*(3), 354–367.

Meikle, M., Wechsler, E., Tupper, A., Benenson, M., Butler, J., Mulhall, D., et al. (1979). Comparative trial of volunteer and professional treatments of dysphasia after stroke. *British Medical Journal, 2,* 87–89.

Mueller, P. B. (1990). A volunteer speech-language facilitation program for communicatively handicapped elders in long-term care facilities. *Adult Residential Care Journal, 4,* 217–225.

National Joint Committee on Learning Disabilities. (1998). Learning disabilities: Use of paraprofessionals. In *Collective perspectives on issues affecting learning disabilities* (2nd ed., pp. 79–98). Austin, TX: Pro-Ed.

No Child Left Behind Act of 2002, 20 U.S.C., § 6311 *et seq.* (2002).

Paul-Brown, D., & Caperton, C. J. (2001). Inclusive practices for preschool children with specific language impairment. In M. J. Guralnick (Ed.), *Early childhood inclusion: Focus on change* (pp. 433–463). Baltimore, MD: Paul H. Brookes.

Paul-Brown, D., & Goldberg, L. R. (2001). Current policies and new directions for speech-language pathology assistants. *Language, Speech, and Hearing Services in Schools, 32,* 4–17.

Phillips, S., Liebert, R. M., & Poulos, R. W. (1973). Employing paraprofessional teachers in a group language training program for severely and profoundly retarded children. *Perceptual and Motor Skills, 36,* 607–616.

Pickering, M., & Dopheide, W. R. (1976). Training aides to screen children for speech and language problems. *Language, Speech, and Hearing Services in Schools, 7,* 236–241.

Pickett, A. L. (1999). *Strengthening and supporting teacher/provider–paraeducator teams: Guidelines for paraeducator roles, supervision, and preparation.* New York, NY: City University of New York Graduate Center.

Pickett, A. L., & Gerlach, K. (Eds.). (1997). *Supervising paraeducators in school settings: A team approach.* Austin, TX: Pro-Ed.

Pickstone, C. (2003). A pilot study of paraprofessional screening of child language in community settings. *Child Language Teaching & Therapy, 19,* 49–65.

Preamble to Federal Regulations. (2004, February 28). *Federal Register,* p. 30585.

Rosenfeld, M., & Leung, S. (1999, July). *A job analysis of speech-language pathology assistants: A study to aid in defining the job of speech-language pathology assistants. A job analysis study conducted on behalf of the American Speech-Language-Hearing Association.* Princeton, NJ: Educational Testing Service, Education Policy Research Division.

Scalero, A. M., & Eskenazi, C. (1976). The use of supportive personnel in a public school speech and language program. *Language, Speech, and Hearing Services in Schools, 7,* 150–158.

Scarr, S., McCartney, K., Miller, S., Hauenstein, E., & Ricciuti, A. (1996). Evaluation of an islandwide screening, assessment and treatment program. *Early Development & Parenting, 3,* 199–210.

Schery, T., & O'Connor, L. (1997). Language intervention: Computer training for young children with special needs. *British Journal of Educational Technology, 28,* 271–279.

Schetz, K. F. (1989). Computer-aided language/concept enrichment in kindergarten: Consultation program model. *Language, Speech, and Hearing Services in Schools, 20,* 2–10.

Shewan, C. M., & Kertesz, A. (1984). Effects of speech and language treatment on recovery from aphasia. *Brain and Language, 23,* 272–299.

Shinn-Strieker, T. K. (1984). Trained communication assistants in the public schools. *Language, Speech, and Hearing Services in Schools, 15,* 70–75.

Suter, A. H. (2002). *Hearing conservation manual* (4th ed.). Milwaukee, WI: Council for Accreditation in Occupational Hearing Conservation.

Swan, I. R., & Browning, G. G. (1994). A prospective evaluation of direct referral to audiology departments for hearing aids. *The Journal of Laryngology and Otololgy, 108,* 120–124.

Thornton, A. (1993). The Cheshire profession. *American Journal of Audiology, 2,* 5.

U.S. Census Bureau. (2010). 2010 Census data. Retrieved from http://2010.census.gov/2010census/data/

U.S. Department of Justice. Civil Rights Division. (2000, August 11). *Executive Order 13166, Title VI of the Civil Rights Act of 1964 (Title VI): Improving access to services for persons with limited English proficiency.* Available from http://www.justice.gov/crt/about/cor/13166.php

Vadasy, P. F., Jenkins, J. R., & Pool, K. (2000). Effects of tutoring in phonological and early reading skills on students at risk for reading disabilities. *Journal of Learning Disabilities, 33,* 579–590.

Van Hattum, R. J., Page, J. M., Baskervill, R. D., Duguay, M. J., Conway, L. S., & Davis, T. R. (1974). The Speech Improvement System (SIS) taped program for remediation of articulation problems in the schools. *Language, Speech, and Hearing Services in Schools, 5,* 91–97.

Wertz, R. T., Weiss, D. G., Aten, J. L., Brookshire, R. H., Garcia-Bunuel, L., Holland, A. L., et al. (1986). Comparison of clinic, home, and deferred language treatment for aphasia. A Veterans Administration cooperative study. *Archives of Neurology, 43,* 653–658.

Werven, G. (1992, August). Training support personnel to provide services to persons with head injury. *ASHA,* 72–74.

Werven, G. (1993). Support personnel: An issue for our times. *American Journal of Speech-Language Pathology, 2*(2), 9–12.

Wright, H. H., Shisler, R. J., & Rau, B. (2003). Maintenance of communication abilities in epilepsy: A clinical report. *Journal of Medical Speech-Language Pathology, 11,* 157–167.

Zeitoun, H., Lesshafft, C., Begg, P. A., & East, D. M. (1995). Assessment of a direct referral hearing aid clinic. *British Journal of Audiology, 29,* 13–21.

Appendix 12-A

Support Personnel in Communication Sciences and Disorders: Key Word Definitions

Aides: Support personnel who have a narrower training base and more limited responsibilities relative to the duties of assistants.

Assistants: Support personnel who perform tasks as prescribed, directed, and supervised by certified and licensed (where applicable) professionals after a program of academic and/or on-the-job training.

Cultural broker: A person who is knowledgeable about the client's/patient's culture and/or speech community and who provides this information to the clinician for optimizing services. Also referred to as cultural guides, cultural informants, or cultural-linguistic mediators.

Direct supervision: On-site, in-view observation and guidance by the professional while an assigned activity is performed by support personnel.

Indirect supervision: Activities performed by the professional that may include demonstrations, record review, review and evaluation of audio- or videotaped sessions, and/or interactive television.

Interpreter: Individual who conveys information from one language to another for oral messages.

Support personnel: Provide activities adjunct to the clinical efforts of certified and licensed (where applicable) professionals with appropriate training and supervision.

Translator: Individual who conveys information from one language to another for written messages.

ACKNOWLEDGMENTS

The authors gratefully acknowledge the expertise, attention to detail, and care of the following ASHA National Office staff in the preparation of this chapter:

Eileen Crowe, Janet Deppe, David Denton, Mark Kander, Pamela Mason, Andrea Moxley, and Sarah Slater. The authors also extend their appreciation to Andrea Castrogiovanni for her assistance with the literature review.

SECTION III

Setting-Specific Issues

13

Health Care Legislation, Regulation, and Financing

Steven C. White, PhD
Ingrida Lusis, BA

SCOPE OF CHAPTER

You are undoubtedly aware of the national conversation concerning health care reform in the United States. This debate affects you as an individual and as a professional. Keep in mind as you read this chapter that if you are to work effectively and proactively within the health care system, and even in educational settings, as an audiologist or speech-language pathologist, you must be knowledgeable and current about health care history, rules, regulations, and reimbursement systems. Your patients and their families will expect you to understand how their services fit into their health care plans and what services can or cannot be covered. Also remember that health care is dynamic and that you will need to continue to keep current on these topics.

The American health care system is complex and ever evolving, and its effect on speech-language pathology and audiology services is substantial. The Patient Protection and Affordable Care Act of 2010 (PPACA) was the first major health care law enacted since the Social Security Act Amendments of 1965 established Medicare and Medicaid. Medicare is the federal health insurance program for older Americans and those with severe disabilities while Medicaid is a joint federal-state program for Americans living in poverty. The PPACA includes relevant sections such as one that establishes habilitation services as an essential benefit in private health plans and creates new approaches for providing Medicare and Medicaid coordinated care. On July 16, 2008, the Medicare Improvements for Patients and Providers Act (MIPPA) of 2008 added speech-language pathologists in private practice to the list of professionals who can directly bill the Medicare program effective July 1, 2009. On October 1, 2013, the United States will require providers and other covered entities to implement the use of the International Classification of Diseases, 10th Revision, Clinical Modification (ICD-10-CM), which expands the number of diagnostic and disorder codes from 14,000 to 68,000.

The federal government continues to search for new ways to slow the growth of Medicare and Medicaid spending and reward quality of care. The Centers for Medicare & Medicaid Services (CMS), formerly the Health Care Financing Administration, an agency in the U.S. Department of Health and Human Services, creates Medicare regulations and coverage determinations based on federal law. The regulations directly affect the practices of speech-language pathology and audiology by both establishing Medicare reimbursement levels and requiring specific elements in documentation such as functional progress. The speech-language pathology and audiology communities continue to adjust to prospective payment systems in all settings including private practice; hospitals; skilled nursing facilities; and home health, rehabilitation, and comprehensive agencies.

The payment systems for outpatient and many inpatient Medicare settings had been remarkably altered with passage of the Balanced Budget Act (BBA) of 1997, a landmark bill that changed the rules for Medicare payment in most rehabilitation provider settings. Consequently, reimbursement based on the cost of rendering inpatient care became prospectively determined rather than reflecting provider-determined charges. Other Medicare laws further altered how health care services are paid. New and revised clinical procedures for the professions were included in annual updates of the American Medical Association's *Current Procedural Terminology* (CPT) (American Medical Association, 2010) while reimbursement rates fluctuated as Medicare revised the outpatient payment system based on medical procedures on an annual basis.

The most positive aspect of the Medicare system has been its ability to ensure accessibility to health care for older Americans and those with severe disabilities who have communication and related disorders. Correspondingly, the growth of the numbers of speech-language pathologists and audiologists in health care over the past 30 years may be attributed, at least in part, to the coverage of services in the Medicare program. This chapter, while providing a chronological account and summaries of pertinent health care legislation, regulations, and financing, updates the Medicare and Medicaid statutes and regulations and examines their impact on speech-language pathology and audiology services. Medicaid becomes more of a concern for speech-language pathologists as states look to contain their health care spending, schools bill Medicaid, and the PPACA mandates the development of health insurance exchanges. This chapter continues its discussion of HIPAA, private health care insurance, and the future of health care. Other forces affecting reimbursement and coverage such as the public policy efforts by the American Speech-Language-Hearing Association (ASHA) and ASHA's new education efforts related to coding, documentation, and advocacy are included.

Note that the number of acronyms appearing in this chapter may at first appear overwhelming. See the list of acronyms at the beginning of this book as a guide to the acronyms used in this chapter and others.

HEALTH CARE LEGISLATION

Medicare

Title XVIII of the Social Security Act, Medicare, which provides health insurance for individuals age 65 and older as well as individuals with disabilities under age 65, was established by the Social Security Amendments of 1965. Congress periodically amends the Medicare statute to add new benefits, create new payment approaches, improve quality of care, and reduce fraud and abuse.

Medicare covers individuals under 65 who have disabilities, including people who have been receiving Social Security disability benefits for at least two years. Disability benefits are paid to people who cannot work because they have a severe medical condition that is expected to last at least one year or result in death. Children are covered under Medicare if they have chronic renal disease, need a kidney transplant or maintenance dialysis, or have amyotrophic lateral sclerosis.

The Medicare program has several distinct parts. Medicare Part A, the hospital insurance benefit, covers the costs of inpatient hospital services, skilled nursing facility services, and most home health services. It is financed by the Medicare payroll tax. Medicare Part B, supplemental medical insurance, is a voluntary program financed by premium payments by enrollees and matching payments from general revenues. Part B benefits include physician services, independent practice diagnostic audiology services, and most outpatient rehabilitation services provided by hospitals, rehabilitation agencies, and comprehensive outpatient rehabilitation facilities and private practitioners. Medicare Part C allows beneficiaries access to managed care programs (e.g., health maintenance organizations) called Medicare Advantage. The Medicare Advantage programs are required to cover standard Medicare benefits such as speech-language pathology and audiology services. A new prescription drug benefit that went into effect on January 1, 2006, is described in Medicare Part D.

Medicare Coverage of Speech-Language Pathology Services

Medicare covers medically necessary services provided by a speech language pathologist. Both assessment and treatment services provided by a speech-language pathologist are reimburseable under the Medicare program. These services may be provided under Medicare Parts A and B and under Medicare Advantage plans. The services were defined in Medicare following enactment of the Social Security Amendments of 1993. To slow the growth in spending for speech-language pathology services, physical therapy, and occupational therapy, Congress placed a financial limit on the amount of outpatient therapy it will pay per patient each year under the Balanced Budget Act of 1997. The legislators used a mechanism that had been in place for private practice physical therapy since the enactment of the Social Security Amendments of 1979. Fortunately, the arbitrary therapy cap has not been consistently in force because Congress approves an exceptions process that allows patients to receive services above the therapy cap if the therapist attests that the services are medically necessary and will allow for continued improvement of the patient. For example, on November 19, 1999, Congress passed the Medicare, Medicaid, and SCHIP (State Children's Health Insurance Program) Balanced Budget Refinement Act of 1999 mandating a two-year moratorium on the $1,500 cap during 2000 and 2001. Congressional repeal of the therapy caps has been unattainable as CMS struggles to find a new payment system to replace it.

What follows is a brief twenty-first-century history of the therapy cap. In 2000, then-President Clinton signed into law the Medicare, Medicaid, and SCHIP Benefits Improvement and Protection Act of 2000, which extended the moratorium on the cap through 2002. CMS delayed implementation of the cap until July 1, 2003, but without congressional action an adjusted cap of $1,590 became effective on that date. Reinforcement did not occur until September 1, 2003. The delay occurred because Medicare beneficiaries needed a proper length of notice that the caps would be in place.

A new moratorium for the cap was put into place from December 8, 2003, through December 31, 2005, when then-President Bush signed the Medicare Prescription Drug Improvement and Modernization Act. Congress failed to act again during the 2004–2005 moratorium, resulting in a new $1,740 cap that went into effect on January 1, 2006. A new approach was included in the Deficit Reduction Act passed on February 1, 2006—an exceptions process. The details of the exceptions process were to be developed by CMS for Medicare beneficiaries needing extended therapy services. The Medicare, Medicaid, and SCHIP Extension Act, signed by then-President Bush on July 15, 2007, provided a brief six-month respite to July 2008 from the therapy cap using the exceptions process. The Medicare Improvement for Patients and Providers Act (MIPPA) then extended the exceptions process through the end of 2009. The therapy cap exceptions process expired on January 1, 2010, and the cap was set at a level of $1,860 for the year. However, President Obama signed the Temporary Extension Act of 2010, and the therapy cap was reinstated until March 31, 2010.

Two more extensions would follow: the Patient Protection and Affordable Care Act signed into law by President Obama on March 23, 2010, extended the therapy cap exceptions process through December 31, 2010, and the president's signing of the Senate Amendment to the Medicare and Medicaid Extenders Act of 2010 prolonged the life of the exceptions process until December 31, 2011. In late December 2011, President Obama signed into law the Tax Cut Continuation Act of 2011, which extended the therapy cap exceptions process until February 29, 2012. Congress passed legislation in late February 2012 to extend the Medicare therapy cap exceptions process through 2012 (Lusis, 2012). The laws just detailed that affected the therapy cap are further described in the Medicare Laws section that follows shortly; that section includes a table of the actions that have had an impact on the cap.

Medicare Coverage of Audiology Services

Audiology services are covered under Medicare when diagnostic tests are ordered by a physician to assist in a medical diagnosis or to determine treatment (section 1861[s][3] or 1861[s][2][C] of the Social Security Act). A section of the *Medicare Benefit Policy Manual* briefly describes the extent of audiology coverage in Medicare (Chapter 15, Section 80.3–Audiology Services). As stated in the *Medicare Benefit Policy Manual,* "Audiological diagnostic testing refers to tests of the audiological and vestibular systems, e.g., hearing, balance, auditory processing, tinnitus and diagnostic programming of certain prosthetic devices, performed by qualified audiologists." Medicare defined the services in the Social Security Amendments of 1993, as it did for speech-language pathology.

CMS and Medicare Administrative Contractors (MACs), that is, Medicare, reimburse for audiology services when the diagnostic testing assists a physician in the development of a treatment protocol or surgery. Medicare excludes coverage of audiology services if they are related to determining the need for a hearing aid. The same holds true for services that are considered routine. Medicare, however, will not deny coverage if the hearing assessment results in the recommendation of a hearing aid evaluation (*Medicare Benefit Policy Manual,* Chapter 15, Section 80.3.C, p. 99). Hearing aids and examinations related to hearing aids are specifically excluded from Medicare coverage. Therefore, if a Medicare beneficiary did not complain of other symptoms related to an illness or syndrome other than a hearing loss, Medicare would not cover the audiology services. If the patient exhibits an asymmetrical or unilateral hearing loss and other symptoms of an illness such as Meniere's disease, then the audiologic services would be covered.

A good example of how the Medicare law is converted to regulations is the hearing aid and hearing aid test exclusion. Section 1862(a)(7) of the Social Security Act states that coverage does not extend "where such expenses are for... hearing aids or examinations therefore...." Chapter 42 of the *Code of Federal Regulations* (42 CFR 411.15[d]) interprets the exclusion policy and includes "hearing aids or examination for the purpose of prescribing, fitting, or changing hearing aids."

Medicare Laws

Medicare, Medicaid, and other federal health care programs are mandated by Congress through laws enacted to provide Americans with access to health care. Although many important pieces of legislation for health care have been in the form of authorizing statutes, much has also resulted from budget reconciliation. Traditionally, the budget process involved setting dollar outlays for broad budget categories or "functions," such as health and education. Specific programmatic changes to achieve those outlays were left to authorizing and appropriate legislation.

However, in the 96th Congress, the "reconciliation" procedure of the Congressional Budget and Impoundment Control Act of 1974 was used to "instruct" the authorizing committees to cut spending in numerous health programs. Since then, reconciliation has become an integral part of the budget process (National Health Council, 1993). Provisions in the following reconciliation laws are of interest to speech-language pathologists and audiologists. These laws illustrate how the federal government develops and revises programs that have a remarkable impact on the coverage of speech-language pathology and audiology services.

Social Security Act of 1965

The Social Security Act was signed into law on July 30, 1965, by then-President Lyndon Johnson and established the Medicare and Medicaid programs. Medicare was instituted as a health insurance program for older Americans, and Medicaid created a federal-state health insurance program for Americans living in poverty.

Social Security Act Amendments of 1967

These amendments added outpatient physical therapy services under Part B of the Medicare program. They also eliminated the requirement that a physician certify the medical necessity of outpatient hospital services. However, periodic examinations by physicians after admission remain a requirement for hospitalized patients.

Social Security Act Amendments of 1972

The 1972 amendments added coverage of speech-language pathology services as part of a subsection of the outpatient physical therapy section pertaining to rehabilitation agencies. As a result of these amendments, regulations were promulgated (effective in 1976) specifying conditions of participation for clinics, rehabilitation agencies, and public health agencies as providers of outpatient speech-language pathology services under Part B. Subsequently, speech-language pathologists independently could obtain a Medicare provider number if they met the requirements for certification as a rehabilitation agency.

The law expanded coverage under Medicare to include another vulnerable population: people with severe disabilities. Individuals who have received cash benefits under the disability provisions of the Social Security Act for at least two years would be eligible for health care benefits under Medicare. Thus, Medicare became the health insurance program for individuals who are 65 and older and individuals who are under 65 and have a severe disability.

Omnibus Budget Reconciliation Act of 1980 (OBRA 1980)

A component of this law had a notable impact on speech-language pathologists providing services to Medicare beneficiaries. ASHA advocated for legislation that was incorporated into OBRA 1980 that eliminated the Medicare requirement that only physicians could develop a patient's plan of treatment for outpatient speech-language pathology services. Effective January 1, 1981, speech-language pathologists, as well as physicians, could write plans of treatment for Medicare beneficiaries.

In the 1979 reports on the Medicare amendments legislation, the Senate Finance Committee and the House Ways and Means Committee stated that, "since speech (-language) pathology services involve highly specialized knowledge and training, physicians generally do not specify in detail the services needed when referring a patient for such services" (House Report 96-588 at p. 15; Senate Report 96-471 at p. 37).

Tax Equity and Fiscal Responsibility Act of 1982

Concern over rapidly rising health care costs led to amendments that changed the way in which Medicare reimbursed hospitals for costs. The Tax Equity and Fiscal Responsibility Act (TEFRA) marked the beginning of a new era in Medicare reimbursement. For the first time, hospitals were paid according to fixed payment levels rather than what they reported as their actual costs. The TEFRA limits were applied to all routine operating costs, costs of special care units, and costs of inpatient services such as speech-language pathology and audiology. Further, the TEFRA limits capped the reimbursement rate of increase for a hospital's Medicare reimbursement per discharge from one fiscal year to the next.

TEFRA offered a strong incentive to providers to contain costs, although Medicare's prospective payment system (PPS) that was enacted in 1983 would offer a stronger incentive. As TEFRA continued and rehabilitation services remained under its limits, providers became increasingly dissatisfied with the effect of the system (National Association of Rehabilitation Facilities [NARF], 1990). According to the National Association of Rehabilitation Facilities (now the American Medical Rehabilitation Providers Association) (NARF, 1990), increases in TEFRA limits were not sufficient to pay for the increasing costs of at least half of all rehabilitation facilities. This led providers to propose changes to the way in which rehabilitation services are reimbursed. Not until 1997 did Congress require a new approach to paying rehabilitation hospitals and rehabilitation units in general hospitals.

TEFRA also added a new Medicare provider setting. Section 122 established coverage for hospice care. The new benefit specifically covers speech-language pathology services for the terminally ill. Section 418.92, Title 42 of the *Code of Federal Regulations* (Office of the Federal Register, 1996) states, "Physical therapy services, occupational therapy services, and speech-language pathology services must be available, and when provided, offered in a manner consistent with accepted standards of practice" (p. 783).

Social Security Act Amendments of 1983

In reaction to predictions that the Medicare program would go bankrupt by the year 2000 without drastic cost controls, the payment methodology of fixed payment levels or cost limits begun under TEFRA was strengthened dramatically in 1983. The Social Security Amendments of 1983 created a new approach to paying for hospital services, the prospective payment system (PPS), in which a flat payment was determined prior to treatment and based on a patient's principal diagnosis or diagnosis-related group (DRG).

PPS was considered to provide strong incentives for hospitals to provide efficient services. Hospitals could keep any savings realized under Medicare DRGs. If the hospital's actual costs to treat a patient were less than the flat amount assigned to that particular DRG, the hospital kept the difference. However, if the hospital's actual costs exceeded the payment assigned, the hospital absorbed the loss.

Although such incentive reimbursement offered strong encouragement to providers for efficiency, it also raised concerns regarding a number of less positive effects. Health care professionals reported that PPS compromised quality of care. They alleged patients were being discharged while still ill after shorter lengths of stay (i.e., "sicker and quicker"). Others raised the concern that hospitals struggling to survive in the health market would learn to "game the system" and simply shift costs to other areas.

Although anecdotal, the fallout of PPS for inpatient speech-language pathology and audiology services consisted of deferred or reduced inpatient referrals, fewer inpatient sessions, downsizing of staff, and reluctance to contract for new services. Moreover, a shift occurred for speech-language pathology inpatient services from language-based disorder services to assessing and treating patients with dysphagia. Physicians and hospital administrators knew the dysphagia services would assist in an earlier discharge.

Rehabilitation hospitals and rehabilitation units were exempt from Medicare PPS (as were children's, psychiatric, and long-term care hospitals), but they remained subject to the TEFRA cost limits because of the unique case mix of patients. During the early period of PPS, the exempt rehabilitation hospitals and units enjoyed unprecedented growth (Wilkerson, Batavia, & DeJong, 1992).

Consolidated Omnibus Budget Reconciliation Act of 1985

Provisions of COBRA 1985, which contained amendments to the Medicare and Medicaid programs, established the Physician Payment Review Commission. This commission was required to make recommendations to Congress regarding changes in the methodology for determining the rates of payment for Medicare Part B services. COBRA led to the implementation of the resource-based relative value scale (RBRVS). The RBRVS is the foundation of the Medicare Physician Fee Schedule, which is described later in more detail because of its implications for audiologists and speech-language pathologists.

Omnibus Budget Reconciliation Act of 1986

OBRA 1986 directed the Health Care Financing Administration (HFCA, now CMS) to proceed with research on a new system of Medicare Part B payments to physicians and other practitioners. The subsequent research, led by Harvard professor William Hsiao, resulted in implementation of the Part B Medicare Physician Fee Schedule, which includes payment rates for speech-language pathology and audiology services. The Omnibus Budget Reconciliation Act of 1989 implemented the resource-based relative value scale.

Omnibus Budget Reconciliation Act of 1987

OBRA 1987, in response to the pervasiveness of substandard conditions in the nation's nursing homes, made sweeping reforms in the care provided by all nursing homes participating in the Medicare and Medicaid programs. This legislation mandates that Medicare- or Medicaid-certified nursing facilities provide each resident the necessary care and services to "attain or maintain the highest practicable physical, mental and psychosocial well-being, in accordance with the comprehensive assessment and plan of care" (*Code of Federal Regulations,* Title 42, Section 483.25, Office of the Federal Register, 1996). The regulations resulting from this legislation further specify that the comprehensive assessment include an assessment of functional status, including the ability to use speech, language, or other functional communication systems (Lubinski & Frattali, 1993; White, 1989).

OBRA 1987 held great potential for improving access to quality care for nursing facility residents with communication disorders and related disorders, such as dysphagia, cognitive deficits, and balance disorders. As a result of this legislation, the Resident Assessment Instrument (RAI) was developed (Morris, Hawes, Fries, & Mor, 1991). The RAI contains a Minimum Data Set (MDS) that requires information on communication/hearing. It was developed with input from ASHA (Lubinski & Frattali, 1993).

Three years after the tool was established in the nation's nursing facilities, survey data collected by the research consortium involved in the development of the RAI documented a 31 percent increase in referrals to speech-language pathology (audiology data were not reported at the time) (Lubinski, personal communication, 1993). Most recently, an MDS 3.0 was released that requires patient involvement when possible and "... requires all members of the SNF care team to include patient goals and to state the intent to facilitate progress toward the patient's discharge from skilled nursing care" (Wisely, 2010). Moreover, Wisely points out that audiologists and speech-language pathologists are the most appropriate professionals to assist SNF administrators "... in properly identifying those with communication disorders and preparing staff for the challenges of MDS 3.0 completion."

Omnibus Budget Reconciliation Act of 1989

OBRA 1989 required Medicare to begin paying for charge-based Part B services by January 1992 using a resource-based relative value scale (RBRVS) with geographic adjustments for differences in costs of practice. This legislation replaced the reasonable charge payment mechanism with a fee schedule based on national uniform relative values for all "physician services," including outpatient physician services. The system was phased in during a four-year period beginning in 1992.

The RBRVS caused concern among audiologists and speech-language pathologists (ASHA, 1992). The RBRVS did not recognize the professional services (e.g., interpretation of test results by audiologists) in the professional component also known as "physician work," but rather under the "technical" component or "practice expense." Under the RBRVS, physicians and other practitioners have an approach that calculates a value for the professional aspect of their services based on intensity of service, time, stress, clinical judgment, and risk to the patient. The value is determined based on a survey of a sample of those who perform the procedure with results submitted by the specialty society and, subsequently, reviewed by a committee of experts known as the AMA/Specialty Society RVU Update Committee (RUC) of the American Medical Association. Services administered solely or primarily by nonphysician practitioners are valued by the RUC Health Care Professionals Advisory Committee (RUC HCPAC) on which ASHA holds a seat. The RUC or RUC HCPAC in turn submits the final values to the Centers for Medicare & Medicaid Services for consideration in the Medicare Physician Fee Schedule (MPFS). The value of the professional component is added to practice expense and the malpractice expense (or professional liability) to give a total RVU (White, 2011a). Conversely, services such as audiology and speech-language pathology had only time values. The time includes preparation for the service before the patient arrives; all time spent with the patient, including preparing the room and counseling the patient and family; report writing; and phone calls. However, it does not take into account the factors included for the professional component. Outpatient Medicare speech-language pathology services were included for reimbursement under the RBRVS in 1999 when the provisions of the BBA 1997 went into effect. ASHA conducts a separate review of audiology and speech-language pathology relative value units in the MPFS and updates it annually. The RBRVS is discussed further in the Medicare Physician Fee Schedule section. In 2010, RUC HCPAC reviewed data presented by ASHA for six speech-language pathology procedures because the profession began billing Medicare directly and services could now be reflected in the professional component. CMS accepted the RUC HCPAC's recommendations for five of the six procedures but lowered the recommended work value for CPT 92508 because the federal agency arbitrarily declared that the typical number of patients in a group was four rather than the three used in the ASHA data presented to the RUC HCPAC.

Another section of OBRA 1989 improved the Medicaid Early and Periodic Screening, Diagnosis and Treatment (EPSDT) program so that proper treatment for communication disorders discovered during screening must be provided. Prior to the law, states avoided providing needed services such as speech-language pathology services, audiology services, and assistive technology (White, 1990). OBRA 1989 mandated coverage of all medically necessary services for children enrolled in the Medicaid program.

Omnibus Budget Reconciliation Act of 1990

OBRA 1990 (Omnibus Budget and Reconciliation Act, 1990) includes Section 4005(b)(1), which states:

> The Secretary of Health and Human Services shall develop a proposal to modify the current system under which [excluded] hospitals receive payment... or a proposal to replace such system with a system under which such payment would be made on the basis of nationally determined average standardized amounts.

Through this provision, Congress made clear its intent to develop a more appropriate payment system for rehabilitation under Medicare (Wilkerson et al., 1992). Interestingly, through the Balanced Budget Act of 1997, Congress had to direct Health and Human Services to implement the system. The 1990 OBRA legislation, as an interim measure, also provided some relief to hospitals in the form of partial payment for differences between the TEFRA cap and actual hospital costs (Wilkerson et al., 1992).

SOCIAL SECURITY ACT AMENDMENTS OF 1993

The Social Security Amendments of 1993 defined Medicare speech-language pathology services and speech-language pathologists and audiology services and audiologists for the first time. Medicare regulations regarding the provision of speech-language pathology services and audiology services must be consistent with the following section of the U.S. Code for Title XVIII of the Social Security Act:

Sec. 1395x. Definitions

(II) Speech-language pathology services; audiology services

(1) The term "speech-language pathology services" means such speech, language, and related function assessment and rehabilitation services furnished by a qualified speech-language pathologist as the speech-language pathologist is legally authorized to perform under State law (or the State regulatory mechanism provided by State law) as would otherwise be covered if furnished by a physician.

(2) The term "audiology services" means such hearing and balance assessment services furnished by a qualified audiologist as the audiologist is legally authorized to perform under State law (or the State regulatory mechanism provided by State law), as would otherwise be covered if furnished by a physician.

(3) In this subsection:

(A) The term "qualified speech-language pathologist" means an individual with a master's or doctoral degree in speech-language pathology who—

(i) is licensed as a speech-language pathologist by the State in which the individual furnishes such services, or

(ii) in the case of an individual who furnishes services in a State which does not license speech-language pathologists, has successfully completed 350 clock hours of supervised clinical practicum (or is in the process of accumulating such supervised clinical experience), performed not less than 9 months of supervised full-time speech-language pathology services after obtaining a master's or doctoral degree in speech-language pathology or a related field, and successfully completed a national examination in speech-language pathology approved by the Secretary.

(B) The term "qualified audiologist" means an individual with a master's or doctoral degree in audiology who—

(i) is licensed as an audiologist by the State in which the individual furnishes such services, or

(ii) in the case of an individual who furnishes services in a State which does not license audiologists, has successfully completed 350 clock hours of supervised clinical practicum (or is in the process of accumulating such supervised clinical experience), performed not less than 9 months of supervised full-time audiology services after obtaining a master's or doctoral degree in audiology or a related field, and successfully completed a national examination in audiology approved by the Secretary.

THE BALANCED BUDGET ACT OF 1997

A Republican-majority Congress and a promise from the Clinton administration to bring the federal budget under control drove the most sweeping changes in the Medicare statute since its inception in 1965. As reported by the Medicare Payment Advisory Commission (MedPAC) of Congress (1998):

> The Balanced Budget Act of 1997 (BBA) enacted substantial changes in Medicare's payment policies. Outpatient rehabilitation providers will be paid according to the physician fee schedule beginning January 1, 1999, and outpatient rehabilitation furnished by non-hospital providers will be subject to annual coverage limits. Skilled nursing facilities (SNFs) will begin transition to a per diem prospective payment system

on July 1, 1998. Prospective payment for home health agencies and for inpatient rehabilitation facilities also is scheduled to be implemented on October 1, 1999, although the units of payment for those systems have not been finalized. (p. 79)

Although there was no mention of "outpatient rehabilitation" as a particular provider in the Medicare statute, there were various rehabilitation providers under the law. Hospital outpatient departments, rehabilitation agencies, and comprehensive outpatient rehabilitation facilities (CORFs) are all providers of rehabilitation services, as are independent practitioners of physical therapy and occupational therapy. Nevertheless, the three major rehabilitation professions are all separately described in the Medicare statute.

The two major areas of the BBA that most affected the practice of speech-language pathology were the requirement to impose a $1,500 annual financial limitation (i.e., therapy cap) per Medicare beneficiary for outpatient speech-language pathology and physical therapy combined and the change to prospective payment systems for inpatient services.

The Medicare, Medicaid, and SCHIP Balanced Budget Refinement Act of 1999 (BBRA)

The BBRA was the first law that responded to the concerns of the beneficiary and provider communities about the problems caused by the Medicare therapy cap. It placed a two-year moratorium on the cap covering calendar years 2000 and 2001. The law also called for CMS to submit a report to Congress about the utilization patterns of outpatient therapy.

The Medicare, Medicaid, and SCHIP Benefits Improvement and Protection Act of 2000 (BIPA)

This federal statute was signed into law in December 2002 and became known as BIPA. BIPA had a positive effect on the provision of speech-language pathology services under Medicare by extending the moratorium on the annual financial cap for outpatient physical, occupational, and speech-language pathology services. Congress thought of the cap as an interim measure to be replaced by a prospective payment approach and, as with BBRA and future laws, BIPA extended the moratorium on the cap through 2002 to add to the two years from the BBRA.

The Medicare Prescription Drug, Improvement, and Modernization Act of 2003 (MMA)

The MMA contains a number of provisions that affect speech-language pathology and audiology services. The most immediate effect of the MMA was a 1.5 percent increase in the Medicare Physician Fee Schedule for services paid under the MPFS provided on or after January 1, 2004. The rates were set to be reduced by 4.5 percent in 2004, and again in 2005, but the MMA reversed the reduction and provided an increase of 1.5 percent in the conversion factor of the MPFS for both years.

A new concept was introduced in the law—a "Welcome to Medicare" preventive screening visit. The new benefit is meant to promote health and detect disease. New beneficiaries of Medicare are eligible for an initial preventive screening visit known as a "Welcome to Medicare" examination. It includes a measurement of height, weight, and blood pressure; a review of the patient's medical and social history; and a review of the individual's risk factors for depression, functional ability, and level of safety. It also includes education, counseling, and referral with respect to screening and preventive services currently covered under Medicare Part B. Hearing acuity is part of the examination but only in an interview format. ASHA recommended that pure-tone screening be used, but CMS stated that an interview between the beneficiary and physician or other qualified health care provider is sufficient for the purpose of the Welcome to Medicare benefit.

As a result of a provision in the Medicare Modernization Act of 2003 (MMA), CMS was charged with significantly altering the way it awards contracts to carriers and fiscal intermediaries—the companies hired by Medicare to process your Medicare claims. The reform efforts were aimed at making Medicare contract awards more competitive and contracts more efficient. CMS is to offer the contracts for bidding at least once every five years. Under the new system, which was completed in 2011, there are 15 new Part A/B Medicare Administrative Contractor (MAC) jurisdictions. This was a significant departure from the replaced system, under which there were 18 carriers for practitioner-based services and 25 fiscal intermediaries for institutional providers.

The legislation also established the Recovery Audit Contractors (RAC) program as a three-year demonstration program for 2005–2008. The demonstration program ran in three states identified to have the largest volume of Medicare claims: Florida, New York, and California. RAC contractors are private entities retained by the government to identify overpayments or underpayments to health care providers under the Medicare program and to recoup underpayments or return overpayments. The focus of RAC audits is the Medicare Part B program. Rather than being paid an up-front fee, the government pays RAC contractors a contingency fee for each inappropriate payment that they identify and recover (Kander, 2009).

The Deficit Reduction Act of 2005 (DRA)

Signed into law by then-President George W. Bush on February 8, 2006, the DRA required that CMS develop an exception process that allows Medicare beneficiaries access to medically necessary outpatient therapy services above the therapy cap for calendar year 2006. Congress extended the use of the therapy cap exceptions process after 2006. Legislation passed in February 2012 allowed the therapy cap exception process to continue through 2012. Speech-language pathologists can use the exceptions process in those situations where medically necessary services above the therapy cap are needed and may include conditions that require both speech-language pathology and physical therapy services or just speech. Moreover, CMS used this approach to collect data to demonstrate the necessity of functional outcomes-based data from providers (Lusis, 2010). Details of the exceptions process are found on the ASHA website.

Tax Relief and Health Care Act of 2006

Section 302 of the Tax Relief and Health Care Act of 2006 made the Medicare Recovery Audit Contractor program permanent and required that the program be expanded to all Part B services in all states by 2010. The RAC program had been established as a demonstration program by the Medicare Modernization Act and was successful in finding errors and recouping money from providers. For example, RACs recovered substantial sums from providers, including audiologists, for overpayment of vestibular function testing in Florida (Romanow & McCarty, 2010). The RACs use Medicare policies, regulations, national and local coverage determinations, and manual instructions when conducting audits and determine whether overpayments or underpayments were made to providers.

Medicare Improvements for Patients and Providers Act (MIPPA) 2008

On July 16, 2008, the Medicare Improvements for Patients and Providers Act (MIPPA) of 2008 was passed, which included a provision that allows speech-language pathologists in private practice to directly bill the Medicare program effective July 1, 2009 (Brown 2008; White 2009). The Centers for Medicare & Medicaid Services began accepting enrollment applications beginning June 2, 2009. Speech-language pathologists can apply for an enrollment number and bill Medicare for their services (Romanow, 2008). Romanow listed the following steps for a speech-language pathologist to follow for Medicare enrollment:

1. Obtain an NPI number. You should prepare to enroll in Medicare by first obtaining a National Provider Identifier (NPI), a unique, 10-digit number required under the Health Insurance Portability and Accountability Act (HIPAA) for covered health care providers. It is required for enrollment and on Medicare claims forms. The NPI application process should be completed well before Medicare enrollment. You may complete an application on the CMS website or request a form by phone. Instructions are available on the ASHA Web site.
2. Identify a Medicare contractor. Next, you should determine the Medicare contractor in the area that will process the application. The contractor will be either a Part B carrier or Medicare Administrative Contractor (MAC). CMS is gradually replacing carriers and fiscal intermediaries with MACs (therefore, a carrier may become a MAC). The contractor will also process Medicare claims. Details on determining your contractor are available on the ASHA website.
3. Submit an enrollment form. Once you have determined the appropriate contractor, the enrollment form may be submitted on or after June 2, 2009. An individual SLP will complete a CMS-855i form to bill for individual services; a business or group practice would also fill out a CMS-855B form. Processing time for the application depends on the Medicare Administrative Contractor.

With speech-language pathologists eligible for Medicare private practice status in mid-2009, the establishment of a Medicare-certified rehabilitation agency became important only to those who wished to bill multiple rehabilitation services to Medicare in a nonfacility setting. There are states that do not allow private speech-language pathologists to establish a group practice that also delivers physical therapy and occupational therapy, where a rehabilitation agency remains a viable alternative.

Several revisions to rehabilitation agency regulations, effective January 1, 2009, facilitate satellite locations and reduce required services not directly related to rehabilitation.

- An on-call physician for emergencies is no longer required.
- Social worker, physiologist, or vocational counselor services are no longer included in the rehabilitation agency definition.
- Extension locations are now defined in regulation (Rehabilitation Agencies as Providers of Outpatient Physical Therapy and Outpatient Speech-Language Pathology Services, 2009) instead of only in the *State Operations Manual.* An extension location is described in the regulation as being "... sufficiently close to share administration, supervision, and services in a manner that renders it unnecessary for the extension location to independently meet the conditions of participation as a rehabilitation agency" (p. 153).
- Thirty-day physician certification/recertification is the single change that is not a reduction of required services. In 2008 CMS revised the physician certification and recertification period for outpatient rehabilitation services from 30 days to up to 90 days if the plan of care covered that duration. For rehabilitation agencies, CMS is reverting to the 30-day period. This time period complies with the conditions of participation that require physician review at least every 90 days.

MIPPA also made changes to the time that records must be maintained. Orders or referrals by physicians, nurse practitioners, or physician assistants must now be retained for seven years from the date of last service. Off-site or electronic storage is allowed as long as the records are readily accessible.

Medicare Regulations: Coverage and Payment Policies

National Medicare policies are described online in Internet-Only Manuals (IOMs). The IOMs have various sections. The information related to the current national coverage determinations (NCDs) for speech-generating devices, electronic speech aids, cochlear implants, tracheostomy speaking valves, and tinnitus maskers are located in section 50 of the Internet manual. Speech-language pathology services for dysphagia and melodic intonation therapy are in the IOM under section 170 of the *Coverage Determinations Manual* (Publication #100-03). An overview of how speech-language pathology services relate to Medicare is found in Chapter 15 of the *Medicare Benefit Policy Manual* (Publication #100-02) sections 220 and 230.

Coding for Reimbursement

Health care coding systems are regulated by the U.S. Department of Health and Human Services (HHS). CMS and the National Center for Health Statistics both oversee the International Classification of Diseases, 9th Revision, Clinical Modification (ICD-9-CM), while CMS alone revises the Healthcare Common Procedural Coding System (HCPCS). The three coding systems are recognized as code sets under HIPAA. ICD-9-CM, CPT, and HCPCS are used by Medicare, Medicaid, and private health plans. Kander (2008) described the relationship of codes to billing. For example, Kander explains how the billing form CMS-1500 is dependent on coding of services and primary and secondary diagnoses.

Current Procedural Terminology

Current Procedural Terminology (CPT) codes are a five-digit system used to describe procedures or services. CMS integrates the CPT codes into its Healthcare Common Procedures Coding System (HCPCS) as Level I codes. The CPT system is maintained and copyrighted by the American Medical Association. Each CPT code has five digits. The American Medical Association (AMA) CPT Editorial Panel reviews and responds to requests for additions to or revisions of the CPT. A member of the ASHA Health Care Economics Committee serves as the ASHA advisor to the AMA CPT Panel Health Care Professionals Advisory Committee.

Healthcare Common Procedures Coding System Level II

HCPCS Level II codes are used to report supplies, equipment, devices, and related procedures provided to patients. A limited number of procedures not otherwise contained in the CPT system are also found here. HCPCS is alphanumeric and is administered by CMS in cooperation with other third-party payers.

CMS includes two levels in its Healthcare Common Procedures Coding System: HCPCS Level I is the CPT coding system; HCPCS Level II is usually referred to as HCPCS codes. Following are examples of HCPCS Level II codes:

- E2504 Speech generating device, digitized speech, using prerecorded messages, greater than 20 minutes but less than or equal to 40 minutes of recording time
- L8501 Tracheostomy speaking valve
- V5244 Hearing aid, digitally programmable analog, monaural CIC

ICD-9-CM (International Classification of Diseases, 9th Revision, Clinical Modification)

Health care professionals use these codes (which have three numeric digits followed by a decimal point) to report diagnoses and disorders. The ICD-9-CM is maintained by the National Center for Health Statistics of the U.S. Public Health Service. The ICD-10-CM is in a revised draft stage but cannot replace ICD-9-CM without a two-year notice of implementation, as mandated by HIPAA. An implementation date of October 1, 2013, has been established by the National Center for Health Statistics, Centers for Disease Control and Prevention, U.S. Department of Health and Human Services.

ASHA is actively engaged in the development of both CPT codes and ICD-9-CM codes. The five audiologists and five speech-language pathologists of the ASHA Health Care Economics Committee (HCEC) monitor these code sets and make recommendations for additions and revisions so that procedures and services performed by the professions can be reported to payers. One ASHA HCEC member serves as an advisor to the AMA CPT Editorial Panel Health Care Professional Advisory Committee while another serves as the alternate advisor. Both audiologists and speech-language pathologists are represented on this committee because of this arrangement. The work of the ASHA HCEC has resulted in new and revised procedure codes that are found in Table 13–1.

Prospective Payment Systems

In 1983, Medicare began its first prospective payment system (PPS) for inpatient hospital services. Reimbursement had been based on the cost of rendering care, but the PPS revised the approach by affixing rates according to the principal diagnosis of the patient. This diagnosis-related grouping (DRG) of patients altered inpatient care so that patients were being discharged early, or "quicker and sicker." Administrators of skilled nursing facilities (SNFs) and home health agencies (HHAs) had to revise their approach to patient care and place more emphasis on rehabilitation services such as speech-language pathology.

It was not until 1997 that the U.S. Congress and the Clinton administration instituted new PPSs. The BBA placed both SNFs and HHAs under unique and, at that time, somewhat unknown PPSs. SNFs began the transition from a cost-based system to a per-diem approach on July 1, 1998, depending on the cost-reporting period to Medicare. HHAs began an interim payment system for cost-reporting periods beginning on or after October 1, 1999. The HHA PPS is based on an assessment instrument known as the Outcome and Assessment Information Set, or OASIS. The SNF PPS system is based on resource utilization groups (RUGs). Other providers scheduled to go under a form of prospective payment system include rehabilitation hospitals and hospital outpatient departments.

The SNF PPS interim final regulations were published by the Health Care Financing Administration (now CMS) in the May 12, 1998 *Federal Register* (Health Care Financing Administration, 1998) and are based on the Nursing Home Case Mix and Quality System, a PPS demonstration project that had been funded by HCFA since 1989. The hallmark of the system is the RUG, which is composed of an assessment, Minimum Data Set (MDS), wage-weighted staff time measurements, and self-performance in activities of daily living (ADLs). SNF patients are assigned to one of 53 RUGs, of which 23 require intensive rehabilitation services. Patients in the 23 rehabilitation RUGs require from 45 minutes to 720 minutes per week of

TABLE 13–1 Speech-Language Pathology and Audiology CPT1 Codes Revised or Established 2003–2011

CPT Code	Descriptor
92506	Evaluation of speech, language, voice, communication, and/or auditory processing
92507	Treatment of speech, language, voice, communication, and/or auditory processing disorder; individual
92540	Basic vestibular evaluation, includes spontaneous nystagmus test with eccentric gaze fixation nystagmus, with recording, positional nystagmus test, minimum of 4 positions, with recording, optokinetic nystagmus test, bidirectional foveal and peripheral stimulation, with recording, and oscillating tracking test, with recording
92550	Tympanometry and reflex threshold measurements
92568	Acoustic reflex testing; threshold
92569	Acoustic reflex testing; decay
92570	Acoustic immittance testing, includes tympanometry (impedance testing), acoustic reflex threshold testing, and acoustic reflex decay testing
92601	Diagnostic analysis of cochlear implant, patient under 7 years of age; with programming
92602	Subsequent reprogramming
92603	Diagnostic analysis of cochlear implant, patient 7 years of age or older; with programming
92604	Subsequent reprogramming
92605	Evaluation for prescription of non-speech-generating augmentative and alternative communication device
92606	Therapeutic service(s) for the use of non-speech-generating augmentative and alternative communication device
92607	Evaluation for prescription of speech-generating augmentative and alternative communication device, face-to-face with the patient; first hour
92608	Each additional 30 minutes
92609	Therapeutic services for the use of speech-generating device, including programming and modification
92610	Evaluation of oral and pharyngeal swallow function
92611	Motion fluoroscopic evaluation of swallowing function by cine or video recording
92612	Flexible fiberoptic endoscopic evaluation of swallowing by cine or video recording
92614	Flexible fiberoptic endoscopic evaluation, laryngeal sensory testing by cine or video recording
92616	Flexible fiberoptic endoscopic evaluation of swallowing and laryngeal sensory testing by cine or video recording

(*Continues*)

TABLE 13–1 Speech-Language Pathology and Audiology CPT1 Codes Revised or Established 2003–2011 (*Continued*)

CPT Code	Descriptor
92620	Evaluation of central auditory function, with report; initial 60 minutes
92621	Each additional 15 minutes
92625	Assessment of tinnitus (includes pitch, loudness matching, and masking)
92626	Evaluation of auditory rehabilitation status; first hour
92627	Each additional 15 minutes
92630	Auditory rehabilitation; pre-lingual hearing loss
92633	Post-lingual hearing loss
92640	Diagnostic analysis with programming of auditory brainstem implant, per hour
98966	Telephone assessment and management service provided by a qualified nonphysician health care professional to an established patient, parent, or guardian not originating from a related assessment and management service provided within the previous seven days nor leading to an assessment and management service or procedure with the next 24 hours or soonest available appointment; 5–10 minutes of medical discussion
98967	11–20 minutes of medical discussion
98968	21–30 minutes of medical discussion
96125	Standardized cognitive performance testing (e.g., Ross Information Processing Assessment) per hour of a qualified health care professional's time, both face-to-face time administering tests to the patient and time interpreting these test results and preparing the report
99366	Medical team conference with interdisciplinary team of health care professionals, face-to-face with patient and/or family, 30 minutes or more, participation by non-physician qualified health care professional
99368	Medical team conference with interdisciplinary team of health care professionals, patient and/or family not present, 30 minutes or more; participation by nonphysician qualified health care professional

Source: 1CPT codes and descriptors are copyright 2011 American Medical Association

speech-language pathology, physical therapy, or occupational therapy services.

The Balanced Budget Act of 1997 (BBA) was an attempt to bring fiscal controls to the Medicare program. A review of the development of Medicare through a series of amendments to the Social Security Act demonstrates the piecemeal approach to revising the program over the past 32 years. Further, the difficulties in creating a logical financing system are compounded by the various settings in which health care is delivered in the United States.

Therapy Caps

As previously noted, the BBA created the arbitrary annual beneficiary cap in response to rapidly escalating expenditures in Medicare outpatient rehabilitation benefits. Costs to the Medicare program for rehabilitation agency services went from $151 million in 1990 to $524 million in 1996 (Medicare Payment Advisory Commission, 1998, p. 80). Corresponding growth in costs for comprehensive outpatient rehabilitation facilities (CORFs) went from $19 million to $115 million in the same time period. Congress chose the cap as a quick fix for a complex issue.

Previously, physical therapists and occupational therapists in independent practice had a $900 cap, and this served as the model for all outpatient services. The outpatient financial limitation became effective on January 1, 1999, for speech-language pathology services, physical therapy services, and occupational therapy services in all Medicare-certified outpatient settings except for hospitals. Occupational therapy has a separate $1,500 cap from the combined cap for speech-language pathology and physical therapy. Advocacy efforts by ASHA and other rehabilitation organizations such as the American Occupational Therapy Association and the American Physical Therapy Association resulted in a revision of the rehabilitation cap. On November 29, 1999, the Medicare, Medicaid, and SCHIP Balanced Budget bill became law (PL 106-113). The Balanced Budget Refinement Act (BBRA) placed a two-year moratorium on the $1,500 cap and required the Secretary of Health and Human Services to report to Congress on a new payment limitation method for outpatient rehabilitation services and on the utilization of services. The moratorium on the cap was a major victory for ASHA and the other professional associations.

CMS contracted with AdvanceMed to review billing practices and investigate the establishment of a payment system related to Medicare Part B rehabilitation services that would obviate the need for a therapy cap. AdvanceMed's Ciolek and Hwang (2004) recommended a global approach to achieve a long-term outpatient therapy payment system solution in the second AdvanceMed report. The global approach would maintain the use of the MPFS, eliminate the therapy cap, and continue medical review to identify targets for utilization review, create utilization thresholds for "medically unbelievable services," use national rather than local coverage decisions, develop a standardized outpatient therapy assessment instrument, and develop a condition-based outpatient therapy payment system.

Several recent (CMS) contracted studies have demonstrated that while the number of beneficiaries receiving outpatient therapy services has increased at a rate of about 2.9 percent per year from 1998 to 2008, Medicare expenditures have increased at a rate of about 10.1 percent per year (fluctuating during capped and not-capped years). While some of the increase can be attributed to inflationary fee schedule price increases, it is uncertain whether the remaining increases were due to necessary services or not.

The growth in outpatient therapy expenditures has surpassed the rate of growth of spending in other Medicare benefits and has been under scrutiny from organizations including the Medicare Payment Advisory Commission (MedPAC), the U.S. Government Accountability Office (GAO), and the Office of Inspector General (OIG) of the U.S. Department of Health and Human Services. These organizations have conducted studies on outpatient therapy services and have provided recommendations for policy changes to better ensure that Medicare pays only for medically necessary services (Ciolek & Hwang, 2010).

To control the growth in outpatient therapy (and other) spending, CMS and its contractors have implemented a variety of different utilization edits in response to perceived overutilization or improper use of certain HCPCS codes. These edits include the following:

- CMS Medically Unlikely Edits (MUEs)
- CMS Deficit Reduction Act (DRA) edits
- CMS National Correct Coding Initiative (CCI) edits (see Kander, 2005)
- Local MAC medical necessity edits including limits per HCPCS, and HCPCS and ICD-9-CM crosswalk edits

In its further review of outpatient therapy services, CMS contracted to develop both short- and long-term solutions to the therapy caps. In 2008, CMS awarded the two-year Short-Term Alternatives for Therapy Services (STATS) project to CSC: to conduct follow-up utilization analysis, to develop new systems capabilities to provide CMS with near real-time utilization trends, and to conduct research. Further, the STATS project allowed CMS to confer with outpatient therapy stakeholders and subject matter experts to develop specific payment policy applications as an alternative to the current outpatient therapy caps that can be used in the short term to limit payments to medically necessary outpatient therapy services. As part of its final recommendations upon completion of the project, CSC recommended that payment be based on function or quality measurements that adequately perform risk adjustment for episode-based payment purposes.

The longer-term solution, Developing Outpatient Therapy Payment Alternatives (DOTPA), will ultimately develop alternatives to the current outpatient therapy payment system and possibly eliminate the need for an exceptions process. To date, DOTPA has developed a tool that will be used to identify, collect, and analyze information related to beneficiary need for and effectiveness of outpatient therapy services. Different versions of the tool have been developed for patients in nursing facilities/day rehabilitation settings and for those in community-based (outpatient) settings. For the past two years, ASHA has provided input to ensure that speech-language pathology services and patient disorders, deficits, and needs are adequately represented in the assessment tool. The DOTPA project is currently collecting data to use in the development of a payment alternative (Romanow, 2010).

Until CMS develops a viable alternative, the therapy cap issue will not recede completely, although federal legislation to repeal the cap has been popular. Legislation for repealing the cap has been introduced by members of Congress who sit on Medicare oversight committees. However, because of the negative budget impact of repealing the cap, the threat of its return persists. Repeal of the cap without a new payment policy may lead to increased utilization of outpatient therapy services and thereby added costs. Table 13–2 lists the extensive legislative and regulatory history of the therapy caps (American Physical Therapy Association, 2011).

TABLE 13–2 Chronological Legislative History of the Therapy Caps

August 1997	Balanced Budget Act of 1997 imposes $1,500 cap on outpatient therapy services including combined speech-language pathology and physical therapy cap.
November 1998	Health Care Financing Administration (now Centers for Medicare & Medicaid Services) publishes 1998 Medicare Physician Fee Schedule implementing the therapy caps in 1999.
January 1999	Therapy caps go into effect.
November 1999	Medicare, Medicaid, and SCHIP Balanced Budget Refinement Act of 1999 mandates a two-year moratorium on caps.
December 2000	Medicare, Medicaid, and SCHIP Benefits Improvement and Protection Act of 2000 extends the moratorium on the cap through 2002.
November 2002	Congress adjourns without passing Medicare reform legislation; Medicare is forced to implement cap effective January 1, 2003.
December 2002	Centers for Medicare & Medicaid Services (CMS) issues a memorandum to Medicare contractors, effectively delaying implementation of therapy caps.
February 2003	CMS issues program memorandum officially delaying implementation of therapy caps until July 1, 2003.
June 2003	Medicare Rights Centers, American Parkinson Disease Association, and Easter Seals bring lawsuit against Secretary of U.S. Department of Health and Human Services in District Court arguing that CMS had not given Medicare beneficiaries proper notice of new caps, and seek a temporary restraining order preventing enforcement of caps.

(*Continues*)

(*Continued*)	
June 2003	CMS enters into a settlement agreement with the plaintiffs that the enforcement of the caps would be delayed for 60 days.
September 2003	CMS begins enforcement of therapy caps.
September 2003	Plaintiffs in lawsuit file motion to enforce partial settlement agreement and to extend moratorium.
September 2003	Federal District Court judge rules that CMS could enforce caps.
December 2003	Medicare Prescription Drug, Improvement, and Modernization Act places moratorium on implementation of cap beginning December 8, 2003, through December 31, 2005, and requires CMS to study therapy cap utilization and alternatives.
December 2005	Congress adjourns without addressing therapy caps, allowing caps to go into effect January 1, 2006.
February 2006	Deficit Reduction Act includes provision allowing CMS to develop an exceptions process for beneficiaries needing medically necessary services above cap through December 31, 2006.
December 2006	Tax Relief and Health Care Act of 2006 extends the therapy cap exceptions process through December 31, 2007.
December 2007	Medicare, Medicaid, and SCHIP Extension Act includes six-month extension of exceptions process.
July 2008	Medicare Improvement for Patients and Providers Act of 2008 provides 18-month extension of therapy cap exceptions process through 2009.
January 2010	Lack of congressional action allows implementation of therapy caps without the exceptions process.
March 2010	Temporary Extension Act of 2010 reinstates the therapy cap exceptions process until March 31, 2010.
March 2010	Patient Protection and Affordable Care Act extends therapy cap exceptions process through December 31, 2010.
December 2011	Temporary Payroll Tax Cut Continuation Act of 2011 extends therapy exceptions process for two months, expiring on March 1, 2012.

Source: Based on information from the American Physical Therapy Association, 2011

Resource-Based Relative Value System

As part of the Omnibus Budget Reconciliation Act of 1989, CMS (then HCFA) was required to develop a physician payment schedule based on a resource-based relative value system (RBRVS) with the goal of integrating the new payment system for practitioner services by 1992. The Medicare agency used the AMA CPT codes for billing so it was logical that such a system use the procedure codes as a variable. The Medicare Physician Fee Schedule (MPFS) has set Medicare Part B prospective payment rates since 1992 for audiologists, physicians, other private practitioners, and medical clinics. Reimbursement for outpatient rehabilitation services (speech-language pathology, physical therapy, and occupational therapy) in facilities such as hospitals, skilled nursing facilities, and rehabilitation agencies was included in the MPFS in 1999. The MPFS includes both facility and nonfacility rates. CMS determined that the higher nonfacility rates apply to audiology and speech-language pathology services (as well as to physical therapy and occupational therapy) even when rendered in a facility.

In 1996, the Administrative Simplification Section of the Health Insurance Portability and Accountability Act (HIPAA) required the Department of Health and Human Services to name national standards for electronic transitions of health care information. The final rule for transactions and code sets identified the CPT codes as the national standard.

Under the Medicare fee schedule, a single fee is paid for each of the more than seven thousand services delivered by physicians, audiologists, speech-language pathologists, and other health professionals eligible to bill independently. The fee is based on a resource-based relative value scale, with each service's total relative value units (RVUs) determined according to three components of resources required to provide each service:

1. The professional component, or physician work, RVU that entails the amount of work for physicians, audiologists, speech-language pathologists, and other practitioners with work composed of time, technical skill, physical effort, stress, and judgment
2. The technical component or practice expense RVU composed of the overhead costs including clinical staff time and the prorated cost of supplies and equipment
3. The malpractice RVU representing the cost of professional liability coverage

Table 13–3 illustrates the three RBRVS components for two frequently reported services: 92507 Individual treatment of speech, language, voice, communication, and/or auditory processing disorder and 92557 Comprehensive audiometry threshold

TABLE 13–3 Selected Audiology and Speech-Language Pathology Procedures and Relative Value Units (RVUs)

CPT Code	Brief Descriptor	Professional Work RVUs	Practice Expense RVUs	Malpractice Expense RVUs	Total RVUs	2011 Medicare Fee (RVUs × Conversion Factor)
92507	SLP treatment; individual	1.30	1.05	0.07	2.42	$61.76
92557	Comprehensive audiometry	0.60	0.56	0.03	1.19	$40.43
92603	Cochlear implant follow-up exam, pt. ≥ 7 yrs. of age	2.25	1.84	0.11	4.20	$142.70
92607	Speech-generating device evaluation; first hour	1.85	3.25	0.01	5.11	$130.42
92567	Tympanometry	0.20	0.24	0.01	0.45	$15.29
92508	SLP treatment; group	0.33	0.45	0.01	0.79	$26.84

evaluation and speech recognition. To contrast the value relativity of those procedures, two more complex procedures are included: 92603 Diagnostic analysis of cochlear implant, age 7 years or older; with programming and 92607 Evaluation for prescription for speech-generating augmentative and alternative communication device, face-to-face with the patient; first hour. Two other procedures are at the low end of the scale: 92567 Tympanometry and 92508 Treatment of speech, language, voice, communication, and/or auditory processing disorder; group, 2 or more individuals. The Medicare fee is for calendar year 2011 and does not reflect a geographic adjustment. The fee is calculated by multiplying the total RVUs times the CMS-determined conversion factor. The 2011 conversion factor was $25.5217. Therefore, the Medicare fee for individual treatment of speech, language, voice, communication, and/or auditory processing disorder was 2.42 RVUs times $25.5217 = $61.76.

The Social Security Amendments of 1994 required the secretary of health and human services to revise the Medicare physician fee schedule by 1998 so that the practice expense RVUs would reflect the resources used rather than historical charges. While the revisions were required to be "budget neutral" so that total Medicare payments to physicians for practice expenses would not change, Medicare payments could increase for some procedures and decrease for others.

In 1999, one of the more dramatic changes that occurred in Medicare was the application of the MPFS to institutional providers for Part B speech-language pathology services, physical therapy services, and occupational therapy services. Previously the MPFS had been confined to billing from physician and audiologist offices or group practices.

The 2008 MPFS marked the first time that audiology professional work was recognized by Medicare in the fee schedule (White, 2007). Speech-language pathology codes included the professional work of speech-language pathologists rather than having only the speech-language pathologist's time represented in the technical component (i.e., practice expense) in the 2011 MPFS. The move for speech-language pathology work was made possible by the change in billing status for private practice speech-language pathologists. The 2011 MPFS rule included a new Multiple Procedure Payment Reduction (MPPR) policy that reduced reimbursement for multiple procedures provided to a single patient on the same day (White, 2011b).

QUALITY INITIATIVES

Omnibus Budget Reconciliation Act of 1989

OBRA 1989 established the Agency for Health Care Policy and Research, renamed the Agency for Healthcare Research and Quality (AHRQ), in 2000. It is one of eight agencies of the U.S. Public Health Service within the U.S. Department of Health and Human Services and replaced the National Center for Health Services Research and Health Care Technology Assessment. AHRQ supports studies on the outcomes of health care services and procedures used to prevent, diagnose, treat, and manage illness and disability (Agency for Healthcare Research and Quality [AHRQ], 2011a). An arm of AHRQ, the National Advisory Council for Health Care Policy, Research, and Evaluation, is charged with improving the quality, safety, efficiency, and effectiveness of health care for all Americans (AHRQ, 2011b).

The Deficit Reduction Act of 2005 (DRA)

The DRA directed CMS to develop a Post-Acute Care (PAC) payment reform demonstration project. The goal of the initiative was to standardize patient assessment information from post-acute care settings (long-term care hospitals, inpatient rehabilitation facilities, skilled nursing facilities, and home health agencies) and to use the data to guide payment policy in the Medicare program. The demonstration was to provide standardized information on patient health and functional status, independent of PAC site of care, and examine resources and outcomes associated with treatment in each type of setting. The DRA required CMS to report on this initiative to Congress in 2011.

The 2006 Tax Relief and Health Care Act (TRHCA) (PL 109-432)

This law required the establishment of a physician quality reporting system, including an incentive payment for eligible professionals who satisfactorily report data on quality measures for covered professional services furnished to Medicare beneficiaries during the second half of 2007 (the 2007 reporting period). CMS named this program the Physician Quality Reporting Initiative (PQRI), since revised to the Physician Quality Reporting System (PQRS) following the adoption of physician quality reporting.

The PQRI was further modified as a result of the Medicare, Medicaid, and SCHIP Extension Act of 2007 (MMSEA) (PL 110-275) and the Medicare Improvements for Patients and Providers Act of 2008 (MIPPA) (PL 110-275). In 2011, the program name was changed to Physician Quality Reporting System (Physician Quality Reporting). Both speech-language pathologists and audiologists are recognized for reporting quality measures to CMS.

Eight of the adult ASHA National Outcomes Measurement System (NOMS) Functional Communication Measures (FCM) have been classified as PQRI quality measures, and NOMS is now approved by CMS as a registry through which eligible SLPs can report on these measures (ASHA, 2010b). The approved FCMs include spoken language comprehension, spoken language expression, motor speech, writing, reading, attention, memory, and swallowing.

ASHA and other members of the Audiology Quality Consortium developed quality measures for use by audiologists. These include referral for otologic evaluation for patients with congenital or traumatic deformity of the ear, referral for otologic evaluation for patients with a history of active drainage from the ear within the previous 90 days, referral or otologic evaluation for patients with a history of sudden or rapidly progressive hearing loss, and otitis media with effusion: diagnostic evaluation—assessment of tympanic membrane mobility (Oyler & Romanow, 2010).

MEDICAID

The Medicaid program was enacted in the same legislation, the Social Security Amendments of 1965, as the Medicare program. Medicaid is Title XIX of the Social Security Act and describes mandatory and optional services that states must provide in order to share in financing of this program with the federal government. The Social Security Act Amendments of 1972 added the Early and Periodic, Screening, Diagnosis, and Treatment (EPSDT) program under Medicaid. This program provides for child health screening, including hearing, speech, and language; hearing aids; augmentative and assistive communication devices; and subsequent treatment. Finally, OBRA 1989 improved the Medicaid EPSDT program so that proper treatment for communication disorders discovered during screening must be provided. Prior to the law, states avoided providing needed services such as speech-language pathology services, audiology services, and assistive technology (White, 1990). OBRA 1989 mandated coverage of all medically necessary services for children enrolled in the Medicaid program.

Medicaid also extended eligibility to include medically indigent persons not on welfare. Under this program, states are to provide at least some of each of five basic services: inpatient hospital services, outpatient hospital services, other laboratory and X-ray services, skilled nursing facility services, and physicians' services. A range of additional benefits, including audiology and speech-language pathology services and assistive technology, also can be offered as optional services by the states.

Medicaid is an entitlement program that is jointly financed by the states and the federal government. Spending levels are determined by the number of people participating in the program and services provided. Federal funding for Medicaid comes from general revenues; that is, there is no Trust Fund for Medicaid as there is for Medicare and Social Security. The federal government contributes between 50 percent and 83 percent of payments for services provided under each state program.

Mandated and optional benefits are described in Table 13–4, adapted from a policy brief by the Kaiser Commission on Medicaid and the Uninsured (2001).

Each state Medicaid program must cover mandatory services identified in the statute and has the option to cover other services. Coverage should be consistent for children because of the Early and Periodic Screening, Diagnosis, and Treatment (EPSDT) program, but statewide use of managed care organizations by some states has had a negative impact on speech-language pathology and audiology services coverage. The Medicaid optional benefit package is defined by each state based on broad federal guidelines. There is considerable variation among state programs regarding not only which services are covered but also the amount of care provided within specific service categories. Note that speech language and hearing services are mandated for children under EPSDT. SLP and audiology are optional services for adults. Table 13-4, from Kaiser Foundation, does not specifically include audiology in its list.

Schools bill Medicaid for speech-language pathology and audiology services required by the Individuals with Disabilities Education Act (IDEA) provided to children in the Medicaid program. Medicaid was authorized by

TABLE 13–4 Mandated and Optional Medicaid Benefits

"Mandatory" Items and Services	"Optional" Items and Services
Acute care	Acute care
• Physicians' services • Laboratory and X-ray services • Inpatient hospital services • Outpatient hospital services • Early and Periodic Screening, Diagnosis, and Treatment (EPSDT) services for individuals under 21 including speech-language pathology and audiology services and assistive technology • Family planning services and supplies • Federally qualified health center (FQHC) services • Rural health clinic (RHC) services • Nurse-midwife services • Certified nurse practitioner services	• Prescribed drugs • Medical care or remedial care furnished by licensed practitioners under state law • Diagnostic, screening, preventive, and rehabilitative services • Clinic services • Dental services, dentures • Physical therapy, occupational therapy, and speech-language pathology services and assistive technology for adults • Prosthetic devices, eyeglasses • TB-related services • Primary care case management services • Other specified medical and remedial care
Long-term care	Long-term care
Institutional Services • Nursing facility (NF) services for individuals 21 or over	• Intermediate care facility for individuals with mental retardation (ICF/MR) services • Inpatient and nursing facility services for individuals 65 or over in an institution for mental diseases (IMD) • Inpatient psychiatric hospital services for individuals under age 21
Home & Community-Based Services • Home health care services (for individuals entitled to nursing facility care)	• Home health care services • Case management services • Respiratory care services for ventilator-dependent individuals • Personal care services • Private duty nursing services • Hospice care • Services furnished under a PACE program • Home- and community-based (HCBS) services (under budget neutrality waiver)

Adapted from *Medicaid "Mandatory" and "Optional" Eligibility and Benefits,* Kaiser Commission on Medicaid and the Uninsured, 2001. Available from http://www.kff.org/medicaid/loader.cfm?url=/commonspot/security/getfile.cfm&PageID=13767.

Congress to reimburse for IDEA-related medically necessary services for eligible children before any IDEA funds are used as a result of the Medicare Catastrophic Coverage Act of 1988. The ASHA Schools Finance Committee has a School Funding Advocacy page on the ASHA website specific to the needs of school-based speech-language pathologists and audiologists.

PRIVATE HEALTH PLANS AND THE STATE ROLE

Speech-language pathology and audiology services have suffered from variable coverage by private health plans. Nevertheless, coverage exists and knowledge of the different kinds of private health plans is necessary for clinical practice. A good source of information that discusses the relationship of speech-language pathology and audiology coverage and health plans is the ASHA *Health Plan Coding & Claims Guide* (McCarty & White, 2010).

Managed care organizations (MCOs) dominate American health plans today. The two major types of MCOs are preferred provider organizations (PPOs) and health maintenance organizations (HMOs). According to the Kaiser Family Foundation and the Health Research & Educational Trust (2005), PPOs now account for 61 percent of employees with health insurance coverage. PPOs contract with networks of providers, predominantly hospitals and physicians, that agree to provide their services according to negotiated reduced payment rates. Most PPOs allow their members to go outside of the network but discourage this behavior with higher copayments (the enrollee's portion of the payment) and deductibles (the amount spent before the health plan pays for services).

HMOs were a force in the health care market because they allowed purchasers to receive a broad range of services, including preventive care, at reasonable premium rates in exchange for a restricted network of providers or a clinical or staff model where the enrolled goes to specific facilities for care. HMO enrollment fell from 25 percent of covered workers in 2004 to 21 percent in 2005. The remainder of employees, 15 percent, remained constant for the past year in point-of-service (POS) plans. These plans, usually an HMO hybrid, allow the enrollee to choose providers outside of the network but with strong PPO-like incentives to stay within the point-of-service plans. The advantage for providers to become a provider for an MCO is inclusion on a restricted provider network list that will improve the number of referrals to your practice.

Speech-language pathologists and audiologists face several problems when claims are submitted to health plans. Most health plans limit coverage to services for health problems related to an accident or illness. They use this limitation to deny coverage of services provided to infants and children with developmental disorders such as a developmental speech disorder. They also limit coverage to physical disorders, thus creating a problem for coverage of speech-language pathology for services rendered to an individual with a fluency disorder. ASHA developed a product to assist speech-language pathologists and their patients facing these types of denials. *Appealing Health Plan Denials* (McCarty, Thompson, & White, 2004) includes sample appeal letters and efficacy papers that assist speech-language pathologists and audiologists in overturning unfair denials. Of course, these may not be successful if the plan has clear language excluding coverage of these services, but the health plan may make an exception if the services have a clear point for termination of treatment.

Audiologists can have other concerns with health plans. Some plans deny coverage of hearing assessment services to physicians and hospitals. State speech-language-hearing associations and ASHA can assist audiologists in presenting a case to a health plan so that private practice audiologists are included in their provider networks.

Historically, states have played an important role in shaping the structure, delivery, and reimbursement of health care services. One of the ways in which states effect change derives from their ability to receive a waiver from a federally prescribed system of implementing a program. Under such a waiver, states can enact systems that are more responsive to the specific needs of their residents while maintaining compliance with the overall goals of the federal program. This action often has an impact far beyond the individual states.

States also affect the structuring and delivery of health care services and the reimbursement for those services through direct authority over a number of health care issues. Those issues include the licensing of health care professionals, health insurance regulation, public health, health care for low-income families, rate setting, and access to health care services within the state.

ADDITIONAL IMPORTANT LEGISLATION RELATED TO PRIVATE HEALTH INSURANCE PLANS

The following laws have had an impact on the private health care system and an individual's access to care.

United States Public Health Service Act (1944)

The Public Health Service Act of 1944 revised and brought together in one statute all existing legislation concerning the U.S. Public Health Service. It set forth provisions for the organization, staffing, and activities of the service. There have been many amendments to this act, including the Health Maintenance Organization Act.

The Health Maintenance Organization Act of 1973

This act amended the Public Health Service Act to provide assistance and encouragement for the establishment and expansion of HMOs. The act added a new title, XIII, Health Maintenance Organizations, to the Public Health Service Act. It required the provision of the following basic medical services for a set, periodic payment fixed under a community rating system: physician services, inpatient and outpatient services, medically necessary emergency health services, short-term outpatient evaluative and crisis intervention mental health services (not over 20 visits), medical treatment and referral for alcohol and drug abuse, laboratory and X-ray services, home health services, and preventive services. Supplemental health services were also to be made available to enrolled members who wished to contract for them. The supplemental health services were intermediate and long-term care, vision care, and dental and mental health services not included under basic services, plus provision of prescription drugs.

Numerous amendments designed to make the requirements under the act less stringent were added to the act over the years. In 1976, an additional provision in the amendments required that HMOs receiving reimbursement from Medicare or Medicaid must be federally qualified. The regulatory language resulting from these provisions also resulted in clarification for the provision of speech-language pathology and audiology services:

> Federally qualified HMOs must provide or arrange for outpatient service and inpatient hospital services (which) shall include short term rehabilitation and physical therapy, the provision of which the HMO determines can be expected to result in the significant improvement of a member's condition within a period of two months. (*Code of Federal Regulations*, Title 42, Section 110.102, 1990)

This section has reportedly had an apparently unintended effect on the length of treatment allowable for speech-language pathology services in HMOs. The regulatory language designates two months or 60 days as a *minimum* limit, at least for rehabilitation services such as speech-language pathology. However, it appears to be used by HMOs as a *maximum* limit, at least for speech-language pathology services. In a 1986 survey of HMOs (Cornett & Chabon, 1986), most reported limitations on speech-language pathology services to a maximum of two months or 60 days.

Technology-Related Assistance for Individuals with Disabilities Act of 1988

The purpose of this act is to provide financial assistance to states for developing and implementing a consumer-responsive statewide program of technology-related assistance for individuals with disabilities. Such programs must be designed, in part, to increase the availability of and funding for the provision of assistive technology devices and services. ASHA worked to include a broad definition of *assistive device* in the act (ASHA, 1990). The term refers to any item, piece of equipment, or product system—whether acquired commercially off the shelf, modified, or customized—that is used to increase, maintain, or improve functional capabilities of individuals with disabilities. The term *assistive technology service* refers to any service that directly assists an individual with a disability in the selection, acquisition, or use of an assistive technology device. It includes evaluation of needs, acquisition of devices, repairing/replacing devices, coordinating services, and training or technical assistance.

The Assistive Technology Act of 1998 reauthorizes the Technology-Related Assistance for Individuals with Disabilities Act of 1988 and includes provisions for low-interest loans for purchasing assistive technology. The 1998 law also supports a national public Internet site and provides training on the need for assistive technology and the rights of people with disabilities to such technology.

Early Hearing Detection and Intervention Act (EHDI)

EHDI grants were first authorized in the Newborn Infant Hearing Screening and Intervention Act of 1999, which was incorporated as Title VI of the Labor, HHS and Education Appropriations Act and signed into law. This law provided federal funds for state grants to develop infant hearing screening and intervention programs. The following year, Congress reauthorized these grants through the Children's Health Act of 2000 (PL 106-310) and included provisions related to early hearing screening and evaluation of all newborns, coordinated intervention, rehabilitation services, and research.

Although great strides have been made, significant work remains to ensure that newborns with hearing loss receive timely and appropriate services. About half of those referred for diagnosis are lost to the system. An estimated one-third of the babies who stay in the system do not receive diagnostic evaluations by three months of age. In addition, more than half of the infants diagnosed with hearing loss are not enrolled in early intervention programs by six months of age. EHDI was reauthorized in 2010 with the passage of the Early Hearing Detection and Intervention Act of 2010. This law calls for an increased emphasis on loss to follow up and intervention.

Health Insurance Portability and Accountability Act of 1996

When the Health Insurance Portability and Accountability Act of 1996 (PL 104-191) amended the Internal Revenue Code of 1986, it was first constructed by Congress to protect the availability of health insurance coverage for workers and their families when they moved from one employer to another. That is, the purpose was to ensure that employees' health insurance was portable, particularly if they changed jobs or a family member had a preexisting medical condition. There were, however, concerns on Capitol Hill with health care record keeping now that the country was in the cyberspace age. As a result, HIPAA has become better known by health care providers for the regulations regarding patient confidentiality and record storage and electronic transmissions of protected health information. Three major regulations have since been developed by agencies within the U.S. Department of Health and Human Services (HHS) as part of the Administrative Simplification section of HIPAA. Those rules are the electronic data interchange (EDI) rule, the privacy rule, and the security rule. Another section of HIPAA was recently released as part of the EDI rule: the National Security Identification Number.

HIPAA was implemented over a period of time. The first transaction standards for the EDI rule of HIPAA had a compliance deadline of October 16, 2002. The deadline for meeting the privacy rule was April 14, 2003, and the deadline for conforming to the security rule was April 2005.

In general, the EDI rule states that any health care provider or insurance entity that maintains or transmits "individually identifiable health information," referred to as *protected information* about a patient, is deemed a "covered entity" and is subject to HIPAA. In addition, business associates who view, manipulate, or otherwise handle this protected information on behalf of a covered entity are also subject to HIPAA. The final HIPAA privacy rule covers all individually identifiable health care information in any form, electronic or nonelectronic, that is held or transmitted by a covered entity. An entity that collects, stores, or transmits data electronically, orally, in writing, or through any form of communication, including fax, is covered under the HIPAA privacy rule. The electronic transmission of this information is governed by the HIPAA EDI format standards. Conversely, if an entity uses a paper-only format, it is not governed by the EDI rules. However, once electronic data interchange is used, there is no going back to escape HIPAA rules.

All identifiable health information generated and transmitted by those in private practice and those practicing in rehabilitation agencies, schools, nursing homes, hospitals, and other institutional settings is considered protected information. Those professionals practicing as employees of covered entities are subject to the policies and procedures of those entities, which must be in full compliance with HIPAA rules. These rules include any provider under contract with a covered entity such as a nursing home or rehabilitation facility. In this situation, the speech-language pathologist or audiologist is a business associate of the facility and is therefore subject to the business associates provisions of HIPAA.

HIPAA is clear regarding the privacy rule and the role of speech-language pathology and audiology students participating in clinical services. Students are among those who are prohibited from disclosing individually identifiable information in any form. If the provider is a covered entity, the student must be educated on and comply with the privacy and security requirements of HIPAA. University clinics are among those providers, and the best approach is to educate students regarding HIPAA before they begin their clinical practicum (White, 2002).

In contrast to the privacy rule, which applies to all forms of protected health information, the security rule applies only to electronic protected health information (EPHI). This includes information that a covered entity creates, maintains, transmits, or receives. All methods of electronic information are covered by the rule, including records on computer hard drives, servers, and CDs. However, the security rule does not mandate the use of any specific technologies.

The new National Provider Identifier (NPI) is required for use by providers that bill electronically, but any health care provider is eligible to apply and receive one (Lusis, 2005). Health plans were required to accept and use NPIs by May 23, 2007.

The security rule has three components. The first component includes the administrative safeguards that assign responsibility of training those who work in the entity about security of information within the entity and ensuring that the entity is secure. The second involves physical safeguards that relate to the actual mechanisms that protect the information. The third focuses on technical safeguards for processes that protect information such as encryption.

Penalties are to be imposed if the HHS Office of Civil Rights determines that an individual's right to privacy has been violated. EDI rule violations will be reported to the secretary of HHS. The rule provides for civil penalties of $100 per violation up to a maximum of $25,000 per year. When violations are with the intent to sell, transfer, or use individually identifiable information for commercial advantage, personal gain, or malicious harm, criminal penalties ranging from $50,000 and 1 year in prison to $250,000 and 10 years in prison may be imposed.

Patient Protection and Affordable Care Act (PPACA or Health Care Reform Act)

On March 23, 2010, President Obama signed into law HR 3590, the Patient Protection and Affordable Care Act. Several critical issues affect audiologists and speech-language pathologists. The law dramatically changed access to and the provision of health care services. These changes affect how individuals can obtain insurance, affect the cost of health care services, and allow CMS to investigate new methods by which individuals will pay for health care services. Specific to audiology and speech-language pathology, the PPACA exempts Class One devices, such as hearing aids, from the medical device tax; includes rehabilitative and habilitative services as part of the basic benefit package that insurance companies must provide; and includes nondiscrimination language that would restrict health insurance companies from discriminating with respect to participation, reimbursement, and coverage of services against any health care provider such as audiologists and speech-language pathologists acting within the scope of their state license.

Medicare The PPACA established a 15-member Independent Advisory Board that would submit legislative proposals to reduce Medicare spending if the spending exceeds an identified target growth rate. This board may not submit proposals that would ration care, increase revenues, or change benefits. The law also created an Innovation Center within CMS to test, evaluate, and expand payment models that would reduce expenditures while improving beneficiaries' quality of care.

In an effort to curb waste, fraud, and abuse in public programs, the PPACA allows CMS to conduct provider screening and creates enhanced provider oversight for initial claims of durable medical equipment suppliers. CMS also could place enrollment moratoria in areas that have been identified to have an elevated risk of fraud and would require Medicare and Medicaid providers to develop compliance programs to reduce risk.

CMS will be required to establish a national Medicare pilot program to develop and evaluate paying a bundled payment for acute, inpatient hospital services; physician services; outpatient hospital services; and post-acute care services for an episode of care that begins three days prior to a hospitalization and includes services provided for the first 30 days after release from the hospital. The goal of the pilot program is to improve quality of services while reducing spending.

Access The PPACA will require most U.S. citizens and legal residents to have health insurance. Those without coverage would be required to pay a tax penalty, phased in over the next six years; at the end of that time, the amount of the penalty will be based on cost-of-living adjustments. The law exempts individuals who can show financial hardship or religious objections (or meet other exemption criteria) from the requirement for mandated coverage.

Health coverage could be obtained by purchasing health care insurance through an individual's employer or through a state-based American Health Benefit Exchange. Individuals and families with income that is 133 to 400 percent of the federal poverty level would be eligible for tax credits. The law also creates a separate exchange through which small businesses could purchase coverage.

Large employers (those with at least 50 employees, at least one of whom is a full-time employee receiving a premium tax credit) that do not offer coverage would be fined $2,000 per full-time employee. Employers with fewer than 50 employees would be exempt from penalties. Companies with more than 200 employees would be required to enroll employees automatically in the health insurance plan they offer; employees, however, may opt out of coverage.

Eligibility Under the PPACA, Medicaid eligibility would be expanded to all individuals younger than the age of 65 whose income is up to 133 percent of the federal poverty level. Medicaid would be required to provide essential health benefits to all newly eligible adults. To finance this expansion, the federal government would provide states with 100 percent funding from 2014 through 2016. In 2017 the rate would begin to decrease progressively until it levels off at 90 percent in 2020.

Medicaid This law also expands Medicaid to all individuals under the age of 65 (children, pregnant women, parents, and adults without dependent children) with incomes up to 133 percent of poverty level. All newly eligible adults would be guaranteed a benchmark benefit package that at least provides the essential health benefits defined in the law.

Coverage The PPACA would create an essential health benefit package that provides coverage for a comprehensive list of services and requires insurance companies to cover rehabilitative and habilitative services and devices. The type and scope of services covered under the health benefit package will be determined through a federal rule-making process, with an effective coverage date of Jan. 1, 2014.

Insurance companies must provide coverage for pre-existing conditions and may not place lifetime limits or unreasonable annual limits on the amount of coverage. Preventive services, identified as either A or B by the U.S. Preventive Services Task Force, would be required to be covered. This would include newborn hearing screening. The Secretary of Health and Human Services will be required to define the benefit package and update it annually.

To allow consumers to review coverage options of various insurance companies, the ACA requires the development of an Internet site; insurance companies also would be required to use standardized language in describing benefits and coverage.

States' Roles in Provision of Health Care Reform States would be required to create health insurance exchanges and provide oversight of health plans with regard to the new insurance market regulations, consumer protections, rate reviews, solvency, reserve fund requirements, and premium taxes and to define rating areas. The new law would also require states to establish an office of health insurance consumer assistance or an ombudsman program to serve as an advocate for people with private coverage in the individual and group markets.

FUTURE OF HEALTH CARE

There has been considerable discussion and debate in Washington, DC, over the Accountable Care Act. Democrats are pleased that health care reform finally occurred and access to health care for the uninsured will improve. Conversely, Republicans are concerned about an increasing government bureaucracy and costs. In 2011, the Republican-controlled House of Representatives voted along party lines to repeal the PPACA, but the Democratic-controlled Senate blocked the repeal with its party-line vote. The PPACA remains viable, and the government agencies charged with implementing the multiple provisions of the law are proposing regulations. The first major proposal is for Accountable Care Organizations (ACOs). The Obama administration is receiving comments from the health care industry that are critical of the creation of ACOs. In other words, the administration and health care providers seem to be at opposite poles at the time this chapter was written. The provider community is saying that the proposed incentives for quality of care are not nearly what are needed to make an ACO viable. From a narrower perspective, ASHA wants to ensure that speech-language pathologists and audiologists who participate in an ACO are appropriately recognized and eligible for quality incentive payments.

States are developing health insurance exchanges as a result of the PPACA. According to Havens (2011) "an exchange is an organized marketplace for the purchase of health insurance. It may be online, accessible by phone, or a physical site where citizens can compare health insurance plans, enroll in a plan, find out about available subsidies, and obtain customer support to access health insurance solutions and fulfill regulatory requirements. The exchanges will initially be offered to individuals and small employers; after 2017, states have the option to expand operation to include larger employers." Havens recommends that speech-language pathologists and audiologists understand the selection of plans, the inclusion of benefits, and the planned growth of the exchanges in the state, and know the unique language of the exchange.

The impact of the PPACA will be felt for some time because of the dramatic attempts to reorganize the health care industry wherein providers become directly reimbursed by government and employers and the health insurance industry are not dominant players. Hope remains high that children with developmental speech and language disorders will have coverage because of the acceptance of habilitation as an essential health care benefit in private health plans.

Two articles that call speech-language pathologists to task make for good reading. The first is a thought-provoking piece by Cornett (2010) in which she points out how health care professionals need to be part of a system driven by results and focus on the treatment delivered rather than the quantity of services provided. She concluded, "Instead of distancing ourselves from other health care professionals or seeking to increase a patient's number of 'visits' with little accountability for communicative outcomes, now is the time to engage in coordination of care with other clinicians to effect change in patients' activities and participation. It is hoped that most speech-language pathologists will accept the increased scrutiny and challenges associated with health care reform and will work closely with others to achieve desired health care outcomes—our consensus goal" (p. 16).

The second article was written by the 2011 ASHA President Paul Rao (2011) who said that audiologists and speech-language pathologists need to understand the impact of the ACA on their services and prepare to take action to make the legislation work for the professions and the individuals served. He recommended that the professions "... champion the use of data to support the services ..." provided and to be "... prepared to show that speech-language pathology and audiology services make a difference" (p. 9).

ASHA heightened its attention to Medicaid in 2009 by appointing an Ad Hoc Committee on Medicaid (ASHA, 2010a). The ad hoc committee submitted a report to the ASHA Board of Directors and is implementing strategies including creating advocacy materials for speech-language pathologists and audiologists.

On another level, there is good news for those new to health care reimbursement and coverage. The ASHA Health Care Economics Committee developed narrated online basic learning modules on coding and reimbursement. They are available with two additional modules that cover related elements of advocacy prepared by the ASHA School Finance Committee and the ASHA Government Relations and Public Policy Board. The online sessions are as follows:

- Module One: Current Procedural Terminology (CPT) – Using Codes to Report Your Services
- Module Two: International Classification of Diseases, 9th Revision, Clinical Modification (ICD-9-CM) – Using Codes to Report Patient Diagnoses
- Module Three: Documentation of Speech-Language Pathology Services in Different Settings
- Module Four: Documentation of Audiology Services in Different Settings
- Module Five: Application Module for Speech-Language Pathology
- Module Six: Application Module for Audiology

Another important document, released in 2011, is the *ASHA Speech-Language Pathology Medical Review Guidelines*, developed by an ad hoc committee chaired by Becky Sutherland Cornett and composed of other speech-language pathologists who are experts in reimbursement matters.

> The purpose of the medical review guidelines for speech-language pathology is to serve as a resource for health plans to use in all facets of claims review

and policy development. The guidelines provide an overview of the profession of speech-language pathology including speech-language pathologist qualifications, standard practices, descriptions of services, documentation of services, and treatment efficacy data (ASHA, 2011).

The reader is referred to the *Medicare Handbook for Speech-Language Pathologists* (Kander, Lusis, & White, 2004b) and the *Medicare Handbook for Audiologists* (Kander, Lusis, & White, 2004a) for a complete explanation of the Medicare program as it relates to either audiology services or speech-language pathology services. The Health Care Economics and Advocacy team at the ASHA National Office can assist speech-language pathologists and audiologists in understanding and interpreting coverage under Medicare and Medicaid. The Health Care Economics and Advocacy team maintains and updates the Medicare, Medicaid, private health plan, and coding reimbursement pages on the ASHA website, and readers are advised to periodically check the site.

The ASHA Strategic Pathway to Excellence now encompasses advocacy for coverage and reimbursement of speech-language pathology services, audiology services, hearing aids, and assistive technology by private health plans. Documents have been produced to assist the requests of speech-language pathologists, audiologists, and patients that private health plans cover these essential services and products. To fulfill its Strategic Objective to increase reimbursement and funding, the Strategic Pathway established a network of ASHA members in the states who serve as leaders for local efforts. The State Advocates for Reimbursement (STAR) network has a listserv, holds periodic conference calls, and assists state associations in efforts to improve private health plan coverage (Jacobson & Thompson, 2005). An example of STAR efforts is the Florida STAR member conducting workshops across the state to enlist more state association members in advocacy (Johnson, 2004). The Strategic Objective allows ASHA to obtain actuarial data illustrating the low cost of speech-language pathology and audiology services to employers and legislators. Another Strategic Objective provides reimbursement advocacy grants such as one to collect state-based data on critical reimbursement issues (Crowe & Swanson, 2011).

SUMMARY

The health care legislation and regulations summarized in this chapter have led to the creation of a complex health care maze that is attempting to meet the needs of all Americans but with the use of myriad payment approaches. Health care reimbursement for audiology and speech-language pathology services is dependent on the variations of major payment approaches such as prospective payment and managed care. The current system imposes layers of both public and private bureaucracies and program limitations that have fed into often-arbitrary decisions about who will provide the services, to whom, and at what cost. Soon you will be competing in a new system, most definitely on the basis of the cost, quality, and availability of your services.

Thus, you must collect and use objective and convincing evidence that demonstrates that what you do makes a difference and is cost-effective and convenient. Change will always be on the horizon. Consequently, speech-language pathologists and audiologists face both obstacles and opportunities. The professions will continue to prepare for the future of health care. You are, however, well advised that the true measure of your success in a reformed health care system will be the ability to compete individually by acting collaboratively and beyond the boundaries of your own discipline.

CRITICAL THINKING

1. How does Medicare cover speech-language pathology services and audiology services in an outpatient setting versus in a hospital?
2. Why did Medicare change from a retrospective to prospective payment system?
3. Describe the chronology of legislation that affects reimbursement of speech-language pathology or audiology services.
4. How has HIPAA affected documentation of our audiology or speech-language pathology services?

5. Describe the relationship between the federal and state governments for Medicaid regulations. What credentials do speech-language pathologists and audiologists require and why? What can you do if you have coverage questions? How would you search for answers beyond the Internet?
6. Privacy and security are major concerns of health care providers and patients. What kind of regulations are in place to ensure that your records are secure and patients do not have to worry about their privacy? Invent a scenario in which a patient's privacy is compromised. What regulations would be brought into play?
7. You are about to open your private practice but want to be prepared for any eventuality related to the Patient Protection and Affordable Care Act. What kinds of issues are involved? What might your state be doing to broaden coverage for those without health insurance?
8. Describe the three components of the Medicare Physician Fee Schedule with particular emphasis on the professional component. Explain why the services you provide belong in the professional component rather than in the technical component.
9. Why should speech-language pathologists and audiologists know about coding systems even if they do not complete the billing forms? How would you keep current on changes in coding systems?
10. You have an opportunity to meet the president of the United States and tell him why speech-language, hearing, and swallowing services should be covered in health care plans. What would you say in three minutes or less?

REFERENCES

Agency for Healthcare Research and Quality. (2011a). *AHRQ at a glance*. Rockville, MD: Author. Retrieved from http://www.ahrq.gov/about/ataglance.htm

Agency for Healthcare Research and Quality. (2011b). *National Advisory Council for Healthcare Research and Quality*. Rockville, MD: Author. Retrieved from http://www.ahrq.gov/about/council.htm#top

American Medical Association. (2010). *CPT 2011*. Chicago, IL: Author.

American Physical Therapy Association. (2011, February). *History of Medicare therapy caps*. Retrieved from http://www.apta.org/FederalIssues/TherapyCap/History

American Speech-Language-Hearing Association. (1990, March). *Federal legislative issues: Current issues of interest to speech-language pathologists, audiologists, and persons with communication disorders*. (ASHA Congressional Relations Division Report). Rockville, MD: Author.

American Speech-Language-Hearing Association. (1992). Strategies for responding to the Medicare resource-based relative value scale (RBRVS). *ASHA, 34,* 63–68.

American Speech-Language-Hearing Association. (2010a, April 27). ASHA forms Medicaid committee. *The ASHA Leader*. Retrieved from http://www.asha.org/Publications/leader/2010/100427/ASHA-Forms-Medicaid-Committee.htm

American Speech-Language-Hearing Association. (2010b, May 18). NOMS approved as quality measure registry. *The ASHA Leader, 15*(6), 7.

American Speech-Language-Hearing Association. (2011). *Speech-language pathology medical review guidelines*. Rockville, MD: Author.

Brown, J. (2008, September 2). SLPs celebrate Medicare victory: Countdown begins to billing change in private practice. *The ASHA Leader, 13*(12), 1, 18–19.

Ciolek, D. E., & Hwang, W. (2004, October 25). *Final project report* (Program Safeguard Contractor [PSC], Outpatient Rehabilitation Services Payment System Evaluation). Retrieved from https://www.cms.gov/TherapyServices/downloads/projectrpt111504.pdf

Ciolek, D. E., & Hwang, W. (2010, June 4). *Short Term Alternatives for Therapy Services (STATS) task order*. Retrieved from https://www.cms.gov/TherapyServices/downloads/STATS_Short_Term_Alternatives_Report.pdf

Cornett, B. S. (2010, August 3). Health care reform and speech-language pathology practice. *The ASHA Leader, 15*(9), 14–16.

Cornett, B. S., & Chabon, S. (1986). *Speech-language pathologists: Winners or losers in the health care revolution?* Paper presented at the meeting of the American Speech-Language-Hearing Association, Detroit, MI.

Crowe, E., & Swanson, N. (2011, April 26). State associations receive advocacy grants. *The ASHA Leader, 16*(5), 28.

Havens, L. A. (2011, April 26). Preparing for health insurance exchanges. *The ASHA Leader, 16*(5), 1, 4.

Health Care Financing Administration. (1998). Medicare program: Prospective payment system and consolidated billing for skilled nursing facilities. *Federal Register, 63,* 26252–26316.

Jacobsen, C., & Thompson, M. (2005, March 1). Advocate for fair reimbursement through the STAR network. *The ASHA Leader, 10*(3), 2, 14.

Johnson, P. (2004, February 17). Developing a statewide strategy to improve reimbursement. *The ASHA Leader, 9*(3), 2.

Kaiser Commission on Medicaid and the Uninsured. (2001). *Medicaid "mandatory" and "optional" eligibility and benefits.* Retrieved from http://www.kff.org/medicaid/loader.cfm?url=/commonspot/security/getfile.cfm&PageID=13767

Kaiser Family Foundation and the Health Research & Educational Trust. (2005). *Employer health benefits: 2005 summary of findings.* Available from http://www.kff.org/

Kander, M. (2005, December 27). Bottom line: Medicare CCI edits extended to all providers. *The ASHA Leader, 10*(17), 3, 20.

Kander, M. (2008, September 23). Bottom line: Billing and coding Medicare services. *The ASHA Leader, 13*(13), 3, 8.

Kander, M. (2009, November 3). Medicare begins audits of claims. *The ASHA Leader, 14*(14), 1, 9.

Kander, M., Lusis, I., & White, S. (2004a). *Medicare handbook for audiologists.* Rockville, MD: American Speech-Language-Hearing Association.

Kander, M., Lusis, I., & White, S. (2004b). *Medicare handbook for speech-language pathologists.* Rockville, MD: American Speech-Language-Hearing Association.

Lubinski, R., & Frattali, C. (1993). Nursing home reform: The resident assessment instrument. *ASHA, 35,* 59–62.

Lusis, I. (2005). Apply for your national provider identification number. *The ASHA Leader, 10*(14), 3.

Lusis, I. (2010, January 19). Good news, bad news on Medicare: Fee cuts averted, but therapy cap exceptions process ends. *The ASHA Leader, 15*(1), 1, 8.

Lusis, I. (2012, March 13). Medicare payments, therapy caps set through 2012. *The ASHA Leader, 17,* 1.

McCarty, J., Thompson, M., & White, S. C. (2004). *Appealing health plan denials.* Rockville, MD: American Speech-Language-Hearing Association.

McCarty, J., & White, S. C. (2010). *Health plan coding & claims guide.* Rockville, MD: American Speech-Language-Hearing Association.

Medicare Payment Advisory Commission. (1998, June). *Report to the Congress for a changing Medicare program.* Washington, DC: Author.

Morris, J. N., Hawes, C., Fries, B. E., & Mor, V. (1991). *Resident assessment instrument training manual and resource guide.* Natick, MA: Eliot Press.

National Association of Rehabilitation Facilities. (1990). ProPAC examines excluded facilities. *Medical Rehabilitation Review, 7,* 1–2.

National Health Council. (1993, July). *Congress and health.* New York, NY: Author.

Office of the Federal Register. (1996). *Code of federal regulations.* Washington, DC: U.S. Government Printing Office.

Omnibus Budget and Reconciliation Act, Pub. L. No. 101-508, Section 4005(b)(1) (1990).

Oyler, A., & Romanow, K. (2010, January 19). Audiology PQRI resources available. *The ASHA Leader, 15*(1), 6.

Rao, P. R. (2011, May 17). From the president: Are you ready to shape the future of health care? *The ASHA Leader, 16*(6), 9.

Rehabilitation Agencies as Providers of Outpatient Physical Therapy and Outpatient Speech-Language Pathology Services, 42 CFR §485.703 (2009).

Romanow, K. (2008, December 16). Private practice regulations released: SLPs can take 4 steps now to enroll as Medicare providers. *The ASHA Leader, 13*(17), 3, 28.

Romanow, K. (2010, November 23). SLPs needed for study on therapy cap alternatives. *The ASHA Leader, 15*(14), 4.

Romanow, K., & McCarty, J. (2010, August 3). When health plans demand repayment. *The ASHA Leader, 15*(9), 1, 8.

Social Security Amendments of 1965, 42 U.S.C. §1818c.

Social Security Amendments of 1983, 42 U.S.C. §1395y.

Social Security Amendments of 1993, 42 U.S.C. §1395x.

Social Security Amendments of 1994, 42. U.S.C. §1395m.

White, S. C. (1989, April). Medicare and nursing home services. *ASHA, 31,* 75, 59.

White, S. C. (1990, June/July). EPSDT: A program you should know. *ASHA, 32,* 77–78.

White, S. C. (2002, July 23). HIPAA essentials: College and university clinics prepare for privacy rule. *The ASHA Leader, 7*(13), 12.

White, S. C. (2007, August 14). 2008 Medicare fee schedule proposed: Professional work values added for audiologists, and 90-day recertification for SLPs. *The ASHA Leader, 12*(10), 1–7.

White, S. C. (2009, April 14). Medicare enrollment for SLPs opens June 2. *The ASHA Leader, 14*(5), 1.

White, S. C. (2011a). Medicare fee schedule: What, why, how. *The ASHA Leader, 16*(1), 3, 29.

White, S. C. (2011b). 2011 Medicare rates, policies finalized. *The ASHA Leader, 16*(2), 3.

Wilkerson, D. L., Batavia, A. J., & DeJong, G. (1992). Use of functional status measures for payment of medical rehabilitation services. *Archives of Physical Medicine and Rehabilitation, 73,* 111–120.

Wisely, J. M. (2010, May 18). Skilled nursing facility assessment tool focuses on patient communication. *The ASHA Leader, 15*(6), 8–9.

RESOURCES

Alliance for Health Reform
http://www.allhealth.org/

American Medical Association
http://www.ama-assn.org/

American Speech-Language-Hearing Association (billing and reimbursement)
http://www.asha.org/practice/reimbursement/

ASHA Medical Review Guidelines
http://www.asha.org/uploadedFiles/SLP-Medical-Review-Guidelines.pdf

ASHA Strategic Pathway to Excellence
http://www.asha.org/about/pathway

Blue Cross and Blue Shield
http://www.bcbs.com/

Coding system table
http://www.asha.org/uploadedFiles/Health-CareCodingSystems(1).pdf

Health Affairs: The Policy Journal of the Health Sphere
http://www.healthaffairs.org/

Henry J. Kaiser Family Foundation
http://www.kff.org/

International Classification of Diseases (9th and 10th eds.)
http://www.cdc.gov/nchs/icd9.htm
http://www.cdc.gov/nchs/icd/icd10cm.htm

Medicare and Medicaid on the Centers for Medicare & Medicaid Services
http://www.cms.hhs.gov/

Medicare audiology site on the Centers for Medicare & Medicaid Services
http://www.cms.gov/PhysicianFeeSched/50_Audiology.asp

Medicare fee schedules and analyses for speech-language pathology and for audiology procedures
http://www.asha.org/practice/reimbursement/medicare/AUDMcareReimbursement.htm

Medicare National Coverage Decisions (NCDs)
http://www.cms.gov/medicare-coverage-database/overview-and-quick-search.aspx?list_type=ncd

Medicare therapy pages on the Centers for Medicare & Medicaid Services
http://www.cms.gov/Medicare/Billing/Therapy-Services/index.html?redirect=/TherapyServices/

News about private health plans from the industry's perspective
http://www.ahip.org/

Appendix 13-A

Common Health Care Acronyms and Abbreviations

PPACA: Patient Protection and Affordable Care Act of 2010. Comprehensive law that, among other health insurance reforms, extends health insurance to most of the uninsured (e.g., provides access to health insurance for those with preexisting conditions) and includes rehabilitation and habilitation as health insurance benefits. Various sections of the law have been put into effect while others will be introduced through 2015.

ACO: Accountable Care Organization. A Medicare provider type described in the Affordable Care Act. It will be a network of physician group practices or hospitals responsible for providing care to patients. An ACO agrees to manage the health care needs of a minimum of 5,000 Medicare beneficiaries for at least three years.

CMS: Centers for Medicare & Medicaid Services. The federal agency that administers the Medicare and the Medicaid programs' aspects not regulated by the states. CMS was known as the Health Care Financing Administration (HCFA) until June 14, 2001.

CORF: Comprehensive Outpatient Rehabilitation Facility. A Medicare provider type that includes coverage for a number of outpatient rehabilitation services, including speech-language pathology, occupational therapy, physical therapy, psychology, and medicine.

CPT: Common Procedural Terminology. A listing of codes and corresponding medical procedures published and maintained by the American Medical Association and used by third-party payers for establishing reimbursement rates.

HCPAC: Health Care Professionals Advisory Committee. Both the CPT Editorial Panel and the AMA/Specialty Society RVS Update Committee (RUC) include a HCPAC composed of representatives from health care professional associations other than those for physicians. The RUC HCPAC serves as a review board for reviewing survey data that will determine relative professional work values for providers such as speech-language pathologists and audiologists.

HCPCS: Healthcare Common Procedural Coding System. The federal government's listing of procedures that incorporates the CPT codes at Level I, codes for devices and durable medical equipment and some procedures used by Medicare and Medicaid not found in the CPT list at Level II.

HIPAA: Health Insurance Portability and Accountability Act. A statute that established requirements for employee mobility without loss of insurance coverage and uniform standards for patient privacy, especially via electronic communications.

HMO: Health Maintenance Organization: A prepaid health plan that includes wellness services; enrollees are required to see a closed panel of providers.

ICD-9-CM: International Classification of Diseases, Ninth Revision, Clinical Modification. A comprehensive list and corresponding codes for diseases and disorders. HCFA and other payers use these codes for identifying the need for medical procedures.

ICD-10-CM: International Classification of Diseases, Tenth Revision, Clinical Modification. The ICD-10-CM is scheduled to be required by the U.S. Department of Health and Human Services on October 1, 2013. Codes will be significantly changed, going from a numerical framework to one that is alphanumeric. For example, presbycusis is coded 388.01 in the ICD-9-CM and is H91.1 in the

ICD-10-CM. Moreover, the number of diseases and disorder codes will expand from approximately 4,000 to 68,000.

IOM: Internet-Only Manual. CMS maintains replicas of official record copies on the Internet. They include CMS program issuances, operating instructions, policies, and procedures based on statutes, regulations, guidelines, models, and directives.

MAC: Medicare Administrative Contractor. Private entities that administer the Medicare program locally to providers and beneficiaries. MACs are usually health insurance plans such as Blue Cross Blue Shield.

MedPAC: Medicare Payment Advisory Commission. A deliberative body composed of appointed experts in Medicare reimbursement and government staff that researches and advises Congress on payment policies and their effect on the budget and patient care.

MPFS: Medicare Physician Fee Schedule. The listing of reimbursement rates by procedural codes for Medicare services billed by physicians and other practitioners. The MPFS was extended to institutional providers for speech-language pathology, occupational therapy, and physical therapy services only.

NCD: National Coverage Determination. A decision by CMS that explains the type of service that is covered under the Medicare program. An NCD usually pertains to a new evaluation or treatment approach.

PPO: Preferred Provider Organization: A health plan that allows enrollees to see providers out of network but with higher cost-sharing responsibilities.

PPS: Prospective Payment System. The federal government's system for determining reimbursement rates based on previous charges and costs rather than current and individual provider charges or costs.

RBRVS: Resource-Based Relative Value Scale. The method for determining payment rates for outpatient medical procedures by comparing the value of procedures with the value of a common procedure. The RBRVS includes the professional component (physician or professional work) relative value unit (RVU), technical component (practice expense) RVU, malpractice component RVU, and total RVU. The MPFS uses the RBRVS.

RUC: AMA/Specialty Society RVS Update Committee. The RUC reviews survey data presented by specialty society representatives and recommends the professional work RVU for CPT procedures to CMS.

SNF: Skilled Nursing Facility. A Medicare-certified nursing facility that meets the conditions of participation developed by HCFA and is reimbursed by Medicare using a PPS. For example, an SNF uses a required patient health and disability screening tool (the Minimum Data Set, MDS) to determine the services required for each patient. The results of the MDS are a major factor in determining the per-diem rate that Medicare will pay.

14

Service Delivery in Health Care Settings

Alex Johnson, PhD

SCOPE OF CHAPTER

This chapter is about professional issues that impact speech-language pathologists and audiologists in health care settings. Professionals from these disciplines serve patients with a variety of health conditions, lead and teach others, promote best and evidence-based practice, advocate for patients and their discipline, and deal with a variety of unique ethical and regulatory issues. At the center of these various activities associated with service delivery in health settings is the primary responsibility of the clinician to provide excellent, safe, affordable care for the patients being served.

The first section of the chapter focuses on a summary of the various "locations" where health care is delivered: acute care, rehabilitation, specialty focused hospitals, extended settings, and outpatient settings. Because the nature of the work and its primary focus and goals change by setting, it is important for current and future practitioners to understand these differences. Much of the information provided applies to both speech-language pathologists and audiologists.

The second part of the chapter examines several complex and dynamic foci of modern health care. Interprofessionalism is an emerging topic of discussion that affects preparation of professionals and behavioral aspects of service delivery by members of various disciplines (including our own), and it competes with traditional (and simplistic) concepts of autonomy with a collective focus on best practice and patient care. Health care disparities are a special concern, well documented in the literature, and the chapter focuses on the historic and contemporary areas of practice that may ignore the needs or welfare of specific groups. Issues of patient safety, health literacy, and documentation are discussed in this section as well.

Finally, the chapter examines trends that will affect and/or drive the future of service delivery in these settings. Preparation of competent and qualified clinicians, degree status and certification programs, and the status of research are some of the topics briefly discussed with the emerging professional in mind.

The concept of evidence-based practice (EBP) is central in almost every discussion of clinical service delivery in audiology and speech-language pathology. Reviewed carefully in Chapter 29 of this text, these principles (using relevant scientific data, focusing on the wishes and needs of the patient, and aligning the data and the patient's wishes with the expertise and experience of the clinician) underlie the discussion that follows. You should assume that in every clinical situation across the health care continuum, the principles and strategies of EBP are relevant and should be applied. Using the highest level of evidence available goes far to protect patients, clinicians, and institutions from faddish or unproven approaches, while ensuring quality, patient-centric care.

HEALTH CARE SETTINGS AND KEY RESPONSIBILITIES

Settings

Speech-language pathologists and audiologists may work in a continuum of health settings. For the individual who is unfamiliar with some of the specific characteristics of each of these settings, this brief introductory description is provided. The key point for consideration is the different typology of each setting and their various purposes in the health care enterprise. A secondary point is consideration of the skill and/or knowledge set that may be most useful in that particular type of setting. It is important to note that experience in one setting may not serve as adequate preparation for another type. Clinicians who move across the continuum need significant flexibility, extensive background preparation, and essential orientation and competency in building programs to be effective and successful. To provide some perspective on the volume of work provided by speech-language pathologists in health care settings, the following data are summarized from the ASHA Health Care Survey (ASHA, 2009a): (1) approximately 36 percent of speech-language pathologists (SLPs) reported working in health care settings; (2) of this group, 24 percent worked in general, pediatric, or acute hospitals; (3) 23 percent worked in skilled nursing facilities; (4) 16 percent worked in home health settings; and (5) 29 percent worked in outpatient clinical settings.

The ASHA Membership Survey (ASHA, 2009b) provides data regarding audiology members of ASHA: (1) about 60 percent of audiologists work in health care, and of this group (2) 19 percent work in hospital settings, (3) 40 percent work in outpatient settings, and (4) 1 percent work in skilled nursing settings.

Acute care hospitals are those hospitals in which patients are admitted for care (typically short term) for an acute illness or for management of problems of such complexity that they cannot be diagnosed or treated in outpatient or other settings. Within the broad category of acute care, several additional descriptors can be helpful in appreciating various roles and differences. Some acute care hospitals provide the most advanced levels of life support, advanced procedures, and surgeries and are able to handle patients with the most complex diseases. These *tertiary care hospitals* are usually located in large metropolitan areas, may be university affiliated or have a significant physician education component, and are staffed and technologically designed to handle the most complex emergencies. These hospitals are typically large, so as to accommodate a large specialty staff of physicians. Typically, these hospitals have a staff of speech-language pathologists who are employed to handle the volume of inpatients and outpatients. When otolaryngology, neurology, or neurosurgery are key specialty components, audiologists may also be employed to provide inpatient and outpatient hearing assessment, vestibular testing, and/or intraoperative monitoring.

A second type of acute care hospital is the *more general community* or *rural hospital.* General hospitals vary in size depending on the geographic area and population served. They may emphasize some aspects of specialty care, are more likely to be staffed by primary care physicians and general surgeons, and have a number of specialists on call. The emergency departments of these hospitals are designed to manage common illnesses and traumas and are typically not organized to receive the most complex cases. A common staffing pattern for speech-language pathology in this setting would be one or two staff SLPs (more in larger institutions). If outpatient services are provided, audiologists may be on staff to provide assessment and rehabilitation services, usually on an outpatient basis.

Another example of an acute care hospital is the *long-term acute care hospital (LTACH).* These hospitals are designed to provide specialty care to patients with acute illnesses who require a longer stay (greater than 25 days) than is typical in many tertiary care hospitals with an average length of stay of 4 to 5 days. Many of these specialty hospitals focus specifically on two populations of great interest for speech-language pathologists: ventilator-dependent individuals and those who have sustained traumatic brain injury. When these are predominant patient populations, skilled SLPs are required to assist in dysphagia and communication management and rehabilitation.

Two more types of acute specialty hospital should be mentioned: *pediatric specialty hospitals* and *designated cancer hospitals.* Most pediatric specialty hospitals in the United States operate in a manner similar to the tertiary care hospitals described previously, serving acute patients with complex diseases and staffed by a variety of specialists. Pediatric hospitals also have the specific mission of being child-centric and family-centric. They are particularly attuned to the illnesses of childhood, to the stressors that are common when a child is ill, and usually have programs and staff customized to address this very important group of patients (and families). Because of the common intersection of communicative/swallowing disorders with childhood illness and disease, it is common for speech-language pathologists and audiologists to be employed as part of a large outpatient or inpatient service in this setting. A second setting, designated *cancer hospitals*, provides care to patients with focus on treatment, management, and end-of-life issues associated with cancer. The federal government has designated a number of cancer centers throughout the country, and it is common for these to be associated with other large medical institutions. In any case, SLPs in these settings are likely to be appointed in order to serve patients with head and neck cancer, brain tumors, or other cancers that affect communication or swallowing in children and adults.

Several *post-acute settings* may also employ SLPs and audiologists. These include *rehabilitation hospitals*, where patients typically have a short post-acute period of rehabilitation, as well as *skilled nursing facilities* where patients may receive less intensive rehabilitation. In each of these settings, SLPs and audiologists may be involved in assessment and treatment, although audiologists are less likely to be included while SLPs are almost always utilized in an attempt to help patients restore function. These settings can be described along the continuum of acuity, complexity of cases, and prognosis. Generally, patients admitted from the acute care setting to the rehabilitation hospital will have significant remaining complications, may have multiple problems needing skilled rehabilitative *and* medical/nursing care, and will have a prognosis that is more positive, even when it is not for full recovery.

When patients cannot tolerate the required three hours per day of rehabilitation, or if they have factors that negatively contribute to their prognosis but could still benefit from rehabilitation, they are typically admitted to a skilled nursing setting that has a rehabilitation component, including speech-language pathology services. It is rare for audiologists to have a full-time appointment in this setting, although contractual arrangements may be in place for individual patient consultation. Patients in skilled nursing settings are seen for post-acute convalescent recovery, with a plan for discharge to home or for transfer to a long-term care environment. In these settings, rehabilitation activities may be slower paced than in the rehabilitation hospital, but this is not necessarily the case and the goals of treatment, as always, are based on the patient's personal goals and capacity. A larger number of patients in these settings are likely to have dementia, and many will have dysphagia and its associated complications with nutrition and feeding.

Another location of post-acute care that is quickly growing is *home care.* Now more than at any other time clinicians are able to serve patients in their home who are more ill or who have complex illnesses. Through the use of new protocols and through advanced technology, patients are being discharged from the hospital earlier than ever. Many SLPs now work primarily in the home setting. Home care organizations may be aligned with specific hospitals or may be independent and accept referrals from many acute or rehabilitation settings. Speech-language pathologists are frequently employed by these agencies as either independent contractors or employees who provide skilled rehabilitation in the home. It is not uncommon for SLPs in this environment to also be asked to provide some routine health monitoring activities and reporting.

A final post-acute setting is that of *hospice care*. Hospice is provided for patients for whom the goals have changed to comfort rather than cure or prolong life. Most hospice care is provided in the patient's home, but approximately 20 percent is provided in inpatient settings (National Hospice and Palliative Care Organization, 2009). The role of speech-language pathologists or audiologists in hospice is limited, given that rehabilitation is not a goal. However, given that comfort and quality of life are particular foci in hospice, the SLP or audiologist has a role in ensuring that communication is maintained with family and staff via external supports and technology, that caregivers understand helpful ways to communicate with the patient, and that the eating process is comfortable and safe. Family and staff may also need education about communication and/or swallowing. Pollens (2004) provides guidance for the SLP interested in working in palliative hospice care.

The third general category of care is the *outpatient setting*. Patients may be seen as outpatients after a hospitalization if further inpatient care is not provided. Commonly, the SLP or the audiologist may see patients with clinical conditions that do not require hospitalization for evaluation and treatment. Examples include patients with a variety of conditions (e.g., dementia, head injury, voice disorders, neurodegenerative diseases). Some outpatient settings are multidisciplinary, rehabilitation-focused programs, while others have services limited to SLP or audiology. In these outpatient settings, it is possible for services to be delivered via a hospital or agency where the clinician is an employee or by a private practitioner who is self-employed.

A final point about the setting in which services are provided should be acknowledged. Regardless of the physical setting where the patient is seen, it is likely that *every* speech-language pathologist will see patients with communication or swallowing disorders that are health related. Frequently, an assumption is made that school-age children have communication disorders that are educationally relevant. In recent years, however, school-based speech-language pathologists have seen children with a variety of physical, emotional, cognitive, and other health-related conditions. Thus, all speech-language pathologists need to develop expertise in serving individuals with health-related communication disabilities, regardless of the setting of their employment.

ROUTINE CONSIDERATIONS FOR SPEECH-LANGUAGE PATHOLOGISTS AND AUDIOLOGISTS IN HEALTH CARE

Although individuals with health-related conditions that affect communication and swallowing may be seen in any of the settings in which clinicians practice, the health settings noted previously, by their nature, have a specific set of concerns that impact the way that the clinician can and should practice. This section focuses on these concerns and their effect on the nature of service delivery in the health care setting.

Health Status of the Patient

For every patient seen in a given health setting, the primary concern is the health status of the patient. When a patient comes for diagnostic services, accurate and timely diagnosis is a critical factor in managing the patient's condition. When a patient comes for speech, language, or swallowing treatment, the clinician should ensure that the patient is safe, make note of any significant changes in behavior that could have medical significance, be cognizant of the overarching medical diagnosis, and understand its implications for rehabilitation. The general medical diagnosis and prognosis are key factors in determining the purpose of the evaluation or treatment referral and contribute to the decision making about the nature of any approach to intervention that will ensue. For example, the young patient with a traumatic brain injury or post-stroke aphasia may be an excellent candidate for rigorous rehabilitation provided by the speech-language pathologist. An approach that is quite different may be appropriate for the individual with progressive deterioration in neurological function, for whom a more palliative approach to assistance may be in order. Thus, the speech-language pathologist is obligated to understand the implications of the patient's health status on communication and swallowing and to also understand the impact of that condition on the communication/swallowing prognosis and potential benefit for rehabilitation.

Safety

A second issue of great concern in all health settings today is patient safety (Institute for Health Care Improvement, 2011). The implications of disorders of speech-language or hearing on patient safety are not well documented. The effects of communication impairments and cognitive, perceptual, or sensory difficulties on compliance with medical or nursing instructions remain undocumented with specific regard to patient safety issues. A growing literature summarizes the effect of low health literacy on patient compliance with such tasks as following medication instructions or other directions from care providers (Davis, Jacklin, Sevdalis, & Vincent, 2007). A logical extension of this literacy concern suggests that the SLP or audiologist should ensure that patients understand and can participate in decision making about their own care. This is especially important in inpatient settings where the pace can be fast and a patient's misunderstanding or lack of hearing can be misinterpreted as cognitive impairment. In these situations, SLPs and audiologists should be conscious of the need for advocacy, provide assistive devices to augment communication or hearing, and advocate for these needs for patients under their care. When patients are knowledgeable about their condition and can obtain the information they need for informed decision making, they are safer. Woods (2006) cites six factors that make communication risky for patients: gender, cultural/ethnic factors, health literacy level, socioeconomic factors, time/urgency factors, and personality/behavioral factors. These categories of concern are well understood by speech-language pathologists and audiologists. Readers from our discipline would also add the impact of the communication disorder as a seventh risk factor to Woods's excellent list.

Another obvious area of safety concern for the clinician occurs when invasive services are necessary or certain patient risk factors are present. Examples of invasive procedures provided by speech-language pathologists include videostroboscopy, insertion and removal of laryngeal prostheses, and a number of swallowing procedures. Also, some speech-language pathologists are involved in intraoperative monitoring during laryngeal, otologic, or neurosurgical procedures. When involved in these types of activities, clinicians should have demonstrated competence in carrying out the task, have documented institutional authorization, and know any risks associated with the procedure. Appropriate precautions and personnel should be available in case of complications. Competency can be established in a number of ways including demonstration and observation over repeated opportunities, clinician testing and interviewing, simulation tasks, or written examinations. Approaches to clinical competency assessment are documented in a publication from ASHA titled *Verifying Competencies in Speech-Language Pathology* (American Speech-Language-Hearing Association [ASHA], 2009c). It is important that those who are engaged in high-risk professional activities (or supervising others in these tasks) have validated competence and that this is documented clearly. This protects the practitioner and the institution from unnecessary complications if an adverse situation arises. Most important, it protects the patient from incompetent or inexperienced practitioners, increasing the probability of a satisfactory clinical outcome.

Infection Control

Clinicians in all settings should be knowledgeable experts in all aspects of infection control, ensuring that they have minimized patient (or staff) risk for exposure to infection. Appropriate procedures for cleaning or disposing of equipment and supplies that have been exposed should be established and followed. All clinicians should know procedures for isolation precaution, hand hygiene, and medical waste disposal. Hospitals require employees to be knowledgeable in this area and are required to provide necessary training. Prevention of disease transmission should be a consideration with every patient and staff contact. Chapter 22 presents a more in-depth discussion of infection prevention.

Measuring Change, Progress, and Outcomes

The benefit to the patient and the family is the centerpiece of all work in communication disorders. Benefit can be measured from multiple perspectives along a continuum from short-term behavioral change to significant change in health status or quality of life. In the various health settings, early changes in communication, cognition, or swallowing can signal the very beginning of recovery. Intermediate levels of progress are seen in recovery of functional skills in listening, attention, understanding, reading and writing, and conversation. The most desired and difficult stages of communication progress are observed when patient's functional abilities are either restored or maximized so that their participation in life activities is enabled rather than disrupted by their communication or swallowing abilities. It is worth noting that rarely are these changes attained in a linear or orderly manner. Patients may show progress in one domain of communication, while experiencing little gain in another aspect. Thus, to document and measure change across the continuum of health care settings (and patient acuity), a number of different tools and approaches are needed.

Measures are critically important to everyone involved in the care process. Evidence of change and outcome is the basis for reimbursement decision making. They also provide guidance for the clinician as to whether treatment is beneficial and should be continued. Conversely, these measures provide support for the decision to stop treatment when minimal benefit is documented. Measures of change or outcome are usually based on assessments of the patient's perceived benefit, the clinician's judgment of change, or objective measures of communication performance.

Patient Self-Assessment Measures Patients are usually the best judges of the benefits of services received. Table 14–1 displays a number of tools that have been developed to help clinicians reliably quantify benefit and/or change from the patient's perspective. Most of these measures are designed to measure the patient's view of the degree of functional impairment or progress, as opposed to improving understanding of the underlying causative mechanisms. Eadie et al. (2006) provide a critical review of the psychometric adequacy of self-report mechanisms in speech-language pathology. In general, with patients who are not significantly impaired in cognition, measures of outcome and progress should include their perspective, ensuring that the clinician and patient agree on the benefit of treatment or other interventions. At times, when a patient cannot respond to the demands of the task, a family member or other caregiver may need to assist with collection of the measurements. While this approach compromises the validity of most assessment tools, it does provide a useful perspective from the view of the patient's "real world."

TABLE 14–1 Tools in Common Use to Measure a Patient's Perspective in SLP and Audiology

Jacobson et al. (1997): Voice Handicap Index
McHorney, Robins, Martin-Harris, & Rosenbeck (2006): SWAL-QOL (Swallowing Quality of Life Measure)
Newman, Weinstein, Jacobson, & Hug (1990): Hearing Handicap Inventory for Adults
Silbergleit, Schultz, Jacobson, Beardsley, & Johnson (2012): Dysphagia Handicap Index

Cengage Learning 2013

Clinician Observation and Measurement Tools Additional outcomes tools have been developed for measuring patient progress in various settings. One of the most widely used measures in rehabilitation settings is the *Functional Independence Measure* (FIM) (Keith et al., 1987). The FIM is a descriptive measure, completed by the clinician and designed to measure change in a number of areas including communication. Because the FIM provides a global measure of communication in the context of other areas of function (walking, eating, etc.), there has been interest in the development of communication-specific tools that provide a more detailed focus on a variety of components of speech-language and swallowing. One set of measures, *Functional Communication Measures* (ASHA, 2003), is now part of ASHA's National Outcomes Measurement System (NOMS). Use of these measures for communication and swallowing allows for assessment of the benefit of treatment services for a given patient, while also measuring the effectiveness of a particular program or service to a group of patients. Thus, the outcomes obtained from these analyses allow for a clinical service to be modified or improved based on results.

As part of their professional preparation, all professionals in speech-language and audiology have been exposed to dozens of specific measurement approaches for diagnosis and assessment. Many of these tools (e.g., standardized tests of language or speech, the modified barium swallow, audiometric testing, vestibular studies, orai mechanism examination, and so on) provide a valuable window to selected functions, allowing careful description of behaviors and some underlying mechanisms as well. While these tools are essential for diagnosis and assessment, they are not always the best measures for studying patient change and progress, especially when the outcomes goal is a change in function rather than specific physiologic, cognitive, or linguistic change. Thus, it is best to use measures that are valid, integrative, and include the combined perspective of the clinician and the patient to assess progress and then document it.

Documentation SLPs or audiologists should address the questions asked by the referring specialist or primary care provider. Responses to referral sources should be clear, direct, timely, and accurate. Good guidelines for report writing and consultation can be found in a number of sources; however, only a few such sources specifically focus on writing reports and notes in health settings (ASHA, 2011; Golper, 2010; Kummer, Johnson, & Zeit, 2007). Johnson and Jacobson (2007) have also written about the errors in patient care attributed to poor or incomplete documentation. Some of the errors associated with documentation are summarized in Table 14–2.

Documentation, as provided by the speech-language pathologist, serves a variety of priorities. These priorities include (1) educating and informing the referral source and other providers, (2) documenting progress toward goals and additional behavioral/clinical observations, (3) reporting on any adverse events or outcomes, and (4) ensuring that information required for compliance or reimbursement is available.

As the first priority, documentation that educates and informs the referral source and others involved in the care of the patient is a critical component of the care process for all patients. Most important, initial speech-language-swallowing consultations should address the question of the referral source. Conley, Jordan, and Ghali (2009) reported that 25 percent of referral notes do not contain a clear question, so SLPs completing initial consultations should be sure to obtain clarity before proceeding with evaluation or treatment. Numerous publications describe good report writing guidelines, and novice speech-language pathologists should review these. In health settings, especially in hospital documentation, reports may be produced using an electronic medical records system that does not allow for the type of writing recommended in common SLP texts. Regardless of the format required, notes should be concise and clear (avoiding SLP terms that the referral source might not know) and should add information that will be helpful in subsequent decision making or in patient care.

Second, when the patient is being seen for treatment beyond the initial consultation, it is important to document the goals and the response to treatment. Again,

TABLE 14–2 Errors Associated with Poor Documentation/Communication

1. Failure to report results of high-risk or invasive procedures in the chart accurately or in a timely manner
2. Failure to document detailed recommendations for communication or swallowing
3. Failure to document supervision of nonlicensed (or noncertified) personnel
4. Failure to document results from evaluations that could have diagnostic significance or could change the medical plan of care
5. Failure to document observation of changes in patient behavior that could signal altered medical or psychological status
6. Failure to document appropriate informed consent for any research activities that include the patient
7. Producing diagnostic statements or interpretations outside the scope of your practice *or* not substantiated with data or observations
8. Failure to ensure confidentiality of patient information

the approach to doing this will be setting dependent; however, the principles of the *SOAP* approach (subjective, objective, assessment, plan) are widely used in clinical SLP settings. This approach, introduced by Weed (1970), has been adapted to many clinical disciplines and is well understood within the health care enterprise. This method, used commonly in medicine, nursing, and other health fields, is one that allows for easy retrieval of relevant information, elimination of irrelevant observations, and clear statement of "next steps," an area that is frequently of great interest to those involved in managing hospital stays for patients. Table 14–3 offers some brief guidance for producing SOAP notes. Chapter 20 discusses documentation issues.

Continuing Professional Development

For the clinical practitioner in the health setting, nothing is more critical than continuous professional education and development, a concept that entails going beyond the traditional idea of continuing

TABLE 14–3 What Are SOAP Notes?

Comment Type	Description	SLP Example
Subjective	Describe patient's emotional, physical, cognitive status; include general observations about patient's mood, appearance, attitude, or conduct.	The patient was lethargic. The patient refused to cooperate with the examination.
Objective	Summarize data related to stated goals; include measurable information. Compare data from current session to previous sessions.	The patient was able to accurately repeat 20 to 30 multisyllabic words today; yesterday he was able to repeat 8 words. The patient was able to sustain vocalization for 12 secs.
Assessment	Interpret the data and observations that have been noted in the current session.	The patient's performance on the oral motor exam showed increased strength. The patient's scores on the test are supported by the increase in intelligibility noted in conversational speech.
Plan	Based on the assessment of what has occurred, describe the "next steps." Changes in goals or recommended activities, changes in therapy scheduling or frequency, and any needed referrals might be included. Also, document any recommendations for family members.	The patient should be referred for laryngological examination. The patient should be considered for discharge from treatment. The patient's family should be encouraged to converse with the patient for several sessions per day focusing on current events.

Based on information from the Center for Connected Health Policy (http://connectedhealthca.org/what-is-telehealth), 2011.

education as attendance at workshops and conferences or occasional reading. Every practitioner should devote a significant amount of time to learning new approaches, technologies, or delivery models that address the issues of cost-benefit to the patient and the system, improving safety for the patient, and enhancing quality of health and life.

Access to such professional development activities is readily available online; in some of the university-affiliated hospitals; through a number of continuing education centers and offerings; and through the American Speech-Language-Hearing Association, American Academy of Audiology, and other professional organizations.

In designing a professional development program that focuses on improving current practice, it is helpful to use a series of self-guided questions to direct selection of activities and information. Following are some questions for planning such a program in a health setting:

1. Are there skills and knowledge that need to be developed to provide services to a specific patient population in a specific setting?
2. For the patient populations that are being served:
   a. What is the core understanding of any disease processes, common symptoms and medications, typical and atypical communication, and swallowing issues needed in order to best manage this group of patients?
   b. What are the resources available to guide "best practice" in managing this group of patients?
   c. Are there special technical procedures or skills that need to be verified before serving this patient population?
   d. What are the expected effects of treatment with this patient population and the range of outcomes that have been reported in the literature?
3. For the specific health setting (e.g., nursing home, acute care, and so on):
   a. What are the service models, regulatory issues, and reimbursement constraints that impact care in this environment?
   b. What are the documentation requirements and what technical or other skills are needed to complete documentation?
   c. What are the collaborative (interprofessional) skills required to work in this setting?
   d. What are the specific desired systematic outcomes associated with this setting? (For example, in acute care, the goals may be rapid assessment, short-term consultation and intervention, and planning for transfer. In hospice care, the goals may be comfort, nutrition, reduced communication effort, and maintaining interaction with caregivers.)

Using these basic questions, a clinician can identify those particular areas of skill and knowledge needed to function as an expert in a given health setting. By identifying these areas, the clinician can then proceed to acquire the information needed through reading, formal education, mentored "hands-on" experience in the clinical setting, and workshop/conference attendance.

Supervision of Others

Speech-language pathologists and audiologists have long been involved in the supervision and mentoring of new professionals in the field. The current educational pathway typically begins in the university clinic and then extends to various practicum and internship experiences, and finally to a clinical fellowship in SLP or a "fourth-year experience" in audiology. Accrediting bodies and certification boards ensure that these clinical experiences are valid, rigorous, and comprehensive. There is a body of literature that addresses the topic of clinical supervision, focusing primarily on the student-clinical instructor/preceptor relationship. Examples of this body of knowledge come from the work of early leaders such as Jean Anderson (1988), who proposed a continuum/developmental model of supervision with an ongoing attempt to encourage independence by the "supervisee." McCrea and Brasseur (2003) continue Anderson's themes. Their work provides a rich discussion of the importance of the supervisory process to the development of professional competence in assistants, in new and advanced students, and in the early years of professional experience. In their book, McCrea and Brasseur encourage a change from the term *supervision* to *clinical education* and refer to the instructional role as *clinical educator*. Moving the focus of discussion to teaching and learning is key to the ongoing development of professionals, especially as they move to levels of advanced practice.

Regardless of the terminology, professional leaders and associations acknowledge that skills and knowledge are required to deliver education to others. In particular, the American Speech-Language-Hearing Association has produced recent consensus documents, *Knowledge and Skills for Supervisors of Speech-Language Pathology Assistants* (ASHA, 2002a) and *Clinical Supervision in Speech-Language Pathology* (ASHA, 2008). There are limited published articles or books that speak specifically to professional education in health settings for speech-language pathologists or audiologists. Guidance for education and professional development in these settings can be attained from two sets of resources. First, ASHA consensus documents (guidelines, technical reports, skills and knowledge statements) are available for a significant number of areas of practice including services to NICU patients (ASHA, 2004a); performing videofluoroscopy (ASHA 2004b); dysphagia (ASHA, 2002b); audiologic services to infants and young children (ASHA, 2006); as well as many others.

A second set of resources that may be useful to those practicing and leading in health settings can be found in literature from other disciplines such as physical therapy, medicine, nursing, and occupational therapy. Many disciplines have struggled with the same issues that have been challenging for those in communicative disorders including teaching clinical problem solving and reflection, learning clinical procedures and psychomotor skills, applying evidence-based approaches, using simulation tasks and/or simulated patient scenarios, and interdisciplinary communication. It is beyond the scope of this chapter to review this literature, but a survey of current educational approaches from a number of disciplines will be enlightening and helpful to those charged with the education of others. See Chapter 25 for a further discussion of supervision and mentoring.

Support Personnel

One area with which the discipline continues to struggle is the use of support personnel, SLP assistants (SLP-A) in the delivery of patient care. While ASHA has long had guidelines for preparation of SLP-As, there are not large numbers of individuals who are employed in this role in health care. Because speech-language pathology service (especially therapy) is often offered on an individual basis, for 60- to 90-minute sessions, over weeks or months, much of the cost of service is associated with the actual time spent with patients. SLP-As may be able to serve as important extenders of quality and quantity of service, while reducing cost. This issue remains contentious within the field. Concerns about the use of SLP-As have been raised regarding potential abuses of the role or the possibility that quality of care will be compromised. In a recent ASHA survey (2009b), approximately 39 percent of SLPs indicated that they supervised an assistant. It is likely that the ever-present discussion about reimbursement, the need to reduce costs of care, and improved efficiency will continue to drive informed discussion of the benefit of SLP-As to the forefront. See Chapter 12 for more discussion of this topic.

Quality and Compliance with Regulatory Processes

The ethical, legal, and other regulatory processes that impact service delivery in the health setting are extensive. Each of these regulations has been put into place to protect patients and institutions, to ensure that best practices are in place and are being used, and to reduce costs. Despite their respectable intent, these goals are competing and produce demands for productivity reports, paperwork, meetings, documentation, site visits by accreditation programs, and so forth. The work associated with compliance is a significant component of delivering modern health care in the United States, and those who choose to work in this setting should understand that their role includes this demanding and sometimes frustrating intrusion into clinical or research goals. Providers in hospitals, nursing homes, health care, and outpatient settings are affected by these various requirements. Administrators in these settings typically provide support for clinicians by completing required paperwork and other activities so that access to service for patients is accomplished most efficiently. ASHA (2002a) has produced a document that will be helpful to speech-language pathologists who need guidance on issues related to compliance. This document, *Knowledge and Skills in Business Practices for Speech-Language Pathologists Who are Managers and Leaders in Health Care Organizations* (ASHA, 2002a), includes many resources that are useful to those trying to understand the myriad responsibilities associated with compliance.

Chapter 13 of this book covers in detail the scope of regulatory issues that are relevant to health care practice and should be reviewed carefully by those interested in practice in the health setting.

Interprofessional Responsibilities and Competencies

Interprofessional practice and collaboration is an important new area of discussion for the discipline. Within the national health care scene, there is widespread interest in the potential impact and professional benefit of interprofessional practice on quality of care, safety, and patient satisfaction. A recent report titled *Core Competencies for Interprofessional Collaborative Practice* (Interprofessional Education Collaborative Expert Panel, 2011) outlines an important discussion from a number of health-related professional organizations representing the disciplines of osteopathic and allopathic medicine, nursing, pharmacy, dentistry, and public health. This document presents four major competency domains for interprofessional practice, including (1) values and ethics, (2) roles/responsibilities, (3) interprofessional communication, and (4) teams/teamwork. The increased prevalence of this topic in the professional literature and in the educational curricula of medical and nursing schools suggests that health professionals from a variety of disciplines, including SLP and audiology, should become familiar with the language and culture of interprofessionalism.

What are and will be the roles of those who work in the discipline of CSD around interprofessional issues? Specifically within the values domain, the role of the clinician in articulating and advocating respectfully for the communication rights and independence of all patients is a key factor. Within the domain of roles and responsibilities, helping colleagues develop a realistic, respectful, and clear picture of the role of the SLP or audiologist is critical. Similarly, SLPs and audiologists need to work diligently to ensure that their understanding of the roles and contributions of other providers is clear. The last two factors—communication and teamwork—are also of critical importance to all professionals caring for a patient. Tools and strategies for effective performance on teams are widely available. These capabilities should become part of the education and practice pattern of every SLP and audiologist who anticipates a successful career in the health care environment.

Historically, speech-language pathology and audiology associations and professionals have worked to establish autonomy in their care of patients and also to achieve recognition for their distinctive contribution to the health care field. Given the number of unique disciplines represented in the arena of health care, it is not surprising that others have challenged these attempts and that occasional turf wars have emerged across disciplines that have common interests. Despite occasional disagreements with colleagues from medical and other health disciplines, the clinical arm of speech-language pathology and audiology has flourished over the past two decades. It is common for these fields to be listed as desirable occupations with demand for speech-language pathology being projected to grow by 19 percent by 2018 and for audiology by 25 percent (Bureau of Labor Statistics, 2011). These statistical predictions for growth exceed the national averages for other occupations. Society, particularly in North America, has become familiar with the knowledge and care provided by certified and licensed speech-language pathologists and audiologists and, in turn, continues to expect expert service from these providers. The recognition and status of the professions of SLP and audiology appear to be moving in the desired direction.

The simultaneous desire for autonomy *and* interprofessional collaboration may seem incongruent. This is not the case. Autonomy in decision making about communication disorders and about training and education needed to serve patients is an essential component of good care. In the interprofessional context, the SLP or audiologist delivers the information about the patient's communication and/or swallowing to the larger discussion of the total care, medical condition, follow-up planning, social and emotional status, and desired outcomes. The assumption is that the patient and the system will be best served when all providers bring their distinctive contribution to the discussion in a respectful manner with an open mind.

Only a few studies have looked carefully at the effectiveness of interprofessional education and care on patient outcomes. In 2009, these results were reported in a Cochrane review ("Education," 2009). From a pool of 56 studies of interprofessional education/practice, the Cochrane group found only six studies that met criteria for further review. Of the six studies, the Cochrane group documented positive or mixed effects in four studies, and no impact in two of the studies.

The positive results found in these few studies were noted to be reduction of clinical errors, patient satisfaction, and development of practitioner competencies. The Cochrane group pointed out, however, that these results should be viewed as inconclusive because of the small number of studies and methodological concerns. It is important to note that the studies to date have included nurses and physicians, physical therapists, and social workers primarily. No SLPs or audiologists were included in the six studies reported in the Cochrane summary.

Because research in the area of interprofessional education and care is just emerging, the intuitive appeal of a cooperative, collaborative, evidence-based model of practice continues to be prominent in health care discussions. Important groups such as the Josiah Macy Foundation and the Robert Wood Johnson Foundation have been strategic in moving this dialogue forward by funding projects and sponsoring dialogues among leaders in education of health professionals. In 2011, the two foundations mentioned previously along with the American Board of Internal Medicine ABIM Foundation, the Health Research Services Administration, and the Interprofessional Care Collaborative (IPEC) sponsored a conference focusing on building team-based competencies for shared foundation in education and practice. It should be noted that the IPEC included representatives from the American Association of Medical Colleges, American Association of Colleges of Osteopathic Medicine, American Dental Education Association, American Association of Colleges of Pharmacy, and the Association of Schools of Public Health. While the other health professions were not included in this dialogue, the results of the deliberations are relevant to all health professionals interested in improving care and reducing costs. Basically, the resultant report summarizes the important aspects of teamwork, collaboration, communication, and respect in delivering care. Another group initiated by the American Physical Therapy Association, the Interprofessional Professionalism Measurement Group, focuses on the development of discussion around health professions and does include ASHA as one of its members. Read Chapter 11 for more information on autonomy and collaboration.

Multicultural Issues and Health Disparities

SLPs and audiologists are well aware of how diverse their patients are. Educational programs in CSD require the development of knowledge and skills around multicultural issues as they affect communication and its disorders. The values associated with respecting differences and valuing the source of these features lies at the heart of being engaged with others in the clinical environment. Thus, skilled clinicians need the interpersonal skills to approach each situation with respect and without judgment. Additionally, differences in behavior or language that are representative of a specific culture should not be treated as abnormal or disordered. Clinicians need to learn about and use appropriate tools for assessment and intervention with the question of the influence of culture as a prominent feature of their patient interactions. Chapter 24 in this text discusses the broad range of issues that come into play when we consider culture in clinical practice settings, and clinicians may find this review helpful as they consider their own background and knowledge in this area.

One area of concern to all who work in the health care environment is that of disparities in access and quality for certain populations. The Centers for Disease Control and Prevention (CDC) describes health disparities as "preventable differences in the burden of disease, injury, violence or opportunities to achieve optimal health that are experienced by socially disadvantaged populations" (Centers for Disease Control and Prevention, 2008). Populations at documented risk are those that are defined by race, ethnicity, income, disability, geographic location, or sexual orientation. Disparities are believed to result from poverty, environmental trends, educational inequalities, or inadequate access to health services. While the topic of disparities is a major area of concern, especially as the distribution of health care is redefined through health reform in the United States, there are specific concerns related to the practice of speech-language pathology or audiology in health settings that should be considered.

Health Literacy

Low health literacy, or difficulty in finding and understanding health information and services, has been documented to be a factor in patient safety and in reduced outcomes. More than 50 percent of Americans exhibit low health literacy (Kirsch, Jungeblut, Jenkins, & Kolstad, 1993). Of particular concern to SLPs and audiologists should be the ability of their patients to comply with instructions (written or spoken) and to access the health system for needed services. Every clinician should learn how to use appropriate levels of communication, always respectfully, and feedback to ensure that the patient (or caregiver) understands necessary instructions. With the use of video, technology, picture systems, and so on, there is ample opportunity to ensure this occurs. Also, when the SLP or audiologist suspects that the patient may be having difficulty accessing the broader health system due to communication disability or due to language differences, it will be useful to assist the patient to ensure that needs are met.

Focusing on an individual patient's ability to understand and comply with health information presented by others is not an area that the field has embraced in a serious manner. This is problematic, as it is likely that many of the tools and approaches used by SLPs and audiologists would be helpful in addressing the huge health literacy problem. An interesting question emerges when one asks the question: How is patients' compliance with critical instructions affected by their lack of comprehension of details provided in written or oral form by a health provider? Given that so much of health improvement requires compliance with such information, it would seem that a likely opportunity for collaboration would be between the provider, the patient, and the specialist in speech-language pathology or audiology.

Communication Disorder as a Risk Factor for Reduced Health Literacy

Many people with language or other communication disorders will have difficulties with health literacy. Beyond their ability to understand and/or comply with clinical instructions regarding self-care or prescriptions, patients with communication disorders are at additional risk. Much of the access to the health care system is driven by patients' perceived health concerns and their ability to ask for assistance. When the symptoms are not obvious, or if patients do not have a reliable caregiver (spokesperson), they may be unable to communicate concerns, particularly patients with aphasia, traumatic brain injury, deafness, or another major communicative disturbance that limits expression. Clinicians should advocate for the health needs of their patients when significant communication deficits are an issue. Studies are badly needed to document the occurrence of preventable illness, mental health problems, and the access to preventive care for those with communication disorders. This is an area where speech-language pathologists and audiologists have a significant opportunity to influence primary care for their patients. Establishing reliable, basic communication strategies and tools for communication between patient and provider, preparing patients for visits with their primary care provider or specialty physician, and following up to ensure that patients understood and can comply with directives are roles that could add value to the scope of care provided by the clinician in communicative disorders.

SOME FUTURE CONSIDERATIONS

In this last section of the chapter, we consider some issues that are just emerging or are on the horizon for the practice of SLP and audiology in health settings.

Health Reform and Cost Control

It is no secret that the portion of the federal budget used to support health care continues to expand, despite attempts to curb these ongoing increases. Regardless of the heavy burden of health care financing in the United States, performance in health outcomes is low when compared with other developed countries. The American public, government officials, and health care providers all express frustration with the cost of care and the extreme variations seen in quality. In 2010, President Barack Obama introduced the Patient Protection and Affordable Health Care Act, with the reported intent of making health care more accessible to everyone and also reducing barriers for individuals who were previously ineligible for insurance coverage (Public Law 111-148). Although no specific analysis has occurred at the time of this writing, the new law appears to offer both threat and opportunity for SLPs and audiologists in health care settings. Additionally, there are concerns for patients with communicative disorders that must be considered, although the intent of the bill is to provide better access to care.

First of all, the attempt to reach out through this bill to those who have not had access to good health care services is landmark. For the first time, most Americans have health care that is available and reasonably affordable. Also, in this new arrangement of service delivery there are prohibitions to keep insurance companies from dropping individuals for preexisting conditions and special considerations for those with disabilities and for children and young families. Young adults will now able to remain covered by their parents' insurance until age 26. Medicaid will be expanded to include all individuals under age 65 with incomes up to 133 percent of the federal poverty level, increasing the availability to many people who are currently underinsured (Kaiser Family Foundation, 2011).

PL 111-148 also expands the primary care workforce by providing loan repayment programs for nurses, physicians, and physician assistants. The bill has significant focus on prevention with particular attention to children and to senior citizens on Medicare. Additionally, there is attention to the development of new models of service to individuals on Medicare and Medicaid through a new Center for Medicare and Medicaid Innovation. Finally, the bill has provided focus on improving care for seniors, especially those at risk after they leave the hospital.

No thorough analysis of the full impact of this new law on the delivery of speech-language pathology and audiology services has been completed to date. However, given that the costs associated with full implementation are significant, it is likely that there is both opportunity and threat for the SLP and audiologist. Professionals should be concerned that there will be further "rationing" of services to reduce overall cost. There will be need for data to support the benefits of care as related to patient safety, prevention, and quality of health and life. Given the strategic emphasis in this bill on the primary care needs of the society, it should be expected that there will be some shifting of payment in the direction of primary care. Fewer funds may be available for speech, language, and hearing services, which have typically been associated with specialty care in rehabilitation, otolaryngology, neurology, and other areas of specialized medicine. Also, with a large cohort of new providers of primary care (nurse practitioners and physician assistants), SLPs and audiologists will need to dramatically increase outreach and education to generate referrals for their services.

The opportunities for individuals who provide services to patients with communication and swallowing disorders may seem less obvious as one reads the law. Helping to work with other health care providers to define communication, hearing, literacy, and swallowing as *primary care concerns* should be paramount. SLPs and audiologists would be wise to describe their work as related to return to the community, patient quality of life, and patient well-being and safety. A need also exists to document and report the relationships among literacy/communication/hearing and ultimate health outcomes.

In conclusion, at the time of this writing, it appears clinicians in the health setting face two broad challenges in light of the implications of health reform and cost containment activities that are under way in the health sector. First, providers need to help referral sources, both traditional and new, to understand the link between their concerns about patient safety and effective care with the appropriate evidence-based approach to management of communicative disorders. Second, SLPs and audiologists need to constantly address the issue of treatment efficiency, ensuring that costs are under control and that patients (and referral agencies) are receiving the most value. The long-term and specific implications of health care reform and its effect on the service delivery, education, and reimbursement in speech-language pathology and audiology remain to be seen.

Trends in Education for Health Settings

Preparation of the next generation of practitioners is always on the mind of those who teach and those who employ new graduates. Education, especially higher education, is a dynamic process that has many stakeholders—students, the public, state and national government, employers, and of course the patients who will be served. A common feature among entry-level graduate programs in the health professions is that they are heavily regulated by many different agencies. All universities participate in regional accreditation, and each of the health professions is subject to specialized accreditations that specify the content and the expected outcomes for graduates.

To address the need for rapid learning and evidence-based care in an interprofessional environment, several new educational approaches are emerging in health professions education. While not readily utilized at this time in communication sciences and disorders programs, they hold promise for providing interesting and helpful solutions to learning integrated clinical skills. Three of these approaches—dedicated education units, clinical simulation, and standardized patients—hold promise for addressing interdisciplinary educational needs, as well as core content in the discipline.

Dedicated (Collaborative) Education Units (DEU) These hospital-based units are designed with two goals in mind: excellent patient care and student-focused education. The DEU developed primarily out of the field of nursing for the purpose of changing the standard approach to nursing education. In this model, faculty members work with staff in the hospital to develop a faculty role and teaching skills. Students are assigned as teams to the unit, and opportunities for education, discussion, and reflection are included as part of the core operation of the unit (Moscato, Miller, Logsdon, Weinberg, & Chorpenning, 2007). Interprofessional practice that focuses on collaboration among nurses, physicians, and social workers in inpatient settings has also been described. While this model is yet to emerge with inclusion of health professionals from rehabilitation disciplines, discussions and planning are beginning at educational institutions and professional associations.

A significant goal of participation in the interdisciplinary DEU is the development of knowledge of and appreciation for the work of each participating discipline in addressing the patient's health concerns. Thus, speech-language pathology students could learn, in some detail, about the roles the nurse and physician play in using medicines to address issues of stabilization and recovery; could appreciate the significance of various test results; could learn from the physical therapist about safety issues in transfers and walking with patients; and could learn strategies for positioning and orientation from the occupational therapist. Evolution of this model, especially in inpatient acute care and rehabilitation settings, has the potential to change the culture of service delivery for the next generation of providers.

Clinical Simulation The use of simulation as a tool for building clinical skills and problem-solving abilities is expanding rapidly in clinical education in the health professions. Simulation allows no-risk practice in aspects of care that previously could only be experienced with live patients (Ziv, Wolpe, Small, & Glick, 2003). The literature on use of simulation for learning procedures in surgery, emergency medicine, anesthesia, and other technically demanding areas of medicine is quite extensive (Gordon, Wilkerson, Shaffer, & Armstrong, 2001). Additional applications of simulation for situations that rely heavily on problem solving, decision making, and communication across disciplines are emerging (DeVita, Schaefer, Lutz, Wang, & Dongill, 2005). Reports of the use of these multidisciplinary approaches rely on clinical scenarios to elicit complex problems that require communication among professionals, an application that will likely be developed to include speech-language pathologists in rehabilitation or pediatric settings. Simulation has been used successfully in audiology settings to teach technical audiology skills in assessment and in amplification (Zurek & Desloge, 2007). There are no reports of technically based approaches to simulation in the educational literature on speech-language pathology. This is an area that is likely to develop in response to the demand for expanded or alternative clinical practicum experience and the need for exposure to patient populations that are inaccessible.

One area of simulation that has significant promise for the health fields is virtual reality. As the technology for this approach becomes more fluid and more "real," it is likely that virtual speech clinics and virtual patients will be readily accessible. Williams (2006) reported on a prototype project in which a virtual immersion center was developed to provide interactive simulation with students or clients in a CSD program at Case Western Reserve University. In this virtual reality setting, students could interact with patients in a 3D environment, and the instructor could control responses of the patient. This example provides a model for clinical education though it may be somewhat unrealistic due to the need for a full room environment and considerable technology support. On the other hand, new technological applications for cellphones, as well as computer-based applications (i.e., "Second Life"), make virtual reality models for simulated clinical experiences, patient/clinician interactions, assessment and treatment scenarios, and interprofessional problem-solving activities a realistic goal for the educational environment.

Standardized Patients Another emerging approach to the development of patient interaction and assessment skills is via the use of standardized patients (SPs). These patients provide a special type of simulation by serving as trained actors. Their use in medicine and nursing education programs is extensive. Several reports in the literature describe the use of standardized patients in speech-language pathology. Zraick, Allen, & Johnson (2003) report on the use of SPs to teach interpersonal skills to new graduate students in SLP, and English, Naeve-Velguth, Rall, Uyehara-Isono, & Pittman (2007) describe a similar application to evaluating students' abilities in counseling the parents of newly identified deaf children. Again, the use of SPs as an innovation in education is likely to continue to develop in clinical settings.

These three emerging approaches to clinical development—dedicated interdisciplinary units, clinical simulation, and standardized patients—will need careful evaluation in the coming years. Determining the effectiveness of these approaches in preparing clinicians to face the "real world" will be essential. However, if it is demonstrated that valuable skills can be acquired efficiently and effectively with generalization to clinical practice, their use will be invaluable as a cost-effective measure for instruction. Additionally, students in early stages of education will be able to benefit from simulated real-world problem solving, integration of clinical and theoretical skills, and risk-free feedback on errors or alternative approaches. While simulated environments using technology or actors may never approach real-world clinical interactions as an effective teaching modality, they do provide a potential bridging experience that new clinicians or those learning advanced skills will find beneficial.

Degrees for the Future An additional concern for the future of the disciplines is the change in requirements for the entry level to practice. Since the mid-1990s, entry requirements for audiology have evolved from a master's degree requirement to a professional doctoral degree, the Doctor of Audiology (AuD). The profession of audiology is not alone in making these entry-level changes. The required professional degrees for other professions include the Doctor of Physical Therapy (DPT), Doctor of Psychology (PsyD), and the Doctor of Pharmacy (PharmD). These degrees are now well established for those choosing to serve as practitioners in these areas. In all of the disciplines mentioned, the PhD (rather than the practice degree) remains the entry-level degree for scientific/research work and academics. The field of advanced practice nursing, which includes the nurse practitioner role, has designated the DNP (Doctor of Nursing Practice) as a "practice doctorate" in nursing, and the profession of occupational therapy has identified an advanced model of education that terminates with the OTD. Thus, there are two major types of degree levels for practice-based professions. The predominant model, entry-level doctoral education, is required in medicine, dentistry, physical therapy, audiology, and pharmacy. The alternative, professional doctoral education after entry into the field (after basic licensure and certification requirements are established) is found in nursing and occupational therapy. It is anticipated by many that in these latter cases, "post-entry" advanced degrees will evolve to entry-level requirements, but this is speculative at this time.

In the 1960s, speech-language pathology and audiology were two of the first nonphysician health professions to require a master's degree for entry-level practice and professional certification. Two to three decades ahead of colleagues in other disciplines, communication sciences and disorders has long been a standard bearer for advancing the highest levels of education and practice. Now, with the entry level as a professional practice doctoral degree in audiology, a significant disparity exists between these two professions, which are part of the same intellectual and disciplinary heritage.

There has been considerable discussion over the years regarding the role of professional doctoral education in speech-language pathology, especially in health care settings. More than 25 years ago Aronson (1987) made a case for the "clinical PhD" as a survival mechanism for communication disorders as a health care profession. He was describing a model, similar to that seen in many clinical psychology programs, where practice is the focus. Since that time occasional references have been made to the professional doctoral model of SLP education. Lubinski (2003) asked for the profession to reconsider its position on the issue and proposes the development of innovative models for implementing professional doctoral education in SLP.

A report from an educational summit held by ASHA documents some support for a model of advanced clinical education resulting in a clinical doctoral degree. The view from this discussion was that the doctoral degree should not become the entry-level requirement. Those who resist the concept have cited practical limitations related to cost, faculty shortages, length of time, and other concerns.

There are currently two post-professional models of professional doctoral entry in the discipline. The first is at the University of Pittsburgh where an ScD is offered and Nova Southeastern University where an SLPD is the degree designator. Alternatively, the University of Washington has established a three-year master's degree with a medical speech-language pathology focus. These innovations in education for practice in medical settings may serve as the basis for further discussion within the profession (via ASHA) and also in academic circles (via the Council of Academic Programs in Communication Sciences and Disorders).

In conclusion, the emerging generation of speech-language pathologists needs to address the following questions regarding education for those who will practice speech-language pathology in health settings:

1. Is there a need for additional professional practice-based education to accommodate the rapidly expanding scope of practice?
2. Is there a need for a new entry-level degree (SLPD?) for practice in the profession (similar to audiology) or for practice in some specific settings?
3. What are the implications for the profession of SLP to be in the minority of health care fields with regard to access to advanced practice-based degrees?
4. If there is consensus on a new professional degree, should it become the entry-level standard (required for licensure and certification) or should it be a post-certification advanced practice degree?

These questions are likely to stir considerable debate about the financial and practical aspects of implementing a new educational model. Those leading the discussion need to ensure that the needs of the discipline and the patients to be served remain central to the discussion as well.

Telehealth

Telehealth is defined as: "the use of telecommunications, health information, and videoconferencing technologies to deliver medical care, health education, and public health services, by connecting multiple users in separate locations." Telehealth encompasses a broad definition of technology-enabled health care services. A 2002 ASHA survey indicated that approximately 10 percent of ASHA members were involved in telepractice (ASHA 2002c). Today, an online search provides extensive listings of therapy services and audiologic services available through a variety of online organizations, hospitals, and private companies. Anecdotal evidence reveals that telepractice can be a useful approach to service delivery, but additional study needs to occur. Published reports (Duffy, Werven & Aronson, 1997; Hill et al., 2006) document success in treatment and diagnosis of communication disorders. To date, there are no documented systematic clinical trials or comprehensive evaluations of this methodology. One could speculate that as technology becomes more familiar to the public and as the quality of the visual and auditory signal improves, the experience of the patient and the accuracy of the clinician would be enhanced.

The implications for the advanced use of portable technology in all of the health professions are significant; however, intensive rehabilitation-oriented services that need face-to-face interaction (i.e., SLP) may also show cost benefits from this technology. A recent online search yielded hundreds of sites that promote the use of this interactive technology with patients representing developmental and acquired communicative disorders. It is clear that the marketability of this technology is high and will need to be evaluated in the context of cost benefit to patients and payers.

SUMMARY

This chapter addresses current and future practice issues related to speech-language pathology and audiology in health settings. First, distinctive characteristics of the various health settings across the continuum of care were reviewed. Next, the critical issues of compliance, documentation, patient safety, and development of clinical skills were discussed as core to the role of the practicing clinician. Finally, exploration of several emerging topics including health reform, evolving professional entry models, and telehealth technologies were also considered.

The health care continuum offers a vibrant and dynamic professional setting for the skilled speech-language pathologist or audiologist. The demand for individuals to join this practice setting with a commitment to excellent patient care and innovation is evident. Advances in technology and practice offer solutions to current disparities in access and quality, as well as address the ever-present need for cost containment.

CRITICAL THINKING

1. What academic and clinical preparation is needed to work effectively as a speech-language pathologist or audiologist in health care settings? What skills are needed in the various types of health care settings?
2. What are the advantages and disadvantages of having a doctoral degree in this type of setting? What type of doctorate would be most useful to you in this setting—a PhD, EdD, SLPD, or other?
3. How can speech-language pathologists and audiologists work more collaboratively in health care settings? How does such collaboration affect our service delivery?
4. How are the current and proposed changes in health care funding likely to affect what you do as a speech-language pathologist or audiologist in a health care setting?
5. What are some nontraditional roles we might develop in health care settings? (Hint: health care literacy)
6. What can practicing speech-language pathologists or audiologists do to provide evidence-based practice data in health care settings?
7. How does technology enhance our roles in health care settings? What technological advances might help us deliver more effective diagnostic and intervention services?
8. It is said, "If you did not write it down, you did not do it." Why is documentation critical in health care centers?
9. You worked as a speech-language pathologist for seven years at a large children's hospital and are now relocating to an area where you can get a position as an SLP in a long-term care facility. Would this be an "easy" transfer of skills from one health care setting to another? How do these skills differ across these medical settings? What would you do to prepare yourself for work in the long-term care setting?

REFERENCES

American Speech-Language-Hearing Association. (2002a). *Knowledge and skills in business practices needed by speech-language pathologists in health care settings*. Available from http://www.asha.org/policy

American Speech-Language-Hearing Association. (2002b). *Knowledge and skills needed by speech-language pathologists providing services to individuals with swallowing and/or feeding disorders*. Available from http://www.asha.org/policy

American Speech-Language-Hearing Association (2002c). *Survey report use on telepractice use among audiologists and speech-language pathologists*. Available from http://www.asha.org/uploadedFiles/practice/telepractice/SurveyofTelepractice.pdf

American Speech-Language-Hearing Association. (2003). *National Outcomes Measurement System (NOMS): Adult speech-language pathology user's guide*. Rockville, MD: Author.

American Speech-Language-Hearing Association. (2004a). *Guidelines for the training, use, and supervision of speech-language pathology assistants*. Available from www.asha.org/policy

American Speech-Language-Hearing Association. (2004b). *Knowledge and skills needed by speech-language pathologists performing videofluoroscopic swallowing studies*. Available from http://www.asha.org/policy

American Speech-Language-Hearing Association. (2004c). *Knowledge and skills needed by speech-language pathologists providing services to infants and families in the NICU environment*. Available from http://www.asha.org/policy

American Speech-Language-Hearing Association. (2006). *Roles, knowledge, and skills: Audiologists providing clinical services to infants and young children birth to 5 years of age*. Available from http://www.asha.org/policy

American Speech-Language-Hearing Association (2008). *Clinical supervision in speech-language pathology*. Available from http://www.asha.org/policy

American Speech-Language-Hearing Association. (2009a). *SLP Health Care Survey 2009*. Available from http://www.asha.org/research

American Speech-Language-Hearing Association. (2009b). *2009 Membership Survey summary report: Number and type of responses*. Rockville, MD: Author.

American Speech-Language-Hearing Association. (2009c). *Verifying competencies in speech-language pathology.* Rockville, MD: Author.

American Speech-Language-Hearing Association. (2011). *Documentation in healthcare settings*. Retrieved from http://www.asha.org/SLP/healthcare/documentation/

Anderson, J. L. (1988). *The supervisory process in speech language pathology and audiology*. Austin, TX: Pro-Ed.

Aronson, A. E. (1987). The clinical PhD: Implications for the survival and liberation of communicative disorders as a health care profession. *ASHA*, *29*(11), 35–39.

Bureau of Labor Statistics, U.S. Department of Labor. (2011). *Occupational outlook handbook* (2010–11 ed.). Washington, DC: Author.

Center for Connected Health Policy. (2011). *What is telehealth*? Available from http://connected-healthca.org/what-is-telehealth

Centers for Disease Control and Prevention. (2008). *Community Health and Program Services (CHAPS): Health disparities among racial/ethnic populations*. Atlanta, GA: U.S. Department of Health and Human Services.

Conley, J., Jordan, M., & Ghali, W. A. (2009). Audit of the consultation process on general internal medicine services. *Quality and Safety in Health Care, 18*, 59–62.

Davis, R. E., Jacklin, R., Sevdalis, N., & Vincent, C. A. (2007). Patient involvement in patient safety: What factors influence patient participation and engagement? *Health Expectations, 10*, 3, 259–267.

DeVita, M. A., Schaefer, J., Lutz, J., Wang, H., & Dongill, T. (2005). Improving medical emergency team (MET) performance using a novel curriculum and a computerized human patient simulator. *Quality and Safety in Health Care, 14*, 326–331.

Duffy, J. R., Werven, G. W., & Aronson, A. E. (1997). Telemedicine and the diagnosis of speech and language disorders. *Mayo Clinic Proceedings, 12*, 1116–1122.

Eadie, T. L., Yorkston, K. M., Klasner, E. R., Dudgeon, B. J., Dietz, J. C., Baylor, C. R., et al. (2006). Measuring communicative participation: A review of self-report instruments in speech-language pathology. *American Journal of Speech-Language Pathology, 15*, 307–320.

Education: Effects on professional practice and health care outcomes (Reprint of a Cochrane review, prepared and maintained by the Cochrane Collaboration and published in the Cochrane Library 2009, issue 4).

English, K., Naeve-Velguth, S., Rall, E., Uyehara-Isono, J., & Pittman, A. (2007). Development of an instrument to evaluate audiologic counseling skills. *Journal of the American Academy of Audiology, 18*(8), 675–687.

Golper, L. (2010). *Medical speech-language pathology: A desk reference* (3rd ed.). Clifton Park, NY: Delmar Cengage Learning.

Gordon, J. A., Wilkerson, W. M., Shaffer, D. W., & Armstrong, E. G. (2001). Practicing medicine without risk: Students' and educators' responses to high-fidelity patient simulation. *Academic Medicine, 76*(5), 469–472.

Hill, A., Theodoros, D. G., Russell, T. G., Cahill, L. M., Ward, E. C., & Clark, K. M. (2006). An Internet-based telerehabilitation system for the assessment of motor speech disorders: A pilot study. *American Journal of Speech-Language Pathology, 15*, 45–56.

Institute for Healthcare Improvement. (2011). *Making care safer*. Available from http://www.healthcare.gov/center/programs/partnership/safer/transitions_.html

Interprofessional Education Collaborative Expert Panel. (2011). *Core competencies for interprofessional collaborative practice: Report of an expert panel.* Washington, DC: Interprofessional Education Collaborative.

Jacobson, B. J., Johnson, A. F., Grywalksi, C., Silbergleit, A., Jacobson, G., Benninger, M.S., et al. (1997). The Voice Handicap Index: Development and validation. *American Journal of Speech-Language Pathology, 6*(3), 66–70.

Johnson, A. F., & Jacobson, B. H. (2007). *Medical speech-language pathology: A practitioner's guide.* New York, NY: Thieme.

Kaiser Family Foundation, (2011). Focus on health reform. Retrieved from http://www.kff.org/healthreform/upload/8061.pdf

Keith, R. A., Granger, C. V., Hamilton, B. B., & Sherwin, F. S. (1987). The functional independence measure: A new tool for rehabilitation. *Advances in Clinical Rehabilitation, 1*, 6–18.

Kirsch, I. S., Jungeblut, A., Jenkins, L., & Kolstad, A. (1993). *Adult literacy in America: A first look at the results of the National Adult Literacy Survey (NALS).* Washington, DC: National Center for Education Statistics, U.S. Department of Education.

Kummer, A., Johnson, P., & Zeit, K. (2007). Clinical documentation in medical speech-language pathology. In A. Johnson & B. H. Jacobson, *Medical speech-language pathology: A practitioner's guide.* New York, NY: Thieme.

Lubinski, R. (2003). Revisiting the professional doctorate in medical speech-language pathology. *Journal of Medical Speech-Language Pathology, 8*(4), li–lxii.

McCrea, E. S., & Brasseur, J. A. (2003). The supervisory process in speech-language pathology and audiology. Boston, MA: Allyn & Bacon.

McHorney, C. M., Robins, J. A., Martin-Harris, B., & Rosenbeck, J. (2006). Clinical validity of the SWAL-QOL and SWAL-CARE outcome tools with respect to bolus flow measures. *Dysphagia, 21*, 3, 141–148.

Moscato, S. R., Miller, J., Logsdon, K., Weinberg, S., & Chorpenning, L. (2007). Dedicated education unit: An innovative clinical partner education model. *Nursing Outlook, 55*(1), 31–37.

National Hospice and Palliative Care Organization. (2009). *NHPCO facts and figures: Hospice Care in America.* Alexandria, VA: National Hospice and Palliative Care Organization.

Newman, C. W., Weinstein, B. E., Jacobson, G. P., & Hug, G. A. (1990). *Ear and Hearing, 11*(6), 395–477.

Pollens, R. (2004). Role of the speech-language pathologist in palliative care. *Journal of Palliative Medicine, 7*(5), 694–702.

Silbergleit, A., Schultz, L., Jacobson, B., Beardsley, T., & Johnson, A. (2012). The dysphagia handicap index: development and validation. *Dysphagia, 27*, 46–52.

Weed, L. L. (1970). *Medical records, medical education, and patient care: The problem-oriented record as a basic tool.* Cleveland, OH: Year Book Medical Publishers.

Williams, S. (2006). The virtual immersion center for simulation research: Interactive simulation technology for communication disorders. Proceedings from the International Society for Presence Conference, Cleveland, OH.

Woods, M. S. (2006, August). How communication complicates the safety movement. *Hospital Safety and Health Networks.*

Ziv, A., Wolpe, P. R., Small, R., & Glick, S. (2003). Simulation-based medical education: An ethical imperative. *Academic Medicine, 78*, 783–788.

Zraick, R. I., Allen, R. M., & Johnson, S. B. (2003). The use of standardized patients to teach and test interpersonal and communication skills with students in speech-language pathology. *Advances in Health Sciences Education Theory and Practice, 8*(3), 237–248.

Zurek, P. M., & Desloge, J. G. (2007). Hearing loss and prosthesis simulation in audiology. *Hearing Journal, 60*, 32–33, 36, 38.

15

Education Policy and Service Delivery

Perry Flynn, MEd
Charlette Green, MS

SCOPE OF CHAPTER

This is an exciting time to be a school-based speech-language pathologist (SLP) or audiologist. According to the American Speech-Language-Hearing Association (ASHA), the majority of its members, 53.5 percent, work in school settings (American Speech-Language-Hearing Association, 2011). The current scope of practice provides many opportunities for these professionals to influence the lives of both regular and special education students in positive ways on a daily basis. Today, opportunities exist for SLPs to work directly in regular education settings as well as in the more traditional "pullout" model. Many SLPs provide services for a wide variety of disorders in classrooms, on playgrounds, in cafeterias, and even in off-campus vocational settings. Your caseload will be diverse, including students who have phonological disorders, language disorders, learning disabilities, autism, apraxia of speech, dysphagia, hearing loss, fluency disorders, or voice disorders. As an educational audiologist, you may be doing hearing screenings, assessing students with hearing loss or auditory processing disorders, or providing collaborative services to students with cochlear implants. You may also be assessing classroom acoustics; assessing and recommending assistive technology; and counseling students, parents, and teachers. Both SLPs and audiologists will be participating in continuing education and hopefully in collecting data for evidence-based practice. Your caseloads will reflect the growing cultural, racial, and ethnic diversity of the United States.

This chapter describes the student population in the United States in grades kindergarten through 12, outlines the federal legislation that governs services to special education students, explains many of the roles and responsibilities of school-based SLPs and audiologists, and describes educational trends across the country. It is hoped that the chapter inspires you to consider the possibilities of training to become a school-based SLP or audiologist.

SETTINGS AND STUDENTS: STATISTICS

The face of education has changed tremendously since the 1999–2000 school year. According to the National Center for Education Statistics (2011b), in 2009–2010 there were 98,816 operating public elementary and secondary schools that enrolled about 49.3 million students. Regular public schools constituted 90 percent of all schools in the United States. The percentage of high-poverty schools, where more than 75 percent of the students are eligible for free or reduced-price meals, increased from 12 percent in 1999–2000 to 17 percent in 2007–2008. Many of these high-poverty schools are in urban areas, though they also exist in suburban and rural areas. During this same decade, the percentage of white students decreased from 68 to 55 percent, and in some school districts minority enrollment has become the majority. For example, in 12 states and the District of Columbia, white students are in the minority. The percentage of Hispanic students has doubled from 11 to 22 percent and has surpassed the enrollment of black students. Most Hispanic students are in urban or urban fringe areas. Twenty-one percent of public school students speak a language other than English at home. Poverty, racial diversity, and limited English proficiency coexist in many schools.

The fact that 13.4 percent of the total enrollment receives special education services is of particular concern to SLPs and audiologists. This represented more than 6.6 million students in the 2009–2010 school year (National Center for Education Statistics, 2010). In 2008–2009, the two major categories of these students were those with specific learning disabilities (38 percent) and those with speech or language impairments (22 percent). Only about 1 percent had hearing impairment. Table 15–1 lists the categories and percentages of students as part of the total school population and by percentage of special education population. Remember that students with a variety of disabilities may also have communication impairments. Interestingly, the percentage of students with autism has increased steadily from 0.1 percent in 1995–1996 to 0.7 percent in 2008–2009. Note, too, that 95 percent of the students who were served under the Individuals with Disabilities Education Act (IDEA) attended regular schools, and only about 3 percent are enrolled in separate schools for students with disabilities. Eighty-six percent of those with speech and language impairments spend most of their day in the regular classroom.

Thus, you as a school-based professional are likely to serve students from a variety of racial and ethnic backgrounds. Many of you will work with students from poverty backgrounds. You will have caseloads that reflect a wide variety of types of problems and degrees of severity. Most of your students will spend most of their day in the regular classroom. Thus, you will need specific skills in the area of cultural competence and educational curriculum to work effectively in today's schools.

LEGAL FOUNDATIONS AFFECTING SERVICES

You will work more effectively in educational settings if you understand the federal legislation that affects public education. Keep in mind that while states and local communities have the major influence on education because of the powers reserved to states, the U.S. Constitution also greatly affects what you do and with whom in the public schools. School-based SLPs and audiologists are expected to know and follow the laws and policies that govern your schools. You have a responsibility to keep current with changes in legislation at federal, state, and local levels. What you do, with whom, and your outcomes all emanate from these laws. Following is a brief discussion of major federal legislation that affects public education.

TABLE 15–1 Types and Percentages of School-Age Students with Disabilities in 2007–2008[1]

Type of Disability	Percentage of Total Enrollment	Percentage of Children with Disabilities
All disabilities	13.4	
Specific learning disabilities	5.2	39.0
Speech or language impairments	3.0	22.0
Mental retardation (intellectual disability)	1.0	7.6
Emotional disturbance	0.9	6.7
Hearing impairments	0.2	1.2
Orthopedic impairments	0.1	1.0
Other health impairments	1.3	9.7
Visual impairments	0.1	0.4
Multiple disabilities	0.3	2.1
Autism	0.6	4.5
Traumatic brain injury	0.1	0.4
Developmental delay	0.7	5.4
Deaf-blindness	#	#

[1]Data abstracted from National Center for Education Statistics. (2011a). *The Condition of Education 2011.*

#Data rounds to zero.

14th Amendment to the U.S. Constitution

Contrary to popular belief, there is no federal constitutional right to a free public education for citizens of the United States. States and local governments are responsible for establishing and financing schools, developing curricula, and determining requirements for enrollment and graduation. Each individual state can guarantee the right to a free public education through the 12th grade in its constitution. However, once a state decides to provide an education to its children, as every state has, the provision of such education must be consistent with the 14th Amendment of the U.S. Constitution. According to the Library of Congress (2010), the 14th Amendment to the Constitution was ratified on July 9, 1868, and granted citizenship to all naturally born or naturalized U.S. citizens and prevents states from denying any citizen "life, liberty or property, without due process of law" or to "deny to any person within its jurisdiction the equal protection of the laws." The 14th Amendment guarantees all citizens equal protections under the law and is often the basis for many of the federal school desegregation legal actions.

Elementary and Secondary Education Act of 1965

In 1965, the Elementary and Secondary Education Act (ESEA) (PL 89-10) was enacted to ensure high standards and accountability and to make certain that the nation's disadvantaged children in poor urban and rural areas had equal access to education. The law authorized federally funded education programs, such as Title I, for primary and secondary schools that are administered by states.

Section 504 of the Rehabilitation Act of 1973

Section 504 of the Rehabilitation Act of 1973 is a national civil rights law that prohibits discrimination against individuals with disabilities. Section 504 ensures that any student with a disability has equal access to an education. Any qualified student with a disability may receive accommodations and modifications under this law. Individuals who have a history of or who are regarded as having a physical or mental impairment that substantially limits a major life function are protected by Section 504. Section 504 uses the Americans with Disabilities Act definition for major life functions where caring for one's self, walking, seeing, hearing, speaking, breathing, working, performing manual tasks, or learning are impaired.

In the school setting, a 504 Plan guarantees that eligible students, who may not require the specially designed instruction that an Individualized Education Program (IEP) affords, will be provided accommodations or modifications to the classroom environment or curriculum. These modifications and accommodations may include a copy of teacher notes, preferential seating, a sound-field amplification system, or teacher training to mention only a few of the possibilities.

Education for All Handicapped Children Act of 1975 (Part B)

The Education for All Handicapped Children Act (EHA) (PL 94-142), a federal law enacted in 1975, was developed to eliminate any exclusion of children with disabilities from education. The Act mandates a free appropriate public school education (FAPE) for children ages 3 to 21 years with disabilities. Free appropriate public education includes special education and related services that are provided at public expense and are based on the student's IEP. Students with disabilities are to be educated in the least restrictive education environment. Parents have the right to participate in decision making regarding evaluations and placements and provide consent in the decision-making process. The law has been amended and reauthorized periodically and is now known as the Individuals with Disabilities Education Act (IDEA).

Education for All Handicapped Children Act of 1986 (Part H)

PL 99-457 extended protection of the EHA to children from birth to age three. It also established early intervention programs for infants and toddlers with disabilities, ages zero to two years, and required an Individualized Family Service Plan (IFSP) for each family with an infant/toddler with disabilities.

Technology-Related Assistance for Individuals with Disabilities Act of 1988

PL 100-407 is also known as the "Tech Act" as it recognizes that students with disabilities might need assistive technology to perform better and more independently. Under the law, states could also create statewide systems of technological assistance to meet those needs. In 1990 this law was followed by PL 101-392, the Carl D. Perkins Vocational and Applied Technology Act, which focused on vocational education for students with disabilities.

Individuals with Disabilities Act of 1990 (IDEA)

PL 101-476 renamed the EHA as the Individuals with Disabilities Education Act (IDEA). The term *handicapped* was replaced with *disability*. Children ages 3 to 21 were entitled to services. Transition services were mandated for students by age 16, and children with autism and traumatic injury were included in the disability categories. Assistive technology was designated a related service in IEPs.

Americans with Disabilities Act of 1990 and Amendments of 2008

The Americans with Disabilities Act (ADA) was enacted in 1990 to protect the civil rights of individuals with disabilities. This civil rights legislation was designed to provide those with disabilities universal access to public services, employment, transportation, and government services (Americans with Disabilities Act, 1990). Also, the ADA Amendments Act of 2008 extended the definition of disabilities to include all physical or mental impairments, even when controlled by medication, treatment, or other aids (such as contact lenses). In the public schools, there could be many students who meet the eligibility for ADA protections due to a medical diagnosis (e.g., attention deficit disorder, diabetes, vision impairment) and who require accommodations without meeting the definition of a child with a disability under IDEA—even if the condition is being successfully managed by medication.

IDEA Amendments of 1997

PL 105-17 increased the rights of students with disabilities by extending the concept of least restrictive environment (LRE), ensured that students who needed assistive technology devices and services had them provided, and added orientation and mobility services as a related service for students who are visually impaired or blind.

No Child Left Behind Act of 2001

Congress amended ESEA and reauthorized it as the No Child Left Behind Act (NCLB) in 2002. NCLB significantly raised expectations for states, school districts, and schools so that all students meet or exceed state standards in reading and mathematics within 12 years. The legislation sought to ensure improved academic progress for all students, focused on prevention versus intervention, and provided a reminder that special education students are first and foremost general education students. Increased accountability accompanied NCLB by requiring highly qualified teachers in all classrooms, high academic standards, and annual academic assessments aligned with the state content standards. Each school, school district, and state is rated on how all students and students within disaggregated subgroups perform on the state assessments to determine adequate yearly progress (AYP). Test scores of students are disaggregated by racial/ethnic categories, limited English proficient, economically disadvantaged, and disability subgroups. The performance of each subgroup is compared to the state target for all students who meet or exceed proficiency in academic areas to determine how well the school, school district, and state educates its students. School districts and Title I schools that do not meet AYP for two consecutive years are placed on a Needs Improvement list and are subject to various forms of federal technical assistance, intervention, and other actions. There are consequences for each year the school or system remains on the Needs Improvement list.

Individuals with Disabilities Education Improvement Act of 2004

The Individuals with Disabilities Education Improvement Act of 2004 (still referred to as IDEA) was signed on December 3, 2004, and became PL 108-446. Within one year of the reauthorization of IDEA, each state was required to have a performance plan evaluating its implementation and describing how the state will improve such implementation. This plan is called the Part B State Performance Plan (SPP) and is required to be posted on the website for each state education agency. Each state must report annually to the U.S. Department of Education Office of Special Education and to the public on the performance of each of its school districts according to the targets in its SPP. This report is called the Part B Annual Performance Report (APR). The law also includes provisions that help align IDEA with the No Child Left Behind legislation particularly in the areas of teacher qualifications and the use of alternative assessments.

EDUCATION FUNDING

Education funding comes from federal, state, and local funds. Federal funds for education in general comprised about 3 percent of the 2011 budget in comparison with 23 percent spent on health care and 25 percent on defense (New America Foundation, 2011). Federal funds come through such programs as ESEA, Title I, IDEA Part B, Improving Teacher Quality Program, 21st Century Community Learning Centers, English Language Learners Program, and Impact Aid (U.S. Department of Education [U.S. DOE], 2005). State legislatures appropriate funds from their general fund. Local governments receive funding from state and federal funds, but the primary source of funding at this level is property taxes within local public school districts. Interestingly, while the federal government gives the least percentage to education as compared with states and localities, it makes most of the rules. For the 2008–2009 school year, about $10,441 was spent per pupil in U.S. public schools (National Center for Education Statistics, 2011b).

In 1975, Congress originally pledged to provide 40 percent of the average per pupil costs to states educating students with disabilities. The federal contribution has not exceeded 17 percent, with the exception of the additional funds from the American Recovery and Reinvestment Act (ARRA) of 2009, provided during the 2009–2010 and 2010–2011 school years (U.S. DOE, 2011). The federal funds that are provided to states, with the exception of 15 percent that can be used for early intervention services, must be used for students who meet the definition of a student with a disability and are in need of specialized instruction in order to participate and progress in the curriculum of age-level peers.

Special education is expensive, and its costs are rising faster than those of regular education because of the increasing number of students enrolled. It is estimated that the cost of educating a student in special education is about 2.08 times that of a regular student (New America Foundation, 2010). According to the New America Foundation, the United States spent $50 billion on special education "support" services and an additional $27.3 billion on regular education for disabled students ($77.3 billion in total) during the 1999–2000 school year. Much of the burden of these costs falls on local districts. In these financially difficult times, a few states are seeking permission to cut the amount of money they give school districts for special education (Samuels, 2010).

Medicaid Funding in Schools

Medicaid is a program cofunded by federal and state governments in which each state develops a plan to support the elderly, disabled, and impoverished. Currently, Medicaid allows for the reimbursement of health claims for services provided to students with disabilities in the public schools and who are eligible for Medicaid. Eligible services currently include audiology and speech-language pathology services that are identified in the student's IEP. These IEP services must meet the Medicaid criteria requirements including amount, duration, scope, comparability, medical necessity, prior authorization, and provider requirements.

ROLES AND RESPONSIBILITIES IN THE SCHOOLS

The roles and responsibilities of school-based speech-language pathologists have undergone significant changes in recent years due to a number of factors. These factors include but are not limited to mandated services in the LRE, increasing numbers of limited English proficient (LEP) students, and increased awareness of the range of knowledge and skills of SLPs. The ASHA (2010b) document *Roles and Responsibilities of Speech-Language Pathologists in Schools* states that "SLPs have integral roles in education and are essential members of school facilities" (p. 1). The following is a discussion of the range of roles and responsibilities of SLPs within the schools. Some of these areas are also pertinent to the educational audiologist.

Range of Roles

School-based SLPs work with a wide range of age levels, from preschool through young adult, including infants and toddlers in some states. Some SLPs serve just one building site, while others serve several and have to travel from site to site. They also serve children with a wide range of communication disorders, including language/literacy, articulation, fluency, voice/resonance, auditory processing disorders, hearing impairment, and swallowing. Each of these disorders may be represented on any given caseload, requiring a broad knowledge base for school-based SLPs. Many SLPs have a specialty area, such as autism spectrum disorders (ASDs) and may serve as a resource to the school district in meeting the needs of a specific population.

The clinician new to schools will quickly discover that services provided in this setting are based on educational relevance. Thus, a clinical or medical model of service is not appropriate in this setting. To be relevant, school-based SLPs need to have a thorough understanding of how treatment goals for students relate to state and local educational goals. See Core Content Standards later in this chapter.

The effective school-based SLP knows how to assist students in accessing the curriculum using specific strategies. These strategies may include integration of the student's curriculum into therapy activities, providing services in the general education setting, and collaborating with classroom teachers. It may also involve serving on curriculum teams with other school personnel, to name a few. The unique knowledge and skills of the SLP working as an effective member of a team may ultimately help all students to learn the curriculum.

Range of Responsibilities

Because school-based SLPs play a critical role in helping students meet state and district performance standards, the range of their responsibilities becomes very broad. These responsibilities may include everything from consulting on the prevention of communication disorders that negatively impact student educational performance, to designing schoolwide curriculum programs that support the needs of all students. The common thread that runs through each of these responsibilities of school-based SLPs is their role as a team member.

General education initiatives designed to support student performance, such as Response to Intervention (RTI), may involve the school-based SLP. Members of an RTI team may request the input of the SLP as they discuss expected levels of student performance related to typical development. See more about RTI later in this chapter. Or, as the need arises for further information about a particular student's performance, the SLP may need to instruct team members in principles of data collection and analysis and/or other research-based, scientifically validated instructional procedures. As members of a team, SLPs play a key role in developing and implementing strategies that are specifically designed to prevent communication disorders that negatively impact student educational performance.

Another area of responsibility for the school-based SLP involves assessment of student performance. Assessments may include both standardized and nonstandardized instruments, including "authentic assessment" of students in their natural environment. Assessments may be for the purpose of determining academic programming for a struggling student, or to determine eligibility for special education. SLPs may also assess the communication skills of teachers to design strategies for improving their own style of communication within the classroom environment.

Providing evidence-based interventions for students typically comprises the bulk of the school-based SLP's day-to-day work. Services may be provided in the traditional, more restrictive "pullout" model, in classrooms, in the lunchroom, on field trips, at off-campus employment sites, or wherever the SLP determines the students' needs will best be met. It is important to remember that it is always in the best interest of the child to provide services in as natural an environment as possible, or wherever communication would typically take place. School-based SLPs can plan appropriate intervention models if they keep in mind that "speech" is not a place where children go, but a service that is provided. Thus, educationally relevant intervention can occur wherever educationally relevant communication takes place.

School-based SLPs and educational audiologists need to familiarize themselves with federal, state, and local mandates related to compliance. These important activities include adhering to time lines for due process, including screenings, evaluations, and development of IEPs and IFSPs; following Medicaid billing procedures; and maintaining appropriate documentation of services. See Chapter 20, Documentation Issues.

Additional responsibilities of the school-based SLP may include supervising graduate students and clinical fellows, providing staff development and teacher training as well as parent education and training, conducting research, and pursuing professional development and continuing education. Working with administrative staff to ensure development and maintenance of high-quality programs at the school and district levels is also a responsibility of the SLP (ASHA, 2010a). While some may view these and other additional responsibilities as an unwanted burden, keep in mind that each of these represents an opportunity for your own professional and personal growth.

Providing services in schools offers SLPs and audiologists unique opportunities to serve a widely diverse range of children with special needs. If you choose to work in this setting, you will learn to define your roles and responsibilities in treating communication disorders related to educational performance. You will be a key player on a team within the school environment, working in partnership with educational staff and families to positively impact the lives of your students.

THE PROCESS OF WORKING IN THE SCHOOLS

As a school-based speech-language pathologist or audiologist, you will be working with students who have been identified for special education in one or more of the 13 primary areas (see Table 15–1). You may be working with some of these identified students who are in regular education classrooms and need only speech-language therapy. These students are, nonetheless, under the umbrella of special education, identified as having speech or language impairments.

These students are sometimes referred to as "speech-only" students since their only special education service is speech-language therapy. For these students, the SLP is typically the case manager.

Additionally, you may be working with those identified students for whom you are providing speech-language therapy as a related service. For instance, a child identified with autism who is in a self-contained special education classroom may be receiving both speech-language therapy and occupational therapy as related services. For such a student, the case manager would typically be the child's classroom-based special education teacher. Thus, speech-language therapy is part of special education, either as a "stand-alone" service or as a related service.

TABLE 15–2 Related Services as Defined by IDEA (2004)

1. Transportation
2. Speech-language pathology and audiology services
3. Interpreting services
4. Psychological services
5. Physical therapy
6. Occupational therapy
7. Recreation, including therapeutic recreation
8. Social work services
9. School nurse services
10. Counseling services, including rehabilitation counseling
11. Orientation and mobility services

Based on IDEA (2004).

General Education versus Special Education

General education is defined by the state's standard course of study. Special education is the adaptation of methodology, content, or delivery of instruction to address the unique needs of a child identified with a disability under state eligibility criteria. These adaptations help identified students access the general curriculum and meet the educational standards within their jurisdiction or public agency.

Identification Procedures

Students who meet the state eligibility criteria in the primary areas receive special education services and can qualify for services in any of the areas in Table 15–1. Special education students do not need to "qualify" for related services (see Table 15–2), as the provision of a related service is an IEP team decision. These data-driven decisions should be based on the student's need for the related service in order to fully benefit from (or achieve the goals in) the primary area of eligibility. Related services may flow in and out of an IEP based on the goals determined by the team for the period of time covered by the document (usually one year). A student may require a related service one year and not the next based on goals stated in the current IEP. *It is important to note that the category of speech or language impaired is the only one that can be both a primary area of special education and a related service.* Although the intent of IDEA (2004) is that goals for a student be written before services and providers are determined, in reality, providers are typically determined first and then goals are written by each provider.

Response to Instruction Intervention

The Individuals with Disabilities Education Improvement Act (IDEA) of 2004 allows for the use of "scientific, research based interventions," commonly known as "Response to Intervention" or "Response to Instruction" (RTI), as one method of identifying students for special education services. This process represents a change from the traditional discrepancy model of identification that is still used in some local educational agencies (LEAs). In the discrepancy model, cognitive scores on educational assessments are compared to achievement scores. If a large enough discrepancy (usually 15 points or more on standard scores) exists, students are placed in special education services. The decision to use this older method for identification is at the discretion of states or LEAs.

States that permit the use of RTI have set careful guidelines for its implementation. According to the National Center on Response to Intervention (National Center on Response to Intervention, 2011), "RTI integrates assessment and intervention within a multi-level prevention system to maximize student achievement and to reduce behavior problems. With RTI, schools identify students at risk for poor learning outcomes, monitor student progress, provide evidence-based interventions, and adjust the intensity and nature of those interventions depending on a student's responsiveness, and identify students with learning disabilities or other disabilities" (p. 1).

RTI has four components according to the National Center on Response to Intervention:

1. A schoolwide, multilevel instructional and behavioral system for preventing school failure
2. Screening
3. Progress monitoring
4. Data-based decision making about instruction, movement within the multilevel system, and disability identification (in accordance with state law)

School systems must consider a number of factors as they move to an RTI model. First, the school districts weigh the advantages and disadvantages of RTI over the discrepancy model. If they choose the RTI approach, the district must write guidelines, policies, and procedures that will govern the practice of RTI. In addition, the district must provide training to all educational personnel, choose universal screening tools to be administered to all students, and identify tiers of progression through the RTI process. A school-based team refers students experiencing failure, implements interventions, monitors student progress, and makes referral to special education.

Eligibility for special education or entitlement under RTI may occur in a variety of different ways. The "tiers" of RTI represent increasing levels of intensity of interventions. Tier 1 typically involves parent and teacher collaboration. Tier 2 typically begins with classroom-based interventions, perhaps with the involvement of the SLP, psychologist, or other exceptional children's teacher. At Tier 3, interventions are increased in frequency and/or intensity. In some states, Tier 3 marks the beginning of the special education process. Each progressive tier is designed to support student success in regular education and prevent entitlement for special education services unless the student is unresponsive to intervention. The following case study is an example of the progression through the tiers of the RTI evaluation system:

Tier 1: All the students in a kindergarten class are administered a universal screening instrument. The kindergarten teacher identifies a student who is well below expectations and is struggling with early literacy skills who also did poorly on universal screening tools. The student displays difficulty forming grapheme/phoneme relationships as indicated by his inability to articulate and write the letters in his name. The teacher alerts the school student assistance team composed of regular education teachers, an administrator, the SLP, and the psychologist. Following the protocol for this school, the assistance team informs the parent and asks for a meeting. The team shares its concerns with the parent and receives consent to begin interventions to support the student in learning. Because the student is minimally responsive to Tier 1 interventions that the teacher and teacher's assistant are incorporating into the classroom curriculum, the team decides to move to Tier 2.

Tier 2: The teacher again collaborates with the assistance of team members including the SLP, learning disabilities specialist, literacy facilitator, and psychologist to plan interventions to target the student's areas of need. The team plans the individualized interventions for the student, the setting (classroom, small group, or individual services in another room), the exact intervention(s), and the personnel who will deliver the intervention(s). The interventionists monitor progress frequently and report to the assistance team. Parents are informed at all stages throughout the process. While the student is making some limited progress, the team concludes that he/she is not responding adequately to Tier 2 intervention so the team decides to increase the frequency and intensity with which the interventions are provided (still at Tier 2). Again, little additional progress is demonstrated on emergent literacy skills including decoding, grapheme/phoneme relationships, and phonemic synthesis. After several weeks of intervention and progress monitoring, the assistance team with input from the parents decides to make a referral to special education.

Tier 3: Data collected from the RTI process in conjunction with psycho-educational testing suggest that the student meets the eligibility criteria for placement in special education. IDEA procedural paperwork and an IEP are initiated, and the student is subsequently placed in special education.

Movement through the tiers of RTI may be both forward and backward depending on the level of support the student requires to be successful. RTI is a promising approach to support learning without identifying students for special education unless their areas of need cannot be met in regular education.

Referral

The referral process to special education serves as the bridge between regular education and special education. After data are gathered through the RTI or a problem-solving process, referral is made to special education if the student has been sufficiently unresponsive to interventions. Although this sequence of events is the typical process, an expedited referral may be appropriate if the student clearly exhibits a disability that interventions in regular education will not change (e.g., blindness, autism). Parents or any member of the school faculty and staff may make a written referral. Whenever a written referral is received by any member of the school staff, a referral team meeting is to be convened in a timely manner. This team is typically composed of the parent, exceptional child's teacher, and/or SLP if speech or language is a concern, a representative of the LEA, and other appropriate school staff. The purpose of this meeting is first to decide if the referral is appropriate and second to determine the evaluation measures that will be used to determine whether the student exhibits a disability warranting placement in special education. Examples of referrals that may be rejected by the team include students who exhibit developmentally appropriate articulation errors or language and reading difficulties that can be managed in regular education. If the referral is appropriate, the team reaches consensus on the evaluation measures that will be used to assess the student, and the procedural safeguards inherent within IDEA commence. According to IDEA, the referral process and eligibility determination must be completed within 60 days unless the state determined a different time line before the federal legislation took effect.

Evaluation and Initial Eligibility

Prior to providing special education and related services to a child with a disability under IDEA, a full and individual initial evaluation must be conducted. The initial evaluation must be conducted within 60 days of receiving parental consent unless the state has a shorter time line (IDEA, 2004). Further, the evaluation must assess all suspected areas of disability and, if necessary, include a description of any nonstandard administration of assessment measures. All evaluations must be conducted in the student's native language or other mode of communication (unless not feasible), free from discrimination and bias, valid, and administered by trained professionals. For limited English proficient (LEP) students, materials should assess disability and special education needs and not English language skills. The evaluation must also include a variety of assessments that are tailored to assess specific areas of educational needs of the student. An assessment is a controlled opportunity to observe and interpret behavior. Assessments are used to gather relevant functional and developmental information, "including information provided by the parent, and information related to enabling the child to be involved in and progress in the general curriculum". The results of the assessment must provide relevant data that directly assists the IEP team in determining the educational needs of the child (IDEA, 2004).

IDEA requires an investigation of the whole child when determining eligibility for special education. This assessment includes more than the results of standardized tests. No single procedure or tool should be the sole eligibility criterion. The team uses the results of the evaluation to write the IEP. Assessments that rely solely on standardized scores are merely a "snapshot" in time—a one-dimensional view of the student over a brief period of time. In the one-dimensional type of evaluation, the assessment is conducted in a separate environment, often the "speech room" with assessors the student has never met, using materials or questions that are unfamiliar to the student.

A comprehensive evaluation includes both qualitative and quantitative data composed of standardized and nonstandard assessments as well as opportunities to observe the student in multiple educational environments. Multiple observers view the student in different settings, focusing on how the impairment may be negatively affecting the student's educational performance. This observational information is required to determine the adverse effect of the impairment on the child's curriculum and is required for initial evaluations. After the evaluation is complete, a team, including the parent, meets to review the results and, using state eligibility criteria, determines whether the student is a child with a disability. This team also decides which category or categories of disability best describe the student's disability. The determination that a child is eligible for special education must be made on an individual basis by the group responsible within the child's school system for making those determinations. If a determination is made that a child has a disability and needs special education and related services, the team develops an IEP.

According to IDEA (2004), speech or language impairment includes communication disorders such as stuttering and impaired articulation, language, or voice that adversely affect a child's educational performance. In a letter to ASHA in 1980, the U.S. Department of Health, Education, and Welfare stated that "meaningful educational performance cannot be limited to showing signs of discrepancies in age/grade performance" (U.S. Department of Health, Education, and Welfare, 1980). In the letter of guidance, requested by ASHA in 2009, the U.S. DOE Office of Special Education Programs affirmed that the 1980 policy on "adverse effect" was still in effect. Further "a child's educational performance must be determined on an individual basis and should include nonacademic as well as academic areas" (U.S. DOE, 2007). The term *adverse effect* is intended to encompass both academic achievement and functional performance.

Individualized Education Programs (IEPs)

The IEP is the blueprint for services SLPs provide students with disabilities and is written to meet the unique needs of each individual child. Every eligible student with a disability must have an IEP in place that is reviewed annually. The IEP is a written statement for each child with a disability that is developed, reviewed, and revised in a meeting that must include the parents of the child; at least one regular education teacher of the child (if the child is, or may be, participating in the regular education environment); at least one special education teacher of the child, or one special education provider of the child; and a representative of the school district who is qualified to provide or supervise the provision of instruction specially designed to meet the unique needs of children with disabilities and is knowledgeable about the general education curriculum and the availability of resources of the public agency. Other required attendees may include an individual who can interpret the instructional implications of evaluation results; other individuals who have knowledge or special expertise regarding the child, including related services personnel as appropriate and at the discretion of the parent or the agency; and whenever appropriate, the child with a disability. Members of the IEP team can serve dual roles. For example, the speech-language pathologist may serve as the special education provider *and* the individual who can interpret the instructional implications of evaluation results.

The purposes of the IEP meeting are to consider the eligible child's strengths and areas of academic, developmental, and functional needs; concerns of the parents; and results of the initial or most recent evaluation and to develop a plan for educating the student. Special factors that the team must also consider include behavioral factors; the language needs of the child with limited English proficiency; whether a child who is blind or visually impaired requires instruction in Braille; communication needs of the child, including opportunities for direct instruction in the child's language and communication mode; hearing impairments; and whether the child needs assistive technology devices and services. The education plan must include measurable goals and accommodations that will allow students to access their curriculum.

Service Delivery Options

Currently a variety of service delivery models are available in school practice. The wide range of service delivery possibilities is one of the many aspects of school-based speech-language pathology and audiology that professionals find appealing in this practice setting.

Curriculum-Relevant Services IDEA intends that all special education be connected to the curriculum. Most states have adopted the Core Content Standards (Common Core State Standards Initiative, 2010) as their curriculum. For SLPs, the intent of IDEA means that all services should be connected to the educational standards of the state. Teachers are the curriculum experts for their grade level. In whatever location students are served, SLPs should be communicating with teachers to connect special education services to the educational standards and classroom instruction. Even when SLPs are pulling students out of classrooms to provide therapy, they often borrow curriculum materials and lessons from teachers to connect the differentiated instruction that is special education to what is being taught in the classroom.

Pullout Services

SLPs can serve students by pulling them out of class to a separate special education environment, which is typically the "speech room." This is a more restrictive environment than the classroom, but it affords the opportunity for drill and practice on concepts one-on-one or in a small group. This service delivery model may represent the least restrictive learning environment for some children as they may require a quieter, more focused setting for optimal learning. SLPs should as much as possible tie pullout services to the curriculum by using concepts or materials that may be provided by classroom teachers. These services are tied to the educational standards that are covered in the classroom. Students often miss classroom content when they are pulled to these sessions. In many cases, these services should continue for a finite period of time before students receive their special education in the less restrictive environment of the classroom or some other educationally relevant location on or off the school campus.

Inclusion/Classroom-Based Services

SLPs may provide services to regular education or self-contained special education students within their classrooms, sometimes referred to as a "push-in" or collaborative model. This often represents a less restrictive environment for many students. Students can also be served at other locations on the school campus including the cafeteria, playground, or gym. Some SLPs serve students off campus at community-based vocational settings. This model often requires planning time with other professionals to best target special education goals embedded in curriculum or classroom-based routines.

Consultative/Collaborative Services

Consultative/collaborative services are those provided on behalf of students and are provided without the student present. They are in collaboration with teachers, assistants, parents, other school personnel, or even other students. This type of service supports the learning environment for a student and may take the form of programming augmented communication devices, teaching other students how to appropriately interact with an augmented communication system user, teaching an assistant a therapy technique, or talking with a teacher to engineer a communication-rich classroom. These activities represent only a few of the possible consultative services that an SLP may provide.

Reevaluation and Continued Eligibility

According to IDEA, children with a disability must have their eligibility considered *at least* every three years to determine whether they continue to have such a disability and to assess their educational needs (IDEA, 2004). If an IEP is in place for a student, the team must review at least every three years existing evaluation data including current classroom-based observations and input from parents and teachers to determine whether additional assessments are required to document the disability. Parental consent is required for any additional assessments that are requested by the IEP team for the purpose of eligibility determination.

Transition Services

IDEA 2004 mandates that transition services be considered for students 16 years and older. The IEP team considers what special education students will do after they leave the public schools by documenting potential interests, hobbies, and the ability to live independently. Both audiologists and SLPs have the opportunity to make insightful contributions during this discussion.

SLPs and audiologists provide services to students as they transition at all stages of their education. Many are involved in transitioning students from preschool settings to kindergarten and from elementary to middle school and middle to high school. SLPs and audiologists can directly affect the successful transition of school-age students by helping them navigate the new challenges of changing classes and interacting with many personalities in middle and high school. SLPs and audiologists can also be instrumental in facilitating successful transitions for students to work and vocational settings. Difficulties with hearing, speech, or language can serve as blocks to success for special education students at vocational sites. SLPs and audiologists are equipped with the knowledge and problem-solving skills to support students in achieving positive outcomes at job sites.

SPECIAL ISSUES IN SCHOOL SETTINGS

Evidence-Based Practice (EBP)

According to IDEA 2004, special education should be "evidence based to the extent practicable." The strategies and techniques described in the IEP should have research validation. EBP is not simply the best researched technique; it is the convergence of researched techniques, parent and student preferences, and clinical expertise. ASHA has a wealth of information on EBP available on its website including a compendium of EBPs in many disorder areas.

The following case study serves to clarify the convergence of the multiple variables of EBP:

Case Study A student has been identified as eligible for special education, and goals have been written in the area of literacy. The parents and school staff have researched the promising practices in literacy intervention and together have found three literacy programs they believe have research validation sufficient to provide good outcomes for the student. However, neither the school staff nor the parents have enough information about any of the programs to be able to suggest one over another. One of the programs (X) incorporates student-produced artwork, and the student in question loves to draw. In addition, the school SLP has been trained in this particular (X) method and endorses its efficacy. The team then agrees that this program (X) will be followed for the particular student. The convergence of the three areas of EBP has led the team to the best decision for this student given all considerations.

Workload versus Caseload

For many years it has been common practice in school districts to measure the SLP's workload by using the caseload approach that simply examines the number of students served. Recently, however, with the multitude of new responsibilities that SLPs perform in the schools, ASHA has endorsed a workload model that considers not only the number of students served but also many other parameters. Other work tasks include committee work, provision of indirect and consultative services on behalf of all students, collaboration with other professionals, and participation in IEP team meetings, to name a few.

Many teachers and other school professionals remain unaware of the knowledge and skills possessed by their SLP colleagues. Thus, they may not be familiar with the myriad roles and responsibilities of the SLP working in their facility. SLPs in the school setting may need to educate their faculty about the variety and number of the assessment, treatment, and collaboration responsibilities that constitute the contemporary SLP workload. A faculty/administration in-service to inform school personnel on the evolving role of the SLP is a worthwhile investment of time and effort. See Resources for more information about the workload analysis approach for establishing caseload standards available on the ASHA website (ASHA, 2002a).

Scheduling

It is difficult to characterize a "typical" daily schedule for a school-based SLP. The responsibilities of these professionals are continuously changing because of the ever-expanding scope of practice for school-based SLPs and the constantly evolving education initiatives at the federal, state, and even local levels. "Scheduling" in the context of school-based SLPs typically refers to the provision of direct services, although these other responsibilities also need to be factored into the overall schedule.

A variety of locations for direct service delivery is represented on the schedule of the present-day SLP. Many school-based SLPs engage in a variety of service delivery models (e.g., in classroom, pullout, consultation) to support the use of least restrictive environment (LRE) and to provide services in the "natural environment" for all students.

Designing a schedule to meet the needs of students, based on their IEPs, requires flexibility and collaboration with staff members. The SLP needs to schedule time for observations and evaluations, consultations, planning and preparation, and, of course, lunch. The master, or "bell," schedule of the individual school is the best template to use in designing a schedule for speech-language services. Once a schedule is in place, it should be shared with appropriate school personnel and, naturally, the student. The effective SLP will remember that the schedule is fluid, with changes to be made as needed throughout the school year.

English Language Learners and Cultural Competence

According to recent statistics, there are approximately five million English language learners (ELLs) in public schools today. That is twice the number from just 15 years ago, and that number is expected to double again by 2015 (National Clearinghouse for English Language Acquisition, 2007). A bilingual speech-language pathologist who is fluent in the student's native language is the most appropriate resource for assessment and treatment of English language learners with speech-language disorders. If an interpreter is needed, however, ASHA's Multicultural Affairs Section and Special Interest Group 14, Communication Disorders and Sciences in Culturally and Linguistically Diverse Populations, has many useful resources for selecting and training appropriate interpreters for working with students who are ELLs. Sources for locating interpreters may include universities, community colleges, court systems, churches, community organizations, and even certain carefully selected school employees. There are several Internet or conference call resources if no one is available in the community.

Speech-language pathologists must carefully select and train people who will assist in assessment and treatment of English language learners. It is crucial that interpreters translate exactly what each party says without using nonverbal cues or rewording the phrasing of the SLP. Interpreters should be familiar with the anticipated tasks and the assessment and intervention materials. Interpreters should take notes as needed as the session proceeds. SLPs and interpreters should allow time after the session to review notes, discuss responses, and address any difficulties that arise in the session. Translators may also be helpful in translating written homework and procedural forms for parents.

SLPs will demonstrate cultural competence when working with students and families if they learn some basic words in the native language of the student. The ability to greet students in their native language creates a positive tone for the session. As mentioned earlier, many Internet resources for translation are available; therefore, it is not difficult to initiate the meeting with a display of respect stemming from knowledge of the student's cultural and linguistic heritage.

To the extent possible, intervention sessions should begin in the student's native language and move toward the language of educational significance, English. Educational performance for purposes of gauging adequate yearly progress (AYP) is assessed in English according to the No Child Left Behind legislation. ELL students have a two-year period of "safe harbor" from AYP testing but eventually are held accountable for mastery of academic goals, ones that are evaluated by assessments administered in English. See Chapter 24 for more information on service delivery to linguistically diverse populations.

Privacy Issues

SLPs and audiologists are obligated to maintain the privacy of all students. Publicly conversing about a particular student, removing confidential files from the facility, or leaving confidential files unattended or unsecured are examples of situations that compromise the privacy of students and their family. The Family Educational Rights and Privacy Act (FERPA) affords parents and students over 18 years of age certain rights with respect to educational records. School-based SLPs and audiologists have a legitimate educational interest in students' educational records, and as such, FERPA permits "disclosure without consent," allowing access to records. With this privilege comes a huge responsibility to keep all records secure, keep all discussions about a student in a private setting, and adhere to standards that respect the confidentiality and privacy of students and their families. See more about FERPA in Chapter 20, Documentation Issues.

Avoiding Conflicts and Maintaining Documentation

The easiest way to avoid due process hearing complaints is to establish professional, communicative relationships with the child's parents at the beginning of the special education process. Acknowledging and addressing parental concerns in a pro-active way often avoids conflict. Many complaints result from lack of timely communication from school staff. Most parental concerns can be effectively addressed through communication, clarification, and/or active listening to the parent concerns. If attempts to resolve parent concerns are unsuccessful, it is critical that the SLP follow established notification procedures of the school district and inform the appropriate school and/or central office staff. The SLP's documentation will frequently be requested and is crucial evidence in due process proceedings.

School districts often choose to compromise or enter into a legally binding settlement agreement with parents to avoid litigation. The best protection for the SLP and school district is to maintain accurate documentation, including summaries of parental contacts, dates of service (including why scheduled services were not provided), session activities, and progress toward attainment of IEP goals. Additionally, it is imperative that SLPs share IEP accommodations, such as preferential seating for a student with a hearing loss, with all the student's teachers and maintain written documentation that accommodations were provided during all classroom activities. Best practice dictates that the SLP communicate regularly with teachers to verify that all parts of the IEP are being implemented as specified. Again, see Chapter 20, Documentation Issues.

Literacy

One of the major functions of the school-based SLP is to serve students who exhibit or demonstrate risk for having literacy disorders. Speaking, listening, reading, and writing are activities that define literate learners. SLPs are uniquely qualified to prevent and remediate literacy disabilities by focusing on prevention and remediation activities that underpin the language functions of literacy. Many SLPs engage in activities that support literate learners in both regular and special education. ASHA's Literacy Gateway listed in the Resources section of this chapter contains much information on the SLP's role in literacy as well as many activities that target the linguistic skills of literate learners.

Authentic Assessment

Checklists, observations, and other nonstandard assessments may save time and be more useful in school-based practice than standardized measures that lack sufficient specificity (Schraeder, Quinn, & Stockman, 1999). Authentic assessments are used to investigate speech and language disorders that manifest themselves in samples of classroom work and are often some of the most curriculum relevant and meaningful data that an SLP can collect (Timler, 2008). These assessment artifacts, which are used to determine how a communication disorder might impact academic achievement, can be useful in determining eligibility for special education as well as in selecting goals that will most affect academic achievement.

Working with Assistants

As a school-based SLP, you may find that a speech-language pathology assistant (SLPA) has been assigned to help you with your day-to-day responsibilities. It is important that you have a clear understanding of the delineation of your roles and responsibilities as the SLP and those of the SLPA. As indicated by its title, the role of an SLPA is to assist, not replace, the SLP. The job description, supervision requirements, and credentialing of these paraprofessionals vary greatly from state to state, as some states have specific credentialing and supervision requirements. You should become familiar with any such requirements within your state. You also need to inform yourself regarding ASHA policy documents pertaining to the use of support personnel as you begin this supervisory relationship.

As noted by Paul-Brown and Goldberg (2001), SLPAs are extenders of speech-language pathology services and not replacements for SLPs (p. 8). According to the ASHA *Guidelines for the Training, Use, and Supervision of Speech-Language Pathologist Assistants* (2004), the tasks delegated to the SLPA by the SLP serve to increase the availability, frequency, and efficiency of services. Such tasks could include but are not limited to assisting with informal documentation, following treatment plans or protocols, documenting client performance, assisting with clerical duties, and performing checks and maintenance of equipment, all under the direction of the supervising SLP. See Chapter 12, Support Personnel in Communication Sciences and Disorders.

Your role as the supervising SLP may be both challenging and rewarding and, like any supervisory relationship, is one that needs to be built on collaboration, trust, and open communication. One final note: If you are supervising an SLPA, you should consider joining ASHA's Special Interest Group 11, Administration and Supervision, and enroll in workshops on supervision. Both of these provide you with opportunities to learn how to work effectively with SLPAs as you learn more about your role as a supervisor. For more information on supervision see Chapter 25.

Supervision of Student Interns and Clinical Fellows

Supervision of student SLPs (interns) and clinical fellows (CFs) is one of the roles and responsibilities of SLPs in the schools. Many SLPs have little or no coursework during their graduate preparation in this area, so you may need to take advantage of the many continuing education opportunities offered on the topic of supervision. By supervising graduate students and CFs, SLPs cultivate the next generation of professionals preparing for school service. By ensuring positive school-based experiences, SLPs encourage students and CFs to choose schools as their work setting.

School-based SLPs may need to reach out to local universities with Communication Sciences and Disorders programs to volunteer to supervise interns. Make sure your licensure and certification are current throughout the period of time you are supervising. Supervision of interns should be a mutually beneficial opportunity. Graduate students bring a wealth of current knowledge on evidence-based practices while SLPs provide the required clinical hours and fine-tuning of skills that students need to become outstanding professionals. Universities may also provide training in supervision to enhance the professional development of school-based SLPs, thus creating well-trained school-based supervisors.

Medicaid Issues

Some school districts rely on Medicaid funding to supplement the provision of speech-language services. As a school-based SLP, you may be required to follow Medicaid billing procedures. Many ethical issues exist in the cost recovery process for Medicaid funds. Therefore, it is the responsibility of SLPs to investigate and adhere to state Medicaid laws in the areas of documentation, use of graduate students for the delivery of reimbursable services, and signatures of supervising clinicians. Medicaid audits have required payback in these areas, so school districts and individual SLPs should carefully adhere to their state Medicaid laws.

Collaboration with Other Professionals

One of the most attractive aspects of the school setting is the opportunity to collaborate regularly with many other professionals. SLPs work closely with occupational therapists, physical therapists, psychologists, social workers, nurses, counselors, and teachers to meet the needs of all students. These collaborative relationships are stimulating to all professionals, ensuring that services are implemented on a regular basis because of this team approach. Collaborative planning time between professionals is critical and may be accomplished in a variety of ways, including electronic and face-to-face meetings (Flynn, 2010).

Dysphagia

According to ASHA (2007), SLPs play a significant role in the management of students with swallowing (dysphagia) and feeding problems in school. The 2006a ASHA Schools Survey reported that 10.2 percent of school-based SLP respondents have an average of four students with dysphagia in their caseload. Even so, uncertainty persists about the educational relevance of dysphagia management.

ASHA's *Guidelines for Speech-Language Pathologists Providing Swallowing and Feeding Services in Schools* provides the following reasons to explain why addressing swallowing and feeding disorders is educationally relevant and part of the school system's responsibility:

1. Students must be safe while eating in school. This includes providing appropriate personnel, food, and procedures to minimize risks for choking and for aspiration during oral feeding.
2. Students must be adequately nourished and hydrated so that they can attend to and fully access the school curriculum.
3. Students must be healthy (e.g., free from aspiration pneumonia or other illnesses related to malnutrition or dehydration) to maximize their attendance at school.
4. Students must develop skills for eating efficiently during meals and snack times so that they can complete these activities with their peers safely and in a timely manner. (ASHA, 2007)

So what is the role of the school-based SLP when it comes to a child with a swallowing and feeding disorder? SLPs in schools may be instrumental in creating dysphagia teams (Anderson & Homer, 2006) composed of SLPs, occupational therapists, child nutrition directors, and nurses. These teams problem-solve to help students gain the hydration and nutrition they need to have sufficient stamina to learn in the least restrictive environment. As part of interdisciplinary decision making, it is also important for school personnel to communicate frequently with medical professionals on issues related to the consistency of food preparation and viscosity of liquid intake provided at school.

The SLP managing the student with dysphagia may need to consider and remain sensitive to cultural factors surrounding food and eating. You should also be aware of legal and ethical issues when addressing feeding and swallowing disorders, including licensure and scope of practice. Your school system may have its own policies and procedures with which you should be familiar, as well as issues pertaining to reimbursement, such as Medicaid.

Performance Appraisal

ASHA's document (2006b) for the appraisal of the school-based SLP's performance of workload duties serves as a model for many states that now have their own evaluation instrument. Some districts are providing additional monetary incentives based on "value added" assessments that are tied to student achievement and are another way to assess the SLP's job performance.

Each school district has its own performance appraisal system, and personnel are typically notified of the process at the beginning of a school year, or upon being hired. Your performance may be evaluated annually or as part of an ongoing process throughout the school year. The evaluation(s) may be performed by an SLP in an administrative role or by a school principal or other school district administrator. In any case, it provides you with an opportunity to share your successes, describe your goals for improvement, and receive constructive feedback to help you grow as a professional. For more information on performance appraisals, see Chapter 10, Building Your Career.

Technology

A wide range of low to high technological advances is currently available in many school settings. Document projectors, Smart Boards, whiteboards, telecommunication, computers, and a rapidly increasing number of computer software programs and applications are now available for use in the disciplines of speech-language pathology and audiology. No longer is technology just for augmented and alternative communication users.

According to the Consortium for School Networking (CoSN), 95 percent of all classrooms nationwide now have high-speed Internet access while computer labs, instead of classrooms, remain the major Internet access points for students. This seems to indicate that schools have yet to fully integrate technology with teaching that takes place in the classroom, and that classroom technology may need to be upgraded, expanded, or replaced. As an SLP, you should have Internet accessibility in your facility, but the availability of a computer for your use varies from district to district. You should determine whether your district is able to provide you with your own computer, and if not, how you will be able to access one in your facility.

One of the promising types of technological advances is telepractice. Telepractice involves the use of telecommunications technology to deliver speech-language pathology services at a distance (Crutchley, Dudley, & Campbell, 2010). The promising practice is gaining in popularity as a means to provide services to underserved or unserved students in school settings. Many rural districts are finding it a viable means of delivering speech-language services. ASHA has developed guidelines for ethical telepractice. Chapter 26 discusses technology in more detail.

AUDIOLOGY SERVICES

Audiological services play a crucial role in supporting students identified for special education and those in regular education. Although these services are widely perceived to be reserved solely for students identified for special education, they should be available to all students in the form of hearing screenings and hearing conservation activities and in the engineering of classroom acoustic environments that are conducive to learning for all students.

ASHA and the Educational Audiology Association provide excellent guidance for the role of audiology in schools (ASHA, 2002b). Audiologists help support a free appropriate public education (FAPE) under IDEA for all students. According to ASHA (2002b), they engage in the following activities in support of FAPE:

- Identification of children with hearing loss
- Determination of the range, nature, and degree of hearing loss, including referral for medical or other professional attention for the habilitation of hearing
- Provision of habilitation activities, such as language habilitation, auditory training, speech reading (lip-reading), hearing evaluation, and speech conservation
- Creation of an administrative program to prevent hearing loss
- Counseling and guidance of children, parents, and teachers regarding hearing loss
- Determination of a child's needs for group and or individual amplification, selecting and fitting of an appropriate aid, and evaluating the effectiveness of amplification

SUMMARY

The evolution of education reform has significantly influenced the roles and responsibilities of the school-based speech-language pathologist and audiologist in recent years. Much of this legislation has enabled school-based SLPs and audiologists to serve a varied and complex caseload of students every day in positive ways. If you choose to work in this dynamic environment, you need to have a wide range of knowledge and skills.

Today's school-based SLPs and audiologists serve as consultants in the prevention of communication disorders through responsiveness to instruction. You are involved in the referral process leading to evaluation and eligibility for special education and related services. As a service provider, you play a key role in the IEP process. You need to demonstrate that your services are relevant to the student's curriculum and facilitate transition across levels of education and to the real-world after graduation.

School-based SLPs and audiologists recognize the importance of evidence-based practices in school settings. In addition to working to improve students' skills in the areas of articulation, language, voice, and fluency, you should know how to serve students exhibiting or at risk for having disorders related to literacy, limited English proficiency, and dysphagia. You will be expected to use technology in the delivery and documentation of services. The effective SLP must demonstrate flexibility when developing and maintaining a schedule and understand issues related to privacy and documentation. You may need to learn more about supervisory processes as you work with assistants, student interns, and clinical fellows. As you work with other staff members as part of a team, you need to know how to collaborate and share your knowledge and ideas. Because your performance will be evaluated, you need to be able to accept constructive feedback and play a role in planning your own professional development.

Schools provide a setting in which both the SLP and the audiologist may acquire, develop, and refine a wide range of knowledge and skills. You have the opportunity to serve as a member of a team of professionals or as a consultant, work with family members, and provide direct services to children of all ages. You may choose to become an expert in a specific area or a generalist in many. In either case, the challenges and the rewards are ever present, and you will play a major role in the future of the children you serve.

CRITICAL THINKING

1. How has federal legislation influenced the practice of speech-language pathology and audiology in the schools of the United States?
2. Discuss how speech-language pathologists and/or audiologists would explain that their services are educationally relevant.
3. Describe the factors that need to be considered by the SLP when developing a schedule for service delivery.
4. What role would the SLP play on a curriculum-planning team developed to support student performance?
5. How is Response to Intervention changing the role of the speech-language pathologist in a school?
6. In what ways might telepractice change the practice of speech-language pathology and audiology in school settings?
7. What skills do you need to work effectively with students and their families from a variety of diverse backgrounds in the schools? Consider the school where you do student teaching or work professionally. What is the cultural and linguistic makeup of the school? What background do you have to meet the needs of these students?
8. What issues might arise in the supervision of speech-language pathology assistants? How might those be different from supervisory relationships with graduate students and clinical fellows in school settings?

9. Suppose you get a professional position in an educational setting in the next year. How do you think your job will change in the next 10 years? What will you do to increase the importance of the speech-language pathologists or audiologists in the educational setting in which you work?

10. You work in a large suburban public school district and have been asked to sit on a committee to evaluate how technology can be used to enhance rehabilitation services. Consider how technology is now used and what your needs are both for students and program management.

REFERENCES

American Speech-Language-Hearing Association. (2002a). *A workload analysis approach for establishing speech-language caseload standards in the schools.* Rockville, MD: Author.

American Speech-Language-Hearing Association. (2002b). *Guidelines for audiology service provision in and for schools.* Rockville, MD: Author.

American Speech-Language-Hearing Association. (2004). *Guidelines for the training, use, and supervision of speech-language pathology assistants.* Available from http://www.asha.org/policy

American Speech-Language-Hearing Association. (2006a). *Professional performance review process for the school-based speech-language pathologist.* Available from http://www.asha.org/policy

American Speech-Language-Hearing Association. (2006b). *2006 Schools Survey report: Caseload characteristics.* Rockville, MD: Author.

American Speech-Language-Hearing Association. (2007). *Guidelines for speech-language pathologists providing swallowing and feeding services in schools.* Rockville, MD: Author.

American Speech-Language-Hearing Association. (2010a). *Guidelines for the roles and responsibilities of the school-based speech-language pathologist.* Rockville, MD: Author.

American Speech-Language-Hearing Association. (2010b). *Roles and responsibilities of speech-language pathologists in schools.* Retrieved from http://www.asha.org/slp/schools/prof-consult/guidelines/

American Speech-Language-Hearing Association. (2011). *Highlights and trends: ASHA counts for year end 2010.* Retrieved from www.asha.org/uploadedFiles/2010-Member-Counts.pdf

Americans with Disabilities Act of 1990, 42 U.S.C. § 1201 *et seq.* (1990).

Anderson, J. C., & Homer, E. M. (2006, September 26). Managing dysphagia in the schools. *The ASHA Leader.*

Carl D. Perkins Vocational and applied Technology Act, Pub. L. No. 101-392. (1990).

Common Core State Standards Initiative. (2010). *Common standards.* Available from http://www.corestandards.org/

Consortium for School Networking. (n.d.). *Positive attitudes mitigate budget threats.* Retrieved from http://www.cosn.org/Resources/CoSNGrunwaldSurvey/PositiveAttitudesMitigateBudgetThreats/IsTechnologyRetrievedtoStudents/tabid/4494/Default.aspx

Crutchley, S., Dudley, W., & Campbell, M. (2010). Articulation assessment through videoconferencing: A pilot study. *Communications of Global Information Technology, 2*, 12–23.

Education of the Handicapped Act Amendments, Pub. L. No. 99-457. (1986).

Elementary and Secondary Education Act, Pub. L. No. 89-10, 79 Stat. 27, 20 U.S.C. ch. 70 (1965).

Flynn, P. (2010, August 31). New service delivery models: Connecting SLPs with teachers and curriculum. *The ASHA Leader.*

Individuals with Disabilities Education Act (IDEA), Pub. L. No. 101-476. (1990).

Individuals with Disabilities Education Act of 1997, Pub. L. No. 105-17. (1997).

Individuals with Disabilities Education Improvement Act of 2004, Pub. L. No. 108-446, 20 U.S.C. § 1400 *et seq.* (2004).

Library of Congress. (2010, July). *Primary documents in American history: 14th Amendment to the U.S. Constitution.* Retrieved from http://www.loc.gov/rr/program/bib/ourdocs/14thamendment.html

National Center for Education Statistics. (2010). *Digest of Education Statistics, 2009.* Retrieved from http://nces.ed.gov/fastfacts/display.asp?id=64

National Center for Education Statistics. (2011a). *The condition of education 2011.* Retrieved from http://nces.ed.gov/pubsearch/pubsinfo.asp?pubid=2011033

National Center for Education Statistics. (2011b). *Number and types of public elementary and secondary schools from the common core of data: School year 2010-2011-First look.* Retrieved from http://nces.ed.gov/pubsearch/pubsinfo.asp?pubid=2012325

National Center on Response to Intervention. (2011.). *The essential components of RTI. What is RTI?* Retrieved from http://www.rti4success.org/whatisrti

National Clearninghouse for English Language Acquisition. (2007). The growing numbers of English Learner Students. Retrieved from http://www.ncela.gwu.edu/files/uploads/9/growingLEP_0708.pdf

New America Foundation. (2010). *Individuals with Disabilities Education Act—Funding distribution.* Retrieved from http://febp.newamerica.net/background-analysis/individuals-disabilities-education-act-funding-distribution

New America Foundation. (2011). *Education in the federal budget.* Retrieved from http://febp.newamerica.net/background-analysis/education-federal-budget

No Child Left Behind Act of 2001, Pub. L. 107–110 (2002).

Paul-Brown, D., & Goldberg, L. R. (2001). Current policies and new directions for speech-language pathology assistants. *Language, Speech, and Hearing Services in Schools, 32,* 4–17.

Rehabilitation Act of 1973, as amended, 29 U.S.C. §701 (1973).

Samuels, C. (2010). States seek federal waivers to cut special education. *Education Week, 29*(1), 31.

Schraeder, T., Quinn, M., & Stockman, I. (1999). Authentic assessment as an approach to preschool speech-language pathology screening. *American Journal of Speech-Language Pathology, 8,* 195–200.

Technology-Related Assistance for Individuals with Disabilities Act, Pub. L. No. 100-407 (1988).

Timler, G. (2008, November 4). Social communication: A framework for assessment and intervention. *The ASHA Leader.*

U.S. Department of Education. (2005). *10 facts about K-12 education funding.* Washington, DC: Author.

U.S. Department of Education. (2007, March 8). Letter from Alexa Posny (Director, Office of Special Education Programs) to Catherine D. Clarke (Director, ASHA Education and Regulatory Advocacy). Retrieved from http://www.asha.org/uploadedFiles/advocacy/federal/idea/RequestClarificationLettertoPosny.pdf

U.S. Department of Education. (2011, February). *The Family Educational Rights and Privacy Act: Guidance for eligible students.* Retrieved from http://ed.gov/policy/gen/guid/fpco/ferpa/for-eligible-students.pdf

U.S. Department of Health, Education, and Welfare. (1980, May 30). Letter from Edwin Martin (Acting Assistant Secretary for Special Education & Rehabilitative Services, Office of Special Education Programs) to Stan Dublinske (School Services Program American Speech-Language Hearing Association). Retrieved from http://www.asha.org/uploadedFiles/slp/schools/prof-consult/LetterPolicyInterpretation.pdf

RESOURCES

American Speech-Language-Hearing Association. (n.d.). *Tips for working with an interpreter.* Retrieved from http://www.asha.org/practice/multicultural/issues/interpret.htm

American Speech-Language-Hearing Association. (2000). *IDEA and your caseload. A template for eligibility and dismissal criteria for students ages 3 to 21.* Available from http://www.asha.org

American Speech-Language-Hearing Association. (2002). *A workload analysis approach for establishing speech-language caseload standards in the schools: Guidelines.* Retrieved from http://www.asha.org/docs/html/GL2002-00066.html

American Speech-Language-Hearing Association. (2005). *Medicaid and third party payments in the schools.* Retrieved from http://www.asha.org/practice/reimbursement/medicaid/thirdparty-payment.htm

American Speech-Language-Hearing Association. (2006, November 2). Letter from Catherine D. Clarke (Director, ASHA Education and Regulatory Advocacy) to Alexa Posny (Director, Office of Special Education Programs). Retrieved from http://www.asha.org/uploadedFiles/advocacy/federal/idea/RequestClarificationLettertoPosny.pdf

American Speech-Language-Hearing Association. (2007). *IDEA series: Developing educationally relevant IEPs.* Available from http://www.asha.org

American Speech-Language-Hearing Association. (2009). *Practical tools and forms for supervising speech-language pathology assistants.* Rockville, MD: Author.

American Speech-Language-Hearing Association. (2010). *Schools Survey report: SLP caseload characteristics trends 1995–2010.* Retrieved from http://www.asha.org/uploadedFiles/Schools10Caseload-Trends.pdf

American Speech-Language Hearing Association. (2011). *Literacy gateway.* Retrieved from http://www.asha.org/publications/literacy/

Americans with Disabilities Act of 1990, 42 U.S.C. § 1201 *et seq*. Available from http://www.ada.gov/

Common Core Standards. Available from http://www.corestandards.org/

McCready, V. (2011). Generational issues in supervision and administration. *The ASHA Leader, 16(*5) 12–15.

Schrag, J., & Schrag, H. (2004). *National Dispute Resolution Use and Effectiveness Study: Executive summary.* Retrieved from http://www.directionservice.org/cadre/pdf/Effectiveness%20Full%20Study.04

State Education Agencies Communication Disabilities Council. http://www.seacdc.org

U.S. Congress. (2004). Individuals with Disabilities Education Improvement Act (IDEA) of 2004. Retrieved from http://idea.ed.gov/explore/view/p/%2Croot%2Cstatute%2CI%2CA%2C602%2C3%2C

U.S. Department of Education. (1990). Americans with Disabilities Act (ADA). Retrieved from http://www.ed.gov/about/offices/list/ocr/docs/hq9805.html

U.S. Department of Education. (2006). *Federal regulations IDEA 2004.* Retrieved from http://idea.ed.gov/explore/view/p/%2Croot%2Cregs%2C

U.S. Department of Education (2010). *Elementary and Secondary Education, No Child Left Behind Legislation and Policies.* Retrieved from http://www2.ed.gov/policy/elsec/guid/states/index.html

U.S. Department of Education. (2011a). *Overview: The federal role in education.* Retrieved from http://www2.ed.gov/about/overview/fed/role.html?src=ln

U.S. Department of Education. (2011b). *Student placement in elementary and secondary schools and Section 504 of the Rehabilitation Act and Title II of the Americans with Disabilities Act.* Retrieved from http://www2.ed.gov/about/offices/list/ocr/docs/placpub.html

U.S. Department of Health and Human Services Centers for Medicare and Medicaid Services. (2003). *Medicaid school-based administrative claiming guide.* Retrieved from http://www.medicaid.gov/Medicaid-CHIP-Program-Information/By-Topics/Financing-and-Reimbursement/Downloads/2003_SBS_Admin_Claiming_Guide.pdf

U.S. Department of Justice. (2010). Highlights of the final rule to amend the Department of Justice's regulation implementing Title II of the ADA. Retrieved from http://www.ada.gov/regs2010/factsheets/title2_factsheet.html

Zirkel, P. (1998, April). Counterpoint: National trends in education litigation: Supreme Court decisions concerning students. *Journal of Law & Education, 27*, 235.

Zirkel, P. (2007). Courtside: 'Higher' education litigation? *The Phi Delta Kappan, 88*(10), 797–799.

16

Service Delivery Issues in Early Intervention

Corey Herd Cassidy, PhD

SCOPE OF CHAPTER

It is every parent's worst nightmare to discover that his/her child has been born with or has been diagnosed with a disability or developmental delay. Parents often experience feelings of fear, anxiety, depression, and helplessness when they do not know where to go for services for their child or support for their family. Early intervention services are specialized services that are designed to meet the needs of infants and toddlers from birth to age three years who have or may be at risk for developmental delays or disabilities and their families. These services are designed to decrease the family's anxiety by providing resources and supports for the child and family to ensure that the child has every opportunity to develop and learn. The Individuals with Disabilities Education Improvement Act (IDEA) is a federally mandated system, of which Part C serves these young children and their families. The system has been restructured several times since its inception in 1997; the most current act was authorized in 2004 and reflects empirically based practices in the arena of early intervention.

In 2008, the American Speech-Language-Hearing Association (ASHA) presented four guiding principles that reflect best practices for speech-language pathologists and audiologists who are providing Part C early intervention services to young children and their families. This chapter presents each of these principles and discusses how each may be effectively implemented by speech-language pathologists (SLPs) and audiologists working as part of a team that includes other service providers and family members within the early intervention system. Family-centered practices, based on the family systems theory, and the importance of considering and incorporating natural environments into the provision of early intervention services are presented and discussed. The concept of cultural competence in the early intervention arena, including the definitions and the considerations that influence the provision of effective and appropriate family-centered services, is defined. This chapter discusses each step of the early intervention process, including considerations regarding eligibility and the creation of the Individualized Family Service Plan (IFSP). In addition, the chapter introduces you to information on different team formats in early intervention programs. Research supporting the fact that the period from birth to age three is a critical time in a child's development is shared and the evidence basis of early intervention is discussed. Finally, the chapter presents general advice for providing best practices within natural environments as well as suggestions for establishing a positive and safe work environment.

WHAT IS EARLY INTERVENTION?

Before 1975, approximately one million children with disabilities were denied pertinent services and were provided only minimal education in separate facilities and institutions. Public Law (PL) 94-142, also known as the Education for All Handicapped Children Act, was passed in 1975 and is considered by many to be the most significant act in the history of education in regard to children with disabilities. This act mandated a free appropriate public education (FAPE) for all children with disabilities from 5 to 21 years of age. Through a series of reauthorizations, FAPE was extended to include children with disabilities from 3 to 21 years of age. PL 94-142 is the predecessor to both the Individuals with Disabilities Education Act (IDEA) and the Individuals with Disabilities Education Improvement Act (IDEIA). The term is often used interchangeably with IDEA and IDEIA, as it also refers to all amendments affecting the 1975 Act.

In 1986, IDEA was passed. This amendment to the original PL 94-142 provided the federal mandate for special education services in each state for children with disabilities from birth to 21 years of age. It outlined the system of funding employed for special education and related services. Provisions were put in place through Part H of IDEA to provide incentives to states to provide services to children from birth to three years of age. Congress established the Part H (early intervention) program of IDEA in recognition of "an urgent and substantial need" to:

- enhance the development of infants and toddlers with disabilities;
- reduce educational costs by minimizing the need for special education through early intervention;
- minimize the likelihood of institutionalization, and maximize independent living; and
- enhance the capacity of families to meet their child's needs.

IDEA Part C

In 1997, IDEA (PL 105-17) was restructured and Part H became Part C—the Program for Infants and Toddlers with Disabilities. IDEA was modified once again in 2004 as the Individuals with Disabilities Education Improvement Act (commonly referred to as IDEA 2004). Federal Part C regulations now require that a statewide policy and system of early intervention services are in effect to ensure that appropriate early intervention services are available to all infants and toddlers with disabilities and/or significant developmental delay and their families. For a state to participate in the program, it must ensure that early intervention will be available to all eligible children and their families. Each state's governor must designate a lead agency to receive the funding and to administer the program. The governor must also appoint an Interagency Coordinating Council (ICC), including parents of young children with disabilities, to advise and assist the lead agency. Currently, all states and eligible territories are participating in the Part C program. Annual funding to each state is based upon census figures of the number of children birth to three years of age in the general population. Part C services may be extended to include children up through six years of age; however, few states have adopted this practice.

Range of Early Intervention Services

Broadly speaking, early intervention services are specialized health, educational, and therapeutic services designed to meet the needs of infants and toddlers from birth to age three years who have or may be at risk for developmental delays or disabilities, and their families. Early intervention services bring families and service providers from many aspects of the community together, including public and private agencies, child care centers, local school districts, and private providers. Supports and services are intended to work together to meet children's unique needs and those of their family in their natural environments. Early intervention services may be simple or complex depending on each child's needs. They can range from prescribing glasses for a two-year-old to developing a comprehensive approach with a variety of services and special instruction for a child, including home visits, counseling, and training for family members. Depending on the child's needs, early intervention services may include family training, counseling, and home visits; special instruction; speech-language pathology services; audiology services; occupational therapy; physical therapy; psychological services; medical services (for diagnostic or evaluation purposes); health services needed to enable the child to benefit from the other services; social work services; assistive technology devices and services; transportation; nutrition services; and service coordination services. Table 16–1 illustrates a sample of the services that may be provided under the scope of IDEA 2004 Part C early intervention services.

Guiding Principles of Early Intervention

Four guiding principles reflect current best practices when providing early intervention for young children and their families (American Speech-Language-Hearing Association [ASHA], 2008a). These principles specifically note that supports and services must be

TABLE 16–1 Examples of Early Intervention Services Provided under IDEA 2004 Part C

- Audiology
- Assistive technology
- Counseling/psychological services
- Family training and counseling
- Medical evaluation (for diagnostic purposes only)
- Nursing
- Nutrition
- Occupational therapy
- Physical therapy
- Prevention education
- Service coordination
- Social work
- Special instruction
- Speech/language intervention
- Transition assistance between Part C and Part B
- Transportation
- Vision

Information from Data Accountability Center (2010)

(1) family-centered and culturally responsive; (2) developmentally supportive and promote children's participation in their natural environments; (3) comprehensive, coordinated, and team-based; and 4) based on the highest-quality internal and external evidence that is available. Each one of these principles is discussed in greater detail throughout the chapter.

FAMILY-CENTERED AND CULTURALLY RESPONSIVE SERVICES

The first guiding principle that reflects current best practices of SLPs and audiologists in the early intervention arena focuses on the delivery of services that are both family-centered and culturally responsive (ASHA, 2008a). These practices involve working collaboratively with families in all aspects of service delivery. It means relating to family members as people, not "patients." A family-centered approach recognizes the importance of all family members, including brothers and sisters, grandparents, and extended family members. It also indicates that you must be sensitive to the cultural considerations and needs of the family members.

Family-Centered Practices

Collaboration between families and providers is the foundation of family-centered services. Figure 16–1 illustrates the principles that help define collaboration and, ultimately, explain the approach and intent of early

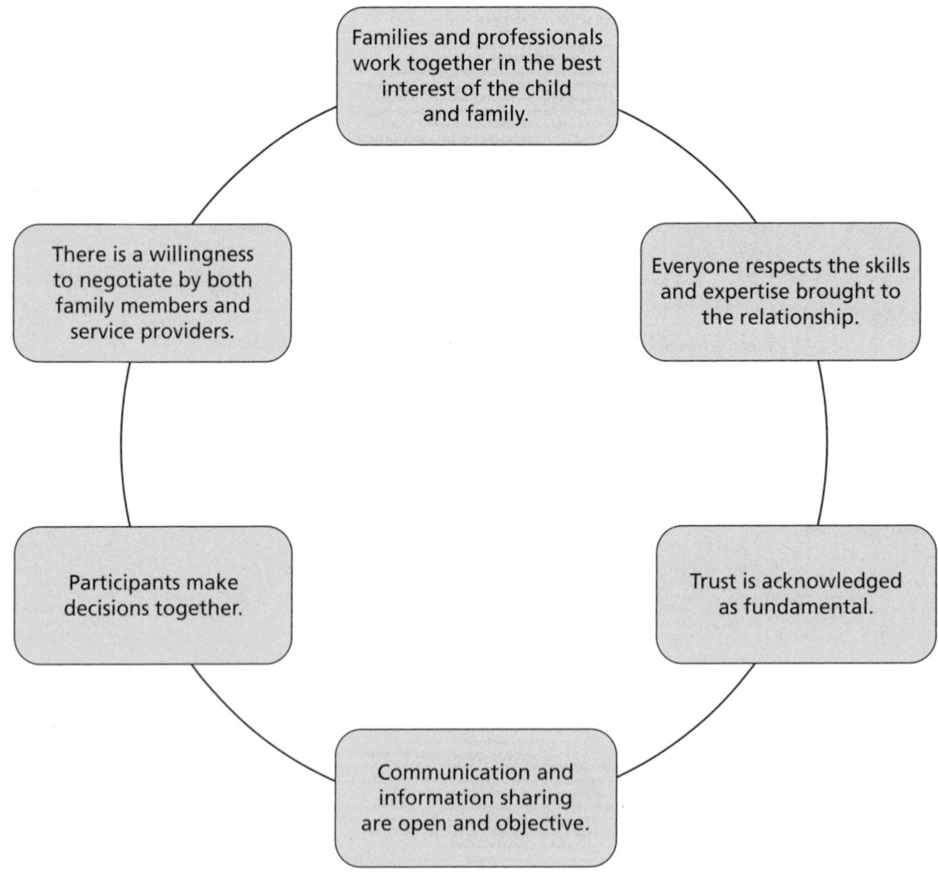

FIGURE 16–1 Principles of Family-Centered Collaboration
Image created based on information from Sandall, S., Hemmeter, M. L., Smith, B. J., & McLean, M. E. (2005)

intervention. To put the principles of collaboration into practice, families and providers must form a partnership. This partnership begins by determining the definitions and roles of both the family and the SLP or audiologist. The term *family* can have many different meanings. Families define themselves by who lives together, who makes decisions, what roles family members play, and how members support each other. Each family operates as a system, and for each child, the family system represents the group of individuals who have the most influence on that child's growth and development. Learning about how a family works is critical to building rapport; working together; and facilitating an individualized, supportive early intervention process. By asking questions about routines, joining their activities, and communicating effectively, early intervention service providers learn about how each family works. These steps also offer families an opportunity to see that this information is vitally important for individualized and meaningful services for their unique child and family (SpecialQuest Multimedia Training Library, 2007).

SLPs and audiologists must learn to adapt their knowledge and expertise to fit the needs of each child and family, ensuring that the family's needs are being addressed and learning is supported. The unique needs of each child and family determine which skills you use, how knowledge is shared, and which strategies are developed. You should combine your professional expertise and activities with the child- and family-specific expertise that the parent brings to the table. Together, you can create intervention that is focused on how the family will encourage the growth, development, and participation of their child when you are not present (McWilliam, 2004).

SLPs and audiologists who use a family-centered approach effectively collaborate with families to share information, strengthen family functioning, empower decision making, and facilitate family participation throughout the early intervention process. Establishing a positive relationship with a family is key to facilitating their participation throughout the early intervention process. You play an important role in developing the relationship and facilitating family participation. Building rapport and trust that lead to a true partnership begins with the first contact and continues through transition (Jung & Grisham-Brown, 2006). Meeting families "where they are"; practicing active listening; and helping them identify priorities, resources, strengths, and needs related to their child's development and their family lay the foundation for a supportive early intervention system.

As SLPs and audiologists, you join the parents, through your relationship, in your common concerns about their infant or toddler. You both observe the child's growth and development and offer developmentally appropriate anticipatory guidance. You, therefore, need to encourage parents to take the lead in the early intervention experience. You also identify the strengths that each parent brings to the relationship with his or her child and identify and support the parent's pleasure in the child. You must take your knowledge and learn to adapt and apply it with each family in each intervention visit. Young children's development occurs within the context of their family and community (Dunst et al., 2001). It is because of the profound influences of family and community that SLPs and audiologists working in early intervention focus on how to support the development of infants and toddlers within these contexts. The guiding principles of Part C recognize that infant and toddler development unfolds during family routines and activities. Supports and services that focus on these routines and activities provide family members with useful, meaningful strategies that can be used daily within the context of those activities that are unique to each individual family (Woods, Kashinath, & Goldstein, 2004).

Cultural Competence

Using the family systems approach, SLPs and audiologists provide early intervention services by supplying knowledge and training to families as they navigate the world of raising their children with disabilities. A 2007 ASHA survey of SLPs indicated that, in all settings, approximately 29 percent of caseloads are composed of culturally and linguistically diverse clients (ASHA, 2007). Results from the National Early Intervention Longitudinal Study, however, indicated that families from diverse ethnic/racial backgrounds and families at lower income levels who had participated in early intervention services were less satisfied with services than Caucasian families and those families at higher income levels (Hebbeler et al., 2007). Therefore, to effectively support families, you must develop a heightened level of sensitivity to the influences of cultural values and beliefs as well as to the strengths that these bring to the family system (Garcia Coll & Magnuson, 2000).

SLPs and audiologists interact with families of many different cultures. Culture is defined as "people's values, religion, ideals, language, artistic expressions, patterns of social and interpersonal relationships and ways of perceiving, behaving and thinking" (Balthrop & Coleman, 2003). Cultural competence is the ability to interact effectively with all people, regardless of their cultures. By becoming more culturally sensitive, you will be able to reduce your own cultural biases and recognize the cultural issues important to each family. Table 16–2 illustrates variables that should be taken into consideration with regard to differences among cultures. For additional information regarding cultural competence in speech-language pathology and audiology, refer to Chapter 24.

Cultural competence is necessary to ensure success in every step of the process when providing early intervention supports and services. The components of the family system are strongly influenced by culture as it influences how a family defines and structures itself (Wayman & Lynch, 1991). Culture influences family functions, the family life cycle, and events that are viewed by the family as stressors. Cultural perspectives that may relate directly to services within early intervention include views of (1) children and child rearing, (2) disability and causation, (3) intervention, (4) medical treatment and healing, (5) family and family roles, and (6) language and communication styles (Hanson & Lynch, 1990). Additionally, according to Hanson and Lynch (1990), several factors regarding the nature of early intervention itself must be considered when working with families from culturally diverse backgrounds. These factors include (1) attitudes regarding intervention, (2) methods used and location of services, (3) qualifications of the service providers, and (4) styles of interaction and communication in the provision of services.

When providing services to families from diverse cultural backgrounds, SLPs and audiologists should consider those factors that affect families' perspectives as well as those considerations that may relate directly to services. By listening to the family and learning about their family system, you can better promote effective intervention. During the initial assessment for the program planning process, you have the opportunity to ask questions and listen to the family members discuss their needs and concerns. Based on their feedback and by collaborating with family members, outcomes should be aligned with family culture, values, needs, and priorities. Additionally, using a routines-based approach to goal selection and intervention may be optimal (Kashinath, Woods, & Goldstein, 2006; Woods et al., 2004). Since intervention activities are built directly into family routines that already exist, this approach builds upon the strengths that are inherent to individual family systems while eliminating cultural mismatches. By determining optimal routines and empowering parents to incorporate opportunities into their own everyday activities, you are able to provide effective services while respecting and considering every family's culture and value system (Peña & Fiestas, 2009).

Establishing and Maintaining Rapport

Building rapport with a family begins with the first contact and affects the relationship throughout the process of intervention. Strong rapport takes time to establish and effort to maintain, but it can be a means of encouraging open communication and learning for everyone involved. Working from a family-centered perspective, SLPs and audiologists are able to build strong relationships with the families that they serve by establishing a positive foundation. By recognizing the family's strengths and perspectives in the first stages of the early intervention process, you are able to consider the demands of intervention in relation to the benefits at each subsequent stage. Keeping an open dialogue with family members and discussing these demands and benefits on a consistent basis are key to maintaining rapport among the team members. Table 16–3 provides suggestions for building positive relationships with families.

Shifting from Direct Services to Indirect Services through the Process of Coaching

Early intervention SLPs and audiologists may find it easier to simply "do it themselves." Effective early intervention clinicians, however, empower families when they coach the parent and child in their natural environments (Hanft, Rush, & Shelden, 2004). During the initiation of the coaching process, the door is opened to engage in a conversation regarding this approach. The SLP or audiologist and the parent develop a plan together that includes the purpose and specific outcomes of the coaching. The purpose within early intervention is typically to support the child's

TABLE 16–2 Variables Regarding Cultural Differences

Personal space	• In some cultures, it is common for people to stand approximately three feet apart when having a personal conversation. • In other cultures, it is typical to stand much closer. • Each distance may feel awkward to someone who is unfamiliar with the other style; the conversational partner may try to move closer or farther away, depending upon his/her own comfort.
Eye contact and feedback behaviors	• In some cultures, individuals are encouraged to look each other directly in the eye and to participate actively in providing feedback behaviors (leaning forward, smiling, nodding, and so on). • In contrast, people from other cultures may show respect or deference by not engaging in eye contact or by participating more passively in their body language and conversation.
Interruption and turn-taking behaviors	• Some cultures have come to expect a conversation to progress linearly (one speaker at a time) while it may be more natural for several people to be talking at once in another culture. • Listening skills that address different cultural rules regarding turn taking in conversation must be developed when considering and accommodating multiple styles.
Gesturing	• Hand and arm gesturing can vary quite a bit in different cultural backgrounds. • In general, extreme gesturing should not necessarily be interpreted as excitement as it may just be an ordinary manner of communication, depending on the speaker.
Facial expressions	• Variance in facial expressions among different cultures is common. • It is important to not assume that someone is cold or distressed based solely on one's own cultural experience.
Silence	• Americans often find it more difficult to tolerate periods of prolonged silence than do others from different cultures and may try to fill the silence with noise.
Dominance behaviors	• In some cultures prolonged eye contact, an erect posture, looking down at someone's hands or hips, looking at someone with lowered lids, and holding the head high are all examples of behavior that may be interpreted as assertive or even aggressive. • The interpretation of these behaviors may vary from one culture to another.
Volume	• Irritation often results when culturally different speakers consider differing levels of volume acceptable. • It is important to remember that each individual may be reacting based on the rules learned in his/her own background and what may be considered normal by his/her peers.
Touching	• Some cultures may perceive someone as cold and aloof if there is not much touching and/or proximity to one another. In other cultures, touching may be perceived as intrusive or rude.

Based on Saldaña (2001)

TABLE 16–3 Suggestions for Building Positive Relationships with Families

- Show genuine interest in the family's life, activities, and interests and in the child's achievements.
- Be sensitive to each family's readiness to share information.
- Facilitate a family member's participation at a level that is comfortable for him or her.
- Include family members in intervention planning.
- Respect the family's time by being on time for visits and offering flexible scheduling.
- Acknowledge the complexities of raising a child with developmental delays or disabilities and offer assistance as needed.
- Provide complete, unbiased information and allow family members time to make informed decisions, even when the family's decisions differ from choices you would have made.
- Respect the family's rights throughout the early intervention process.

Based on information from SpecialQuest Multimedia Training Library (2007)

participation and development in ordinary family and community life. Following the initial discussion, the SLP or audiologist may choose to observe the parents as they use an existing strategy, try out a new skill, or demonstrate a skill that has been used between visits. The SLP or audiologist may also observe the parent engaging in an activity with the child. When the SLP or audiologist has an opportunity to see the parent and child interact, it allows you to (1) see what the parent or family member is doing well and (2) offer additional suggestions and/or modifications. Such active guidance provides an opportunity to build partnerships with families. These partnerships enhance the family members' effectiveness as they engage in everyday learning opportunities with their children (Shelden & Rush, 2001).

DEVELOPMENTALLY SUPPORTED SERVICES IN THE NATURAL ENVIRONMENT

Effective early intervention services meet the family where they are, at the level of their needs, and in the environments in which they find themselves. Each family exists within a system that includes the people with whom they interact, the supports and resources they have, and the places they go. The primary purpose of early intervention is to support family efforts and to build their confidence and competence in meeting the needs of their children. With that purpose in mind, intervention visits that are provided within each family's support system and natural environment may be best suited to positive developmental outcomes for children and families (ASHA, 2008b).

According to Part C of IDEA 2004, a "natural environment" is defined as a setting that is natural or normal for a child's peers who have no disabilities. Natural environments include the home as well as other settings in which children without delays and disabilities participate in their communities. Natural environments are not places where children go because of their disabilities, the convenience of the SLP or audiologist, or access to a special place or equipment. Natural environments are, instead, those settings and activities in which each individual child's family participates or in which they would like to participate.

SLPs and audiologists must determine not only *where* the supports are provided but also *how* they will provide them. Children learn best when they learn in context and have multiple opportunities to practice the skills and abilities throughout the day. It is much easier for infants and toddlers to generalize their newly learned skills when they have learned them during meaningful, functional activities as they happen naturally, rather than learning them in contrived situations in a clinical setting. It is your job to provide parents with this perspective.

SLPs and audiologists must learn to think beyond the traditional "home visit." You must consider the multitude of activities that occur outside of your scheduled block of time (Hanft et al., 2004). Thinking beyond the typical home visit requires a shift in how early intervention has been provided in many localities. Therefore, to help your teams move forward, you need to understand the similarities and differences between traditional "home visiting" and intervention that is provided when incorporating each family's priorities, routines, and activities. Services provided through traditional "home visits" tend to be limited to what can be accomplished during the span of time the SLP and family have allotted for the visit. Specific skills may be addressed in isolation, and activities may be discussed but not practiced because they do not coincide with the scheduled time. In contrast, supports and services that consider the concept of natural environments use that allotted "home visit" time much differently. The time is used to explore a variety of family routines and activities to find out how they can be enhanced to address IFSP outcomes, both during and between early intervention visits. Since SLPs and audiologists may join the family in those activities, the intervention visit is scheduled in response to the activities being explored and is flexible with regard to day and time.

Intervention provided in the home or other natural settings and environments gives SLPs and audiologists the opportunity to see what daily life is like for the family. These interactions may include learning what goes well for each family and where assistance is needed. By becoming familiar with the specifics of each family's routines and activities, SLPs and audiologists can help parents develop individualized outcomes and intervention strategies based on those activities that are meaningful and useful to the family during their routine daily life.

COMPREHENSIVE, COORDINATED, AND TEAM-BASED SERVICES

One of the four guiding principles of early intervention (ASHA, 2008a) states that supports and services should be "comprehensive, coordinated, and team-based." Regardless of state or local programming methods, however, all young children and their families follow the same basic steps as they enter into and move through the early intervention system in order to receive these supports and services. The process begins with referral for assessment and follows the child and family while they are receiving services through the Part C system. This process is often called the *supports and services pathway*. The supports and services pathway describes the early intervention process that assists in the identification of eligible families and delivery of early intervention services. It consists of seven distinct components of service delivery, including referral, intake, eligibility determination, assessment for service planning, Individualized Family Service Plan (IFSP) development, implementation and reviews of the IFSP, and transition activities. Embedded in each of these processes is the legal acknowledgment of the child's and family's procedural rights and safeguards. Figure 16–2 provides the typical sequence that a family follows while involved in Part C services.

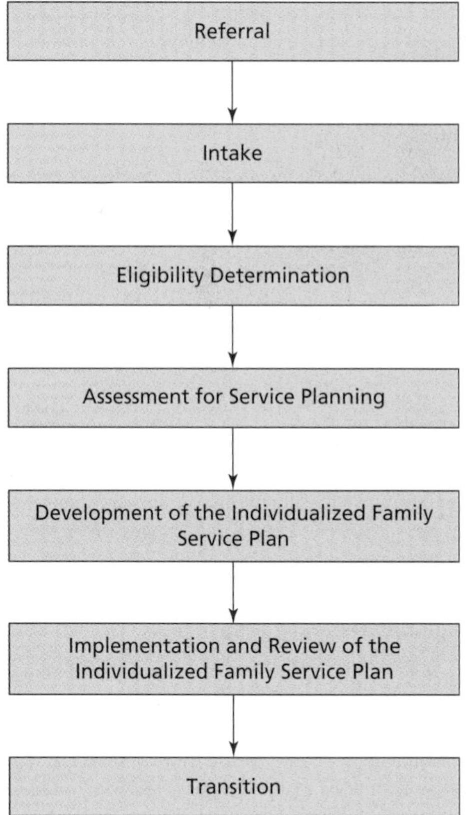

FIGURE 16–2 The Sequence of Early Intervention

Referral

A primary referral source, such as a parent, pediatrician, or health department representative, identifies a child who may have a developmental delay or may be in need of further assessment. Referral sources often have concerns based on results of developmental screenings, observations, or a diagnosis indicating a potential developmental delay. Anyone in the community can make a referral of a child who might be eligible for Part C services as long as parent/guardian permission is secured. The referral is made to the Part C local Central Point of Entry. The Central Point of Entry collects the referral information and assigns a service coordinator to meet with the family. During the referral process, information regarding the local or statewide early intervention process is shared with the family, and initial information regarding the child and family is gathered. Each local lead agency develops policies and procedures in the community to ensure quick response from the Central Point of Entry and to move quickly toward the next step in the early intervention process.

Intake

Intake involves face-to-face and/or phone meetings with the family to continue gathering information to determine eligibility. Such information includes developmental history, medical history and medical home information, family routines, schedules, and activities of interest as well as the completion of a developmental screening, if needed. In-depth information is shared with the family regarding the Part C system including eligibility criteria, IFSP development if the child is eligible, family cost share participation, and child and family procedural rights and safeguards. At this point, the Central Point of Entry, or a service coordinator who has been assigned to the family, begins the process of eligibility determination.

Eligibility Determination

Eligibility determination is the process of determining whether a child meets the system's eligibility criteria to receive early intervention services. This process includes the evaluation of the child's skills and needs through a review of information, including medical/developmental reports, assessment reports, observations, and parent report. Eligibility determination is based on the child's needs within the child's natural environment, which may include the home or any community setting in which children without disabilities participate (e.g. child care centers, public playgrounds). All areas of a child's development are considered to determine whether the child has a delay and/or differences in development that might make him/her eligible for Part C services. This information is reviewed by a multidisciplinary team, which includes providers of various disciplines, to determine whether a child meets one of the criteria for eligibility. Part C of IDEA 2004 states that systems must provide services to any child "under 3 years of age who needs early intervention services" (IDEA 2004, § 632(5)(A)) because the child "(i) is experiencing developmental delays, as measured by appropriate diagnostic instruments and procedures in one or more of the areas of cognitive development, physical development, communication development, social or emotional development, and adaptive development; or (ii) has a diagnosed physical or mental condition which has a high probability of resulting in developmental delay" (IDEA 2004, § 632(5)(A)).

A state may also provide services, at its discretion, to at-risk infants and toddlers. States have some discretion in setting the criteria for each of these variables. As a result, definitions of eligibility differ significantly from state to state. Evaluation procedures used to determine developmental delay involve determining the status of the child in each of the developmental areas.

A multidisciplinary evaluation team typically consists of at least two early childhood professionals who are appropriately qualified in their areas of expertise (i.e., speech-language pathologist, occupational therapist, developmental specialist), at least one of whom is qualified in the primary area(s) of concern. The service coordinator works with the multidisciplinary evaluation team to facilitate the evaluations, ensuring that all of the appropriate procedures are completed and properly documented. At a minimum, a multidisciplinary evaluation team gathers information from a review of pertinent records related to a child's current health status and medical history, family report, and the results of appropriate diagnostic methods. These methods may include additional reports from other sources, criterion-referenced instruments such as developmental checklists, a developmental history, language samples, norm-referenced instruments, observation of the child, play-based evaluations, and routine-based interviews. When you are working with families for whom English is not the native language or when there is a language barrier, an interpreter must be involved. The evaluation must be completed in the native language of the family.

Developmental Delay Each state has the opportunity to determine criteria for developmental delay in its own way. Many states determine criteria quantitatively, including (1) the difference between chronological age and actual performance level expressed as a percentage of chronological age, (2) delay expressed as performance at a certain number of months below chronological age, or (3) delay as indicated by standard deviation below the mean on a norm-referenced instrument. There is wide variability in the type of quantitative criteria states use to describe developmental delay, and there also is a wide range in the level of delay states require for eligibility. Common measurements of level of delay are 25 percent delay or two standard deviations (SD) below the mean in one or more developmental areas, or 20 percent delay or 1.5 SD in two or more areas. Traditional assessment instruments, yielding scores in standard deviations or developmental age in months, may not adequately address some developmental domains or may not be comparable across developmental domains or across age levels (Benn, 1994; Brown & Brown, 1993). For this reason, some states have included qualitative criteria for determining developmental delay. Qualitative criteria include delay indicated by atypical development or observed atypical behaviors.

Atypical Development Children are considered to have atypical development if they demonstrate abnormal or questionable sensory-motor responses (such as abnormal muscle tone, poor quality of movement patterns, or oral-motor skills dysfunction such as feeding difficulties) or have an identified affective disorder (such as a delay in achieving expected emotional milestones, a persistent failure to initiate or respond to most social interactions, or distress that does not respond to comforting by caregivers).

Diagnosed Physical or Mental Condition A diagnosed physical or mental condition refers to a child who has a diagnosed physical or mental condition that has a high probability of resulting in a developmental delay if early intervention services are not provided. This includes conditions such as chromosomal abnormalities; genetic or congenital disorders; severe sensory impairments; inborn errors of metabolism; disorders reflecting disturbance of the development of the nervous system; congenital infections; disorders secondary to exposure to toxic substances, including fetal alcohol syndrome; and severe attachment disorders.

At Risk An at-risk infant or toddler is defined under Part C as "an individual under 3 years of age who would be at risk of experiencing a substantial developmental delay if early intervention services were not provided to the individual" (IDEA 2004, § 632(1)). Although many states are interested in serving children at risk, they also fear increasing the numbers of eligible children because of escalating costs. Three categories of risk that are frequently described by states that do serve these children include conditions of established risk, biological/medical risk, and environmental risk. States that do not serve children at risk under their guidelines for eligibility typically indicate that they will monitor the development of these children and refer them for early intervention services if and when delays are manifested.

Assessment for Service Planning

This is a multistep process that includes identification of the family's resources, priorities, and concerns through family-centered assessment, multidisciplinary team observations, and assessment of eligible children. In addition to assessing the family, assessment is also an opportunity to determine the child's strengths and needs in all areas of development. The assessment process provides the IFSP team with an opportunity to identify early intervention supports and services that may be necessary to address the child's unique needs. Although assessment tools may vary, ASHA (2008b) recommends combining formal and informal assessment tools that include both standardized and nonstandardized measures to provide the most comprehensive picture of the child. This combination of assessment tools provides information regarding the communication skills of the child in comparison to same-age peers. Conducting an assessment with a comprehensive battery is more conducive to encouraging family and team member participation and collaboration and to guiding the IFSP development. Some local and statewide systems have implemented specific requirements regarding the choice and use of assessment tools for the purposes of both eligibility determination and assessment for service planning.

Development of the Individualized Family Service Plan

Based on the assessment for service planning, the Individualized Family Service Plan is developed. The IFSP is a written plan for providing early intervention services to eligible children and their families. The plan is developed jointly by the family, the service coordinator, and others who may be providing early intervention services to the child and family. The IFSP is based on the multidisciplinary evaluation and assessment of the child and the assessment of the resources, priorities, and concerns of the child's family. The plan includes outcomes, strategies, and services that are necessary to enhance the development of the child and the capacity of the family to meet the special needs of the child (IDEA 2004, § 303.340(2)). Part C of IDEA mandates that the IFSP meeting must be conducted in settings and at times that are convenient to the family. The meeting and the documents must also be in the native language of the family. An interpreter must be involved if the native language of the family is not English. The SLP or audiologist must work collaboratively with the interpreter to ensure that families fully understand their rights and role in the early intervention system.

There are eight required components of the IFSP:

1. A statement of the infant's or toddler's present levels of physical development (including fine motor, gross motor, vision, hearing, and health status), cognitive development, communication development, social or emotional development, and adaptive (self-help) development based on objective criteria. This can be listed as an age level or a range.
2. A statement (with the family's permission) of the family's resources, priorities, and concerns related to enhancing the development of the family's infant or toddler with a disability. Priorities may include the hopes and dreams of the family for their child. This statement may also include information about how the family would like its child to more fully participate in family and community activities. Resources include people in the family's life with whom they rely and interact.
3. A statement of the measurable results or outcomes expected to be achieved for the infant or toddler and the family. The statement should include emergent literacy and language skills that are developmentally appropriate for the child. The statement should also include the criteria, procedures, and time lines used to determine the degree to which progress toward achieving the results or outcomes is being made. Any modifications or revisions of the results/outcomes/services that may be necessary should be included. Outcomes are statements about what the family wants its child to learn or do. For example, an IFSP outcome may focus on the child learning to sit at the table with the family at dinner and eat with a spoon, walk around the block to the playground with the family in the evening, or say new words to tell the family what toys the child wants. Outcomes should be individualized for each child and family. As such, they should be contextualized, functional, and discipline-free. Outcomes should be relevant to the family and focused on the whole child and his or her participation in activity settings that are important to the family (Infant & Toddler Connection of Virginia, 2003).
4. A statement of specific early intervention services based on peer-reviewed research, to the extent possible, necessary to meet the unique needs of the infant or toddler and the family. This statement should include the frequency, intensity, and method of delivering services. Supports and services should be individualized. If a group of IFSPs are reviewed within a local system, the reviewer should see this individualization reflected with varying services and supports being provided from IFSP to IFSP. Early intervention services include, but are not limited to, service coordination, speech therapy, physical therapy, occupational therapy, special instruction, and assistive technology. All children must receive service coordination. Additional services are dependent upon many variables and often change over the course of the child's involvement in early intervention.
5. A statement of the natural environments in which early intervention services will appropriately be provided. If the services will not be provided in a natural environment, a justification must be presented. Natural environments include locations where children live, learn, and play, and how they learn in those natural places.

6. The projected dates of initiation of services and the anticipated length, duration, and frequency of the services. Projected start dates must include the month, date, and year.
7. The identification of the service coordinator from the profession most immediately relevant to the child's or family's needs (or who is otherwise qualified to carry out all applicable responsibilities under this part). All families in early intervention have a service coordinator who is responsible for overseeing the IFSP, ensuring that all the IFSP services are provided and that changes in the IFSP are made when necessary.
8. The steps to be taken to support the transition of the toddler with a disability to preschool or other appropriate services. This transition plan must be individualized for each child. (PL 108-446, Sec. 636(d))

IFSP Implementation and Review

Implementation and review of the IFSP involves the coordination and monitoring of the delivery of IFSP supports and services. Periodic reviews are held to facilitate IFSP changes as necessary. These changes may reflect the child's development and any changes, including those that may be medical in nature, that occur in regard to a family's priorities and concerns. IFSP reviews must take place at least once every six months. Annual reviews must be within 365 days of the initial or previous annual IFSP meeting.

Transition

Transition is the entry and exit of children and families to and from early intervention services. This is an ongoing process that begins with the child and family as they enter the system and ends when they transition to another public or private community system when the child turns three years of age. The service coordinator tends to be the provider who is primarily responsible for assisting families through the transition process. All service providers, however, including the SLP and audiologist, should be knowledgeable about the transition process. Transition should be discussed at every IFSP meeting. As the child approaches 30 months of age, the service coordinator should increase the level of detail of these discussions in preparation for the child "aging out" of the early intervention system at the age of three years. Children transitioning from early intervention include those who no longer qualify for Part C supports and services prior to the age of three years, children who are turning three years and whose parents do not want to pursue Part B services, and/or children who are between two and three years of age and are preparing to transition to Part B services.

Transition plans look different for each child and are dependent on the child's and family's needs. Regardless of where the child transitions, there may be an adjustment for the child and family when leaving the Part C system. You may be able to help the family with this adjustment by discussing the process and being prepared to answer any questions about the transition from Part C services to preschool services (IDEA Part B).

Service Coordination

Under IDEA 2004 Part C, service coordination is defined as an active, ongoing process that assists and enables families to access services and ensures their rights and procedural safeguards. Part C mandates that every family in the early intervention system receives service coordination at no cost. It is the responsibility of the service coordinator to ensure that children and their families receive the following:

- A multidisciplinary evaluation and assessment
- An IFSP
- Provision of services in natural environments
- Service coordination

In some states, the speech-language pathologist or audiologist, as a member of the IFSP team, may assume the functions of the service coordinator. When you are not responsible for the service coordination role, it is still imperative that you have an understanding of this role within the system to effectively collaborate with the service coordinator.

The service coordinator's primary function is to serve as the single point of contact for the family throughout the early intervention process. Service coordinators help the family identify and obtain needed services and assistance. Often, the service coordinator also acts as the initial point of contact and may therefore play the important role of assisting the family as they begin to understand and process the nature of their child's disability and needs. The family's first interactions with the service coordinator may have a significant influence on their level of trust and expectations of the early intervention system as a whole (Dunst, 2002).

Once a referral has been made for early intervention services, a service coordinator is assigned to the family as quickly as possible and becomes actively involved in the IFSP process. Table 16–4 illustrates the tasks that a service coordinator must accomplish efficiently and effectively.

The service coordinator supports the family members as they develop, implement, and monitor their intervention plan based on the IFSP. Service coordinators help families develop the knowledge and skills necessary to advocate for their children in the future. Service coordinators also access and coordinate resources and services for families. Ultimately, the service coordinator must ensure that the early intervention services are family-centered and collaborative among the multidisciplinary team members. When service coordination is not effective, families may not have a strong understanding of their child's strengths or needs. They may be left to coordinate information and services from multiple sources on their own. In this case, intervention and transition are likely to be fragmented, and the family may be unaware of all available resources (ASHA, 2008b). All service providers must communicate regularly with assigned service coordinators to ensure cohesion between their services and the needs of the children and families.

TABLE 16–4 Initial Service Coordination Tasks

- Families are informed of their rights, procedural safeguards, and various time lines as specified by Part C of IDEA 2004.
- Families are informed that a primary purpose of early intervention is to assist them as they support their child's development.
- A collaborative relationship is initiated with the families.
- Information about family priorities, resources, and concerns, as well as daily routines and activities, is collected.
- The family's problem-solving skills are supported as a course of action begins to develop.
- Families and other team members plan the developmental evaluation/assessment, formulate questions that reflect the family's concerns, and consider state eligibility standards.
- Information from various sources is compiled and integrated in order to develop a comprehensive developmental profile of the child.
- Communication among and between the various team members and the family is facilitated in order to develop functional and meaningful outcomes based on the family's and child's daily routines and activities.
- Communication and collaboration among team members are maintained to ensure that outcomes are being addressed.
- Services are monitored to ensure that functional and natural activities are being utilized to address outcomes.
- Consistent evaluation and review of the IFSP ensure that the services specified in the IFSP are being conducted.
- The transition plan from the early intervention system (IDEA 2004 Part C) to the school-based system (IDEA 2004 Part B) is coordinated.

Based on information from ASHA (2008b)

The Team Approach

The early intervention system relies heavily on a team approach to service delivery. In addition to working closely with family members, SLPs and audiologists need to collaborate with service coordinators, specialists within other domains, and educators. Regardless of the level of severity of a child's or family's needs, services in early intervention include all types of resources or supports that the child needs and is eligible to receive (ASHA, 2008b). When team members communicate well with one another, all participants reap the benefits from the comprehensive services. Access to all necessary supports and services, the provision of skills and resources from multiple agencies, and the sharing of information and opinions across areas of expertise are just a few of the benefits of teams collaborating within the system.

The integration of services, including the coordination of the team members, is critical to the effective nature of early intervention. Effective coordination and collaboration among team members are essential elements of family-centered practices (Dinnebeil, Hale, & Rule, 1996). As discussed earlier, the roles and responsibilities of the service coordinator are central to successful communication among the early intervention team members. Part C of IDEA 2004 requires that members of the IFSP team coordinate their approaches, consult with one another, and recognize that the child and family outcomes are a responsibility to be shared by the entire team. Collaboration is dependent upon the type of team model that is used, the lead agency's program guidelines, and the knowledge and skills of the individual team members (ASHA, 2008b). Although collaboration among team members may vary, professional communication with the family is essential.

Part C of IDEA 2004 uses the term *multidisciplinary* to describe the early intervention team approach. Other team models may be applied, however, depending on the needs of the child and family. Three team models are commonly used within early intervention. In addition to multidisciplinary teams, interdisciplinary and transdisciplinary team models may be options within the local and/or state service delivery systems. Each one of these teams is different in regard to the amount of communication and coordination required among team members (Paul-Brown & Caperton, 2001). Regardless of the model chosen, SLPs and audiologists are often integral members of early intervention teams.

Multidisciplinary Teams In a multidisciplinary approach, service providers from different disciplines (i.e., physical therapy, occupational therapy, and audiology) assess and/or provide intervention to the family and child separately. Each provider completes an evaluation and/or assessment and makes recommendations independently of the other disciplines. Although several providers may be involved with the family, each professional works distinctly and separately in providing services. Team members therefore focus on their own disciplines and subsequent perspectives and do not tend to engage in collaborative planning or service provision. The service coordinator is typically a designated position within this type of team. Unfortunately, because collaboration among team members is often limited, cohesion of services may be affected (Paul & Roth, 2010).

Interdisciplinary Teams Interdisciplinary teams have a greater focus on collaboration and communication. Typically, providers from various disciplines conduct the evaluation and/or assessment with the child and family individually; occasionally, an "arena" method of evaluation, in which multiple team members are present during the evaluation and/or assessment, may also be conducted. The team members then communicate with one another and integrate the findings to determine the needs, recommendations, and services for the child and his/her family (Paul & Roth, 2010).

Transdisciplinary Teams The transdisciplinary team model involves a greater degree of collaboration among team members than the other service models. This approach is often more difficult to implement because of the need for increased collaboration and communication. It is the model, however, that is identified in IDEA for the design and delivery of services for children with multiple needs and their families (Paul, Blosser, & Jakubowitz, 2006).

The transdisciplinary approach requires the team members to share roles and systematically cross discipline boundaries. The purpose of the approach is to pool and integrate the expertise of team members so that more efficient and comprehensive assessment and intervention services are provided. Communication among team members involves continuous give and take between all members on a consistent basis. Evaluation and assessment, as well as intervention services, are typically conducted jointly by designated members of the team family; one team member will then serve as the primary service provider and will provide direct services that relate to all of the developmental disciplines for the child and family (Paul & Roth, 2010; Paul et al., 2006).

SERVICES BASED ON EVIDENCE

Part C services under IDEA were created to enhance the development of infants and toddlers with disabilities, to minimize potential developmental delay, and to reduce educational costs to society by minimizing the need for continuing special education services as children with disabilities reach school age (IDEA 2004, § 1400(20)). Children grow and develop differently and at their own pace. Decades of research support the fact that the period from birth to age three is a critical time in a child's development and an important time for parents to have accurate information and consistent support close at hand (Center on the Developing Child at Harvard University [CDCHU], 2008, 2010).

Research has shown that a child's earliest experiences play a critical role in brain development. It is therefore crucial that services are provided during these early years (CDCHU, 2008). According to the CDCHU (2008, 2010), neural circuits, including those that create the foundation for learning, behavior, and health, are the most flexible during the first three years of life. The findings also indicate that early social/emotional development and physical health provide the foundation upon which both cognitive and language skills develop. Positive early experiences that involve stable relationships with responsive adults within safe and supportive environments and appropriate nutritional opportunities are all key elements of healthy brain development (CDCHU, 2010). Services have been shown to positively influence outcomes across developmental domains, including health, language and communication, cognition, and social/emotional well-being of infants and toddlers who have disabilities or are at risk for developmental delays (ASHA, 2008b; Branson & Demchak, 2009; CDCHU, 2010; Hebbeler et al., 2007; Joint Committee on Infant Hearing, 2007; Landa, Holman, O'Neill, & Stuart, 2010; McLean & Cripe, 1997; Ward, 1999).

Benefits of Part C services to society also include reducing economic burden through later academic success and a decreased need for special education in the school years (Hebbeler, 2009). Therefore, intervention is likely to be more effective and less costly when it is provided earlier rather than later in life. These research findings underscore the importance of intervention in the earliest years and support the impact of IDEA 2004 Part C services on children, families, and society as a whole.

OTHER CONSIDERATIONS FOR EARLY INTERVENTION SERVICES IN NATURAL ENVIRONMENTS

When intervening with families, SLPs and audiologists must be able to establish and maintain rapport as well as professional boundaries; gather information; and handle difficult situations, including reporting suspected child abuse and neglect. SLPs and audiologists must also be flexible in their approaches to these activities, as each family requires a unique approach to benefit from early intervention.

General Safety

Providing best practices and quality intervention is your priority as an SLP or audiologist in early intervention. Since these best practices mean providing services primarily in families' homes and community settings, it is important for you to consider your personal safety and other issues unique to providing services outside of clinic or center-based settings. Visiting families in natural environments means that you are often on your own in unfamiliar locations. Be sure to let others know your schedule, including when you will be at specific locations. It is also a good idea to keep your cell phone with you on intervention visits for safety purposes; remember, however, to keep the ringer turned off in respect for the family that you are visiting. Visit families with another staff person in certain situations, when you find that you are uncomfortable on your own or as deemed appropriate. Maintaining your own safety ensures that you will have the opportunity to share your knowledge and skills with families. Table 16–5 provides additional safety tips for early intervention visits in natural environments.

TABLE 16–5 Safety Tips for Visits in Natural Environments

- Always keep a cell phone with you on visits in natural environments.
- Be aware of your clothing, avoiding heels and revealing clothing, and limit jewelry.
- Do not take a purse into a family's home. Put your purse or any personal belongings in the trunk of the car prior to arriving at your destination.
- Clearly document your visits, particularly if anything or anyone makes you uncomfortable or causes you concern. Discuss these concerns with your supervisor immediately.
- Make early intervention visits in pairs to areas where safety is a concern.
- If unidentified people are in the environment, ask the family members what their relationship is to the child. If you are uncomfortable in their presence, ask the familiar family member(s) to request that they leave.
- Avoid making visits on Friday afternoons or on the first or last day of the month to areas where safety is a concern (as the arrival of paychecks or federal aid checks may cause an increase in the number of people in the area). Consider morning visits to these areas whenever possible.
- Survey the area thoroughly before leaving the car or the home; look all around for any signs of danger.
- Park on the street rather than in the driveway (to ensure that you will not be blocked in).
- When walking to your car, have your keys available.
- Make eye contact and be friendly with people as you walk to/from a family's home; become a familiar face in the neighborhoods in which you provide services.
- Be aware of your limits and ask for help when needed. Trust your instincts; if you feel uncomfortable in a home or in a situation, excuse yourself and leave.

Based on information from Partnership for People with Disabilities (2010)

Maintaining Professional Boundaries

Establishing and maintaining a relationship with families while upholding professional boundaries can be tricky for the SLP and audiologist. To build rapport, sharing some personal information can be helpful when getting to know the family. Knowing what is appropriate to share, how much, and how to handle situations when families want more information about you are important considerations when working closely with families. Another aspect of maintaining professional boundaries involves knowing how far to become involved in a family member's personal life. Parents often share a great deal about their lives with the SLP or audiologist, particularly when under challenging circumstances. It is ultimately your responsibility to know when you are becoming too involved. When professional boundaries are crossed, it becomes difficult to serve the family objectively and in a manner that makes them feel empowered to help themselves.

Reporting Child Abuse and Neglect

Early intervention personnel, including SLPs and audiologists, are mandated reporters of suspected child abuse or neglect in most states. Therefore, it is important that you become familiar with how to make a report in your area, what information Child Protective Services (CPS) needs, and any documentation required when making a report. You should also be aware of internal policies within your agency for making CPS reports. Refer to Chapter 23 for additional considerations regarding child abuse and neglect.

TABLE 16–6 Considerations to Increase Comfort in an Unclean Environment

- Wear dark clothing that can be easily laundered.
- Keep a change of clothing in the car.
- Keep hand sanitizer in the car and approved disinfecting wipes in the trunk to clean any toys or materials after the visit.
- Sanitize all toys between visits. Avoid using toys or materials that cannot be cleaned easily.
- Bring a small blanket or table cloth to spread out on the floor, providing an area on which everyone can play.
- Remember that you are in someone's home, and although it may not be as clean as your standards, it may suit the family's standards.
- Recognize that if the unclean environment is truly a health hazard to the child (i.e., roaches in the child's bedroom or spoiled formula in the infant's bottle), you will need to communicate with the family about the issue and offer to assist in finding a solution. If the family is unable or unwilling to take action to correct the health hazard, you may need to file a CPS report.

Based on information from Partnership for People with Disabilities (2010)

Managing an Unclean Environment

Each environment in which you provide services may present a different level of cleanliness. The challenge that faces you is to maintain the balance between respect for the family and comfort for yourself while providing services in these environments. Table 16–6 provides some considerations to increase your comfort while providing family-centered services.

SUMMARY

Early intervention is a federally mandated system that operates under the Individuals with Disabilities Education Improvement Act (IDEA). The system, which has been restructured multiple times since its inception in 1997, authorizes services to meet the needs of infants and toddlers, from birth to age three years who have been or may be at risk for developmental delays or disabilities, and their families. In 2008, ASHA presented four guiding principles that reflect best practices for SLPs and audiologists who are providing early intervention services to young children and their families. This chapter presented each of these principles and discussed how each may be effectively implemented by the SLP and audiologist within the early intervention system. Cultural competence, including the definitions and the considerations that influence the provision of effective and appropriate services, was addressed. This chapter defined family-centered practices, based on the family systems theory, and presented the importance of considering and incorporating natural environments into the provision of early intervention services. Each step of the early intervention process, including considerations regarding eligibility and the creation of the IFSP, was also presented and discussed. The chapter also outlined the team approach to early intervention and the different team formats, including the basic considerations of each type of team. Finally, the chapter offered general advice for providing best practices within natural environments and suggestions for establishing a positive and safe work environment.

CRITICAL THINKING

1. Discuss the four guiding principles that reflect current best practices in early intervention. How does each principle impact the role of the speech-language pathologist and the audiologist in the early intervention arena? Provide a scenario of how each one can be implemented in practice.
2. Describe a speech-language pathologist's or audiologist's role and level of involvement in regard to each of the seven components of the early intervention process.
3. The speech-language pathologist or audiologist may occasionally be responsible for coordinating an IFSP meeting. What extra duties will the speech-language pathologist or audiologist be responsible for in this situation?
4. Provide an example scenario based on the eight suggestions (other than active listening) for building positive relationships with families in the early intervention system.
5. In your own words, explain the differences between multidisciplinary, interdisciplinary, and transdisciplinary team approaches. Which one is the most effective when providing family-centered early intervention services? Explain.
6. Why do speech-language pathologists and audiologists need to be familiar with cultural competence? Provide a scenario in which a speech-language pathologist or audiologist is *not* demonstrating cultural competence with a child and family. What can the speech-language pathologist or audiologist do differently to correct the situation?
7. Speech-language pathologists and audiologists with the best intentions often have difficulty designing services that are both family-centered and routines-based. Read the following scenarios and answer the following questions for each one:
    a. What is missing from each of these situations? What else should be considered?
    b. How would you change these practices to make them more family-centered?
    c. What would you do to ensure that these sessions are routines-based?

    Scenario 1: As Joey's mom works on a few chores in the kitchen, the speech-language pathologist explains and demonstrates how Joey's sitting can be supported when he is watching television in the evenings with his family.

    Scenario 2: Jenna's father, Tony, has a neatly organized home, is systematic in accomplishing daily tasks, and is quite directive in his interaction style with Jenna. During the initial home visit, the speech-language pathologist suggests that Tony consider using more open-ended questions and arranging Jenna's toys on shelves in various rooms throughout the house to promote communication initiations from Jenna.

    Scenario 3: Candace has bilateral cochlear implants and uses both sign language and vocalizations to communicate. Her parents have requested that the audiologist visit her at home as well as at her child care center; they want both services to be coordinated to ensure that the routines and coaching strategies are consistent across the natural environments. Her child care teacher believes in a child-directed play approach and does not believe in coaching or adult direction. She wants Candace to be pulled out of her classroom to receive special education services with the audiologist and speech-language pathologist because, as she states, she "doesn't have time to work with her individually during every routine."
8. As a clinician doing early intervention, you are likely to go into homes from a variety of cultures and with varying child-rearing practices. What should you do to prepare for this experience?
9. You are likely to be working with a variety of other professionals when you provide assessment and therapy services to children and families through early intervention. Who are these other professionals? What are their roles in EI? What should you do to work effectively in a team context?
10. What ethical dilemmas might you face in working as a professional in an early intervention context? How would you resolve these?

REFERENCES

American Speech-Language-Hearing Association. (2007). *ASHA SLP Health Care Survey 2007: Caseload characteristics.* Rockville, MD: Author.

American Speech-Language-Hearing Association. (2008a). *Core knowledge and skills in early intervention speech-language pathology practice.* Available from http://www.asha.org/policy

American Speech-Language-Hearing Association. (2008b). *Roles and responsibilities of speech-language pathologists in early intervention: Guidelines.* Available from http://www.asha.org/policy

Balthrop, C., & Coleman, W. (2003, March). *Why is Suzy so weird? Understanding cultural differences in the classroom.* Paper presented at the meeting of the Virginia Association for Early Childhood.

Benn, R. (1994). Conceptualizing eligibility for early intervention services. In D. M. Bryant & M. A. Graham (Eds.), *Implementing early intervention* (pp. 18–45). New York, NY: Guilford Press.

Branson, D., & Demchak, M. (2009). The use of augmentative and alternative communication methods with infants and toddlers with disabilities: A research review. *Augmentative & Alternative Communication, 25*, 274–286.

Brown, W., & Brown, C. (1993). Defining eligibility for early intervention. In W. Brown, S. K. Thurman, & F. Pearl (Eds.), *Family-centered early intervention with infants and toddlers: Innovative cross-disciplinary approaches* (pp. 21–42). Baltimore, MD: Paul H. Brookes.

Center on the Developing Child at Harvard University. (2008). *InBrief: The science of early childhood development.* Retrieved from http://developingchild.harvard.edu/download_file/-/view/64/

Center on the Developing Child at Harvard University. (2010). *The foundations of lifelong health are built in early childhood.* Available from http://developingchild.harvard.edu/library/reports_and_working_papers/foundatins-of-lifelong-health/

Data Accountability Center. (2010). *Part C child count: 2009.* Available from https://www.IDEIAdata.org/arc_toc11.asp#partcCC

Dinnebeil, L. A., Hale, L. M., & Rule, S. (1996). A qualitative analysis of parents' and service coordinators' descriptions of variables that influence collaborative relationships. *Topics in Early Childhood Special Education, 16*, 322–347.

Dunst, C. J. (2002). Family-centered practices: Birth through high school. *Journal of Special Education, 36*(3), 139–147.

Dunst, C. J., Bruder, M. B., Trivette, C. M., Hamby, D., Raab, M., & McLean, M. (2001). Characteristics and consequences of everyday natural learning opportunities. *Topics in Early Childhood Special Education, 21*(2), 68–91.

Garcia Coll, C., & Magnuson, K. (2000). Cultural differences as sources of developmental vulnerabilities and resources. In J. P. Shonkoff & S. J. Meisels (Eds.), *Handbook of early childhood intervention* (2nd ed., pp. 94–114). Cambridge, UK: Cambridge University Press.

Hanft, B. E., Rush, D. D., & Shelden, M. L. (2004). *Coaching families and colleagues in early childhood.* Baltimore, MD: Paul H. Brookes.

Hanson, M. J., & Lynch, E. W. (1990). Honoring the cultural diversity of families when gathering data. *Topics in Early Childhood Special Education, 10*(1), 112–132.

Hebbeler, K. (2009). *First five years fund briefing.* Presentation given at a Congressional briefing on June 11, 2009, to discuss *Education that works: The impact of early childhood intervention on reducing the need for special education services.* Retrieved from http://www.sri.com/neils/pdfs/FFYF_Briefing_Hebbeler_June2009_test.pdf

Hebbeler, K., Spiker, D., Bailey, D., Scarborough, A., Mallik, S., Simeonsoon, R., et al. (2007). *Early intervention for infants & toddlers with disabilities and their families: Participants, services, and outcomes. Final report of the National Early Intervention Longitudinal Study (NEILS).* Retrieved from http://www.sri.com/neils/pdfs/NEILS_Report_02_07_Final2.pdf

Individuals with Disabilities Education Improvement Act of 2004, Pub. L. No. 108-446, § 632, 118 Stat. 2744 (2004).

Infant & Toddler Connection of Virginia. (2003). *Individualized Part C early intervention supports and services in everyday routines, activities and places*. Available from http://www.infantva.org

Joint Committee on Infant Hearing. (2007). Year 2007 position statement: Principles and guidelines for early hearing detection and intervention programs. *Pediatrics, 120*(4), 898–921.

Jung, L. A., & Grisham-Brown, J. (2006). Moving from assessment information to IFSPs: Guidelines for a family-centered process. *Young Exceptional Children, 9*(2), 2–11.

Kashinath, S., Woods, J., & Goldstein, H. (2006). Enhancing generalized teaching strategy use in daily routines by parents of children with autism. *Journal of Speech, Language, and Hearing Research, 49,* 466–485.

Landa, R., Holman, K., O'Neill, A., & Stuart, E. (2010). Intervention targeting development of socially synchronous engagement in toddlers with autism spectrum disorder: A randomized controlled trial. *Journal of Child Psychology and Psychiatry, 52*(1), 13–21.

McLean, L., & Cripe, J. (1997). The effectiveness of early intervention for children with communication disorders. In M. J. Guralnick (Ed.), *The effectiveness of early intervention* (pp. 349–428). Baltimore, MD: Paul H. Brookes.

McWilliam, R. A. (2004). Early intervention where it counts: Natural environments. *All Together Now! 10*(3), 3–6.

Partnership for People with Disabilities. (2010). *Kaleidoscope: New perspectives in service coordination* [Trainer's notebook]. Virginia Commonwealth University: Author.

Paul, D., Blosser, J., & Jakubowitz, M. (2006). Principles and challenges for forming successful literacy partnerships. *Topics in Language Disorders, 26*(1), 5–23.

Paul, D., & Roth, F. (2010). Guiding principles and clinical applications for speech-language pathology practice in early intervention [Electronic version]. *Language, Speech, and Hearing Services in Schools,* Article 10.1044/0161-1461(2010/09-0079).

Paul-Brown, D., & Caperton, C. J. (2001). Inclusive practices for preschool-aged children with specific language impairment. In M. J. Guralnick (Ed.), *Early childhood inclusion: Focus on change* (pp. 433–463). Baltimore, MD: Paul H. Brookes.

Peña, E., & Fiestas, C. (2009). Talking across cultures in early intervention: Finding common ground to meet children's communication needs. *Perspectives on Communication Disorders and Sciences in Culturally and Linguistically Diverse Populations, 16,* 79–85.

Saldaña, D. (2001) *Cultural competency: A practical guide for mental health service providers*. Austin, TX: Hogg Foundation for Mental Health.

McWilliam, R. A. (2005). DEC recommended practices: Interdisciplinary models (Introduction). In S. Sandall, M. L. Hemmeter, B. J. Smith, & M. E. McLean (Eds.), *DEC recommended practices: A comprehensive guide for practical application in early intervention/early childhood special education.* Missoula, MT: DEC.

Shelden, M. L., & Rush, D. D. (2001). The ten myths about providing early intervention services in natural environments. *Infants and Young Children, 14*(1), 1–13.

SpecialQuest Multimedia Training Library. (2007). *Creating bright futures: Building relationships with families* [Facilitator's guide]. Retrieved from http://ncoe.pointinspace.com/trainingmaterials/searchsessions_resultsdetail.lasso?-Search=Action&-Table=webpackages&-Database=NCO_Hilton_TrainingMaterials&-KeyValue=6

Ward, S. (1999). An investigation into the effectiveness of an early intervention method for delayed language development in young children. *International Journal of Language & Communication Disorders, 34*(3), 243–264.

Wayman, K., & Lynch, E. W. (1991). Home-based early childhood services: Cultural sensitivity in a family systems approach. *Topics in Early Childhood Special Education, 10*(4), 56–76.

Woods, J., Kashinath, S., & Goldstein, H. (2004). Effects of embedding caregiver-implemented teaching strategies in daily routines on children's communication outcomes. *Journal of Early Intervention, 26*(3), 175–193.

17

Service Delivery Issues in Private Practice

Kenneth E. Wolf, PhD

SCOPE OF CHAPTER

Private practice, regardless of the profession or discipline, at one time was fairly easy to understand, namely working independently for oneself in one's own office. That simple definition has been broadened over the past 20-plus years. Currently, private practice describes those who work for themselves, work full or part time for others and then for themselves after hours, contract with other professionals and work in a variety of locations, have a single business location, supply professional staff to other agencies and corporations that require services, and serve as consultants. And the list goes on. Just about any type of service offered by a speech-language pathologist or audiologist may fall within the realm of private practice. The common denominator is the person(s) who owns the business and is ultimately responsible for all of its aspects, including business, professional services, practice standards, and obligations.

Private practice appeals to those of you who desire employment autonomy—being your own boss and taking the ultimate risk and responsibility for economic and professional success. Private practice has often been associated with the health care environment, as that was the primary focus of the service delivery base. Today, however, private practice goes beyond health care, extending into the educational arena as well. Therefore, many of the service delivery issues described in the health care and education settings need to be fully understood and may have significant implications for the private practitioner. You are referred to other chapters in this text for additional information regarding other work settings.

A recent survey by the American Speech-Hearing-Language Association (ASHA, 2009a) revealed that 15.8 percent of its members were engaged in private practice at the end of 2009 (6.3 percent full time and 9.5 percent part time). Those who are employed in such settings will likely face issues similar to those faced by other health care and education employees. Owners of private practices, although confronted with comparable issues, have even greater responsibility, with prosperity and survival the overriding concerns.

This chapter cannot address all aspects of private practice. ASHA (1991a, 1991b, 2004a, 2010a, 2011b, 2011f), the American Academy of Audiology (AAA), and the American Academy of Private Practice in Speech-Language Pathology and Audiology (AAPPSLPA) provide valuable information about initiating and working in a private practice (see the Resources section). Rather, this chapter provides you with an overview of key issues to be considered by those who work in private practice environments. Included is a discussion of the practitioner confronting business and professional issues and how these issues may differ from those in other work settings. The chapter concludes with consideration of issues that have emerged or are about to emerge that will influence speech-language pathologists and audiologists in private practice.

SERVICE DELIVERY ISSUES IN PRIVATE PRACTICE

Although private practice offers many alluring features, it also holds some obvious and hidden pitfalls (Currie, 2004). Entering private practice requires speech-language pathologists and audiologists to actively and honestly self-evaluate their personal skills, talents, likes and dislikes, and knowledge of business and the business climate, all in addition to addressing the challenges of their profession (American Academy of Audiology [AAA], 2008b; ASHA, 2003c; Currie, 2004; Dougherty, 2008; Goffinet, 2005). Table 17–1 offers some basic questions about oneself and business in general that should be approached honestly

TABLE 17–1 Basic Questions Before Starting a Private Practice

Questions to Ask Yourself

- Do I enjoy working alone?
- Do I have the knowledge and skills to work independently?
- Do I have the skills to manage the stress of owning my own practice?
- Do I understand the people whom I will serve and the community in which I will have my practice?

Business Questions to Ask

- Do I know the need for private practice in the community in which I will work?
- Do I know the financial climate in the community in which I will work?
- Are there small-business support groups in the community that I can turn to for advice?
- What are the financial requirements for starting and maintaining a private practice?
- What types of payments and reimbursement schedules are available and needed to support the practice?
- What are my long-term financial needs?

Adapted from *Starting a Private Practice,* by P. S. Currie, 2004. Available from http://www.audiology online.com/

before the audiologist or speech-language pathologist commits to starting a private practice. Then speech-language pathologists or audiologists who decide to enter private practice will understand that they immediately assume a role greater than that of service provider. They must think and perform as a businessperson, an administrator, a clinician, probably a supervisor, and possibly a teacher and/or researcher as well. As such, establishing a private practice requires advanced thinking and questioning.

Private Practice Options

One of the first decisions a professional must make is whether to enter private practice on a full-time or part-time basis. The percentage of speech-language pathologists and audiologists working in full-time private practice had been relatively stable for nearly 20 years: 6 to 8 percent of the speech-language pathologists and 20 to 30 percent of the audiologists. During the same period (1986–2003), there was a slight downward trend in the percentages engaged in part-time private practice: 10 to 22 percent of the speech-language pathologists and 7 to 16 percent of the audiologists (Zingeser, 2005). Comparisons of the *ASHA Counts for 2004* (reported by Wolf, 2007) with the most recent *ASHA Year End 2009* show a slight decrease of about 2 percent in those participating in private practice (about 1 percent decline for audiologists and speech-language pathologists each). Unfortunately, the data that identify those who limit their work activity to part time versus those engaged in part-time private practice as a supplement to their primary or other employment are not available.

The important issue is that private practice may offer greater flexibility for the individual who cannot work full time. Some professionals may want or need flexible scheduling, and others may wish to "moonlight" to generate additional income. Regardless of full- or part-time status, those who enter private practice must treat such a venture with the same dedication and commitment as they would any business venture. Such commitment is critical to the individual's success and to the way one is viewed by peers and professional colleagues. Respect will only come from exhibiting the highest level of professionalism. The remainder of this chapter addresses issues from the perspective of the full-time practitioner-owner; however, the information may easily be applied to those who engage in part-time private practice.

Private practice offers professional and business autonomy, without the requisite accountability to a boss or supervisor. However, accountability of performance may be even greater than that of an employee. As a private practitioner, the final responsibility for all decisions and performances rests with the practitioner. Income is dependent on services being delivered in a timely and appropriate manner, and thus all absences (e.g., illness, vacation, or other emergency) must be covered, just as they would in any other employment setting. Financial obligations (e.g., monthly bills, salaries, taxes, other expenditures) associated with the practice must be honored. This often means additional work for private practitioners beyond their clinical service delivery hours or the hiring of employees to perform these functions. In short, a successful private practice entails numerous nonbillable activities.

Solo or Affiliated Practice One of the first decisions to be made is the type of business structure that the practice will assume. A private practice assumes one of four legal organizational structures: sole proprietorship, partnership, limited liability company (LLC), or corporation (ASHA, 2011b; U.S. Small Business Administration, 2011). *Sole proprietorship* is a business run by one individual for his or her own benefit and does not exist apart from the owner. *Partnership* is a business owned by two or more people and may be either general or limited. General partnership is an agreement between two or more people to join together to carry on a business venture for profit, with each partner contributing money, property, labor, or skill and receiving equal shares of profit or loss and unlimited personal liability for the debts of the business. Limited partnerships limit personal liability for the debt of the business to the amount invested by the partner. *Limited liability company (LLC)* is a hybrid between a partnership and a corporation. Members of an LLC have operational and income benefits that are similar to a partnership, but with limited liability. *Corporation* is a legal entity whose scope of activity and its name are restricted by its charter and must be granted permission to operate under the laws of that state. The corporation, not the owners and the managers, is liable for the debts and taxes. In a C corporation, there are taxes on the profits and taxes on the stockholders' dividends, commonly called double taxation. An S corporation is a special closed corporation to provide small businesses a tax advantage (if certain regulations are met) to avoid the double

TABLE 17–2 Primary Advantages and Disadvantages of Four Types of Business Entities

Sole Proprietorship	Partnership	Limited Liability Company	Corporations
Advantages	**Advantages**	**Advantages**	**Advantages**
• Simple • Minimum legal restrictions • Ease of discontinuance • Owner is truly the boss	• Greater availability of capital • Greater resources for decision making, support, and creative activity	• Greatest flexibility for customizing the structure • Limits member liability • In states allowing only one member, benefits of sole proprietorship but limited liability	• Limited liability to stockholders • Perpetual life of the corporation • Ease of transferring ownership • Ease of expansion of the corporation
Disadvantages	**Disadvantages**	**Disadvantages**	**Disadvantages**
• Difficult to raise capital • Limited life of the business • Unlimited liability	• Unlimited liability in general partnership • Divided authority among the partners	• Comprehensive operating agreement because of high degree of variability and flexibility	• Government regulations • Higher costs to organize • Corporation is limited to operate in state chartered unless permission granted from other states • Double taxation (corporate and personal) unless S corporation

Adapted from *Frequently Asked Questions about Business Practices*, American Speech-Language-Hearing Association, 2011b. Available from http://www.asha.org/

taxation. Dougherty (2008) shares her experiences with the different types of entities and strongly recommends consulting with an attorney and/or accountant before choosing a business structure. The advantages and disadvantages of each entity are summarized in Table 17–2. ASHA (2011b) offers a discussion of business practices on its website.

One of the first issues to be considered is the decision between solo practice or affiliation with another professional(s) either as a partnership or other working agreement. Such an affiliation may be with another speech-language pathologist, audiologist, physician, health care provider, or educator, assuming the affiliation does not violate any legal statutes of a particular state. Such a decision is based, at least in part, on other factors described in this chapter, but also on one's own goals, objectives, personality, and answers to the basic questions posed in Table 17–1. Equally important is to know when a partnership is not successful (professionally, philosophically, financially) and needs to be terminated for the sake of all concerned. Zingeser (2005) reported that 60 percent of speech-language pathologists in private practice were solo, and those in group practices were nearly equally divided between group practices that were exclusively communicative disorders professionals or included other disciplines. Audiologists were less likely to be in solo practices (48 percent), but those in group practices tended to be with other audiologists or speech-language pathologists. Solo versus affiliated practice must be considered fully in business terms and based on legal and professional advantages and disadvantages.

Location The location of the practice is important. Will it be a freestanding independent practice or located within another practice site? If it is to be an independent practice, should it be in a specific type of building with potential referral sources as tenants, or might the goals and objectives of the practice be equally or better accomplished in another location that offers a greater degree of traffic (self-referral), easier patient/client access, or lower rent? For example, if the primary objective is to sell hearing aids, the practice should be located in an accessible area, preferably on the first floor, with appropriate signage and visibility for walk-up traffic to maximize opportunities for self-referrals. Lower rents at a strip mall may be more advantageous than a more expensive medical building. Conversely, if the practice is expected to focus more on diagnostic audiology, then a location in a medical building in reasonable proximity to referring physicians may be necessary. Zingeser (2005) reported that speech-language pathologists in private practice were most likely to provide services in their clients' homes (59 percent) or in a freestanding clinic or office (34 percent). On the other hand, audiologists in private practice overwhelmingly provided services in a freestanding clinic or office (75 percent) or in a health care setting (25 percent).

If the practice is to be located within another practice, additional considerations are warranted. Will this practice function autonomously within that larger practice, simply renting space or perhaps equipment and/or staff? This is often a way of establishing a practice, building it to a level for eventual relocation or merger with the preexisting practice. The advantage of such an agreement is that some assistance is usually offered, if no more than the affiliation with an ongoing successful practice. Other private practitioners have no physical office space of their own for serving patients/clients, but work as independent contractors providing a service in another professional's facility. In this case, the work activities and responsibilities must be distinct from those of an employee. Practitioners who are independent contractors must at least minimally set their own working hours; have an established rent agreement and/or fee schedule that is charged to the existing practice; carry their own insurances; and meet all other local, state, and federal requirements. The independent contractor and the owner of the practice site must agree on responsibility for equipment ownership and maintenance, supplies, and staff. These agreements are found between audiologists or speech-language pathologists, other health care professionals, or educational facilities.

Business Plan A business plan that details the whats and the hows must be established during the initial development of a private practice. This plan will tell the story of the business (Goffinet, 2005), describing the practice and how it will be financed, marketed, and managed. In other words, the plan will drive what the practice is intended to do and how those intentions will be accomplished. The major elements of a business plan are outlined in Table 17–3. The plan typically delineates such areas as physical, personnel, and financial needs, resources, and strategies. It describes the space, professional and office equipment, supply needs, and personnel requirements. Each item in the plan has some financial implication (cost) that needs to be identified. Pro forma income projections will be needed. Revenue streams and access to patients should also be identified in the plan along with strategies for attracting and building a solid referral base. Without a continuous source of patients/clients, the practice cannot be maintained. This plan should be used in each phase of practice development and should be revisited periodically, at least annually to ensure progress is being achieved in a measurable way. The U.S. Small Business Administration (2011) provides an excellent and comprehensive overview and tutorial for preparing a business plan and how to get started. Business students at a local college or university who are seeking to gain business planning experience may also be a valuable resource (Dougherty, 2008).

Most businesses require start-up capital to launch. That capital is usually acquired through financing and loans. Private practices are indeed businesses, and as such, carry a degree of risk. Commercial lenders, therefore, rarely capitalize 100 percent of a new business, especially in a tight financial atmosphere. At one time, private practices in the health care environment (including medical practices) were considered relatively

TABLE 17–3 Core Elements of a Business Plan

Introduction
- Description
- Ownership and legal structure
- Skills and experience you bring to the business
- Advantages over competitors

Marketing
- Services to be offered
- Customer demand
- Market
- Public relations, planned advertising, and marketing
- Pricing strategy

Financial Management
- Source and amount of equity capital
- Monthly operating budget for first year
- Expected return on investment
- Monthly cash flow for first year
- Projected income statements for first year
- Break-even point
- Methods of compensation
- Maintaining accounting records

Operations
- Day-to-day management
- Personnel
- Insurances and agreements
- Equipment

Concluding Statement
- Summarize goals and objectives
- Review with colleague or consultant
- Approach a lender

Adapted from *Thinking About Starting,* U.S. Small Business Administration, 2011. Available from http://www.sba.gov/category/navigation-structure/starting-managing-business/starting-business/thinking-about-starting

low risk. However, at least in some markets, health care practices have been viewed as a greater risk to lenders than in the past. Funding for loans of all types has become more difficult to secure and does not look to ease in the near future. As a result, lenders are expected to apply greater scrutiny to the review and analysis of the business plan and, where applicable, other documents such as affiliation agreements and/or partnership agreements. Most important, lenders demand evidence of financial commitment and risk sharing on the part of the practitioner. In other words, is the practitioner placing any of his or her finances into the project? Typically, commercial lenders require that the practitioner enter such a venture with at least 10 percent (sometimes 20 percent) of the up-front capital needed to launch the practice.

Licenses, Certification, and Insurances It is understood that practitioners, and those who provide services on their behalf, will hold valid and current licenses to practice their profession as required by the laws of the state(s) in which they are performing services. All 50 states plus the District of Columbia regulate audiologists and speech-language pathologist (ASHA, 2012). Board certification in audiology from the American Board of Audiology (ABA) is recognized for the purpose of expedited licensure in 9 states (Colorado, Florida, Illinois, Ohio, Maryland, Michigan, Minnesota, Virginia, and Washington) (AAA, 2008a). In states where there is no licensure, ASHA certification is the only national credential available. Additionally, ASHA certification is recognized by the Centers for Medicare and Medicaid Services (CMS) as the credential for the provision of speech-language pathology and audiology services. In states with licensure, ASHA certification may not be required. However, the private practitioner is always in competition with other providers to gain access to patients/clients and referral sources. The more credentials you have, the more attractive your practice may be to potential and actual patients/clients and/or referral sources. Thus, even if ASHA certification is not required, it may be viewed as a characteristic that positively distinguishes one practitioner from another. Additional licenses may be required to own, name, and/or operate a business. These licenses may vary depending on the exact nature, structure, and location of the practice and on municipal and/or state regulations.

Insurances are also required. Not only do practitioner-owners need professional liability insurance, but each clinical service provider in their employ does as well. Many provider contracts also proscribe the minimum limits of insurance. Typically, liability insurance in the range of $1 million per occurrence and $3 million to $5 million aggregate are common minimum limits of liability. Proof that liability insurance is currently in effect is a common requirement. Workers' compensation and unemployment insurances are required for all employees. Health and disability insurance will be available only if the practitioner purchases them. Independent contractors are often required to show proof of their own workers' compensation as part of their contractual agreement. Additional insurances are also advisable to protect the practice and its contents from loss due to fire, theft, accident, or other liability.

Specialization It is difficult for individual practitioners to be an expert in all aspects of their profession. Therefore, many elect to limit their practice to a specific area such as dysphagia, aphasia, voice, or stuttering or to a specific age group such as geriatrics or neonatal assessment. Those who limit their practices within these narrowly defined areas often maintain that only those with specialized training and experience can provide the best and most competent services, and such an argument may be valid. Currently, three areas have established Specialty Recognition Boards: child language, fluency, and swallowing and swallowing disorders. Specialty Board recognition is beyond ASHA certification. Holders of such recognition may identify themselves as a *Board Recognized Specialist* in that specialty if they so desire, and such individuals often believe that this label provides a potential marketing advantage over those who are not so recognized (ASHA, 2011f). However, acquisition of specialty recognition is voluntary and is not required for practice in any area or with any specific population group. Other specialty groups outside of ASHA have established their own requirements and offer specialty certification (i.e., the Academy of Neurologic Communication Disorders and Sciences, the American Board of Audiology specialty certification in cochlear implants). Nevertheless, the ASHA Code of Ethics (Principle of Ethics II, Rule B) requires that all clinicians be trained, competent, and experienced in any area of clinical service they perform (ASHA, 2010b). See Chapter 3 for more information on certification and licensure.

Specialization may be desirable for some, but it may also have some disadvantages, particularly as the structures of health care coverage and payment continue to evolve. Regardless, most managed care organizations (MCOs) want to provide services to the greatest number of patients with the least amount of administrative effort, support, and complication (i.e., cost). If an individual or group practice is capable of providing quality and competent services to a broader and more diverse population than those competing for the same contract, the generalists may be viewed more favorably. The advantage to the MCO is a single contract covering all of its needs in a given service area, as opposed to multiple smaller contracts that in the aggregate provide the same total coverage as the single larger contract. The more contracts the MCO must manage, the greater its administrative costs. In other words, restricting specialization too severely may limit access to contracts, patients/clients, and referrals, depending on the market served. If a narrowly defined service area is desirable, specialization definitely should be considered. However, early in the development of a private practice, general practice may be required to facilitate its growth.

Referral Base Practice sites cannot exist without patients/clients who require services. Publicly funded programs, such as public schools and public hospitals, may have greater access to patients/clients, especially for those individuals who cannot or elect not to pay for services out of pocket. Private practices, however, are totally dependent on those who can and will pay for services or who have someone else (e.g., a third party) pay all or the majority of the expenses associated with that service. Thus, the private practice is in competition with the publicly funded service providers and other private group and individual practices. The successful practice must have a plan and mechanism for sustaining patient/client referrals. This should include access to such populations to assess quality of services and effectiveness of marketing strategies.

The changes in funding of health care services over the past 25 years have resulted in access to patients becoming a much larger issue than it once was, especially in markets with high managed care penetration.

The health care industry has evolved from largely individual and solo practices to various configurations of groups and networks to secure access to patients and ensure payment for services. Health maintenance organizations (HMOs), independent practice associations (IPAs), and preferred practice organizations (PPOs) have generally been grouped under MCOs to manage access to and payment for care. The newest iteration is called the accountable care organization (ACO), which like its predecessors manages patient care and payment for services but also adds quality improvement and efficacy metrics for the population as a key component of reimbursement structure. The focus is on value rather than units of service. It is anticipated that there will be only 150 of the new ACOs during the initial three years. At the time of this writing, these new ACOs are in their infancy and will require the test of time to determine effectiveness, but they will influence professionals' access to patients.

When indemnity insurance was the predominant health care coverage mechanism, patients were able to seek services from almost any licensed provider, and their insurance company would reimburse at a reasonable rate. Under the current systems, patients may be obligated to seek services only from paneled or approved providers if they want to receive the maximum coverage benefit. If services are provided by other than a paneled provider, the patient's financial responsibility for that service increases, sometimes dramatically. However, most MCOs do not allow for any willing provider and limit the number of providers per profession as a way of maintaining efficient management of their group. The fewer number of providers they have to deal with in terms of record keeping and payments, the less expensive their administrative costs. Thus, there is competition among providers to be paneled, and without such status, access to patients may be severely compromised (Klontz, Napp, White, & Wolf, 1997; Kreb, 1997; Wolf, 1995).

Private practitioners may join provider networks to maintain or increase their access to patients/clients. Sometimes, there is a fee associated with being a network provider. Some network affiliations (paid for or not) actually mean little more than being listed in a larger book of acceptable providers. None of these affiliations guarantee referrals, only access and possible referrals. One strategy used by some private practices for maintaining access to patients/clients is to form their own provider networks and offer the network to the MCO as a single provider (e.g., Kreb et al., 1995; Napp, 1997). The network maintains its own administrative structure, making referrals, collecting payments, and distributing payments to the providers. A provider network may also offer broader geographic coverage for that profession or specialty, a greater range of subspecialties, faster service, increased ease, and greater flexibility to the patients/clients. These advantages are often reflected in patient/client satisfaction. Additionally, the MCO may still maintain cost containment, having multiple service providers from the network, but only having to maintain and manage a single account to the network. In other words, a significant segment of the administrative overhead is shifted to the network. One disadvantage to the providers within the network is the cost of its maintenance. These costs may require significant monthly fees to the network or still greater reduction in the net reimbursement to the provider. Regardless of the type of network affiliation, without it, access to patients, and possibly the viability of the practice, may be compromised in the current health care environment (ASHA, 2011b).

Staff and Consultants Maintaining a smooth functioning practice requires good business practices and performance. As stated earlier, this often means additional work for private practitioners beyond their clinical service delivery hours (work that is not billable to patients or MCOs) or hiring employees to perform those functions. If the practitioner-owner is devoting most of the working day to providing patient services, no one is available to answer telephones, schedule patients, greet the public, and provide nonpatient-related services. Today's society is dependent on technology. Practice websites and voice mail are the most common technologic applications. However, a high proportion of the public, particularly patients in need of service, prefer to talk to a live person, especially if they are contacting a small business. Patient/client satisfaction is critical to continued patient/client access. Remember, the front door to the practice for the rest of the world is that initial telephone contact, and it provides a lasting impression. Thus, one staff position that should be considered is an office receptionist.

Depending on the size and needs of the practice, other full- or part-time employees may be needed such as a billing clerk or office manager. A trustworthy and knowledgeable accountant and attorney, at least on a part-time or as-needed consulting basis, are also necessary. A banker who works specifically with that particular practice is also valuable. Other consultants to be considered might include a general business manager, marketing and public relations professionals, and investment consultants.

As the practice expands, the professional obligations to provide services may exceed the abilities of a single practitioner-owner. At that time, additional professional colleagues must be considered. If an additional partner is neither planned nor desired, then the only other option is to consider professionals who are either employees or independent contractors. Both have advantages and disadvantages in terms of costs and responsibility to the practice. Employees may be slightly less costly in terms of salary, but they may expect benefits and have other associated costs such as health, workers' compensation, and professional liability insurances; taxes; and holiday, sick leave, and vacation time. Independent contractors may be more expensive for the services they render, but they have none of the other associated costs. In addition, the practice pays contractors only when there is enough work to generate income.

Whether the additional personnel are employees or independent contractors, the practitioner-owner must determine if the additional services are cost-effective. If the additional caseload is to be handled by existing personnel, and there are ample existing resources to do so through excess capacity, then the additional caseload is sound. If the cost of expansion will not cover the additional expenses associated with it or be reasonably justified indirectly, it would seem prudent to forestall such activities and possibly reconsider in the future. If the additional patient/client services produce enough revenue to just meet the additional expenses associated with the expansion, then it becomes a decision for the practitioner-owner to determine if the additional work and responsibility are justified for little or no immediate net economic gain. One factor to consider is the potential gain in terms of goodwill with referral sources and probability of economic gain in the future. Finally, if the expansion is revenue positive and a sound business and professional move, it should be implemented (Wolf, Cohen, & Arnst, 1994). Growth simply for the sake of growth or undertaken too rapidly has been catastrophic and sometimes fatal to small businesses, and private practices are no exception.

Productivity Productivity standards have not been developed for speech-language pathologists and audiologists. The ASHA Omnibus Survey was retired in 2003, but its last issue addressed caseloads in both professions. At that time, speech-language pathologists across health care settings averaged about 5.8 hours (out of 8 hours) per day in patient/client services (ASHA, 2003a). Audiologists average slightly more time: 6.6 hours (out of 8 hours) per day in patient care (ASHA, 2003b). Although these are only averages, they provide an indication of the amount of work expected to maintain a practice. These figures indicate how hours of the workday are allocated but may not be a true indication of productivity. Likewise, the most recent survey reports caseload characteristic trends and distribution of services across disorders and ages rather than on accountability and productivity (ASHA 2009b; ASHA 2010a).

Another aspect of productivity that is almost never mentioned in relation to speech-language pathology and audiology is the ratio of revenue generated to cost to provide that service. In some businesses, this ratio is the major, if not the only, indicator of productivity. The impact of a negative ratio is obvious; no business can survive if it costs more to provide a service than can be generated from providing it. But how large must that ratio be for the service (or employee) to be worthwhile to the practitioner-owner? In some financial businesses and professions, it is not unrealistic to expect and demand employees to generate revenues that are four to eight times their annual salary (i.e., 4:1 or 8:1). An informal survey of some speech-language pathology practice sites, including private practices, indicated that the ratio of revenue generated to cost expenditures is more likely to be less than 2:1. Those types of productivity ratios are critically important to the financial viability of a small business such as a private practice (Wolf, 2007). Another type of productivity indicator will be examined later in the chapter under the discussion of evidence-based practice and benchmarks.

Other Issues

Other issues that affect your ability to run an effective, efficient, and productive private practice include payment for services, evidence-based practice, implementation science, information technology, the creation of value for clients, cultural competence, ethical values, research and education, and volunteerism.

Payment for Services The structure of the health care payment landscape has changed drastically over the past four decades. Presidents dating back to Nixon and then Clinton have tried and failed to bring about health care reform. The existing public/private system resulted in an estimated 46 million Americans without health insurance coverage and an additional 23 million who were underinsured. The United States spends approximately twice as much per capita on health care as any other industrialized nation while ranking low in terms of health outcomes. The first comprehensive health care reform bill, the Patient Protection and Affordable Care Act (PPACA), was signed into law on March 23, 2010. As it is phased in over the next few years, it promises to expand health care coverage, increase consumer choice, and ban insurance discrimination for preexisting conditions (Connors & Gostin, 2010).

Historically, the traditional system was based on a retrospective payment model, in which services were provided and the practitioner received payment for those services *after* the fact—thus, the term *retrospective fee-for-service reimbursement.* The financial risks for health care fell mainly on the payer in a retrospective fee-for-service model, even with significant preestablished discounts. Although it began earlier, the 1990s witnessed a strong movement toward a prospective payment or capitated system. Under capitation, the provider agrees to accept a flat or fixed per-member, per-month (PMPM) premium, paid in advance, for a guaranteed number of covered lives or enrollees, usually for several thousand lives. The provider also agrees that any member of that covered population group who needs such services, regardless of the actual cost to the provider, will receive such services in a timely manner. In other words, there is a shift in the financial risk. Under the prospective capitated system, more of the risk is shared between the payer and the provider. For a more detailed discussion of prospective payment systems, see Wolf, 2001.

Most providers remain under a retrospective reimbursement system, whereas networks and some Medicare and Medicaid programs may contract with MCOs under capitated agreements. The providers within the network bill the network retrospectively for services rendered. Often those services require prior authorization from the network for payments to be made in a timely manner. Further, since the capitation that the network receives is usually discounted from full fee-for-service, the reimbursement rates to the providers are further discounted, sometimes severely. Private practitioners must know their costs and required reimbursement rates before affiliating with any provider network, if at all (Wolf & Kreb, 1996; White, 2010).

On the other hand, insurance and provider network reimbursements may not be adequate to sustain the practice. Foehl (2009a, 2009b) raised the question of moving to an insurance-free practice. Such practices hold the patient financially responsible for services, and patients must deal directly with their own insurance carrier. Practices that accept third-party payment should periodically evaluate their payer mix and patient mix to seek maximum balance and avoid dependence on a single type or disproportionate mix of payers. Such imbalance could lead to unintended vulnerability for the practice.

Understanding their own price structure, diagnostic and procedural coding, and payer fee schedules is imperative for practitioner-owners. Private practitioners must also know the reimbursement sources and the underlying structures for their profession and practice. For example, Zingeser (2005) reported that private pay (out-of-pocket) was the largest source of payment for both audiologists (49 percent) and speech-language pathologists (41 percent) in private practice, followed by private insurance (25 percent for audiologists, 15 percent for speech-language pathologists) and Medicare/Medicaid (21 percent and 20 percent for audiologists and speech-language pathologists, respectively). Understanding and adjusting the payer mix for the practice is important for sustenance and sustainability of the practice (Foehl, 2009b).

Evidence-Based Practice The concept of evidence-based medicine began to emerge in the United Kingdom and Canada throughout the 1990s. The process quickly became applicable to all aspects of health care delivery, evolving into evidence-based health care (EBHC) (McKibbon, Eady, & Marks, 1999) and today is referred to as *evidence-based practice* (EBP). Evidence-based practice is used to establish practice guidelines, clinical pathways, and benchmarks for quality of care (Wolf, 1999). An evidence-based approach to care communicates to the professions, consumers, and payers that best practices are rooted in data with the expectation of accuracy (diagnostics) and benefit (therapy) (Plante, 2004).

The transition to an evidence-based approach to clinical decision making is not without challenges

(Dollaghan, 2004; Sackett, Straus, Richardson, Rosenberg, & Haynes, 2000). EBP deemphasizes practitioner intuition, opinion, and unsystematic clinical experience. Instead, EBP requires that decisions are reached through the systematic examination of evidence from clinical research. It is dependent on the scientific method (Evidence-Based Medicine Working Group, 1992; Sackett et al., 2000). EBP does not ignore clinical experience but instead considers it in context against high-quality evidence that meets a priori standards (McKibbon et al., 1999; Sackett et al., 2000). As such, EBP demands that practitioners be efficient and effective searchers of the literature. Once that literature is identified, it must be critically appraised, not only for its scientific and clinical merit but also for its applicability to the target patient or population.

The need for clinical trials in communication sciences and disorders has emerged within the past decade (Logemann, 2004). However, evidence garnered from other types of studies (e.g., meta-analyses or case studies) or from publications in non-peer-reviewed journals may be helpful (Kent, 2004). Therefore, it is critical that clinicians learn how to use EBP and interpret it. A more extensive discussion of EBP is beyond the scope of this chapter. Over the past several years, ASHA has embraced the concepts of EBP, first with a technical paper and position statement (ASHA, 2004c; 2005a) and then with a National Center on Evidence-Based Practice in Communication Disorders. ASHA also has an extensive website on the topic (ASHA, 2011a) including web-based tutorials, a compendium of clinical practice guidelines and systematic reviews, and evidence maps to guide professionals in evidence-based decision making. See Chapters 28 and 29 for further discussion of research and evidence-based practice.

An old problem has been the underutilization or nonutilization of new knowledge. Underutilization of evidence-based research is often described as a gap between "what is known" and "what is currently done" in practice settings. *Knowledge translation* (KT) is a relatively new term that emerged in Canada to describe the transition of new knowledge into practice (e.g., Davis et al., 2003). Also known as *implementation science*, the objective is to change practitioner behaviors to use research findings in routine health care in both clinical and policy contexts. Evidence-based decision making, therefore, goes beyond knowledge acquisition. Rather, contemporary practitioners must be able to apply that new knowledge to effectively and efficiently yield clinical outcomes comparable to community standards and expectations.

Benchmarks may be useful in terms of productivity standards. Instead of measuring productivity based on hours of service, as has been used in the old paradigm, comparisons with established benchmarks may be a more meaningful standard (Wolf, 1999). In other words, standards and rewards are based on achieving outcomes rather than number of hours worked. Productivity standards also are valuable when competing for a contract with a managed care organization. The private practice that can demonstrate outcomes data and benchmarks has an advantage over those that cannot and is likely to be more appealing to MCOs and other contractors. For several years, Congress has debated linking reimbursement to quality measures and indicators. Those that cannot or do not report such measures may receive lower reimbursements compared to those that do. Outcomes, quality, and accountability are fundamental to the new ACOs and are deeply imbedded in the new Patient Protection and Affordable Care Act (i.e., health care reform). Ideally, the new ACOs will align networks of providers with the emphasis on clinical care integration for the population.

What do payers want? Payers want the best possible outcome. They do not want a test score. They want to know if a patient can be discharged, go home, recover, and get back to work. Payers want that outcome for the least amount of money and in the least amount of time. Practitioners who can provide data related to outcomes, time, and cost are in the best position to succeed. In other words, providers need to keep costs down and quality high, achieve maximum patient satisfaction, and be able to measure it and prove it (Wolf, 1999). Health care delivery has become a process that balances cost and risk and that also affords an acceptable outcome and level of quality (Wolf et al., 1994). See Chapter 29 for further discussion of this topic.

Information Technology The use of information technology has become a mainstay in health care delivery. Computers are used not only to facilitate a smooth-functioning office by integrating scheduling, billing, inventory, and payroll but also for marketing, promotion, scientific, and clinical purposes. Many practices have developed websites to describe and market their practice (Dougherty, 2008; Weimann, 2009), schedule appointments, provide access to patients for their questions, and serve as a source of information and educational materials about communication disorders. Patients are turning to the Internet to gather information about the professions and about potential providers before ever making an appointment. Patients are also seeking knowledge about diagnosis and treatment and bringing that information to their health care providers. Providers must know what the patients are reading and whether that information is or is not a viable option.

Additionally, providers are turning to the Internet for literature searches and information applicable to their practices and to receive their professional literature via electronic publishing. Some are also using e-mail and social networking sites to stay in communication with their patients (collectively or as individuals) with announcements and electronic newsletters. Clinically, electronic health records (EHRs) have become common but are still undergoing refinement. Computers are making it possible to go paperless, improving record storage demands and retrieval efficiency as well as providing an accurate and efficient way to collect practice data on many variables for business and/or clinical analysis and benchmarking (Krebs, 2008). Practices that move to electronic billing and patient record transfers, however, must comply with the Health Insurance Portability and Accountability Act (HIPAA) privacy and security rules (Lusis, 2008). Many practices and MCOs are requiring that patient data be submitted electronically not only for billing but also for building databases, leading to internal benchmarks.

The use of health information technology (HIT) goes beyond eliminating or even just reducing paper. The "meaningful use of health information technology" is focused on transferring information and providing the new measures of quality. The EHR now plays a critical role in achieving and documenting higher-quality, safer, more effective health delivery, thereby improving the health care system. Meaningful use of health information technology is expected to provide the mechanism for clinicians to know more about their patients, make better decisions through the use of evidence-based practice, and therefore save money (U.S. Department of Health Services, Office of the National Coordinator for Health Information Technology, 2011). The use of computers now makes collecting, retrieving, and analyzing treatment outcomes data for an individual practice more practical, when it was simply overwhelming for most practitioners in a paper-based system. The new ACOs will, therefore, be the point of interface between implementation science and the meaningful use of health information technology with expectation of documented cost-effective, high-performance (as opposed to high-volume), outcome-based health care as the basis for reimbursement. See Chapters 1 and 26 for further discussion of technology in the professions.

Creating Value Speech-language pathology and audiology services are beneficial to those who receive them, but if those services are to be paid for, the consumer (and the payer) must perceive a value from those services. In other words, patients/clients must perceive that services are worth reaching into one's own pocket and paying for them, if they are not covered by insurance, the schools, the government, or some other third-party payer (Kreb & Wolf, 1997). Marketing speech-language and hearing services to those who receive them and pay for them has been a frequent topic and objective for many professionals and organizations. The real and perceived value of those services, however, must be constructed before there is any chance of generating a successful marketing program. The creation of value begins at the level of the individual provider-to-patient/client relationship.

To illustrate the creation of value, Kreb (personal communication, 1998) uses the example of orthodontia. Huge numbers of children and young adolescents receive orthodontia annually in the United States. How many of them truly require such services for functional purposes? How many believe they need such services because of cosmetic reasons? At costs typically over $3,000 per child, how many parents are willing to pay for these services themselves, as insurance companies rarely, if ever, cover orthodontia? The answer is simple. In almost all cases, orthodontia is paid for by the consumer, actually the parents, because they perceive a value in those services, whether functional or cosmetic. When there is perceived value, it is much easier to market services.

On the other hand, Cohen (1993) described an example of an elderly couple he observed dining in a restaurant. Coffee and dessert were desirable, if included in the price. However, when they learned that dessert and coffee were a la carte, they declined. In other words, if there is no additional out-of-pocket expense, they want it, but if it means added cost, there is question of the desire and value of the additional items.

Although these two examples appear to be dated, they actually represent extremely relevant and contemporary scenarios. Are speech-language pathology and hearing services perceived by the education and health care consuming public like orthodontia or like dessert and coffee at a restaurant? Are the services desired and perceived to hold value only if someone else is paying for the services, or are consumers willing to forgo other valued services and products to pay for speech-language or hearing services? The professions, the services offered, the outcomes to be gained, and the return on investment (dollars spent for services) need to be viewed in such positive light that individuals are willing to undergo some financial sacrifice to receive services, creating a high degree of value. Until that perceived value is achieved, marketing efforts are at risk of being compromised and falling short of their objective.

The burden of creating value and marketing cannot be placed solely on the professions and their professional associations. Practitioners must be actively involved in the process by marketing their own practices and establishing their value. These activities include public relations, marketing, advocacy, and educating individuals at all levels of health care, education, government, politics, and the corporate worlds (Dougherty, 2008; Nelson, La Puma, & Wolf, 1998;Weimann, 2009). Time, energy, and resources need to be planned for and dedicated to these efforts. Remember that every time you talk to a client or patient, families, colleagues, and others about what you do, you are marketing. ASHA has developed many marketing tools and offers workshops that may be a vital stepping-stone for you as a private practitioner. See the ASHA website for the most current information.

Cultural Competence The United States has become increasingly diverse. Racial and ethnic minorities are 36 percent of the current population and their numbers are increasing (U.S. Census Bureau, 2010). The 2000 U.S. Census found that about 18 percent of people over the age of 5 years spoke a language other than English at home (Moxley, Madhendra, & Vega-Barachowitz, 2004). Some communities are changing more rapidly than others, but all are undergoing shifts in demographic composition. Diversity is reflected in attitudes, customs, and expectations about health care, illness, disease, and healing, and it presents challenges to the health care system (Wolf & Calderon, 1999). Further, diversity in education parallels that of health care (Medrano, 2003). Thus, clinicians and educators need to be competent to offer services that are responsive to and effective for myriad populations (ASHA, 2004b). To abide by the Code of Ethics, speech-language pathologists and audiologists may need additional or continuing education. Therefore, maintaining or developing new knowledge and skills to be culturally competent is a requirement of not only good, but also ethical, practice (ASHA, 2005b; Crowley, 2004).

Success as a practitioner-owner in the twenty-first century may depend on the ability to develop cultural competence as well as clinical competence, to ensure that any cultural differences that may exist between the practitioner and the patient/client do not bias or affect clinical outcomes (Wolf, 2004; Wolf & Calmes, 2004). ASHA has developed guidelines (ASHA, 2004b) as well as ethical statements (ASHA, 2005b) for delivering culturally competent services. The reader is encouraged to visit the ASHA website for access to many additional tools and references (ASHA, 2011d; ASHA, 2011e). Also see Chapter 24 for further discussion of diversity as a professional issue.

Ethical Practices Every day, the practitioner-owner will be faced with clinical, business, and personal decisions that are likely to have competing values and interests. Ethical considerations guide that decision-making process (Chabon & Morris, 2005). The ASHA Code of Ethics clearly and succinctly delineates appropriate behaviors for its members (ASHA, 2010b), and all members are bound by this code. The Principles of Ethics and the Rules of Ethics describe the fundamental aspects of ethical conduct as related to service delivery, research, scholarly activity, and those who are served by speech-language pathologists and audiologists. The Principles of Ethics form the underlying moral basis, whereas the Rules of Ethics are statements of minimally acceptable behaviors. The Code of Ethics clearly delineates members' responsibilities to hold paramount the welfare of the people they serve; responsibility to achieve and maintain the highest level of professional competence; responsibility to the public; and responsibility to the professions and to colleagues, students, and members of other professions. ASHA maintains an active ethics education program, including publications (e.g., Chabon, Denton, Lansing, Scudder, & Shinn, 2007; Denton, 2009), educational presentations, and periodic development of Issues in Ethics statements (ASHA, 2011c). The Board of Ethics processes and adjudicates formal ethics complaints from members or the general public and provides ethics education for the members. Chapter 5 discusses ethical issues in more detail.

Research and Academic Affiliations Individuals in private practice, just as any other clinically competent professionals, must be consumers of research and the application of new knowledge. The private practice setting also offers an ideal environment to translate the basic science discoveries of our professions into clinical application. In fact, a great deal of the data used to generate databases, practice guidelines, benchmarks, and overall knowledge translation will have to emerge from the private practice milieu to be meaningful and representative. This need creates an extraordinary opportunity for collaboration with researchers and university training programs. Additionally, university training programs often seek a broader range of practicum sites in which to train their students, and the private practice site offers a rich teaching environment that may not be paralleled in other clinical speech-language pathology or audiology venues. Further, academic and teaching responsibilities provide another mechanism for the practitioner to remain current. Finally, an academic affiliation, even as an adjunct instructor, often adds market value to the practitioner in the eyes of the public and/or other professional colleagues. For these reasons, like colleagues in medicine, some private practitioners are carving out a segment of their time for teaching and affiliating with academic institutions.

Continuing Education Mandatory continuing professional development for maintaining ASHA certification began in 2003 for audiologists and in 2005 for speech-language pathologists. The requirements were based on trends in client demographics, emerging issues, changes in practice patterns, skills validation studies, independent research on consumer advocacy, and extensive internal peer review comments. Maintaining ABA Board certification in audiology also requires continuing education, with the required number of hours divided into advanced (Tier 1) and standard (Tier 2) categories (AAA, 2008a). Tier 1 continuing education activities must be of a minimal length and require some form of outcome measure (e.g., an examination or self-assessment). Tier 2 activities do not have length or outcome measure requirements. Some states also require participation in mandatory continuing education programs to maintain licensure. Additionally, many hospital credentialing committees require annual evidence of continuing professional development to maintain hospital privileges. Continuing education is necessary regardless of the mandatory status and is the cornerstone for performance improvement for every professional. The ASHA Code of Ethics, Principle of Ethics II Rule C (ASHA, 2010b), states that practitioners shall engage in lifelong learning to maintain and enhance their professional competence and performance. Maintaining a continuing education transcript demonstrates that these professionals have a commitment to lifelong learning, without the need to do so by mandate. Regardless of mandate or voluntary participation, the individual who is engaged in private practice needs to dedicate time and resources to maintaining currency and improving performance through continuing education.

Volunteerism

Volunteerism is the backbone of any national, state, or local professional organization. However, individuals in the later part of the 1990s were volunteering less than any previous generation (Blanken & Liff, 1998; Ellis, 2005). Unfortunately, speech-language pathologists and audiologists are no different from the rest of society, and there is greater competition for their volunteer time to ASHA and other groups. As a result, decisions, regulations, practice guidelines, and advocacy and position papers are being drafted and approved by those willing to volunteer their time to do so. The voice of the private practice community needs to be heard if it is to influence any such actions. That means practitioners need to be involved and participate, giving more of their time for which they cannot be reimbursed. However, this investment of time and effort may have significant rewards, personally and professionally.

SUMMARY

This chapter presented some of the issues facing the individual who elects to enter the private practice environment. Although some who enter private practice are employees or part-time practitioners, the information was presented from the perspective of the practitioner-owner. Options and advantages of private practice were discussed, along with the business considerations unique to a practitioner-owner. Included were topics such as development and maintenance of a business plan, funding and loans, licenses and insurances needed to practice, referral bases and networks, and the use of staff and consultants. Additional topics not unique to the private practitioner, but that affect the delivery of speech-language pathology and audiology services in the private practice arena, were also discussed. Those issues include retrospective versus prospective payments systems, treatment outcomes, accountability, evidence-based practice and implementation science, the use of information technology, the need to create value for speech-language pathology and audiology services, the need to participate in education and advocacy activities, the need for cultural competence, the potential to participate in research and affiliate with an academic institution, a commitment to lifelong learning and continuing education, ethical practice, and finally a call for increased volunteerism. Some issues are shared with other delivery environments such as health care and education, and readers are referred to those chapters for more information.

No single article, chapter, or book can adequately provide all of the information to describe the service delivery issues in private practice. Professional organizations such as ASHA, AAA, and AAPPSLP are tremendous resources. Individuals who elect the world of private practice need to network with colleagues, participate in professional development, and dedicate themselves to a commitment that goes beyond serving patients/clients. Private practice requires involvement in the business, practice, and professional issues of speech-language pathology and audiology service delivery.

CRITICAL THINKING

1. You have been working in the public schools for the past four years, occasionally providing evening, weekend, and vacation coverage for some colleagues in hospitals. Now that you have experienced work in both the education and health care environments, you think you would like to start your own practice. Describe the process you will undertake to help you decide if private practice is appropriate for you.
2. Your business is competing with two others of about the same size and scope of services for a contract to provide services. Discuss how evidence-based practice might be used to help you win that contract.
3. Describe how you as a private practitioner will participate in the creation of value for our services and why it is important.
4. Owner-practitioners must participate in several activities that are nonbillable and may actually detract from their profit. Therefore, explain why it is important for private practitioners to participate in ASHA, AAA, and other state and national professional organizations.
5. How might you as a private practitioner benefit from an affiliation with a research and academic facility?
6. What are the disadvantages of establishing a private practice in either speech-language pathology or audiology?
7. You and your best friend from graduate school now have about five years of professional experience and want to pursue your mutual "dream" of opening a private practice together. What are the advantages and disadvantages of working with a best friend in a professional practice? How would you make this work?
8. You decided to establish the private practice with your friend (question 7) and went to the local bank for a loan. You were asked for a "business

plan." What is this document? What is included in it? Where would you go to get information about a business plan in speech-language pathology or audiology?

9. You will rely on a number of other people to make your private practice effective, efficient, and profitable. Who are these people? What characteristics would you look for in people you hire?

10. Marketing is an important part of establishing and maintaining a private practice. What goes into a marketing plan? How would you make your marketing plan work for you in a private practice?

REFERENCES

American Academy of Audiology. (2008a). *ABA board & specialty certification: 2008*. Available from http://www.audiology.org/

American Academy of Audiology. (2008b). *Private practice checklist*. Available from http://www.audiology.org/

American Speech-Language-Hearing Association. (1991a). Considerations for establishing a private practice in audiology and/or speech-language pathology. *ASHA, 33* (Suppl. 3), 10–21.

American Speech-Language-Hearing Association. (1991b). Report on private practice. *ASHA,* 33 (Suppl. 6), 1–4.

American Speech-Language-Hearing Association. (2003a). *2003 Omnibus Survey: Caseload report: SLP*. Rockville, MD: Author.

American Speech-Language-Hearing Association. (2003b). *2003 Omnibus Survey: Practice trends in audiology*. Rockville, MD: Author.

American Speech-Language-Hearing Association. (2003c). Knowledge and skills in business practices needed by speech-language pathologists in health care settings. *ASHA Supplement, 23*, 87–92.

American Speech-Language-Hearing Association. (2004a). Knowledge and skills in business practices for speech-language pathologists who are managers and leaders in health care organizations. *ASHA Supplement, 24*, 146–151.

American Speech-Language-Hearing Association. (2004b). Knowledge and skills needed by speech-language pathologists and audiologists to provide culturally and linguistically appropriate services. *ASHA Supplement, 24*, 152–158.

American Speech-Language-Hearing Association. (2004c). *Evidence-based practice in communication disorders: An introduction*. Rockville, MD: Author.

American Speech-Language-Hearing Association. (2005a). Web-based tutorials. Available from http://www.asha.org/

American Speech-Language-Hearing Association. (2005b). Cultural competence. *ASHA Supplement, 25*, 1–2.

American Speech-Language-Hearing Association. (2009a). *Highlights and trends: ASHA counts for year end 2009*. Available from http://www.asha.org/

American Speech-Language-Hearing Association. (2009b). *ASHA SLP Health Care Survey 2009: Caseload characteristics trends, 2005–2009*. Available from http://www.asha.org/

American Speech-Language-Hearing Association. (2010a). *Audiology Survey 2010: Private practice*. Available from http://www.asha.org/

American Speech-Language-Hearing Association. (2010b). Code of ethics (revised). *ASHA Supplement, 23*, 13–15.

American Speech-Language-Hearing Association. (2011a). *Evidence-based practice (EBP)*. Available from http://www.asha.org/

American Speech-Language-Hearing Association. (2011b). *Frequently asked questions about business practices*. Available from http://www.asha.org/

American Speech-Language-Hearing Association. (2011c). *Issues in ethics statements*. Available from http://www.asha.org/

American Speech-Language-Hearing Association. (2011d). *Office of Multicultural Affairs and Resources*. Available from http://www.asha.org/

American Speech-Language-Hearing Association. (2011e). *Resource guide for audiologists in private practice*. Available from http://www.asha.org/

American Speech-Language-Hearing Association. (2011f). *Specialty recognition: FAQs*. Available from http://www.asha.org/

American Speech-Language-Hearing Association. (2012). *ASHA state-by-state*. Retrieved from http://www.asha.org/advocacy/state/

Blanken, R. L., & Liff, A. (1998). Facing the future: Preparing your association to thrive. Washington, DC: Foundation of the American Society of Association Executives.

Chabon, S. S., Denton, D. R., Lansing, C. R., Scudder, R. R., & Shinn, R. (2007). *Ethics education*. Rockville, MD: American Speech-Language-Hearing Association.

Chabon, S. S., & Morris, J. (2005). Raising ethical awareness in the practice of speech language pathology and audiology: A 24/7 endeavor. *CSHA, 35*(1), 6–8.

Cohen, M. (1993). Planes, trains, and speech therapy. *CSHA, 20*(2), 12–13, 16.

Connors, E. E., & Gostin, L. O. (2010). Health care reform—A historic moment in U.S. social policy. *Journal of the American Medical Association, 303*(24), 2521–2522.

Crowley, C. J. (2004). The ethics of assessment with culturally and linguistically diverse populations. *The ASHA Leader, 9*(5), 6–7.

Currie, P. S. (2004). *Starting a private practice*. Available from http://www.audiologyonline.com/

Davis, D., Evans, M., Jadad, A., Perrier, L., Rath, D., Ryan, D., et al. (2003). The case for knowledge translation: Shortening the journey from evidence to effect. *British Medical Journal, 327*(7405), 33–35.

Denton, D. (2009, August 11). Watch out for these ethical traps in private practice. *The ASHA Leader*. Retrieved from http://www.asha.org/Publications/leader/2009/090811/090811j/

Dollaghan, C. A. (2004). Evidence-based practice in communication disorders: What do we know, and when do we know it? *Journal of Communication Disorders, 37*(5), 391–400.

Dougherty, D. (2008, September 02). Transitioning to private practice. *The ASHA Leader*. Retrieved from http://www.asha.org/Publications/leader/2008/080902/f080902a/

Ellis, S. J. (2005). Tracking volunteer trends. *Association Management, 57*(1), 72–74.

Evidence-Based Medicine Working Group. (1992). Evidence-based medicine: A new approach to teaching the practice of medicine. *Journal of the American Medical Association, 268*(17), 2420–2425.

Foehl, A. (2009a, January 20). Making a move away from insurance contracts. *The ASHA Leader*. Retrieved from http://www.asha.org/Publications/leader/2009/090120/090120e/

Foehl, A. (2009b, August 11). Payer and patient mix: Keys to a healthy private practice. *The ASHA Leader*. Retrieved from http://www.asha.org/Publications/leader/2009/090811/090811i/

Goffinet, M. (2005). Private practice: Where do you begin? *Access Audiology, 4*(4). Available from http://www.asha.org/

Kent, R. D. (2004). Science in the courtroom and the clinic. *The ASHA Leader, 9*(16), 33.

Klontz, H. A., Napp, A. C., White, S. C., & Wolf, K. E. (1997). *The competitive edge for audiologists negotiating with managed care*. Rockville, MD: American Speech-Language-Hearing Association.

Kreb, R. A. (Ed.). (1997). *A practical guide to applying treatment outcomes & efficacy resources*. Rockville, MD: American Speech-Language-Hearing Association.

Kreb, R. A., Swigert, N. B., Conoway, J., Markus, G., von Unwerth, F. H., & White, S. C. (1995). PPOs: Are they good for ASHA members? *ASHA, 37*, 39–41.

Kreb, R. A., & Wolf, K. E. (1997). *Successful operations in the treatment outcomes driven world of managed care*. Rockville, MD: National Student Speech Language Hearing Association.

Krebs, J. M. (2008, September 2). Paper, paper everywhere? How to go paperless in your private practice. *The ASHA Leader.* Retrieved from http://www.asha.org/Publications/leader/2008/080902/080902e/

Logemann, J. A. (2004). Clinical trials: CSDRG overview. *Journal of Communication Disorders, 37*(5), 419–423.

Lusis, I. (2008, September 2). Bottom line: Private practice and HIPAA. *The ASHA Leader.* Retrieved from http://www.asha.org/Publications/leader/2008/080902/bl080902/

McKibbon, A., Eady, A., & Marks, S. (1999). *PDQ: Evidence-based principles and practice*. Saint Louis, MO: B.C. Decker.

Medrano, M. A. (2003). *Affirmative action: Challenges and opportunities in creating a diverse health care workforce*. Paper presented at the Association of American Medical Colleges, Washington, DC.

Moxley, A., Madhendra, N., & Vega-Barachowitz, C. (2004). Cultural competence in health care. *The ASHA Leader, 9*(7), 6–7, 20–22.

Napp, A. (1997). Developing networks at state and regional level for negotiating empowerment. In H. A. Klontz, A. C. Napp, S. C. White, & K. E. Wolf (Eds.), *The competitive edge for audiologists and speech-language pathologists.* Rockville, MD: American Speech-Language-Hearing Association.

Nelson, J. A., La Puma, J., & Wolf, K. E. (1998). When the patient's health plan limits care: An ethics roundtable. *ASHA, 40*, 48.

Plante, E. (2004). Evidence-based practice in communication sciences and disorders. *Journal of Communication Disorders, 37*(5), 389–390.

Sackett, D. L., Straus, S. E., Richardson, W. S., Rosenberg, W., & Haynes, R. B. (2000). *Evidence-based medicine: How to practice and teach EBM* (2nd ed.). New York, NY: Churchill Livingstone.

U.S. Census Bureau. (2010). *U.S. Census 2010.* Available from http://www.census.gov/

U.S. Department of Health Services, Office of the National Coordinator for Health Information Technology. (2011, February 9). *Electronic health records and meaningful use*. Retrieved from http://healthit.hhs.gov/portal/server.pt?open=512&objID=2996&mode=2

U.S. Small Business Administration. (2011). *Thinking about starting a business*. Available from http://www.sba.gov/category/navigation-structure/starting-managing-business

Weimann, G. (2009, August 11). Marketing during an economic downturn. *The ASHA Leader.* Retrieved from http://www.asha.org/leaderissue.aspx?id=2009-08-11&year=2009

White, S. C. (2010, October 12). Audiology health care plan contracting. *The ASHA Leader*. Retrieved from http://www.asha.org/Publications/leader/2010/101012/Audiology-Health-Plan-Contracting.htm

Wolf, K. E. (1995). What audiologists need to know about managed care. In S. Holzberger (Ed.), *Meeting the managed care challenge: Strategies for professionals and the professions.* Rockville, MD: American Speech-Language-Hearing Association.

Wolf, K. E. (1999). Preparing for evidence-based speech-language pathology and audiology. *Texas Journal of Audiology and Speech Pathology, 23*, 69–74.

Wolf, K. E. (2001). Service delivery issues in private practice. In R. Lubinski & C. M. Frattali (Eds.), *Professional issues in speech-language pathology and audiology* (2nd ed., pp. 301–315). Clifton Park, NY: Delmar Cengage Learning.

Wolf, K. E. (2004). Cultural competence in audiology. *The ASHA Leader*, *9*(7), 8–9.

Wolf, K. E. (2007). Service delivery issues in private practice. In R. Lubinski, L. A. C. Golper, & C. M. Frattali (Eds.), *Professional issues in speech-language pathology and audiology* (3rd ed., pp. 371–386). Clifton Park, NY: Delmar Cengage Learning.

Wolf, K. E., & Calderon, J. L. (1999). Cultural competence: The underpinning of quality health care and education services. *ASHA, 28*(2), 4–6.

Wolf, K. E., & Calmes, D. (2004). Cultural competence in the emergency department. *Topics in Emergency Medicine, 26*(1), 9–13.

Wolf, K. E., Cohen, M. S., & Arnst, D. J. (1994). Managed care: Costs and risks. In B. S. Cornett (Ed.), *Managing managed care: A practical guide for audiologists and speech-language pathologists.* Rockville, MD: American Speech-Language-Hearing Association.

Wolf, K. E., & Kreb, R. A. (1996). Actuary data: What's in it for you? *ASHA, 38*(2), 33–36.

Zingeser, L. (2005). Trends in private practice among ASHA constituents, 1986–2003. *The ASHA Leader,* 10–11, 14.

RESOURCES

American Academy of Audiology
11730 Plaza America Drive, Suite 300
Reston, VA 20190-4798
Telephone: 800-AAA-2336
Website: http://www.audiology.org/

American Academy of Private Practice in Speech-Language Pathology and Audiology
Website: http://www.aappspa.org/

American Speech-Language-Hearing Association
2200 Research Blvd.
Rockville, MD 20850
Telephone: 301-296-5700
Website: http://www.asha.org/

For ASHA's overview of state associations, regulatory agencies, state laws, and other relevant information, see http://www.asha.org/advocacy/state/state-policy.htm.

Marsh U.S. Consumer, a Service of Seabury and Smith
P.O. Box 14576
Des Moines, IA 50303-3576
Telephone: 800-503-9230
Website: http://www.proliability.com

U.S. Small Business Administration
See local white pages for address and telephone number.
Website: http://www.sba.gov

U.S. Small Business Administration. (2011). *Thinking about starting*. Available from http://www.sba.gov/category/navigation-structure/starting-managing-business/starting-business/thinking-about-starting

18

Strategically Promoting Access to Speech-Language Pathology and Audiology Services

Brooke Hallowell, PhD
Bernard P. Henri, PhD

SCOPE OF CHAPTER

Access to quality speech-language pathology and audiology services for people who need them is most threatened at a time when the number of people throughout the entire age range needing such services is increasing steadily. To best position ourselves to counteract strategically the forces that threaten access to our services, we must have a clear understanding of the barriers to access and a sound rationale for the need for speech-language pathology and audiology services. In this chapter, we discuss the factors that impede access despite a dire and growing need for services. We then discuss strategic means of enhancing access through optimizing reimbursement for clinical services, finding alternative ways to fund clinical services, pursuing legislative channels to enhance access, engaging in advocacy, using care extenders, taking advantage of technology, educating the public, and modifying our service-providing environments.

BARRIERS TO ACCESS

Reimbursement and funding problems constitute the greatest barriers for access to audiology and speech-language pathology services. An emphasis on cost containment in all areas of health care delivery is at the root of many of those problems (Reaven & Rosenbloom, 2009; Segal, Pedersen, Freeman, & Fast, 2008). Children and adults with disabilities face unique difficulties as they attempt to obtain services through our progressively more unwieldy health care system (White, 2002). Overall, access to our services is being reduced by the coverage and reimbursement limitations imposed by managed care and health maintenance organizations (MC/HMOs), Medicare's Prospective Payment System (PPS), Medicare's on-again off-again reimbursement caps, increasing discrimination on the part of insurance companies against people with preexisting conditions, and the ongoing efforts in many states to transfer control of public education to local school boards (ASHA, 2006a; Frymark & Mullen, 2005; Grabowski, 2008; National Joint Committee for the Communication Needs of Persons with Severe Disabilities, 2002; O'Callaghan, McAllister, & Wilson, 2010; Rosenbaum, 2009; Rodwin, 1995; Shulman et al., 2010).

Physician referrals are decreasing, authorizations for evaluations and treatment are slow in coming, denials are increasing, and the appeals process is cumbersome and lengthy. Additionally, public and private health insurance carriers' reimbursement rates are commonly well below the actual cost of providing services (Lim, McManus, Fox, White, & Forsman, 2010; McManus et al., 2010). As a result, some health care employers are eliminating positions or are placing clinicians on as-needed schedules, actions that further jeopardize access to services. Primary care physicians are more aggressively guarding scarcer financial resources to ensure the availability of basic health care for their patients. Many physicians see audiology and speech-language pathology services as a low priority or a service that should be paid for by other entities, such as school districts, public service organizations, or clients themselves. Insurance companies are following suit.

Additional common barriers to access to our services relate to literacy limitations. Understanding today's medical literature and health insurance materials can be a daunting challenge for even the most sophisticated person. For those with major literacy problems, difficulties are substantial and, as a result, differentially impact access and related needs for patient advocacy. Those who live in geographic areas remote from service delivery sites are also disadvantaged in terms of access.

THE NEED FOR SERVICE

Why is it critical that an individual obtain services for communication disorders? What are the consequences to a child or adult of diminished communicative effectiveness when services are inaccessible or otherwise unavailable? The answers to these questions must be addressed and elaborated upon continuously by members of our professions if we are to substantiate the need for our services to consumers, third-party payers, legislators, and other professionals in health care and education. Likewise, the effectiveness of our interventions must be documented and promoted continuously.

The need for health care services, including those provided by audiologists and speech-language pathologists, is expected to increase up to 19 percent by 2018 (U.S. Department of Labor, 2010). There are several reasons for this growing need:

- There is a greater emphasis on health promotion and disease prevention (Novelli, 2008; Pelletier, 2009).
- The elderly population is growing, with corresponding increases in hearing loss and neurologically based speech-language problems (U.S. Department of Labor, 2010).
- Advances in medical technology are saving lives and increasing the life span (U.S. Department of Labor, 2008, 2010).
- The bilingual/multilingual population, which has a proportionately greater need for speech and language diagnostic and intervention services, is expanding (Centeno & Kohnert, 2009).
- There is a greater emphasis on early identification and diagnosis, as well as increased referrals of students to professionals (Pelletier, 2009; U.S. Department of Labor, 2010).
- There are increased enrollments in elementary and secondary schools, including enrollments in special education (U.S. Department of Labor, 2010).

Another factor affecting the need for services for people with communication disorders is the accelerating worldwide dependence on information technology, requiring people to have ever more effective communication abilities. On a daily basis, we are required to manage greater amounts of complex language-based information. Those who have untreated communication challenges risk becoming marginal participants in our society, observers standing on the sidelines. Reading abilities, particularly in the country's large urban school districts, are plummeting (Rouse & Kemple, 2009). Nationwide, 43 percent of fourth graders in urban areas are failing basic reading proficiency tests (Hemphill & Tivnan, 2008). Many of the parents and guardians of children with low literacy levels, especially those with low income, are unable to provide basic reading support due to their own low education levels. Recent research demonstrates that children who are poor readers, particularly those raised in poverty, often experience careers of academic failure and may eventually become trapped in lives of generational poverty, accompanied sometimes by teenage parenthood and criminal behavior (Maughan et al., 2009; Snow & Powell, 2008).

The prevalence of language learning disabilities and illiteracy in state prisons provides dramatic evidence of the cost of not providing speech-language pathology and audiology services. Up to 75 percent of individuals remanded to adult correctional facilities have significant communication disorders, which are vitally linked to literacy (Shippen, Houchins, Crites, Derzis, & Dashaunda, 2010). Likewise, teenage mothers raised in poverty have a high prevalence of speech-language and literacy problems. Such problems may affect not only their own economic and social futures but also those of their children, who may not benefit from literate environments or from competent speech-language models (Noria, Borkowski, & Whitman, 2009). Additionally, in high-technology industries, employers report difficulty recruiting candidates with even minimal literacy and mathematical abilities. For many individuals, access to our services is crucial for establishing the communication skills necessary for success in school, employment, and social interaction.

Despite worldwide efforts to improve the ways individuals with disabilities are treated and regarded, the social consequences of communication disorders remain fundamentally challenging. Many individuals with communication disorders face "attitudinal barriers, marginal social status, rejection, distrust, stigmatization and loss of esteem" (Hallowell & Chapey 2008, p. 12).

OPTIMIZING REIMBURSEMENT FOR CLINICAL SERVICES

Unless the financial viability of service providers and their institutions is ensured, there will be limited or no access to speech-language pathology and audiology services. The primary means by which financial viability can be maintained is through the enhancement of clinical revenues, that is, earned income. In today's managed care environment, multiple sources of reimbursement for evaluations, treatment, and consultation must be identified and developed. Contractual agreements with managed care organizations can be carefully negotiated to ensure clinical revenues and minimize financial risk. One must know in detail the policies and procedures of multiple payers and stay abreast of changes in policies and procedures of each payer. This requires unprecedented amounts of communication with payers and monitoring of follow-up to those communications by the provider.

One especially effective approach to optimizing an organization's payer reimbursements is to identify the six most common reasons for authorization and/or treatment denials an organization experiences and then develop action plans that address each reason. Generally, the most common reasons for denials include the following:

- There is insufficient documentation.
- An appropriate physician referral was not obtained.
- The service provided was not covered by the client's health insurance plan.
- The service was deemed "not medically necessary."
- The authorization period had lapsed.
- The patient was no longer improving.

Given that these causes typically make up 80 percent to 90 percent of the reasons for denial by public and private insurance companies, clinical professionals and administrators may best use their time and resources by proactively addressing the causes of each of these problems. By implementing careful documentation strategies, along with ongoing verification procedures to ensure attention to each of these potential pitfalls, service providers may greatly reduce the percentage of reimbursement claims that are denied. Many service-providing organizations have implemented automated denial management processes for a systematic approach for analyzing claim problems, tracking denials and appeals, and preventing future denials.

Also essential to predictable clinical revenue flow is a sound understanding of the diagnosis and treatment classification coding systems that are the basis for reimbursement—that is, the International Classification of Diseases (ICD-10) and Common Procedural Terminology (CPT) codes, as they relate to speech-language pathology and audiology services. Failure to keep abreast of variations in coding and billing procedures from one insurance carrier to another and to use current ICD-10 and CPT coding can be costly (McManus et al, 2010; White, 2008). Fortunately, more universal implementation of the Health Insurance Portability and Accountability Act (HIPAA) is helping reduce problems of inconsistency in billing codes accepted by various payers through required use of uniform coding processes. Medicare administrative contractors, such as National Governmental Services (NGS), are required to meet regularly with providers to identify coding, billing, and documentation problems that bring about denials. Working with providers, NGS strives to eliminate these problems, thus saving resources for providers and payers.

Educating administrators, payers, and physicians about possible health care cost savings associated with speech, language, swallowing, and hearing services is an additional means of enhancing access to these services. Consider an important example provided by Dr. Alex Johnson (personal communication, 2011). In efforts to reduce payments for treatment under its own health maintenance organization, representatives at Henry Ford Hospital in Detroit proposed to eliminate reimbursement for several speech-language pathology services that had long been covered. Johnson, who was overseeing those services at the time, reports that he was able to demonstrate that eliminating the coverage for these services would conservatively cost the hospital approximately $1.6 million in revenue. As a result, the proposal to restrict coverage was withdrawn.

Another approach to enhancing clinical revenues is offering services for which clients or their employers pay directly. Direct payment is the usual form of reimbursement for some services, such as accent modification and individualized coaching for professional speakers. Patients and clients may also pay out-of-pocket for most clinical services. Emphasizing the possibility of direct payment to those who can afford it is an alternative route to accessing care that is not dependent on insurance coverage and helps to enhance providers' clinical revenues.

Rebutting Denials Based on "Medical Necessity"

As managed care and health maintenance organizations attempt to rein in health care costs, the loosely defined and yet broadly and inconsistently applied concept of medical necessity is frequently being used to deny authorizations or reauthorizations for care (Granger et al., 2009; Ireys, Wehr, & Cooke, 2000). Strictly defined, medical necessity relates to treating conditions proceeding from illness, injury, or disease. First-level claims reviewers, whose purpose it is to protect health insurance company funds, typically apply this restricted definition, leading to denied claims.

In most instances, claims reviewers have minimal to no understanding of speech-language pathology or audiology and thus are poorly prepared to render informed decisions concerning the medical necessity of these services. Because of their inexperience with the services provided by our professions, third-party payers are often more easily convinced of the necessity for the treatment of physical disabilities than they are of the need to treat problems associated with cognitive and communication disorders. Further, reviewers in commercial insurance companies tend to implement medical necessity requirements based on cost, predictable outcomes, and the medical nature of conditions being treated, not on knowledge specific to audiology and speech-language pathology (Fox & McManus, 2001). Clinicians must be able to provide substantive arguments demonstrating how most of our services do, in fact, meet definitions and criteria of medical necessity.

The following perspectives, drawn from the medical literature, offer guidance concerning the rebuttal of denials based on an apparent lack of demonstrated medical necessity. Berman (1997) states that, because medical necessity has no standardized definition, its inclusion in contract language gives the health plan considerable discretion determining the use, scope, and duration of covered benefits. He recommends the following criteria be used to guide decisions concerning medical necessity:

- Is the service appropriate for the age and health status of the individual?
- Will the service prevent or ameliorate the effects of a condition, illness, injury, or disorder?
- Will the service aid the overall physical and mental growth and development of the individual?
- Will the service assist in achieving or maintaining functional capacity? (p. 858)

Sindelar (2002) provides substantial detail about court decisions that are useful in challenging medical necessity denials specific to state Medicaid programs, including services required under Early Periodic Screening, Diagnosis, and Treatment (EPSDT). An exemplary denials mitigation process described by Olaniyan, Brown, & Williams (2009) illustrates a strategic approach to denials management useful in overturning denials based on an application of medical necessity. Briefly, their approach includes three components:

1. Ensuring proper prior authorization/notification
2. Conducting concurrent review to ensure that the health insurance company has the necessary information to support medical necessity
3. Having a clear understanding of the insurance carrier's appeals process

The American Academy of Pediatrics (2005) expanded the scope of the medical necessity definition to address health problems, evidence of effectiveness, and value for children. Perkins and Olson (1998) propose a model definition of medical necessity for physical care contracts. They state that medically necessary care is the care that, in the opinion of the treating physician, is reasonably needed to:

- prevent the onset or worsening of an illness, condition, or disability;
- establish a diagnosis;
- provide palliative, curative, or restorative treatment for physical and/or mental health conditions; and/or
- assist the individual to achieve or maintain maximum functional capacity in performing daily activities, taking into account both the functional capacity of the individual and those functional capacities that are appropriate for individuals of the same age. (p. 1)

Kahan and colleagues (1994) declare that a procedure is medically necessary if the following criteria are met:

- The procedure is appropriate.
- It would be improper care not to recommend this service.
- There is sufficient likelihood that the procedure will benefit the patient, especially in light of associated risks.
- The benefit to the patient is not "minor." (p. 359)

Finally, ASHA (2005c) has published *Medical Necessity for Speech-Language Pathology and Audiology Services,* a comprehensive document providing additional information supporting why our services meet the definition of medical necessity.

Evidence-Based Practice

Evidence-based practice (EBP) is a concept being applied increasingly by many payers to further restrict access and reduce care and, thus, their payments. This topic is discussed in depth in Chapter 29. EBP represents an approach to clinical care in which decision making is based on an analysis of the data from clinical research (Ellrodt, Cho, & Cush, 1997). As defined by Sackett et al., 1996 (in Dollaghan, 2004), evidence-based practice is "... the conscientious, explicit, and judicious use of current best evidence in making decisions about the care of individual patients... [by] integrating individual clinical expertise with the best available external clinical evidence from systematic research" (pp. 71–72). Simply stated, health insurance companies now tend to permit authorizations and reimbursements only for those interventions for which efficacy and effectiveness are supported by published research. While laudable in principle, implementation of strict EBP rules reduces access to all health care disciplines for minorities and underrepresented groups (women, children and adolescents, people of color, and the elderly) who generally are disproportionately excluded from clinical effectiveness studies (Epstein, 2008; Kneipp, Lutz, & Means, 2009; Nolan & Bradley, 2008). As a result, these groups suffer disproportionately when an insurance company's coverage is dependent on published evidence of a treatment's effectiveness.

Despite recent concerted efforts to address treatment efficacy and outcomes research in communication sciences and disorders, work to develop a solid foundation in EBP through our own disciplines lags behind the implementation of EBP requirements imposed by the insurance industry and by state and federal policymakers (Lerner, Gesek, & Adams, 2003; Siobhan & Catharine, 2009). ASHA and members of several of its affiliated special interest divisions, as well as the Academy of Neurologic Communication Disorders and Sciences (ANCDS), have prepared extensive bibliographies summarizing treatment efficacy in various clinical areas such as stuttering, cognitive and communicative problems associated with traumatic brain injury, feeding and swallowing disorders, hearing loss, hearing aids, audiological rehabilitation, aphasia, child language disorders, autistic spectrum disorders, phonological disorders, and dysphagia. This information has been developed to help support claims of effectiveness and to reverse denials based on the concepts of medical necessity and evidence-based medical necessity. It may also be used advantageously when negotiating contracts with insurance companies. These resources can be accessed online through ASHA and ANCDS. The *Preferred Practice Patterns for the Profession of Audiology* (ASHA, 2005e) and the *Preferred Practice Patterns for the Profession of Speech-Language Pathology* (ASHA, 2005d) offer especially helpful guidance to support clinicians' assertions that services are medically necessary and appropriate.

ALTERNATIVE FUNDING APPROACHES

In the face of dramatic cuts in reimbursement rates, organizations typically must enhance access to services by systematically developing funding alternatives that supplement clinical revenues. These alternatives have long been central to the operation of most not-for-profit organizations, which are commonly required to provide services to clients regardless of their ability to pay. In the midst of grave reductions in clinical revenues in the current service delivery arena, alternative funding sources are now more critical than ever. Even for-profit agencies are developing their own not-for-profit foundations or are partnering with extant foundations that will help support the provision of services to clients whose access might otherwise be curtailed.

Service-providing agencies can best support their nonclinical revenue base by strategically developing a funding plan consisting of several possible revenue sources (Henri & Hallowell, 1999a). Essential components include the following:

- Ensuring a fundraising-oriented board of directors and chief executive officer or executive director, an experienced development professional, staff, volunteers, and any additional "friends" of the organization.
- Developing a case statement that describes the agency's mission and vision and details why donors should invest their resources in its programs and services.
- Establishing a resource development or fundraising team, including members of the organization's donor base of individuals, patients/clients, foundations, and corporations that support programs and services for people with communication disorders. The donor base may include, but should not rely solely on, federated donor bases, such as United Way, United Black Fund, or Easter Seals Society.
- Engaging in specific fund-raising activities. These may include the following:
    - An annual fund campaign—This is typically conducted during the last quarter of a calendar year to take advantage of contributions that individuals and corporations make to reduce their income tax liability.
    - Special events—Examples are benefit concerts, special recognition dinners, golf outings, fashion shows, marathons, and evenings at the theater. In addition to raising operating revenue for the organization, these events generate publicity, media attention, and community goodwill. They also introduce potential donors to the organization and its mission.
    - Online fundraising is a relatively new way to generate contributions. Most organizations' websites now have links on their home pages to guide potential donors on how to support the organization in a private and safe manner (see Adair, 2009).
    - Planned and deferred giving programs—These long-range funding programs typically yield

benefits in an average of five to seven years. They include bequests, gift annuities, charitable remainder annuity trusts, charitable remainder unitrusts, pooled income funds, charitable life insurance, and gifts of real estate and goods (e.g., works of art). Guidance from professionals with expertise in planned giving, estate planning, law, and accounting is essential to successful planned and deferred giving programs.

- Corporate partnerships—Partnerships between corporations and not-for-profit organizations serving people with communication disorders may help to augment client access through agencies' improved fiscal stability. Corporations are most likely to "adopt" a charity or one of its programs in communities where corporations have a significant presence (e.g., in areas where their corporate headquarters are located).
- Fraternal organizations and sororities—Community fraternal organizations such as the Eagles, Elks, Junior League, Kiwanis, Lions, and Rotary are all sources of usually client- or program-specific funding. SERTOMA and Scottish Rite, though present in only certain regions of the United States, are also fraternal organizations with long-standing histories of support for audiology and speech-language pathology services. Delta Zeta sororities have historically supported programs that serve people who are deaf or hard-of-hearing. Most of these entities entertain proposals to fund services, equipment, or materials needed by individuals unable to afford these.
- Research funding to support clinical services—Clinical research funding from local, regional, state, and federal agencies may strengthen a service-providing agency's fiscal stability. Often, research instrumentation and materials purchased through grant funds (e.g., diagnostic equipment, published tests, treatment materials, computers, and software) enrich not only the research environment but the organization's clinical environment as well. Also, indirect cost or "overhead" monies provided by funding agencies can be used to support an organization's general operational costs, thus enhancing clinical access.

Agencies that do not have in-house development expertise can contract with fundraising consultants for specific resource development projects and/or long-range planning. In many instances, these arrangements are more cost-effective and further allow the organization's staff to concentrate on more profitable activities, such as acquiring major gifts.

LEGISLATION IMPROVING ACCESS

Several pieces of federal and state legislation have been passed to ensure that children and adults with special conditions have access to adequate and appropriate levels of service. Knowledge of federal laws, their state equivalents, and the rules and regulations that guarantee access to special services, including speech-language pathology and audiology, is essential. The Social Security Act, for example, contains several "titles," that is, chapters or subsections, that ensure reimbursement for speech-language pathology and audiology services, including the following:

- Title 5, the Crippled Children's Act, the funding base for states' Bureaus for Children with Medical Handicaps
- Title 18, Medicare, which provides for speech-language pathology and audiology coverage (Medicare coverage is also available for those under the age of 65 who have disabilities lasting longer than two years, such as chronic neurological conditions)
- Title 19, Medicaid, which also includes Aid to Aged, Blind and Disabled; Early Periodic Screening Diagnosis and Treatment (EPSDT); and state-contracted Medicaid HMOs
- Title 20, the Social Services Subsidy, which in some instances supports social work services and, in turn, can help families access speech-language pathology and audiology services
- Title 21, Children's Health Insurance Program (CHIP), a new funding source for speech-language pathology and audiology services, usually administered by a state's Department of Human Services, Medicaid Division
- Individuals with Disabilities Education Improvement Act (2004), the primary funding vehicle for states' preschool early intervention, elementary, and secondary special education programs

- Rehabilitation Act, which funds rehabilitation services, including audiology and speech-language pathology, for individuals ranging in age from 16 and up

Many of these reimbursement mechanisms have mixed histories in terms of their effectiveness in supporting services for populations with special chronic or degenerative conditions (Smith & Ashbaugh, 1995). Several other pieces of federal legislation indirectly support our services. The Americans with Disabilities Act (ADA), for example, does not ensure funding per se but may require employers to make available certain resources in cases in which communication disorders have a demonstrated impact on an individual's ability to perform job duties. Likewise, the Rehabilitation Act is a national law that prohibits discrimination against qualified people with disabilities for employment in the federal sector. Additionally, the No Child Left Behind Act (NCLB) is intended to support education of all children, including those with disabilities, in the public schools, through high standards, an emphasis on school and teacher accountability, and selective funding programs. However, the effectiveness and legitimacy of many of the principles guiding NCLB remain areas of concern as varied aspects of this law are implemented (e.g., Hock & Deshler, 2003).

ADVOCACY AND PROFESSIONAL ASSERTIVENESS

The goals of improved access and quality of care of most current health insurance companies are often in direct conflict with their goals of cost containment (Henri & Hallowell, 1999b; Hiller & Lewis, 1995; Rodwin, 1995). Improving access for speech-language pathology and audiology services requires that action plans for advocacy be thoughtfully developed and executed at various levels of governmental bureaucracies, in the public and private reimbursement arenas (ASHA, 2004a; Henri & Hallowell, 1996; Henri, Hallowell, & Johnson, 1997; White, 2008).

People coping with communication disorders are often at a disadvantage when the need arises for personal advocacy concerning access or reimbursement. Many individuals with communication disorders find it difficult to advocate vigorously for their own needs. This problem may be further compounded by difficulties related to communication infrastructure, travel, distance from legislators in rural areas, and literacy. Furthermore, individuals who would benefit from our services often do not have the knowledge necessary to confront a complex bureaucratic system to obtain coverage for needed services. Audiologists and speech-language pathologists thus have numerous opportunities to initiate or support consumers' advocacy efforts. These opportunities require that we professionals be knowledgeable about the content and the process required for an effective advocacy effort (Henri, 2010).

Historically, most audiologists and speech-language pathologists have had little experience, and often little inclination, to participate in the arena of public policy development, political advocacy, and lobbying. Given the ongoing dramatic challenges to consumer access and the consequent fiscal instability of service-providing agencies, though, it is no longer possible for clinicians, administrators, educators, and consumers to remain passive, adopting a "let someone else do it" attitude. Together, professionals and consumers must participate in coordinated efforts aimed at educating and influencing decision makers about the value of audiology and speech-language pathology services and especially about the societal consequences of not providing these services. Information related to access issues must be disseminated and used as a basis for action. Specific actions for advocacy are described here and are outlined in Table 18–1.

Advocacy among Clinicians and Clinical Administrators

Specific action steps in which clinicians and clinical administrators may make solid contributions to advocacy efforts to improve consumer access are summarized here.

Continuing Education Clinicians who consistently and attentively read current publications and participate in seminars and workshops to improve their knowledge concerning managed care and its impact upon our services will be most effective as advocates. ASHA and the American Academy of Audiology (AAA) offer resources to assist members in their efforts to stay attuned to heath care policy changes and maintain current understanding of coding and billing procedures. The reader is encouraged to visit the ASHA and AAA websites regularly and read reimbursement-related articles that routinely appear in *The ASHA Leader*,

TABLE 18–1 Actions for Advocacy and Professional Assertiveness

Advocacy among Clinicians and Clinical Administrators	Advocacy among Consumers and Their Significant Others
• Continuing education • Consumer education and mobilization • Addressing literacy and non-native speaker challenges • Marketing to and education of referral sources • Appealing denials of treatment authorization and reimbursement • Promoting access to people with geographic and transportation challenges • Financial support • Active writing to legislators • Inviting legislators to work settings • Visiting legislators in their local offices or on Capitol Hill • Engaging in quality assurance	• Active pursuit of coverage for speech-language pathology and audiology services • Reporting of health care policy coverage inconsistencies • Education of employers • Mobilization of consumer groups **Advocacy among Educators and Students** • Continuing education concerning modes of service delivery and health policy and about the effects on people with communication and swallowing disorders • Curricular revision • Education of medical students and their professors • Engagement in concerted legislative advocacy

an online ASHA publication. State associations may also be excellent resources for continuing education related to enhancing consumer access.

Consumer Education and Mobilization Clinicians must take advantage of the direct access they have to consumers to provide counseling and education that will motivate consumers and their families to appreciate:

- the complex relationships between an individual's communication abilities and the success one experiences in other life arenas, such as progress in school or independent living;
- any restrictions consumers' insurance companies place on the treatment of communication and/or swallowing disorders; and
- specific means by which consumers may become more involved in advocacy.

Addressing Literacy and Non-Native Speaker Challenges Case managers, volunteers (e.g., retired insurance specialists and law students), and community members with shared cultural and linguistic backgrounds may be enlisted to help those with literacy problems to navigate and understand health care and health insurance information. All written materials should be written in what the Institute of Medicine calls plain language. This includes organizing the most important action-focused information first, breaking information into understandable units, avoiding jargon, and making the pages easy to read. Also, ensuring that materials are translated and published in multiple languages is important for those who are less proficient in English than another language.

Education of and Marketing to Third-Party Payers Providers must convince insurance representatives of the need to include speech-language pathology and audiology services in health care plans (Henri, Hallowell, & Johnson, 1997; Lim et al., 2010). We must also convince physicians of the necessity of our services.

Marketing to and Education of Referral Sources Many of the decision makers who have the greatest potential for making an impact on patient access are often unaware of the issues faced by people with communication and swallowing problems and of the vital role that SLPs and audiologists play. It is important that decision makers such as physicians, discharge planners, and directors of student services and special education programs be educated about the link between communication abilities and one's success in life.

Appealing Denials of Treatment Authorization and Reimbursement Providers must work with their clients to appeal vigorously all decisions denying coverage of services. A concerted appeals process in a service-providing agency helps improve access to services in that agency, as success rates for concerted appeals are high (Henri, Hallowell, & Johnson, 1997). To support these efforts, ASHA published in 2002 a helpful document, *Appealing Health Plan Denials*. This resource provides model letters that can be sent to health insurance companies to reverse authorization and reimbursement denials as well as treatment efficacy statements that can be appended to an appeal letter as a supporting document. The American Academy of Audiology also provides guidance to its membership on issues related to reimbursement.

Promoting Access to People with Geographic and Transportation Challenges It is important that service providers develop and promote telehealth services to enhance access for those who have limited access to on-site services. Clinical agencies should also provide their clientele with information on how to access public transportation, senior citizens transportation available within a community, and the option of home health care if possible.

Financial Support Contributions to ASHA's Political Action Committee (ASHA-PAC) help to advance concerted professional advocacy efforts at state and federal levels. The purpose of the PAC is to provide financial support to "candidate committees for the U.S. House and Senate that recognize the importance of speech-language pathology and audiology services and who demonstrate concern for the rights of all citizens to receive these services" (ASHA, 2012). Similarly, the AAA supports its own political action committee and hosts an online legislative action center to assist its members in advocating for hearing health services.

Writing to Legislators As they want to remain in office and be reelected, legislators have a vested interest in knowing their constituents' concerns. Without the strong voice of professionals who understand the impact of policy decisions on consumers, legislators are unlikely to be sensitive to and knowledgeable about critical issues important to informed decision making. Professionals do not need to be sophisticated about legislative processes to join in legislative campaigns to address the numerous challenges to patient access. National, state, and local organizations offer ample guidance.

Taking advantage of ASHA's grassroots advocacy resources, free of charge, allows professionals to read concise descriptions of issues that need to be addressed and specific actions professionals may take. These actions almost always involve calling, writing, or e-mailing legislators. At annual ASHA and AAA conventions, congressional affairs staff members offer hands-on help with letter writing and related advocacy projects. Further assistance is available through the "Professionals" segments of ASHA's website and the "Practice Management" section of the AAA website. Additional guidance can be found in an ASHA publication edited by Golper and Brown (2004), in which advocacy processes are analyzed and discussed as critical to business practices within the profession.

Inviting Legislators to Work Settings Hosting a member of Congress in the clinical environment allows clinicians to directly discuss and demonstrate problems of access, the need for access, and the ways in which speech-language pathology and audiology services improve the quality of life of legislators' constituents.

Visiting Legislators in Their Local Offices or on Capitol Hill The Governmental Affairs staff of ASHA arranges appointments for professionals visiting Washington, DC, and provides in-person briefings and other materials. Because legislators have temporary terms, it is a good idea to visit and write to elected officials on a yearly basis to keep them informed about critical access and service delivery issues confronting children and adults in their districts.

Participating in Clinical Research Given the dire need for empirical research to support EBP, clinicians' roles in research are more important than ever. For those not having skills, time, training, or resources to initiate or oversee research programs, there are ample possibilities for collaboration with university-based researchers.

Engaging in Quality Improvement By maintaining ongoing quality improvement programs, providers continue to demonstrate cost-effective, functional treatment outcomes, which are essential to local, state, and national advocacy efforts. Again, ASHA has developed a number of resources to assist its membership in developing and maintaining quality improvement programs.

Advocacy among Consumers and Their Significant Others

Consumers and their significant others are among the most powerful and credible advocates in improving access to audiology and speech-language pathology services. As there are often limitations due to consumers' communication disorders, support from family and from clinicians in encouraging consumer advocacy is essential. Specific ways in which consumers and their significant others may make solid contributions to advocacy efforts to improve access to services include active writing to legislators and visiting legislators in their local or Capitol Hill offices, as described previously under "Advocacy among Clinicians and Clinical Administrators." Additional steps are described briefly here. Backing by the SLP or audiologist in each of these efforts may be helpful, as may be the support of the consumer's primary care physician.

Active Pursuit of Coverage for Speech-Language Pathology and Audiology Services It is important that consumers pursue adequate coverage by health insurance companies. Consumers often are unaware of the coverage provided by their health care policies and restrictions that many place on speech-language pathology and audiology services. Careful study of a health plan's coverage and policies is the first step toward proactively seeking greater access to services. For those covered by employer-sponsored plans, staff members of the employer's human resources department may offer assistance in checking on specific coverage issues. Referring an insurance case (or "utilization") reviewer to a particular policy document may easily resolve some coverage issues. In cases in which needed services are not covered, consumer appeals to third-party payers regarding the need for services to enhance independence, educational status, medical management, and/or overall quality of life may help to shape future policy modifications.

Reporting of Health Care Policy Coverage Inconsistencies When there are discrepancies between what an insurance company purports to cover, through its promotional materials and policy documentation, and its actual practice in terms of authorizing and/or reimbursing for services, appeals brought by consumers are critical. Discrepancies can be reported at a variety of levels. Working through a hierarchy of contacts is recommended, beginning with insurance case reviewers, thereon to consumer liaisons, and up to CEOs. If necessary, state insurance commissioners may be contacted. If reporting at each of these levels fails, contacting your United States congressperson or senator often helps. Other avenues for advocacy in the face of restricted services include letters to the editor in newspapers and professional journals and carefully constructed press releases that may lead to newspaper, radio, and/or television coverage of access problems. If aired constructively, such media coverage may help to foster public education about access issues while exerting due pressure on insurance companies.

Education of Employers Organizations that pay for insurance coverage for their employees should be urged to reconsider contracts with companies that have a pattern of limiting or violating their coverage policies or of not covering critically needed services. Consumer feedback to employers' human resources departments helps raise awareness of a plan's effectiveness and worth and has been found to be especially effective.

Mobilization of Consumer Groups The advocacy power of individual consumers may be compounded exponentially through consumer groups. Personal and political advocacy efforts among members of local, state, and national organizations for people with specific communication disorders may be especially effective in the retention and expansion of access to services.

Advocacy among Educators and Students

Before they enter the clinical workforce, it is important that students gain awareness and knowledge of professional practice issues and how they may work to foster positive changes within their profession. Such preparation is especially essential in medical, rehabilitation, and skilled nursing contexts, where supervisors and other experienced practitioners are increasingly called to engage in billable clinical service as opposed to training and supervisory activity related to issues of insurance coverage (i.e., coding, authorizations, documentation, billing, appeals, and marketing). Graduates who are savvy about these issues and about productive actions for advocacy will have a distinct advantage over others in the job market and in their initial stages of clinical practice. An additional advantage to having students get involved in professional practice issues is that students are capable of achieving significant advocacy work while they are still in school.

Specific actions in which faculty members and students may engage to advance advocacy for clinical access are addressed here.

Continuing Education Concerning Modes of Service Delivery and Health Policy and about the Effects on People with Communication and Swallowing Disorders Because of the recency of the gravest challenges accompanying the expansion of managed care and major federal health care policy changes, few university faculty members have practiced in environments in which there have been significant threats to consumer access. Still, it is essential that all faculty members obtain an understanding of managed care principles and their ramifications for the practice of speech-language pathology and audiology. Such an understanding, in turn, helps foster students' potential for strategic advocacy as well as effective future professional practice (Hallowell & Henri, 1996; Whitmire, Reder, Ralabate, & White, 2006). Continuing education is available through current publications, Internet resources, conferences, seminars, and workshops. Three methods of advocacy by educators and students are curricular revision, education of medical students, and engagement in concerted legislative advocacy.

Curricular Revision Coursework emphasizing the interconnections among functional clinical outcomes, cost-effectiveness of intervention, reimbursement, and consumer access will help to foster professional advocacy for years to come. Infusing such concepts throughout the curriculum will help students to see the import of such concepts in their current and future professional roles (Hallowell & Henri, 1996; Vekovius, 1995).

Education of Medical Students and their Professors In universities with medical schools, faculty members may take advantage of opportunities to engage medical students in preceptorships related to our field, and clinical observation of audiological and speech-language services, thus enhancing appreciation of our services to future physicians. Likewise, presenting lectures or workshops to medical students and their professors may elevate the medical community's understanding of the impact of communication disorders upon a person's life trajectory and how these conditions may be beneficially addressed.

Engagement in Concerted Legislative Advocacy Students and faculty have clout as political constituents whose voice may have an impact on legislators. It is important that faculty and students be encouraged to participate in advocacy efforts sponsored by ASHA, the National Student Speech Language Hearing Association (NSSLHA), AAA, the Student Academy of Audiology (SAA), and state and local student and consumer groups. Academic classes or student groups may organize letter-writing campaigns involving significant numbers of participants.

CARE EXTENDERS

One way to cope with limitations in access to professional specialized care that many people with communication and swallowing disorders are facing is to expand the reservoir of individuals who may provide needed care. "Care extenders" consist of individuals who are not certified or licensed SLPs or audiologists, but who nevertheless are involved in helping to further the development or rehabilitation of communication and swallowing skills. Ideally, they are trained and monitored by a fully certified clinician. They may be "support personnel" (aides, technicians, or assistants), clinicians in training, family members, or community volunteers.

Support Personnel

Many SLPs and audiologists find the use of professional aides, technicians, and assistants to be essential for ensuring clients' access to care (Bloom, 2009; Lizarondo, Kumar, Hyde, & Skidmore, 2010; McNeilly, 2009). Support personnel may help in the handling of large caseloads, such that more clients are treated and/or more treatment time per client is offered than would otherwise be possible (Keane & Rogers, 2009). Support personnel may also allow fully credentialed clinicians more time to treat individuals with severe and complex communication disorders, thus improving overall quality of care. An additional advantage is that the level of care needed by an individual may be more closely matched with the level of training and experience of an aide or assistant. For example, individuals who use alternative and augmentative communication (AAC) devices have been shown to benefit from assistants specially trained to facilitate AAC use (Beukelman, Ball, & Fager, 2008).

Services once thought to be within the sole domain of the speech-language pathologist or audiologist, but that do not require the skills and expertise of professionals with all the training and experience required for clinical certification, may now be offered by people whose services are far less costly. Support personnel vary widely in their level of academic and on-the-job training. Speech-language pathology aides, for example, generally have training in specific areas of practice and have more limited responsibilities than assistants. The increase of support personnel in speech-language pathology and audiology has led to further proliferation of regulations and standards (Ross & Harding, 2010; Montgomery, Dodd, Giess, & Barnes, 2010). Within the United States, states vary in the use of terms used to refer to the various levels of training and/or licensure required of support personnel (ASHA, 2004b; 2005a; 2005b; 2012a). State laws also vary in terms of the tasks in which support personnel are permitted to engage; some states do not permit the use of support personnel (ASHA, 2009).

Examples of tasks that speech-language pathology assistants may perform under the supervision of an SLP, according to ASHA's *Guidelines for the Training, Use, and Supervision of Speech-Language Pathology Assistants* (ASHA, 2012a), include conducting speech-language screenings and participating in treatment plans or protocols that have been established by a certified speech-language pathologist. Examples of tasks that audiology technicians may perform under the supervision of an audiologist include conducting hearing screenings, application of electrodes for electronystagmography testing, and calibration checks for audiological equipment. Support personnel may perform clerical duties; document test results and patient/client progress; prepare diagnostic and treatment materials; schedule diagnostic and treatment activities; and participate in research projects, in-service training, and public relations programs. Examples of tasks that support personnel are generally not permitted to perform include diagnostic testing or interpretation of test results, hearing aid fitting, patient/client or family counseling, development or modification of a patient/client's individualized treatment plan, and discharging a patient/client from services. Regardless of specific duties performed, an ongoing supervisor relationship by a fully licensed and certified speech-language pathologist or audiologist is critical (McCready, 2007).

Despite the advantages mentioned, the use of support personnel remains controversial in the field of communication and swallowing disorders. Those opposing support personnel maintain that the quality of care rendered to patients is diminished, that time savings through services provided do not merit the increased time demands for supervision, and that the job security of licensed professionals is threatened (McCartney et al., 2005). There is also concern that cost-minded health care and educational administrators will abuse the use of support personnel by compelling them to provide services outside their scope of practice and by implementing cost-saving hiring practices in which ideal supervisor-to-support staff ratios are exceeded. An additional disadvantage is that many health insurance companies still do not recognize support personnel as qualified service providers and therefore do not pay for treatment delivered by these people. See Chapter 12 for more discussion of this topic.

Graduate Students

The provision of supervised evaluation and treatment services by graduate students in speech-language pathology and audiology has long been a source for extending care to clients/patients. In many university clinics, ample free and low-cost services are made available to surrounding communities while providing diverse clinical learning opportunities to student clinicians. Additionally, networks of student volunteers may be helpful in extending services beyond clinical and diagnostic treatment sessions. Examples are students serving as communication partners (Lyon, 1992), in-home respite caregivers (Hallowell, 2000), or as volunteers in a wide array of clinical educational contexts.

Trained Volunteers

Trained volunteers can be effective care extenders. As no compensation is involved, and as these individuals are clearly identified to clients/patients as volunteers, there are fewer legal and licensure-related problems than in the use of multiskilled professionals. Volunteers provide additional opportunities to practice and maintain developing communication skills (Kagan, Black, Duchan, Simmons-Mackie, & Square, 2001; Lyon, 1992). Before their direct involvement with patients or clients, volunteers may be required to observe treatment sessions and then may be guided by the clinician in the provision of treatment-reinforcing activities such as repetitive drills. Volunteers may also be trained to handle other tasks, such as clerical work, scheduling, and equipment maintenance, allowing skilled clinicians more time to spend with clients/patients.

Family Members and Other Caregivers

Given the current health care service delivery climate, family members are now often required to assume greater responsibilities in caring for their significant others (Dexter et al., 2010; Teng et al., 2003). As with trained volunteers, coaching and training by the skilled clinician are essential. Treatment-complementing activities provided by a properly guided caregiver can be highly effective. With increased family member involvement, it will become necessary to identify the unique variables that minimize or prevent successful caregiver follow-through at home or elsewhere (Chan, 2010; Jorgensen et al., 1999; Thomas et al., 2002).

Multiskilling of Professionals

Multiskilling is the cross training of professionals to enable them to perform functions that have been exclusively within the scope of practice of a profession other than their own (ASHA, 1996). Multiskilling is one more means by which patients' access to care may be enhanced because it ideally enables more professionals to provide needed services. Multiskilling also has cost-saving implications in that it is less expensive to hire one individual to perform a series of tasks that traditionally have required multiple professionals.

Consider a home health patient recovering from a stroke. The patient may have a speech-language pathologist visit three times per week to work on compensatory swallowing strategies for dysphagia, an occupational therapist visit five times per week to work on activities of daily living, a physical therapist visit five times per week to work on mobility and strength, and a nurse visit once per week to obtain a blood sample and record vital signs. Under a multiskilling model, a home health agency may have each of those specialized professionals conduct initial diagnostic evaluations and develop care plans based on contact with the patient. Then, rather than each professional repeatedly visiting the patient, one multiskilled professional would carry out the multiple plans of care specified by the group of specialists.

The cost-saving implications for multiskilling are evident. Likewise, it is clear that multiskilling may increase patient/client access to services through the sheer number of professionals trained to offer a service. Still, if not implemented carefully, with respect to the training needed to perform skilled services, multiskilling poses a serious threat to the integrity of the specialized health care professions (ASHA, 2006b). Also, job security of some certified clinical professionals may be threatened. In some contexts, the responsibilities and required skills of multiskilled professionals are unclear (ASHA, 1996; Pietranton & Lynch, 1995). The regulations for the training, experience, licensure, and certification required for each specialty may be breached in many contexts where multiskilled personnel perform in areas beyond their scope of practice.

ASHA's position statement on multiskilling (ASHA, 1997) indicates that it is acceptable for multiskilled providers to perform basic activities that do not require professional-level skills, such as taking blood pressures or assisting with bed-to-wheelchair transfers. It is unacceptable to provide cross-training of clinical skills.

TECHNOLOGICAL ACCESS

Advances in technology improve and augment the clinical services of speech-language pathologists and audiologists. For many individuals, these advances improve access to services, particularly for those with limited physical accessibility to evaluations or intervention. Technology also may be a cost-effective support for clinicians wishing to access current information to improve their clinical skills. See Chapter 26 for continued discussion of technology as a professional issue.

Telehealth

Telehealth is the use of electronic information and communications technologies to provide and support health care services when there is a distance between participants. The term *telehealth* is sometimes used interchangeably with *telemedicine,* although many authors and practitioners in health professions prefer the connotation of the former term, as it is more inclusive of professions outside of primary medical practice. The term *telerehabilitation* is also used by some. Audio, visual, and text media are generally combined in telehealth applications. From its inception, one of the most promising aspects of telehealth has been the improvement of access to care in remote areas where skilled service providers are scarce or absent (Swanepoel et al., 2010; Wick, 2010). In addition to the lack of geographic access to service providers, other barriers to care might be alleviated by telehealth. As aptly summarized by Field (1996), these barriers include the following:

- Distance from primary, secondary, and tertiary medical services
- Poor transportation (e.g., lack of automobile, limited or nonexistent bus service), even for relatively short distances
- Inadequate financial resources, particularly insurance coverage or directly subsidized services
- Family, educational, and cultural factors (e.g., illiteracy, distrust of technology)
- Delivery system characteristics, including poor coordination of care, long waiting times for appointments, inadequate numbers or kinds of specialists, and bureaucratic obstacles to services
- Gaps in our knowledge about how these factors interact to affect the use of services and what can be done to overcome or eliminate barriers to access (p. 174)

In addition to expanding access for disadvantaged populations and patients in rural areas, opportunities are emerging for expansion of home health services through technology (Bloch, 2008; Sanberg, 2010). As home health care remains one of the most rapidly expanding forms of service delivery, it is essential that professionals in our disciplines stay abreast of telehealth mechanisms that may allow replacing some home visits with video visits, checking up on carryover of treatment activities, and furthering patient and family education (cf., Hard, 2010). An additional advantage of providing care through distance technology is that it may expand clinicians' availability to people who live in areas that are considered unsafe, such as some urban neighborhoods, correctional facilities, and even within active international war zones (Doolittle, Otto, & Clemens, 1998; Khazei, Jarvis-Sellinger, Ho, & Lee, 2005; Hart, 2010).

In conjunction with the expansion of digital technology, enabling image capturing, compression, transmission, and interpretation, interest in telehealth is expanding rapidly across a vast array of health care professions. High-speed, high-bandwidth telecommunication systems are expanding globally. In addition to improved access, advantages reported by evaluators of some rural telemedicine programs include reduction of duplicative diagnostic services, improved consumer confidence in local medical personnel and facilities, reduced need for referral to service providers outside the local area, improved recruitment and retention of health care personnel, and improved continuing education for service providers (Brown, 2005). Clinical applications in telehealth are found in virtually every health specialty (Kairy, Lehoux, Vincent, & Visintin, 2009; Wakefield, Holman, Ray, Morse, & Kienzle, 2004). Much of what we know about possibilities for remote service delivery for diagnosis and treatment in communication and swallowing disorders is derived from research and applications from other disciplines (cf., Burtt, 1997). For example, research in long-distance interpretation of radiographic imaging (e.g., Pauly, 1993) may have important implications for diagnostic interpretation of videofluoroscopic studies of swallowing. On a regulatory level, cases in which state regulations have been developed to control the delivery of services from medical practitioners between states may also be applied to SLPs and audiologists.

A growing number of published empirical studies directly address the effectiveness of telehealth delivery in audiology and speech-language pathology. Studies involving comparisons of face-to-face and telehealth assessments support the feasibility, reliability, and acceptability of telehealth evaluations of acquired speech and language disorders (Duffy, Werven, & Aronson, 1997; Glykas & Chytas, 2004; Kairy, Lehoux, Vincent, & Visintin, 2009; Mashima et al., 2003; Sicotte, Lehoux, Fortier-Blanc, & Leblanc, 2003; Theodoros & Russell, 2008; Wertz et al., 1992; Wilson & Onslow, 2004).

Access to the Internet has had profound impact on people living in more remote regions and can significantly minimize or even remove barriers to access resulting from geographic isolation. Increasingly, health insurance companies, including state Medicaid programs, are acknowledging the merits of services rendered remotely by SLPs via software such as Skype, a voice-over Internet protocol. Computers, whether laptops or desktops, now typically come equipped with video cameras as standard features. Tablets and smart phones are similarly equipped. Creative SLPs across the globe are developing applications ("apps") that facilitate remote intervention with meaningful content.

New developments in technological access to care will be shaped by ongoing developments in health policy as it affects telehealth. The following factors will be most influential in continuing efforts to expand service delivery options for professionals in our disciplines:

- Licensure issues, especially for services provided among states
- Training in the use of telehealth technology
- Establishment of standards
- Reimbursement issues
- Patient confidentiality issues
- Attitudes of providers and patients
- Means of ensuring quality of clinician-patient relationships
- Potential cost savings
- Demonstration of clinical outcomes
- Telecommunications infrastructure and cost (Hibbert et al., 2004; Hill & Theodoros, 2002; Ostbye & Hurlen, 1997; Yoo et al., 2004)

Information Technology

Given that access to care involves more than direct contact with a skilled clinician, the notion of technological access also includes the use of telecommunications and information technology to improve access to information that may allow consumers and potential consumers to learn about communication problems, diagnostic and treatment options, and prevention strategies. For those who remain without computers and connection to the Internet and/or telephones, access to information resources is tenuous. Funding for technology through regional clinics and public facilities, such as libraries, is highly variable across the country, and is often subject to changes in tax or grant allocations and annual budgets. Deficits in language and literacy skills may impose further obstacles to care for disadvantaged populations. Gaps in access may actually widen if information services are improved only for those with the means, education, and skills to pursue those services (Field, 1996). See Chapter 26 for more information on telepractice and technology in the professions.

EDUCATING THE PUBLIC

Most individuals take communication for granted and are frequently unaware of the link between one's communication abilities and one's success in life. To improve access to speech-language pathology, audiology, and swallowing services, it is increasingly more critical to improve the general public's and consumers' awareness and knowledge about speech-language pathology and audiology services.

ADJUSTMENTS IN SERVICE-PROVIDING ENVIRONMENTS

Certain environmental and operational adjustments must be made to improve client access to speech-language pathology and audiology services. Flextime and compressed workweeks are rapidly becoming the norm. Recognizing the value of schedules that are more convenient for their consumers, organizations are expanding their daily work hours and days of operation and, as a result, improving their revenues. Speech-language pathology and audiology providers must follow suit. In environments where traditional appointment schedule models create significant client/patient hardships, creative, nontraditional scheduling approaches have been found helpful. To improve attendance rates, for example, some organizations are experimenting with "fluid" appointment schedules wherein a client's treatment appointment can occur anytime between certain times, such as 9 a.m. to noon or 1 p.m. to 4 p.m. As clients arrive during these time periods, they are integrated into an ongoing three-hour session to receive their treatment, whether it be 30, 45, or 60 minutes. They leave when their time period ends.

Another tactic being used to improve access and attendance is the development of interagency collaborations in which several agencies contribute to fund a minibus to bring clients to their locations. Other environmental adjustments must be explored to ensure maximum access to our services. To improve geographic access, satellite offices (leased, shared, or donated space) should be considered. Finally, while more expensive, home visits have been useful as one avenue for improving access for individuals with limited resources and mobility challenges.

SUMMARY

In this chapter, we identified significant barriers that influence access to audiology and speech-language pathology services and stressed the broad and serious consequences of current service delivery trends on our field. We also emphasized the growing need for our services throughout the age continuum. Access to audiology and speech-language pathology services can be significantly enhanced through comprehensive, focused strategies that remove or minimize barriers and maximize the use and impact of health care and educational resources, both financial and human. With this in mind, we described effective strategies to improve revenues, decrease costs, and increase clinical outcomes. To subsidize diminishing reimbursements, strategies to create alternative funding sources were presented. More than ever, it is today the responsibility of all audiologists and speech-language pathologists to ensure that barriers are eliminated and resources are maximized. To accomplish these goals, our roles in educating the public and in advocacy were described in detail.

CRITICAL THINKING

1. What are the key factors that have led to a growing need for services in speech-language pathology? What are the key factors that have led to decreased access to those services?
2. Imagine that you are the CEO of a not-for-profit center for the treatment of communication disorders. What are the key steps that you would take to maximize your center's (a) clinical revenues and (b) nonclinical revenues?
3. When justifying your services to a managed care organization, how would you defend the treatment for each of the conditions listed below as "medically necessary"?
   a. Adult dysphagia
   b. Infant dysphagia
   c. Adult aphasia
   d. Adult acquired neurogenic motor speech disorders
   e. Child language delay
   f. Child articulation disorder
   g. Child hearing impairment
   h. Adult hearing impairment
   i. Child central auditory processing disorder

   In addition to your own descriptions of medical necessity, what other information and references might you include in your documentation to third-party payers regarding the medical necessity of your services?
4. In what specific actions for advocacy might you engage in your current educational or work context to enhance access to service in speech-language pathology and audiology for people who need them? Write an action plan for achieving one or two of those actions within the next month, either alone or with students or professional colleagues. Include specific dates for each activity in which you would need to engage to achieve that action.
5. What is the role of local, state, and national professional organizations in improving access to audiology or speech-language pathology services?
6. Suppose you have a client who needs a hearing aid but has no health insurance or financial means to purchase the device. Do you have a responsibility to help the client find financial aid? What sources might help in this situation?
7. Consider possible options for delivering audiology and speech-language pathology services to people who are financially, geographically, or otherwise limited in access. Choose one example of such means, and describe a hypothetical scenario in which an individual would be best served through that mode of service delivery. Include details about the geographic region, socioeconomic context, and the individual's clinical profile (age, diagnosis, symptoms, services needed, etc.) as well as details about how the individual would benefit in terms of enhanced access to care.

8. You are employed at a large university hospital and have been asked by a medical school professor to give a talk on either speech-language pathology or audiology to the medical students. What would be your goals in this presentation? Write out an outline for your presentation.

9. You are director of a large urban speech and hearing center that serves clients across the age span, and you just heard that one of your federal legislators will be visiting your agency for a two-hour morning visit. What would you want to accomplish on this visit? What aspects of your program would you want to showcase and how would you do this?

REFERENCES

Adair, A. (2009). *How to raise money online for family and friends with limited or no medical insurance.* Retrieved from http://voices.yahoo.com/how-raise-money-online-family-friends-with-4675421.html

American Academy of Pediatrics. (2005). Policy statement: Model contractual language for medical necessity for children. *Pediatrics, 116*(1), 261–262.

American Speech-Language-Hearing Association. (1996). Technical report of the ad hoc committee on multiskilling. *ASHA, 38* (Suppl. 16), 1–9.

American Speech-Language-Hearing Association. (1997). Position statement: Multiskilled personnel. *ASHA , 39* (Suppl. 17), 13.

American Speech-Language-Hearing Association. (2002). *Appealing health plan denials.* Prepared by the Health Care Economics & Advocacy Team. Rockville, MD: Author.

American Speech-Language-Hearing Association. (2004a). *Advocacy in action: Negotiating for increased Medicaid rates and coverage.* Rockville, MD: Author.

American Speech-Language-Hearing Association. (2005a). *Frequently asked questions about speech-language pathology assistants.* Available from http://www.asha.org/

American Speech-Language-Hearing Association. (2005b). *Guidelines for the training, use, and supervision of speech-language pathology assistants.* Available from http://www.asha.org/

American Speech-Language-Hearing Association. (2005c). *Medical necessity for speech-language pathology and audiology services.* Available from http://www.asha.org/

American Speech-Language-Hearing Association. (2005d). *Preferred practice patterns for the profession of speech-language pathology.* Available from http://www.asha.org/

American Speech-Language-Hearing Association. (2005e). *Preferred practice patters for the profession of audiology.* Retrieved from http://www.asha.org/docs/html/PP2006-00274.html

American Speech-Language-Hearing Association. (2006a). Medicare caps back & fees cut, pending Congressional action. *The ASHA Leader.*

American Speech-Language-Hearing Association. (2006b). *Preferred practice patterns for the profession of audiology.* Available from http://www.asha.org/

American Speech-Language-Hearing Association. (2009). *ASHA's support personnel trends.* (2009). Available from http://www.asha.org/

American Speech-Language-Hearing Association. (2012). *ASHA-PAC: Your voice on Capitol Hill.* Retrieved from http://www.asha.org/advocacy/federal/pac/

Berman, S. (1997). A pediatric perspective on medical necessity. *Archives of Pediatric Adolescent Medicine, 151*, 858.

Beukelman, D., Ball, L., & Fager, S. (2008). An AAC personnel framework: Adults with acquired complex communication needs. *Augmentative and Alternative Communication, 24*(3), 255–267.

Bloch, C. (2008, December 21). *VA telehealth in the spotlight.* Retrieved from http://telemedicinenews.blogspot.com/2008/12/va-telehealth-in-spotlight.html

Bloom, S. (2009). The audiologist's assistant: Assessing a growing trend in practice management. *The Hearing Journal, 62*(1), 19–20, 22, 24–25.

Brown, N. A. (2005). Information on telemedicine. *Journal of Telemedicine and Telecare, 11*, 117–126.

Burtt, K. (1997). Nurses use telehealth to address rural health care needs, prevent hospitalizations. *American Nurse, 29*, 21.

Centeno, J., & Kohnert, K. (2009). Serving linguistically and culturally diverse adults with communication disorders: Multidisciplinary perspectives and evidence. *Seminars in Speech and Language, 30*(3), 137–138.

Chan, S. (2010). Family caregiving in dementia: The Asian perspective of a global problem. *Dementia and Geriatric Cognitive Disorders, 30*(6), 469–478.

Dexter, P., Miller, D., Clark, D., Weiner, M., Harris, L., Livin, L., et al. (2010). Preparing for an aging population and improving chronic disease management. *AMIA Annual Symposium Proceedings*, 162–166.

Dollaghan, C. A. (2004). Evidence-based practice in communication disorders: What do we know, and when do we know it? *Journal of Communication Disorders, 37*, 391–400.

Doolittle, G. C., Otto, F., & Clemens, C. (1998). Hospice care using home-based telemedicine systems. *Journal of Telemedicine and Telecare, 4*, 58–59.

Duffy, J. R., Werven, G. W., & Aronson, A. E. (1997). Telemedicine and the diagnosis of speech and language disorders. *Mayo Clinic Proceedings, 72*, 1116–1122.

Ellrodt, A. G., Cho, M., & Cush, J. J. (1997). An evidence-based medicine approach to the diagnosis and management of musculoskeletal complaints. *The American Journal of Medicine, 103*, 3S–6S.

Epstein, S. (2008). The rise of "recruitmentology": Clinical research. Racial knowledge, and the politics of inclusion and difference. *Social Studies of Science, 38*(5), 801–832.

Field, M. J. (Ed.). (1996). *Telemedicine: A guide to assessing telecommunications in health care.* Washington, DC: National Academy Press.

Fox, H. B., & McManus, M. A. (2001). A national study of commercial health insurance and Medicaid definitions of medical necessity: What do they mean for children? *Ambulatory Pediatrics, 1*(1), 16–22.

Frymark, T. B., & Mullen, C. (2005). Influence of the prospective payment system on speech-language pathology services. *American Journal of Physical Medicine & Rehabilitation, 84*(1), 12–21.

Glykas, M., & Chytas, P. (2004). Technology assisted speech and language therapy. *International Journal of Medical Informatics, 73*, 529–541.

Golper, L., & Brown, J. (Eds.). (2004). *Business matters: A guide for speech-language pathologists.* Rockville, MD: American Speech-Language-Hearing Association.

Grabowski, D. (2008). Medicare and Medicaid: Conflicting incentives for long-term care. *The Milbank Quarterly, 85*(4), 579–610.

Granger, C.V., Carlin, M., Diaz, P., Dorval, J., Forer, S., Kessler, C., et al. (2009). Medical necessity: Is current documentation practice and payment denial limiting access to inpatient rehabilitation? *American Journal of Physical Medicine and Rehabilitation, 88*(9), 756–765.

Hallowell, B. (2000). A student-run respite network for caregivers of persons with dementing illness. *Communication Connection, 14*(1), 10.

Hallowell, B., & Chapey, R. (2008). Introduction to language intervention strategies in adult aphasia. In R. Chapey (Ed.), *Language intervention strategies in adult aphasia* (5th ed., pp. 3–19). Baltimore, MD: Williams & Wilkins.

Hallowell, B., & Henri, B. P. (1996). Preparing students for the realities of health care changes: Incorporating concepts of managed care and health care financing into clinical training programs. *HEARSAY: Journal of the Ohio Speech and Hearing Association, 11*, 40–42.

Hard, J. (2010). Expanding access to telespeech in clinical settings: Inroads and challenges. *Telemedicine Journal and E-Health, 16*(9), 922–924.

Hart, J. (2010, November). Medical connectivity: Expanding access to telespeech in clinical settings: Inroads & challenges. *Telemedicine Journal and E-Health, 16*(9), 922–924.

Hemphill, L., & Tivnan, T. (2008). The importance of early vocabulary for literacy achievement in high-poverty schools. *Journal of Education for Students Placed at Risk, 13*(4), 426–451.

Henri, B. P. (2010). Business: At the table or on the table: It's our choice. *American Speech-Language-Hearing Association Special Interest Division 11 Perspectives on Administration and Supervision, 21*, 3–8.

Henri, B. P., & Hallowell, B. (1996). Action planning for advocacy: Issues for speech-language pathologists and audiologists in the face of the expansion of managed care. *HEARSAY: Journal of the Ohio Speech and Hearing Association, 11*, 61–64.

Henri, B. P., & Hallowell, B. (1999a). Funding alternatives to offset the reimbursement impacts of managed care. *Newsletter of Special Interest Division 2, Neurophysiology and Neurogenic Speech and Language Disorders*. Rockville, MD: American Speech-Language-Hearing Association.

Henri, B. P., & Hallowell, B. (1999b). Relating managed care to managing care. In B. S. Cornett (Ed.), *Clinical practice management in speech-language pathology: Principles and practicalities*. Gaithersburg, MD: Aspen Publishers.

Henri, B. P., Hallowell, B., & Johnson, C. (1997). Advocacy and marketing to support clinical services. In R. Kreb (Ed.), *A practical guide to treatment outcomes and cost effectiveness* (pp. 39–48). Rockville, MD: American Speech-Language-Hearing Association Task Force on Treatment Outcomes and Cost Effectiveness.

Hibbert, D., Mair, F. S., May, C. R., Boland, A., O'Connor, J., Capewell, S., et al. (2004). Health professionals' responses to the introduction of a home telehealth service. *Journal of Telemedicine and Telecare, 10*, 226–230.

Hill, A., & Theodoros, D. (2002). Research into telehealth applications in speech-language pathology. *Journal of Telemedicine and Telecare, 8*, 187–196.

Hiller, M. D., & Lewis, J. B. (1995). Managed health care benefit plans: What are the ethical issues? *Trends in Health Care, Law & Ethics, 10*, 109–112, 118.

Hock, M. F., & Deshler, D. D. (2003). "No Child" leaves behind teen reading proficiency. *The Education Digest*, 27–35.

Ireys, H. T., Wehr, E., & Cooke, R. E. (2000). Defining medical necessity. *The Exceptional Parent, 30*(3), 37–39.

Jorgensen, H. S., Reith, J., Nakayama, H., Kammersgaard, L. P., Raaschou, H. O., & Olsen, T. S. (1999). What determines good recovery in patients with the most severe strokes? The Copenhagen Stroke Study. *Stroke, 30*, 2008–2012.

Kagan, A., Black, S. E., Duchan, J. F., Simmons-Mackie, N., & Square, P. (2001). Training volunteers as conversation partners using "supported conversation for adults with aphasia" (SCA): A controlled trial. *Journal of Speech, Language, and Hearing Research, 44*, 624–638.

Kahan, J. P., Bernstein, S. J., Leape, L. L., Hilborne, L. H., Park, R. E., Parker, L., et al. (1994). Measuring the necessity of medical procedures. *Medical Care, 32*, 357–365.

Kairy, D., Lehoux, P., Vincent, C., & Visintin, M. (2009). A systematic review of clinical outcomes, clinical process, healthcare utilization and costs associated with telerehabilitation. *Disability & Rehabilitation, 31*(6), 427–447.

Keane, L., & Rogers, L. (2009). Using what you have: Training teacher assistants as speech-language assistants. *ASHA Perspectives on School-Based Issues, 10*(1), 19–22.

Khazei, A., Jarvis-Selinger, S., Ho, K., & Lee, A. (2005). An assessment of the telehealth needs and health-care priorities of Tanna Island: A remote, under-served and vulnerable population. *Journal of Telemedicine and Telecare, 11*, 35–40.

Kneipp, S. M., Lutz, B. J., & Means, S. (2009). Reasons for enrollment, the informed consent process, and trust among low-income women participating in a community-based participatory research study. *Public Health Nursing, 26*(4), 362–369.

Lerner, J. C., Gesek, J., & Adams, S. (2003). Will using evidence-based approaches to a standards development process improve Medicaid policy making? Report on a promising effort. *Journal of Ambulatory Care Management, 26*(4), 322–333.

Lim, S., McManus, M., Fox H., White, K., & Forsman, I. (2010). Ensuring financial access to hearing aids for infants and young children. *Pediatrics. 126*(1), S43–S51.

Lizarondo, L., Kumar, S., Hyde, L., & Skidmore, D. (2010). Allied health assistants and what they do: A systematic review of the literature. *Journal of Multidisciplinary Healthcare, 3*, 143–53.

Lyon, J. G. (1992). Communication use and participation for adults with aphasia in natural settings: The scope of the problem. *American Journal of Speech-Language Pathology, 1*, 7–14.

Mashima, P. A., Birkmire-Peters, D. P., Syms, M. J., Holtel, M. R., Burgess, L. P. A., & Peters, L. J. (2003). Telehealth: Voice therapy using telecommunications technology. *American Journal of Speech-Language Pathology, 12*, 432–439.

Maughan, B., Messer, J., Collishaw, S., Pickles, A., Snowling, M., Yule, W., et al. (2009). Persistence of literacy problems: Spelling in adolescence and at mid-life. *Journal of Child Psychology and Psychiatry, 50*(8), 893–901.

McCartney, E., Boyle, J., Bannatyne, S., Jessiman, E., Campbell, C., Kelsey, C., et al. (2005). 'Thinking for two': A case study of speech and language therapists working through assistants. *International Journal of Language & Communication Disorders, 40*(2), 221–235.

McCready, V. (2007, May 8). Supervision of speech-language pathology assistants: A reciprocal relationship. *The ASHA Leader*. Available from http://www.asha.org/

McManus, M. A., Levtov, R., White, K. R., Forsman, I., Foust, T., & Thompson, M. (2010). Medicaid reimbursement of hearing services for infants and young children. *Pediatrics, 126*, S34–S42.

McNeilly, L. (2009). Speech-language pathology assistants current state of affairs. *ASHA Perspectives on School-Based Issues, 10*(1), 12–18.

Montgomery, J., Dodd, J., Giess S. A., & Barnes, K. (2010). A 21st century communication sciences and disorders program. *ASHA Perspectives on School-Based Issues, 11*(2), 66–70.

National Joint Committee for the Communication Needs of Persons with Severe Disabilities. (2002). *Adults with learning disabilities. Access to communication services and supports; Concerns regarding the application of restrictive "eligibility" policies* [Technical report], pp. 205–206. Available from http://www.asha.org/docs

Nolan, P., & Bradley, E. (2008). Evidence-based practice: Implications and concerns. *Journal of Nursing Management, 16*(4), 388–393.

Noria, C. W., Borkowski, J. G., & Whitman, T. L. (2009). Parental influences on self-regulation and achievement in children with adolescent mothers. *European Journal of Development Psychology, 6*(6), 722–745.

Novelli, W. (2008). Transforming the healthcare system: A focus on prevention. *Healthcare Financial Management, 62*(4), 94–99.

O'Callaghan, A., McAllister, L., & Wilson, L. (2010). Experiences of care reported by adults with traumatic brain injury. *International Journal of Speech-Language Pathology, 12*(2), 107–123.

Olaniyan, O., Brown, I. L., & Williams, K. (2009, August). Managing medical necessity and notification denials. *Healthcare Financial Management*, 62–67.

Ostbye, T., & Hurlen, P. (1997). The electronic house call: Consequences of telemedicine consultations for physicians, patients, and society. *Archives of Family Medicine, 6*, 266–271.

Pauly, A. (1993). Telemedicine permits long-distance diagnosis. *Diagnostic Imaging, 15*, 57–59.

Pelletier, K. (2009). A review and analysis of the clinical and cost-effectiveness studies of comprehensive health promotion and disease management programs at the worksite: Update VII 2004–2008. *Journal of Occupational and Environmental Medicine, 51*(5), 822–837.

Perkins, J., & Olson, K. (1998). The threat of evidence-based definitions of medical necessity. *Health Advocate*. Los Angeles, CA: National Health Law Program.

Pietranton, A. A., & Lynch, C. (1995). Multiskilling: A renaissance or a dark age? *ASHA, 36*, 37–40.

Reaven, N., & Rosenbloom, J. (2009). Commentary on the reimbursement paradox. *Critical Care Medicine, 37*(7 Suppl.), S285–S289.

Rodwin, M. A. (1995). Conflicts in managed care. *The New England Journal of Medicine, 332,* 604–607.

Rosenbaum, S. (2009, Fall). Insurance discrimination on the basis of health status: An overview of discrimination practices, federal law, and federal reform options. *Legal Solutions in Health Reform,* 103–120.

Ross, S., & Harding, M. (2010). Regulating the use of support personnel in schools. *ASHA Perspectives on School-Based Issues, 11*(4), 149–155.

Rouse, C. E., & Kemple, J. J. (2009). Introducing the issue. *Future of Children, 19*(1), 3–15.

Sanberg, P. (2010, November 4). *Telehealth offers technological solution to caregivers.* Department of Veterans Affairs Captain James A. Lovell Federal Health Care Center. Retrieved from http://www.lovell.fhcc.va.gov/LOVELLFHCC/features/Telehealth_offers_technological_solution_to_caregivers.asp

Segal, M., Pedersen, A., Freeman, K., & Fast, A. (2008). Medicare's new restrictions on rehabilitation admissions: Impact on the elderly. *American Journal of Physical Medicine & Rehabilitation, 87*(11), 872–882.

Shippen, M. E., Houchins, D. E., Crites, S. A., Derzis, N. C., & Dashaunda, P. (2010). An examination of the basic reading skills of incarcerated males. *Adult Learning, 21*(3/4), 4–12.

Shulman S., Besculides, M., Saltzman, A., Ireys, H., White K. R., & Forsman, I. (2010). Evaluation of the universal newborn hearing screening and intervention program. *Pediatrics, 126*(1), S19–S27.

Sicotte, C., Lehoux, P., Fortier-Blanc, J., & Leblanc, Y. (2003). Feasibility and outcome evaluation of a telemedicine application in speech-language pathology. *Journal of Telemedicine and Telecare, 9*, 253–258.

Sindelar, T. (2002). *The "medical necessity requirement" in Medicaid.* Boston, MA: Disability Law Center.

Siobhan, O., & Catharine, P. M. (2009). The barriers perceived to prevent the successful implementation of evidence-based practice by speech and language therapists. *International Journal of Language & Communication Disorders, 44*(6), 1018–1035.

Smith, G., & Ashbaugh, J. (1995). *Managed care and people with developmental disabilities: A guidebook.* Alexandria, VA: National Association of State Directors of Developmental Disabilities Services, Inc.

Snow, P. C., & Powell, M. B. (2008). Oral language competence, social skills and high-risk boys: What are juvenile offenders trying to tell us? *Children & Society, 22*(1), 16–28.

Swanepoel, D., Clark, J., Koekemoer, D., Hall, J. W., III, Krumm, M., Ferrari, D. V., et. al. (2010). Telehealth in audiology: The need and potential to reach underserved communities. *International Journal of Audiology, 49*(3), 195–202.

Teng, J., Mayo, N. E., Latimer, E., Hanley, J., Wood-Dauphinee, S., Cote, R., et al. (2003). Costs and caregiver consequences of early supported discharge for stroke patients. *Stroke, 34*, 528–536.

Theodoros, D., & Russell, T. (2008). Telerehabilitation: Current perspectives. In R. Latifi (Ed.), *Current principles and practices of telemedicine and e-health* (pp. 191–209). Amsterdam, Netherlands: IOS Press.

Thomas, P., Chantoin-Merlet, S., Hazif-Thomas, C., Belmin, J., Montagne, B., Clement, J., et al. (2002). Complaints of informal caregivers providing home care for dementia patients: The Pixel study. *International Journal of Geriatric Psychiatry, 17*, 1034–1047.

U.S. Department of Labor, Bureau of Labor Statistics. (2008). *Occupational outlook quarterly, 2008 edition, healthcare.* Retrieved from http://www.bls.gov/opub/ooq/2008/spring/art03.pdf

U.S. Department of Labor, Bureau of Labor Statistics. (2010). *Occupational outlook handbook, 2010–2011 edition, speech-language pathologists.* Retrieved from http://www.bls.gov/oco/ocos099.htm

Vekovius, G. T. (1995). Managed care 101: Introducing managed care into the curriculum. *ASHA, 37*, 44–47.

Wakefield, B. J., Holman, J. E., Ray, A., Morse, J., & Kienzle, M. G. (2004). Nurse and patient communication via low- and high-bandwidth home telecare systems. *Journal of Telemedicine and Telecare, 10,* 156–159.

Wertz, R. T., Dronkers, N. F., Bernstein-Ellis, E., Sterling, L. K., Shubitkowski, Y., & Elman, R. (1992). Potential of telephonic and television technology for appraising and diagnosing neurogenic communication disorders in remote settings. *Aphasiology, 6*, 195–202.

White, P. H. (2002). Access to health care: Health insurance considerations for young adults with special health care needs/disabilities. *Pediatrics, 110*(6), 1328–1335.

White, S. (2008). Bottom line. Coding and reimbursement for auditory rehabilitation. *The ASHA Leader, 13*(16), 3.

Whitmire, K., Reder, N., Ralabate, P., & White, S. (2006). The regulatory context for public education. *Seminars in Speech & Language, 27*(2), 119–128.

Wick, J. L. (2010, October 1). *Army's tele-health program provides continuity of care*. U.S. Army Medical Department Walter Reed Army Medical Center. Available from http://www.veteransbenefitsinformation.com

Wilson, L., & Onslow, M. (2004). Telehealth adaptation of the Lidcombe program of early stuttering intervention: Five case studies. *American Journal of Speech-Language Pathology, 13*, 81–93.

Yoo, S. K., Kim, D. K., Jung, S. M., Kim, E., Lim, J. S., & Kim, J. H. (2004). Performance of a web-based, realtime, tele-ultrasound consultation system over high-speed commercial telecommunication lines. *Journal of Telemedicine and Telecare, 10*, 175–179.

RESOURCES

See the reference list for specific guidelines from ASHA pertaining to clinical practice issues discussed in this chapter. AAA's website at http://www.audiology.org and ASHA's website at http://www.asha.org include numerous resources for those wishing to learn more about access, funding, and legislative and advocacy issues discussed in this chapter. For hands-on help with letter writing to legislators, contact the governmental affairs section of ASHA's website or call ASHA's Action Center at 800-498-2071.

Internet links for learning about and contacting consumer groups related to a wide variety of communication and swallowing disorders may be easily accessed through Dr. Judith Kuster's website "Net Connections for Communication Disorders and Sciences" at http://www.communicationdisorders.com. Also available through this site are additional resources related to technology.

SECTION IV

Working Productively

19

Policies and Procedures

Paul Rao, PhD

SCOPE OF CHAPTER

Despite whatever practice setting you find yourself in, never in my 40 years in the profession of speech-language pathology (SLP) or 25 years in administration has the need for clear and concise departmental policies and procedures been more critical and necessary. A current and comprehensive set of policies and procedures is a manager's coat of armor for risk management and the compass for one's standard operating procedures. There was a day when a policy and procedure (P&P) manual might have gathered dust or served as a bookend in your bookcase. Today, immediate access to all P&Ps is an absolute sine qua non for managing by the book and knowing when and how to administer a program. There is no course in our curriculum on P&Ps, but they are as an important a component of practice management as your billing system and office equipment. When I became the inaugural director of SLP at the National Rehabilitation Hospital in Washington, DC, the first task I had to complete before we opened our doors in 1986 was to draft a P&P manual. I stress the word *draft* since once our doors opened many policies and procedures were noted to be either too unwieldy, unclear, or unenforceable. We needed to fine-tune, revise, delete, and tweak continuously to make sure our P&Ps were accessible to our staff, understandable, clear, and nondiscriminatory. As all readers now know, the bar for all such criteria is constantly being raised. This chapter is an effort to reach that bar.

This chapter familiarizes you with what commonly constitutes a P&P manual and answers the following questions: What is a policy and procedure? What should be included in a P&P manual? When, why, how, and by whom are P&Ps written? After reading this chapter, you will have a clearer idea of what is entailed in "managing by the book" in a variety of speech-language pathology and audiology employment settings. According to Rizzo and Trudeau (1994), in establishing an Audiology and Speech-Language Pathology Department, the development of clear policies and procedures can serve a vital function by defining expectations and standards of performance. As my expertise is in the area of hospital-based speech-language pathology, many illustrations will be derived from that area of clinical practice. However, much of the rationale, principles, and operational procedures discussed here may be applied to audiology as well, and to universities, schools, private practices, and other settings.

DEFINING TERMINOLOGY

Before we can discuss the topic of P&Ps, we need to lay the groundwork for delving into this multifaceted topic. Each of us comes to the topic with a seemingly high degree of familiarity. All of us are required to follow P&Ps in our workplace. As parents, we likely have undocumented P&Ps in the home to maintain order. Clearly one must differentiate between a policy, a procedure, a plan, and a guideline. P&Ps may be considered a set of documents that describe an organization's policies for operation and the procedures necessary to fulfill the policies. P&Ps usually are written because of some external requirement, such as environmental compliance or other government regulations. For example, the Centers for Medicare & Medicaid Services (CMS) require a policy on patient rights to fulfill the Conditions of Participation requirements prior to becoming an approved Medicare provider. In communication disorders, two recent rules are particularly germane to our discipline and require explicit policies:

- Hospitals that participate in Medicare must now allow inpatients to designate who may visit them under new visitation regulations that went into effect January 18, 2011. The SLP must know the policy and abide by this new regulation with visitors who may present themselves to your door to observe the patient's treatment or otherwise participate in care decisions.
- Health care organizations that have earned accreditation by The Joint Commission (TJC) are now required (2011), under the TJC Chapter on Rights and Responsibilities of the Individual, to have a policy and evidence of performance "respecting the patient's right to and need for effective communication."

Regardless of practice setting or client population, clinicians need to improve how they—and their colleagues—communicate with patients and address cultural and linguistic differences. Besides being ethical and appropriate, patient-centered communication is also—or soon will be—a requirement under new and pending laws, regulations, and standards (American Speech-Language-Hearing Association [ASHA], 2011, pp. 24–25).

What Is a Policy?

According to the Commission on Accreditation of Rehabilitation Facilities (CARF) (2009), a policy is a "written course of action or guidelines adopted by leadership and reflected in actual practice" (p. 271). Organizations seeking CARF accreditation may consult the CARF glossary when determining their conformance with standards that require a policy. The key word in the CARF definition is *leadership* and its inferred responsibility and overall accountability. According to the Society of Human Resources Management (SHRM) (2011), a policy is a "broad statement that reflects an organization's philosophy, objectives, or standards concerning a particular set of management or employee activities." For example, a policy may describe what an employee is entitled to in terms of vacation days and how many days may be retained in one's leave bank from year to year. The policy statement provides a basis for management practices, and a framework within these practices is established.

The human resources function of an organization should review organizational policies periodically and revise those that are obsolete so that they no longer influence decision making. A policy is thus an organization's guide to be followed under a given set of circumstances. A good policy will not force a manager into narrow or rigid decision making. Rather, it will provide guidance for handling a wide range of organizational issues and will establish a framework for both management and staff decision making. For example, a P&P on documentation in a medical setting may state, "It is the policy of the Speech-Language Pathology Department to document a comprehensive evaluation in the medical record within 48 hours of the first patient contact." This statement is an explicit and measurable guide to policy, and all clinical staff members should be cognizant of what the policy is. An example of a policy from a university setting might be a statement of the quality point average that must be maintained to continue graduate study.

The Bureau of Business Practice (BBP) (1988) describes good policies as "broad, current, comprehensive, inviolate, written to specify responsibility for action, and used frequently" (p. 11). These attributes are essential ingredients of P&Ps if they are to be user-friendly and convey the mission, philosophy, and goals of a given program, department, or organization. Kaluzny, Warner, Warren, and Zelman (1982) stress that P&Ps are an organization's written rules and regulations that describe the values of the organization and thus define specific directions, goals, and expectations. Rao (1991) notes that a P&P manual can also be used as a management tool and a training aid for employees to avoid misunderstanding and errors. If you were to conduct a web search using the words *policies* and *procedures,* you would obtain more than 38 pages of references on the web in a variety of industries that provide timely illustrations of P&Ps. For example, the very first link you would find is to Johns Hopkins Hospital's entire, fully accessible online policy and procedure manual.

WHAT IS A PROCEDURE?

According to CARF (2009), a procedure is a "how to" description of actions to be taken. They do not need to be written unless specified (p. 271). Here again, the organization may wish to determine if a given procedure needs to be formally documented based on CARF's specification in the relevant standards. According to SHRM (2011), a procedure "is a detailed, step-by-step description of the customary methods of handling activities." Using an example mentioned previously, a procedure for vacation pay may establish necessary actions for a planned absence. The employee must request the absence at least one week in advance of the vacation, and no more than a specific number of employees can be off at the same time. A procedure may outline the manner in which a particular policy is to be implemented, but it cannot take the place of that policy. According to Rizzo and Trudeau (1994), procedures should be written to reflect the most efficient method for carrying out a task. They should reflect current regulations and standards of relevant accreditation programs. Recall that a good policy is inviolate. Policies change slowly and infrequently. Procedures, on the other hand, change often, as dictated by any number of factors, such as funding, staffing, equipment, space, accreditation standards, and technology. The steps necessary for a graduate student to be advanced to candidacy, for example, constitute an academic procedure.

What Are Institutional, Departmental, and Programmatic P&Ps?

All organizations should have an *institutional* P&P manual that applies to all employees. Such a manual includes a host of P&Ps that need not necessarily be restated in a departmental manual (e.g., the institution's policy on sexual harassment or dress code). Many institutions are organized by *departments* (e.g., Dietary or Medicine in a health care setting; Early Childhood Education or Speech-Language Pathology and Audiology in a university setting). Each department is required to have its own P&P manual, including those P&Ps specific to the department. For example, in a hospital setting, only Audiology and Otorhinolaryngology may have a P&P on cerumen removal, whereas *all* patient care policies have a P&P on documentation and infection control. Other agencies and institutions may be organized along *programmatic* or product lines. In a rehabilitation facility, for instance, product lines such as a stroke program or a brain-injury program commonly exist. The people served with a given diagnosis (e.g., stroke) are admitted to a special geographic area in the facility (e.g., stroke unit). A number of professional disciplines, including nursing, physical therapy, occupational therapy, and speech-language pathology, form an interdisciplinary team to treat people with stroke. The services the stroke team provides constitute the stroke *program.* CARF (2009) requires the various rehabilitation programs within an institution to have P&Ps, such as admission criteria (how a person served enters a given program), continued stay criteria (how long a person served remains in the program), discharge criteria (when and how a patient leaves the program), and exit criteria (when a person served is no longer followed by the program). Thus, each program must also have a P&P manual to guide the interdisciplinary team in delivering the desired programmatic care. Following is the index of CARF (2009) required policies for Accreditation in 2010:

- Advance Directives
- Confidentiality and Handling of Records
- Contractual Relationships
- Corporate Compliance
- Financial
- Informed Consent
- Personnel (including background checks and students and volunteers)
- Persons Served (including complaints, funds, resuscitation, and rights)

What Is a P&P Manual?

For ease of access and use, all P&Ps for a given institution, department, or program should be kept together in a central manual either in hard copy or on an electronic database or disc. Frequently, this manual takes the form of a large three-ring binder, from which outdated P&Ps can be removed readily and into which new or revised ones can be inserted easily. Today, a manual copy is likely to be necessary for disaster recovery and to provide the crucial backup that is necessary when the server is down or Internet and intranet access is disrupted. Increasingly, organizations are supporting "computer kiosks" throughout a given environment where all employees can access company policies as well as any other need-to-know employee resource (e.g., the employee handbook).

In addition to the P&Ps themselves, several requisite components facilitate consistent, efficient, and effective use. The first of these, according to the BBP *Personnel Policy Manual* (BBP, 1988), is a complete and detailed table of contents that lists major areas of policy and, under each major heading, the specific P&Ps in that area. In conjunction with a table of contents, the BBP suggests the use of a simple numbering system, in which each major heading is assigned a corresponding section number (e.g., Clinical Policies = Section 200), and each subordinate P&P within that section has an individual subsection number (e.g., Client Referral and Assignment = 200.01). This system enhances an employee's or manager's ability to identify and locate the necessary P&P at a glance. As a CARF surveyor, the author has had an opportunity to examine and review hundreds of P&Ps, and most use a numbering format as just described. However, many institutions also organize their P&Ps alphabetically under macro categories.

Other P&P manual components recommended by the BBP (1988) include a written explanation of the relationship between the P&P manual and other manuals, handbooks, and documents in existence within the organization; a statement of the purpose of the P&P manual; and a statement of the organization's practice with regard to ensuring compliance with its policies and procedures. For example, at my place of employment, I chair the institutional P&P Committee and report that *plans* have been separated from P&Ps. Thus, the plan manual includes the organization's required plans such as performance improvement, information management, safety, patient safety, infection control, and plan of care. Organizations may also publish rules and guidelines that are separate from the P&Ps but have managerial approval. The Society for Human Resources Management (SHRM) (2011) states that rules "reflect management decisions that actions be taken—or avoided—in a given situation" (p. 6). For instance, most companies want to ensure that alcoholic beverages are not consumed during work hours. Management may therefore establish a rule that alcoholic beverages cannot be brought onto or consumed on company property.

NECESSITY AND VALUE OF POLICIES AND PROCEDURES

As a manager, you need show up in court only once to defend a personnel action to fully appreciate and then embrace the potent and prerequisite nature of P&Ps in any organization. The P&P manual can be a manager's "best friend."

Accrediting and Regulatory Requirements

A P&P manual is required by accrediting, certifying, licensing, and regulatory bodies such as The Joint Commission (TJC), CARF, state licensing boards, state education agencies, and the American Speech-Language-Hearing Association's Council on Academic Accreditation in Audiology and Speech-Language Pathology (CAA). These organizations establish and promote minimal standards that must be met by an institution seeking accreditation. Many of these standards must be translated into P&Ps for dissemination and implementation throughout the institution or practice setting. For example, TJC (2011) requires that all institutional policies be reviewed and approved at least every three years except the human resources P&P, which must be updated annually. Without a P&P manual, it is likely that the responsible program would be cited by CAA, TJC, CARF, or other accrediting or licensing agencies for noncompliance with a standard.

For example, when reviewing the CARF 2010 (2009) standards, the reader is cognizant of what is required for each standard. Section #1, Criterion I, Accessibility L of CARF's *2010 Standards Manual* dealing with Business Practices in Medical Rehabilitation notes that the organization "must have an accessibility *plan* that addresses barriers in the following areas:

a) Architectural;
b) Environmental;
c) Attitudinal;
d) Financial;
e) Employment;
f) Communication;
g) Transportation; and
h) Any other barrier identified by the:
   1. person served;
   2. personnel; and
   3. other stakeholders" (p. 13).

However, in Section #1, Criterion I, Rights of Persons Served, K, the standard states that "the organization implements policies promoting the following rights of the person served:

a) Confidentiality of information;
b) Privacy; and
c) Freedom from the following:
   1. abuse;
   2. financial or other exploitation;
   3. retaliation;
   4. humiliation; and or
   5. neglect" (p. 74).

Finally in the same section and criterion, CARF requires the organization to "implement a policy and written procedure by which the person served may make a formal complaint, file a grievance, or appeal a decision made by the organization's personnel or team members" (p. 75). Although the presence of a P&P manual is no guarantee of quality, without it an organization cannot become accredited (Rao, 1991).

According to Golper and Brown (2004), "while accrediting standards address a broad range of areas (e.g., provision of care, ethics, leadership, human resources, information management, environment of care), individual clinicians will be most affected by the organization's policies and procedures, the requirements for 'qualified providers,' and the need to maintain competencies to practice with the population with which they are working (e.g., age range and disorder types)" (p. 64). Golper and Brown (2004) present a sample of a department-specific policy and procedure on staffing.

Legal Considerations

We live in a litigious society in which nearly every decision can be called into legal question. In addition, government oversight of Medicare and Medicaid waste that began in 1993 with new money and power granted by Congress has empowered the Office of the Inspector General in the U.S. Department of Health and Human Services (2005) to require every health care provider to establish a corporate compliance plan to prevent, detect, and correct any violations of federal and state fraud and abuse laws. In audiology and speech-language pathology, there is no shortage of potential litigants: clients, payers, and professionals. The P&P manual is a prerequisite for documenting compliance with existing laws. According to Applegate (1991),

> You want your policy manual to be as clear as possible because it often plays a key role in court if any employee sues you for wrongful termination or any other labor dispute. Many courts around the country have ruled that a policy handbook often serves as a contract between employees and employer. (p. C-8)

The legal and regulatory climate alone has changed so rapidly during the past decade that a host of new policy areas have emerged. The Family and Medical Leave Act, which is intended to provide employees equal opportunity to take time off from work to care for a child or parent, has resulted in a number of new legal requirements for employers and service providers. The law thus mandates a number of changes in the human resource function of the P&P manuals of many organizations.

The Health Insurance Portability and Accountability Act (HIPAA) (2003) is the most significant recent federal law that compels organizations to have in place a host of new, explicit policies and procedures. HIPAA encompasses three major rules and regulations: (1) privacy, (2) transactions, and (3) security. HIPAA was designed specifically to ensure that health care providers make every effort to ensure that protected health information (PHI), or a patient's medical records, is kept private. The final rule applies to all information, whether electronic, written, or oral. Today when you enter a health care institution, you will receive a privacy notice, and you may observe new procedures that reflect a culture of confidentiality. Providers are now required to train all staff in the specifics of the HIPAA rules and regulations. Provisions of the HIPAA statute generally carry significant penalties. Civil penalties range up to $100 per person, per violation, up to $25,000 per year. Criminal penalties apply as well—up to $50,000 in fines and a year in prison for knowingly disclosing PHI; up to $100,000 in fines and 5 years in prison if the disclosure is under false pretenses; and, finally, up to $250,000 in fines and 10 years in prison if the disclosure is for commercial advantage. Thus, it is imperative that providers have in place the P&Ps to address all three components of HIPAA and have evidence of training all staff on relevant policies and procedures.

Identification and Definition of Relevant Rules and Regulations

The P&P manual is a comprehensive compendium of all relevant rules and regulations with which an organization must comply. Accreditation standards aside, a manager cannot operate effectively without written P&Ps. Although control of all management decisions may not be possible, a framework for managerial and clinical decision making is necessary. The P&P manual should not be designed to establish a rigid set of rules but should enable managers to (1) appreciate how far the impact of their decisions might reach, (2) encourage logical and consistent thinking, and (3) provide an opportunity for all employees to operate in a cohesive manner (Rao, 1991). Many P&Ps are management protocols designed for the smooth and efficient operation of a department. The P&P manual should be the last word on what is required of an employee. It is designed to equip both employer and employee with a means to ensure compliance with all relevant rules and regulations.

WHAT TO INCLUDE IN A POLICY AND PROCEDURE MANUAL

A variety of administrative, clinical, and professional policies and operational procedures for audiology and speech-language pathology must be considered when gathering, expanding, or revising a policy and procedure manual. Standards set forth by accrediting bodies, as well as legal requirements at the federal, state, and local levels, also serve as guidelines for many of the items to be incorporated as standard components of a P&P manual. Beyond these standards, requirements, and general areas of consideration, the content of a P&P manual is determined by the individual needs of a given program or department and by those of the institution in which it operates.

Accrediting Body Requirements

Anyone in health care realizes that there is increasing attention being paid to safety and quality and a host of federal compliance initiatives. When one "opens shop," usually the very first order of business is to document all the policies required by accreditation bodies. If you wish to admit patients and be paid, usually the ticket that must first be punched to enter the health care arena is meeting the various stringent regulatory requirements. Schools and universities must first ensure that they have the correct policies and procedures in place prior to any admissions.

ASHA Council on Academic Accreditation (CAA) in Audiology and Speech-Language Pathology Following are the core standards considered essential by ASHA CAA

(ASHA, 2011) for the provision of quality services and instruction in the university setting:

- Standard 1.0 Administrative Structure and Governance
- Standard 2.0 Faculty/Instructional Staff
- Standard 3.A Curriculum (Academic & Clinical Education) in Audiology
- Standard 3.B Curriculum (Academic & Clinical Education) in Speech-Language Pathology
- Standard 4.0 Students
- Standard 5.0 Assessment
- Standard 6.0 Program Resources

Specifically, ASHA CAA standards include the need for a written mission statement that describes the department's purpose and scope of practice and that remains up to date in relation to changing needs by means of periodic and systematic review. ASHA's CAA requires that the administration of an audiology and speech-language pathology university department be based on established P&Ps that are consistent with the department's stated mission and goals. ASHA maintains that any policies related to clinical decision making in the field must be established in consultation with individuals holding a current ASHA Certificate of Clinical Competence (CCC) in the respective profession.

Sample Mission Statement This following mission statement, as well as corresponding measurable and attainable goals and objectives, is located in the first section of our department's SLP P&P manual and may drive a number of core policies such as admission and discharge criteria. The National Rehabilitation Hospital's (NRH) Speech-Language Pathology Service mission statement (National Rehabilitation Hospital [NRH], 1998a) is:

> The mission of the Speech-Language Pathology (SLP) Service of National Rehabilitation Hospital's Medical Rehabilitation Network is to apply state-of-the-art theory and knowledge in the realm of communication sciences and disorders to the quality of care of persons with communication/swallowing disorders in order for them to achieve maximum independence and optimum functioning within the community. The SLP Service is committed to the assessment and treatment of individuals exhibiting communication/swallowing disorders; to educating and counseling patients and their families regarding the nature, cause, treatment, and prevention of conditions which may result in a communication &/or swallowing disturbance; to educating the NRH network and community at large regarding current concepts in the application of communication sciences to the communicatively impaired population; to expanding the knowledge base of the communication sciences through clinical research; and to serving as an advocate for persons with communication impairments. A continuous performance improvement and outcomes management program is the foundation of the SLP Service's efforts to render the highest quality of care in an effective and efficient manner. All activities of the SLP Service will be in accordance with the Scope of Practice and Code of Ethics of the American Speech-Language-Hearing Association and with legal and professional standards established for certification, licensure, accreditation, and protection of patient and staff rights. (p. 1)

SOURCE: Reprinted with permission from the National Rehabilitation Hospital.

The Joint Commission (TJC) (2011) requires that certain P&Ps be established for specific functions such as patient rights and organizational ethics, assessment and care of patients, special procedures, performance improvement, leadership, environment of care, human resources, infection control, medical affairs, and nursing leadership within health care organizations seeking TJC accreditation. These include P&Ps regarding documentation in the medical record, fire and safety, infection control, equipment inspection and preventive maintenance, and special procedures (e.g., the P&P for responding to a medical emergency). Other TJC requirements of particular import to the SLP manager/supervisor include a policy on the following: orientation of new employees; age-based competencies; evidence of a performance improvement plan with appropriate indicators addressing important aspects of care; a comprehensive staffing model and a care plan that ensures one level of care; the presence of an organizational chart and explanation of the relationship of the SLP department to other hospital departments; and a statement of the scope of services/plan of care provided.

CARF (Commission on Accreditation of Rehabilitation Facilities) has developed its own set of standards for rehabilitation organizations that wish to obtain CARF accreditation. Evidence that these standards are met must be present at the organizational level and also at the individual program level (e.g., brain-injury program) if the organization seeks specialty program accreditation. To the extent that audiology and speech-language pathology departmental policies and procedures may complement or reinforce organizational or specialty program P&Ps in meeting the standards of this and other accrediting bodies, you should consider them for inclusion in a departmental P&P manual. CARF standards (2009) in their "requested survey resource documents" that may have relevance for the audiology and speech-language pathology departmental P&P manual include, but are not limited to, the following:

- Documentation of the program's or department's role in the continuum of care
- Measurable criteria for the initiation and termination of specific treatments
- Policies and procedures that promote safety and security
- Procedures for filing grievances and appealing decisions
- Policies for advance directives and resuscitation orders
- Admission, continued stay, discharge, and exit criteria per department and program
- Policies that address confidentiality of records, release of records, records retention, records storage, and protection of records from fire and water damage
- Policies for electronic records that address protection of records, privacy of records, and security of records
- Policies concerning ethical conduct
- Policies and procedures related to taking and reporting disciplinary actions against practitioners
- Procedures for handling vehicle accidents and road emergencies
- Administrative policies and procedures

P&Ps that identify the functions and the responsibilities of rehabilitation physicians providing treatment

Federal, State, and Local Requirements In addition to the components of a P&P manual required by accrediting bodies, laws and regulations at the federal, state, and local levels may also dictate organizational and departmental P&Ps. The presence of and compliance with these P&Ps are not always regularly monitored through formal site visits or surveys. However, when compliance with the law is called into question in the form of litigation or other civil action, your ability to demonstrate the presence of and adherence to federal, state, and local regulations is of paramount importance. With the advent of corporate compliance to combat fraud and abuse, it is imperative that your staff is familiar with and compliant with your organization's plan, policies, and procedures that ensure compliance with all federal, state, and local laws.

Federal Requirements In the past decade, a relevant example of a federal law that has been enacted and that has significant impact on P&P requirements is HIPAA (2003), previously described in detail. In the early 1990s, another landmark federal law that has had dramatic impact on the American scene is the Americans with Disabilities Act (ADA) (1990). This law prohibits discrimination on the basis of disability in employment, public services and transportation, privately operated public accommodations and services, and telecommunication services. P&Ps regarding recruitment, employment, promotion, and termination of employees; job descriptions, performance standards, and performance appraisals for staff; access to job training and continuing education opportunities; access to services provided; physical accommodations; and telecommunications, to name a few, must reflect compliance with the law by removing barriers to people with disabilities through the provision of reasonable accommodations.

State and Local Requirements Local requirements obviously vary among jurisdictions but frequently have significant impact on P&Ps in areas such as fire safety, infection control, and/or the parameters of employees' entitlement to family/medical leave. State licensure requirements for audiology and speech language pathology have been adopted in all states. Specific exemptions to these requirements sometimes exist. For example, school speech-language pathologists in South Dakota, which currently has no SLP licensure, must possess their ASHA CCCs or demonstrate equivalent completion of these CCC requirements in order to provide and bill for Medicaid services. Many states are also enacting laws to deal with speech-language pathology assistants. All such state and local requirements must be incorporated into the P&P manual.

Other Necessary Policies and Procedures

Beyond the P&Ps dictated by accrediting bodies and federal, state, and local licensing agencies, P&Ps should be documented for a variety of administrative and mission-driven rationales.

Administrative Issues Administrative issues for which you may want to develop and maintain P&Ps include staff vacation, sick, and administrative leave; dress code for the workplace; access to secretarial support; staff productivity levels; staff meetings; and management reports. One essential element is the establishment and annual review of *job descriptions* that delineate duties and responsibilities; requisite language and mathematical skills; reasoning ability; physical demands; lines of authority; work environment; any equipment, aids, tools, materials, or vehicles used; certificates, licenses, and registrations; and required education and experience. Likewise, you should consider establishing the department's P&P regarding development and utilization of *performance standards* to be used to objectively measure performance within the critical components established for each job title.

Sample performance standards for a staff speech-language pathologist are illustrated in Table 19–1 and for audiologists in Table 19–2. Another pressing issue in today's health care environment revolves around unions, bargaining units, and labor issues. Do you have a no solicitation policy? If you do not have a clear policy on this issue and a clear history of practicing this policy, a union could argue that it should be permitted to post union activity notices on your company bulletin boards along with "Girl Scout cookie" solicitations and notices of "apartments for rent." Do you have a dress code policy that prohibits logos or nonbusiness identifiers? If you do not have a clear dress code that is enforced, individuals who may support a bargaining unit in a campaign to organize, may wear buttons and logos and other insignia of the labor union. Management will be unable to prevent such open displays. Do you have a clear policy on paying overtime for nonexempt employees and a consistent leave policy for

TABLE 19–1 Sample Performance Standards for Staff Speech-Language Pathologists

A. Quality of Work

1. Accurately evaluates communication abilities of assigned patients and plans and organizes treatment to achieve functional outcomes.

Outstanding: Consistently and independently reaches projected functional outcomes as a result of providing superior evaluation and treatment.

Commendable: Consistently and independently reaches functional outcomes as a result of providing appropriate evaluation and treatment.

Competent: Consistently reaches projected functional outcomes with supervisory input.

2. Accurately documents diagnostic and treatment services in a timely fashion in accordance with SLP and Program policies and guidelines.

Outstanding: Consistently and independently.

Commendable: Consistently with occasional supervisory input.

Competent: Consistently with more than occasional supervisory input.

From "National Rehabilitation Hospital Performance Standards for Staff Speech-Language Pathologists," by P. Rao and T. Goldsmith, 1998a, *National Rehabilitation Hospital Speech-Language Pathology Service Policies and Procedures Manual,* p. 220.04–0. Copyright 1998 by the National Rehabilitation Hospital. Reprinted with permission.

TABLE 19–2 Sample Performance Standards for Staff Audiologists

A. Quality of Work

1. Accurately provides assessment and (re)habilitation of auditory and/or vestibular function of assigned patients to enhance communication and functional competence.

Outstanding:	Consistently and independently evaluates and enhances abilities as a result of providing superior evaluation and treatment.
Commendable:	Consistently and independently evaluates and enhances abilities as a result of providing appropriate evaluation and treatment.
Competent:	Consistently evaluates and enhances abilities with supervisory input.

2. Accurately documents diagnostic and treatment services in a timely fashion in accordance with Audiology and Departmental policies and procedures.

Outstanding:	Consistently and independently.
Commendable:	Consistently with occasional supervisory input.
Competent:	Consistently with more than occasional supervisory input.

3. Appropriately incorporates age, cognitive level, and communication skills into evaluation, treatment, and patient education.

Outstanding:	Consistently and independently.
Commendable:	Consistently with occasional supervisory input.
Competent:	Consistently with more than occasional supervisory input.

Based on information from "Washington Hospital Center Competency Standards for Staff Audiologists," by T. Wilson-Bridges and C. Surowicz, 2005, *Washington Hospital Center Hearing & Speech Center Clinical Procedures & Protocols Manual*, p. 200.30.

exempt employees? If you have exempt employees such as SLPs, but you hold them to hourly time requirements that you hold nonexempt employees to, the SLPs may be included in a union campaign as part of the bargaining unit that is focused on hourly nonexempt employees. These are questions that may put an organization at risk of an unfair labor practice were a bargaining unit to attempt to organize your facility or practice.

Clinical Issues As stipulated by TJC, CARF, and CAA, another essential P&P should provide for a program of continuous evaluation and improvement of the quality of clinical care rendered to consumers. This particular P&P defines the parameters within which a performance improvement (PI) program can be developed to support the PI plan outlined by the leadership of the organization. Other clinical issues for which you may consider developing a P&P include patient referral and assignment; general and/or specific evaluation and treatment protocols; treatment planning, implementation, and discontinuation; department-specific medical record documentation standards (for a concise review of this topic, refer to Paul-Brown, 1994); education and counseling of those who are served and their families; and maintenance of standards of ethical practice.

Additional P&Ps related to clinical issues may be largely determined by the individual needs of a particular clinical setting, perhaps more than any other area of practice. For example, with prospective payment in place in all postacute settings since 2002, a P&P addressing the Minimum Data Set 3.0 (MDS) (Rand Health Corporation, 2008), the outcome system designed for long-term care, or a P&P regarding completion of the Inpatient Rehab Facility-Patient

Assessment Instrument (Inpatient Rehabilitation Facility Prospective Payment System, 2009) would appear to be an obvious priority.

Professional Issues Beyond strictly administrative or clinical issues, examples of other areas for which you may develop written P&Ps include continuing professional education, student training, research activity, and professional presentations and publications. When issues arise requiring an administrative decision about these activities, or when questions of appropriateness, equity, or protocol are raised, it is extremely helpful to have ready and consistent access to clearly articulated P&Ps with regard to these areas of professional practice.

HOW TO WRITE POLICIES AND PROCEDURES

Now it is appropriate to address the mechanics of drafting and approving P&Ps. It takes nearly a village to get consensus on many of your draft policies. However, many P&Ps are so transparently obvious and required that authors frequently "borrow" standard P&Ps. For example, many CARF surveyors whose organizations are eventually surveyed have a penchant for finding "best practices" in a given facility and asking for permission to copy same back at their facility. The dictum seems to be for the more obvious P&Ps, "do not re-create the wheel."

Components and Format

Specific P&P components and format will vary from organization to organization, but within an organization or department, each P&P should reflect consistent documentation and presentation of policies, practices, and procedures. A sample format, as well as component definitions, utilized at National Rehabilitation Hospital in Washington, DC, follows:

Title/Section/Department/Effective Date

Section 1.0 Purpose: A positive statement of the intention or aim of the policy conveyed to the reader in as few words as possible.

Section 2.0 Policy: A brief descriptive statement articulating the policy.

Section 3.0 Procedure: A sequence of prescribed steps for implementing the policy.

Section 4.0 Responsibilities: An explanation of the policy and expectations of personnel implementing it.

Section 5.0 Applicability: A statement of those personnel to whom the policy and procedure apply.

Section 6.0 Signature Approval: Evidence of approval by the designated authority.

Section 7.0 References: Other existing documents or policies and procedures which are cited in, or related to, the policy and procedure. (NRH, 1998b, #213.3)

The original effective date and latest revision date should be documented and clearly visible on each P&P within a department or organization. At NRH, revised P&Ps are disseminated to staff with an attached memo via e-mail. This e-mail draws the reader's attention to the specific revisions made to the P&P. A computerized format is becoming increasingly necessary with efforts of organizations to become paperless. The computerized format was adapted from the Windows version of Policies Now (Knowledge Point, 2011), which permits the author to write customized personnel policies in minutes. The Society of Human Resources Management (2011) has established a policy handbook from a variety of sources on its web page, wherein the person who accesses the web page can click to view and download any one of the following P&P related materials:

- A complete handbook
- At-will employment policies
- EEO/Affirmative Action
- Exempt/nonexempt
- Overtime
- Drug/alcohol policies
- Sexual harassment
- Electronic communication
- Voluntary/involuntary separation

A number of proprietary companies are also in the P&P business (see Resources). Medical Consultants Network, Inc. (2011) customizes P&Ps for client organizations and provides web access. The available manuals cover all of the key TJC functions and other health care policy needs. Its marketing mantra is "Why reinvent the wheel?" A similar venue can be found at

Hospital and Physician Publishing, Inc. (2011), which provides updated documents on a continuous basis to subscribers. This publisher offers more than 350 P&P manuals and 100 medical books in electronic form and highlights its currency with TJC standards and breadth of topics. A manager starting from scratch in a new facility might be well served to investigate these off-the-shelf, state-of-the-art options.

NRH has attempted to reduce its reliance on a paper manual and to take advantage of computer technology. Besides the hard copy of the "heavy" P&P manual, which is centralized in administration for backup purposes when computer systems shut down or crash, NRH had also automated its P&Ps in 1998 on Lotus Notes and disseminated them on a local area network (LAN). Consistent with the goal of performance improvement, the NRH P&P Committee elected to simplify the process and eliminate redundancy. As NRH has expanded to more than 40 sites over a 25-year institutional history, the organization needed to arrive at a network policy on policies and procedures that provided the required P&Ps for each site, program, and department. However, the former organization policies that were applicable under one roof, such as the fire and safety policy, were no longer applicable at the outpatient sites that had no inpatients and were under the rules and regulations of local jurisdictions and the fire code of the particular building in which the site was housed.

NRH P&Ps are organized under the following categories: Patient Care, Care Coordination, Pharmacy, Dietary, Medical Affairs, Admissions, Infection Control, Quality Improvement, Administration Communications and Development, Human Resources/Employee Health, Accounting/Budget and Reimbursement, Patient Financial Services, Materials Management, Medical Records, and Safety Policies.

The search is made easy via a keyword approach. For example, if you are interested in the policy on restraints, the computer will call up all policies that deal with restraints. If you are interested only in site-specific policies, the computer will organize only those P&Ps dealing with outpatient sites. There are specific security protocols for "read only" versus "contributing editor" versus "author only." Anyone who has access to the NRH LAN can connect to the P&P pages then read, and if desired, print. This e-site is password protected and has an organizational firewall in place to prevent unauthorized access as well as the site being hacked by damaging viruses.

Style P&Ps should be written in clear, concise language that can be easily and quickly understood by all employees to whom the P&Ps apply. Technical or professional jargon and ambiguous statements should be avoided to minimize the possibility of misinterpretation. The BBP (1988) recommends use of active voice when possible and suggests that exclusive passive voice use makes P&Ps sound "dull and pompous." The BBP also suggests that short, but not choppy, sentences enhance P&P readability. See the appendix for a sample P&P.

WHO SHOULD WRITE POLICIES AND PROCEDURES

Normally, there is not a long line of employees wishing to be responsible for P&Ps in a given department and organization. The want ad would suggest that the prospective individual is computer literate with excellent organizational and detail-oriented skills. In addition, the "czar" or "czarina" of your P&Ps must be skilled in grammar, patience, and persistence. Finally, this individual must be able to access all accreditation and licensure resources applicable to your organization.

Primary Responsibility

In most cases, the department director has primary responsibility for drafting and revising departmental P&Ps. This task may be delegated to subordinate staff in some instances, but the responsibility for final review remains with the director. Other director-level responsibilities include ensuring appropriate dissemination of and ready access to all applicable P&Ps as well as ensuring compliance with and enforcement of both department-specific and organizational P&Ps.

Solicitation of Input

In many organizations, employees are encouraged to recommend new P&Ps and to suggest revisions to existing P&Ps. An example of employee persuasion and input in the author's experience involved staff suggestions regarding the employee dress code. In 1999, NRH embarked on a cultural transformation titled "New Value" (Rao, 2002) that was modeled after the Disney Corporation. Disney has an extremely strict dress code and a "zero tolerance" policy for noncompliance with the dress code policy. When NRH implemented its revised dress code more than a decade ago with an accompanying "style book," NRH Team Members felt dictated to and controlled with little to no input on the policy and apparently no degrees of freedom in complying with the strict dress code policy. The SLP Service opted to be creative in its advocacy for a less stringent dress code policy. During one of the senior management staff meetings, the SLP Service provided an impromptu breakfast of homemade pastries with each serving topped with a toothpick and a flag like '"jean" fabric. The obvious message was that employees would really appreciate senior management's approval of a trial "jean therapy day." After little discussion, an exemption to the strict dress code was approved with an allowance of a quarterly "dress down/jean therapy" day that could be thematic and fun (e.g., Halloween/Freaky Friday Dress Down Day). A regular practice of soliciting staff input on a P&P manual's usefulness and on suggestions for additions or changes to the manual is one grassroots mechanism of ensuring that your manual is the current, accurate, relevant, and authoritative resource it is intended to be. NRH hosts an annual town hall for staff to provide input on current and proposed policies, practices, and guidelines as well as to inform staff of important policy changes during the past year.

Administrative Review and Approval

Although generally developed and/or approved at the department director level, department-specific P&Ps also frequently require review and approval by a member of an organization's senior management staff before dissemination and implementation. For P&Ps that involve or have an impact on departments other than the one initiating the policy, review and approval by other affected department directors are also needed. Interdisciplinary clinical procedures, such as modified barium swallow studies, provide such opportunities for interdepartmental collaboration. The originating department director is responsible for obtaining all necessary authorizations and signatures in accordance with the organization's policy.

WHEN SHOULD POLICIES AND PROCEDURES BE WRITTEN?

The need for P&Ps may be prompted by a number of factors. Updates in the standards manuals of TJC, CARF, and CAA may include new or additional requirements that prompt P&Ps. P&Ps may also be dictated by federal, state, or local regulations.

New Policies and Procedures

For all of the previously cited reasons, new policies may be required of an organization as well. In 2009, our corporate parent prohibited any smoking of tobacco products on the hospital campus, and in addition no employees could possess a tobacco odor on their person while on duty. Violations of the policy were subject to the NRH disciplinary policy including termination. Thus, a campus policy on smoking was instituted. Then, in 2010, with the Centers for Disease Control data on the contagion of the flu readily available, our corporate parent again required that *all* employees have an annual flu vaccine. Very few exceptions to this immunization requirement were granted (e.g., religious or allergic to eggs). The rationale for the dramatic change in policy is, given that patient and employee safety is really our No. 1 priority, then the risk of flu and transmitting the virus to others should be minimized as much as possible. Protecting the employee's own family and the community was also considered an indirect benefit. Hence, another policy needed to be written and implemented.

Development of an entirely new program or service within the department may be further grounds for development of a new P&P. If your department, which formerly treated only adolescents and adults, embarks on the management of children, for instance, the department would clearly require new P&Ps regarding a number of critical areas that are unique to children (e.g., age-based competencies, revised and adapted testing and treatment protocols, and manner of obtaining informed consent). In 2005, NRH was licensed to operate 12 pediatric rehabilitation beds. A number of new policies had to be developed and approved before pediatric patients could be admitted to the newly built unit. Obviously, issues such as "medical emergency" in a six-year-old differ from those of an adult in terms of equipment, protocol, and practice. Finally, evolving societal standards may prompt a P&P. One example in this area is a pre-employment drug screening, which has become an increasingly common employment prerequisite because of the prevalence of drug use in society. If a drug screening practice is adopted, a corresponding P&P must be in place.

Policy and Procedure Review and Revision

Most organizations establish a schedule of P&P review, which is at least as frequent as the minimum P&P review schedules mandated by accrediting and licensing bodies. TJC, for example, requires P&P review every three years. CARF requires an annual review of all job descriptions in the organization. Such review schedules are designed to ensure that necessary and appropriate revisions to P&Ps are reflected in an organization's current manual. Factors that might prompt the revision of a given policy are the same factors one would consider when drafting a new policy. For example, the NRH SLP Service recently revised its policy on documentation of progress notes. Originally, SLPs were responsible for writing inpatient progress notes every two weeks. However, because of a national trend toward shortened lengths of stay (LOS) for rehabilitation patients, along with a change in local standards (managed care companies were requiring more frequent notes), the SLP Service revised the policy from documenting progress every two weeks to documenting a daily "log" note and a weekly progress note. The SLP Service has modified a number of other policies for a variety of reasons. Table 19–3 details that process, stating the nature of the policy, the nature of the change, and the primary reasons for revision of sample P&Ps.

P&P revision may also result from the performance improvement data of the institution, program, or department. Our compliance audits revealed challenges with scheduling patients to comply with the CMS Three-Hour Rule and scoring of the required outcome measures. As a result of these audits and therapist feedback, a capital request was

TABLE 19–3 Original Policy, Revised Policy, and Reason for Revisions in NRH SLP'S 1998 P&P Manual

Original Policy	Policy Revision	Reason for Revision
Biweekly inpatient progress summaries	Weekly inpatient progress summaries and daily logs	Shortened length of stay (LOS)
Discharge Summary within 48 hours of discharge	Discharge Summary within 24 hours of discharge	Referring institutions request more timely data. Physicians request data for medical discharge summaries. Case Managers request more timely reports to enhance continuity of care.
Written Evaluation Report within 5 working days of initial contact	Written Evaluation Report within 2 working days of initial contact	Shortened LOS & External Case Managers' request
Uniform staff working hours from 8:00 A.M. to 4:30 P.M.	Establishment of flexible schedule options	Staff retention & expand tour of duty to reach patients' families
Modified Barium Swallow studies conducted off-site	Modified Barium Swallow studies conducted on-site	New equipment at NRH precluded the need to go off-site

From *The National Rehabilitation Hospital Speech-Language Pathology Service Policies and Procedures Manual*, by P. Rao and T. Goldsmith, 1998a, pp. 220.01–220.40. Copyright 1998 by the National Rehabilitation Hospital. Reprinted with permission.

submitted and approved for an electronic rehabilitation documentation system. This very expensive software product made a huge difference in compliance and documentation but also required a host of detailed new policies and procedures. When the new e-system was installed, clinical and scheduling staffs were trained, and the revised P&P was documented and disseminated hospitalwide.

ACCESS TO POLICIES AND PROCEDURES

It should be clear from this chapter that the P&P manual is intended to be a dynamic management tool—consulted often, revised periodically, and available to all staff. Familiarity with the P&P manuals of an institution, program, and department can be accomplished by following several steps.

Orientation

All new employees should be provided an opportunity to access and read the P&P manual and to ask questions about its contents during the probationary period of employment (typically the first three or four months of employment). Written verification by the employee that he or she has read the P&Ps and agrees to abide by them is standard practice in many organizations. In addition to this initial orientation to existing P&Ps, new or revised P&Ps must be circulated through all current staff, and written verification of an awareness and understanding of the new and/or revised P&P should be obtained.

LOCATION

In sites that do not have an electronic version, the hard copy of the P&P manual must be located where all staff within a given program, site, or department have free and easy access. It is suggested that a sign-out sheet for the P&P manual be maintained in a central location so that the manual can be readily located if it is in use. Clearly, access to the P&Ps on the LAN is dependent on available computers and the individual's authorization to read versus edit the P&P. With today's wireless technology and the prevalence of laptops and iPads, most clinical personnel should be able to access e-versions of all organizational policies from wherever wireless connections can be made. A firewall protecting unauthorized access must also be provided.

Promulgation

In addition to orienting new employees to the entire P&P manual, and current employees to new and revised P&Ps, the department, program, or site manager is strongly encouraged to regularly highlight or note important policy issues in staff meetings. If the manager has observed confusion about a given P&P, an informational review and discussion is a necessary first step in promulgating the policy. Another method of updating employees on P&Ps is to write a "Did You Know?" column as a regular feature in your institution's newsletter. Such a column can highlight certain P&Ps and clarify any common problems of misinterpretations. Managing *by* the book is easier if staff members know what is *in* the book. Finally, if the institution holds regular all-staff meetings, this is a perfect forum for stressing a compliance issue with a given P&P.

SUMMARY

A policy and procedure manual is perhaps the single most important tool a manager can have, as long as it accomplishes the following:

1. Clearly articulates the department's and the organization's mission, philosophy, and goals
2. Documents compliance with all applicable laws, rules, regulations, and standards
3. Provides a sound framework for logical and consistent decision making

This chapter defined the terms *policy* and *procedure*; argued for the necessity and value of P&Ps; and offered suggestions regarding what to include in a hard-copy and computerized version of a P&P manual. Because a P&P manual is useful only to the degree that it is *used,* recommendations were also made for the regular review and revision of P&P manuals, as well as the promulgation of P&Ps to all applicable staff.

CRITICAL THINKING

1. Why establish a P&P manual rather than simply maintain a notebook of memoranda and guidelines?
2. You have been hired to establish a new audiology and speech-language pathology clinic. What P&Ps would you develop first and why?
3. What commercial resources are available to help you construct policies that conform with national accrediting groups?
4. In your current academic and/or clinical setting, is there a new P&P that needs to be established and a current one that needs to be revised? Why does it need revision? Practice formulating a new one.
5. Recall one instance in your practice when a disagreement or debate ensued over a particular institutional practice. Was the P&P instrumental in resolving this conflict? How could the conflict be avoided?
6. Why and how should staff be involved in creating new policies and procedures? What are the advantages to seeking staff input?
7. What four media forms could you use to disseminate information regarding new or revised P&Ps in your organization?
8. Why is it important for a private practitioner to have a "policy and procedures manual"? Write an outline for the policies that a private practitioner should include in this document.
9. Upon reviewing the *2012 Standards Manual* for The Joint Commission, what new standard that applies to hospitals would you feel requires a corresponding hospital policy and why? Once you have justified the new policy and procedure, draft your P&P for your community hospital using the chapter format. Finally, discuss the steps you would take to disseminate the policy to your staff.

REFERENCES

American Speech-Language-Hearing Association. (2011). *Standards manual for CAA accreditation.* Rockville, MD: Author.

Americans with Disabilities Act of 1990, Publ. L. No. 101-336, *Federal Register.* Retrieved from http://www.hhs.gov/od/about/fact_sheets/adafactsheet.html

Applegate, J. (1991, September 23). Succeeding in small business. *Baltimore Evening Sun,* p. C8.

Bureau of Business Practice. (1988). *Personnel policy manual.* Englewood Cliffs, NJ: Prentice Hall.

Commission on Accreditation of Rehabilitation Facilities. (2009). *2010 Standards manual for CARF accreditation.* Tucson, AZ: Author.

Golper, L. A., & Brown, J. E. (2004). *Business matters: A guide for speech-language pathologists.* Rockville, MD: American Speech-Language-Hearing Association.

Health Insurance Portability and Accountability Act. (August 2003). Complete Privacy, Security, and Enforcement (Procedural) Regulation Text (45 CFR Parts 160 and 164), December 28, 2000 as amended May 31, 2002, August 14, 2002, February 2003, and April 17, 2003. Available from http://www.hhs.gov/ocr/hipaa/finalreg.html

Hospital and Physician Publishing, Inc. (2011). *Policy and procedures manual.* Marion, IL: Author.

Inpatient Rehabilitation Facility Prospective Payment System. (2009, August 7). Final Rule (42 CFR Part 412). Retrieved from http://www.gpo.gov/fdsys/pkg/FR-2009-08-07/pdf/E9-18616.pdf

(The) Joint Commission. (2011). *Comprehensive accreditation manual for hospitals.* Oakbrook Terrace, IL: Author.

Kaluzny, A. D., Warner, D. M., Warren, D. G., & Zelman, W. N. (1982). *Management of health services.* Englewood Cliffs, NJ: Prentice Hall.

Knowledge Point. (2011). *Policies now!* Petaluma, CA: Author.

Medical Consultants Network, Inc. (2011). *Policy and procedure manual.* Englewood, CO: Author.

National Rehabilitation Hospital. (1998a, August). *Speech-language pathology policy and procedure manual.* Washington, DC: Author.

National Rehabilitation Hospital. (1998b, September). *Policy and procedure on policy and procedures, #700.00.* Washington, DC: Author.

National Rehabilitation Hospital. (2005, November). Hand hygiene. *The National Rehabilitation Hospital policy and procedures manual.* Washington, DC: Author.

Office of the Inspector General, Department of Health and Human Services. (2005). *Work plan: Fiscal year 2005.* Washington, DC: U.S. Government Printing Office.

Paul-Brown, D. (1994). Clinical record keeping in audiology and speech-language pathology. *ASHA, 36,* 40–43.

Rand Health Corporation. (2008). *Development and validation of a revised nursing home assessment tool: MDS 3.0.* Baltimore, MD: Centers for Medicare & Medicaid Services.

Rao, P. (1991). The policy and procedure manual: Managing by the book. In C. Frattali (Ed.), *Quality improvement digest.* Rockville, MD: American Speech-Language-Hearing Association.

Rao, P. (2002, May). *Cultural shift happens: A new value framework.* Course presented to the Maryland & D.C. Health Information Management Association.

Rizzo, S. R., & Trudeau, M. D. (1994). *Clinical administration in audiology and speech-language pathology.* Clifton Park, NY: Delmar Cengage Learning.

Society for Human Resources Management. (2011). *Policy handbook on the web.* Alexandria, VA: Author. Available from http://www.shrm.org

RESOURCES

American Speech-Language-Hearing Association
CAA Accreditation Manual, Standards Manual for CAA Accreditation
10801 Rockville Pike
Rockville, MD 20852-3279
Telephone: 888-498-6699
Website: http://www.asha.org/

Commission on Accreditation of Rehabilitation Facilities (CARF)
Standards manual for 2012 CARF accreditation
4891 East Grant Road
Tucson, AZ 85712
Telephone: 800-444-8991
Website: http://www.carf.org

Hospital and Physician Publishing, Inc.
P.O. Box 158, Ordill Area #7, Bldg. 2-1
Marion, IL 62959
Telephone: 618-997-9375

The Joint Commission
One Renaissance Blvd.
Oakbrook Terrace, IL 60181
Telephone: 630-792-5000
Fax: 630-792-5005
Website: http://www.jointcommission.org

Joint Commission Resources
One Renaissance Blvd.
Oakbrook Terrace, IL 60181
Telephone: 630-792-5000
Website: http://www.jcrinc.com

Knowledge Point
1129 Industrial Avenue
Petaluma, CA 94952
Telephone: 707-762-0333
E-mail: kp@knowledgepoint.com

Medical Consultants Network, Inc.
3191 South Broadway
Englewood, CO 80110-2423
Telephone: 800-538-6264
Website: http://www.medconnetwork.com

Society for Human Resources Management
606 North Washington Street
Alexandria, VA 22314-1997
Telephone: 703-548-3440
E-mail: shrm@shrm.org

Appendix 19-A

Sample P&P

NRH Policies & Procedures

Title:	**Hand Hygiene**	**Section:**
Purpose:	This policy outlines the procedure for maintaining hand hygiene, which is the most effective way to prevent transmission of disease.	**Scope:** **Number:**
Forms:		**Effective Date of This Version:**

1. **Policy:** All team members must follow the guidelines for hand hygiene.
2. **Procedure:**
   A. To reduce the number of organisms on the hands, use the following guidelines:
      1. When hands are visibly soiled or contaminated, wash with soap and water.
      2. If hands are not visibly soiled, use an alcohol based hand-rub.

   B. Decontamination of hands is required for, but not limited to the following:
      1. Before having direct contact with patients
      2. Before performing procedures such as catheter insertion, peripheral vascular catheter, or other invasive devices that do not require a surgical procedure
      3. After contact with patient's intact skin (e.g. when taking pulse or blood pressure and lifting patients)
      4. After contact with body fluids or excretions, mucous membranes or dressings
      5. After removing gloves
      6. When moving from a contaminated body site to a clean body site during patient care
      7. After eating, drinking or using the bathroom

   C. Dispensers
      1. Liquid soap dispensers are replaced or cleaned and filled with fresh product. Liquids are not added to a partially filled dispenser.
      2. Alcohol-based hand rub containers are replaced as needed.
      3. Dispensers are located in every patient room and in patient care areas or close proximity.

   D. Soap and water handwashing steps
      1. Apply soap to wet hands.
      2. Lather and briskly rub hands together over all surfaces of hands, fingers, and fingernails for at least 15 seconds.

3. Rinse thoroughly under a stream of warm water.
4. Dry completely with a paper towel.
5. Turn off water with paper towel.

E. Alcohol-based hand rub steps for decontamination
1. Ensure hands are free of visible debris prior to using the alcohol-based hand rub.
2. Dispense product into palm of one hand and place fingernails of other hand into the foam and rotate. Repeat procedure for opposite hand. Then rub product over both hands.
3. Rub until the alcohol has evaporated.
4. Wash hands with soap and water after 7–8 alcohol uses, and/or when there is a build up of the emollients on the hands.
5. Alcohol-based hand-rub is flammable. Do not use near electrical outlets or oxygen.

F. Gloves
1. Wear gloves when in contact with blood or other potentially infectious materials, mucous membranes and non-intact skin.
2. Change gloves during patient care when moving from a contaminated body site to a clean one.
3. Remove gloves after having contact with a patient. Do not wear the same pair of gloves for the care of more than one patient.

G. Nails
1. Nails must be clean, short and natural.
2. Artificial nails, extenders, nail wraps or other nail applications may not be worn by staff providing direct patient care.
3. Polish, if worn, will not be chipped.

Reference: Guidelines for Hand Hygiene in Healthcare settings: Recommendations of the Healthcare Infection Control Practices Advisory committee and the HICPAC/SHEA/APIC/IDSA Hand Hygiene Task Force (2002)

CDC: Guidelines for Hand Hygiene

Approved By: ______________________________

Edward A Eckenhoff President/CEO

Additional Signature Information:

From *The National Rehabilitation Hospital Policy and Procedures Manual.* Copyright 2005 by the National Rehabilitation Hospital. Reprinted with permission.

20

Documentation Issues

Barbara Moore, EdD

SCOPE OF CHAPTER

No matter the profession, complaints about paperwork are part of the common culture. A necessary evil of our times, paperwork creates the evidence, the record that shows we have followed the law and completed our work in accordance with requirements set forth by government, associations, and other regulatory agencies. Through documentation, we prove compliance, design plans, present a rationale, justify recommendations, and submit financial remuneration requests. This chapter outlines the various types of documentation common to speech-language pathologists and audiologists in the variety of work settings in which we practice, including schools, private practice, and medical settings. As this chapter shows, accurate completion of documentation is essential for speech-language pathologists and audiologists, regardless of the setting, because "if it's not documented, it didn't happen" (Hapner, 2008; Moore, 2010b).

GENERAL PRINCIPLES OF DOCUMENTATION

Speech-language pathologists and audiologists provide services in a variety of settings: schools, hospitals, clinics, universities, private practice offices, telepractice, and possibly others. With the exception of fee-for-service arrangements in private practice, where a client pays directly for the service rendered, the vast majority of our professional services are funded through third-party payers, generally either government funding or insurance. As a result, there are requirements for documentation to demonstrate that requirements are met. The ASHA Code of Ethics (American Speech-Language-Hearing Association [ASHA], 2010), Principle I, Rule M requires that "Individuals shall adequately maintain and appropriately secure records of professional services rendered, research and scholarly activities conducted, and products dispensed, and they shall allow access to these records only when authorized or when required by law" (p. 2). This requirement, then, applies to all work settings.

Third-party payers set forth eligibility requirements for services. The laws for education and the requirements for insurance, including Medicaid and Medicare, establish the foundation on which documentation requirements are built. The professional community of communication sciences and disorders establishes the expectations within the discipline that will form the content of what is documented. Paul and Hasselkus (2004) state, "Clear and comprehensive records are necessary to justify the need for treatment, to document the effectiveness of that treatment, and to have a legal record of events" (p. 1).

In graduate school, you may think that report writing is the biggest part of documentation in the work world. In fact, it is far more. Learning to document correctly and adequately is a skill that is necessary and must be practiced, just like clinical skills. Speech-language pathologists and audiologists should always be attentive to their own documentation, as well as learning procedures from other clinicians. Throughout a career, you should actively seek information about documentation practice. For example, before you submit a report, you might consult writing manuals, review other approved reports, select appropriate procedural terminology, use a spell-checker, and ask others to review your completed work.

Regardless of the work setting, you will be expected to use a formal writing style in your documentation, which means the use of standard American English as well as the formal conventions of written language. Certainly abbreviations and codes will be used, as appropriate to the type of documentation. Keeping to the standards of the field is vital not only because the documentation drives the actions of the reader but also because it is a reflection on you, the writer, and on your program.

Although schools and medical settings are funded by different sources, the basics of clinical documentation remain the same. Clinicians in any setting must remember Hapner's (2008) warning: "If the record is not clear, concise, and comprehensive, then the therapeutic process is at risk" (p. 33). Many individuals who are lax in their paperwork justify their transgressions by stating that the burden of paperwork is "too much" or that "it doesn't matter." In fact, the documentation is the record on which decisions about eligibility and services are made. The documentation guides teams, other professionals, and funding decision makers about how to do their jobs in relation to the student, client, or patient. Poor documentation can lead to funding denials, eligibility uncertainty, and inappropriate diagnosis and treatment. It also can lead to professional consequences, when colleagues and others question why inappropriate documentation was completed and/or are challenged to make service and placement decisions based on inadequate documentation. This can not only reflect on a clinician's professional reputation but also result in incorrect clinical and service decisions.

To ensure that paperwork is completed correctly, it is helpful to understand the funding source and reasons for the documentation requirements. In both medical and educational settings, the "how to" of documentation may change periodically. It is an expectation that the clinician will keep up with such requirements to avoid denials, delays, or legal action.

DOCUMENTATION IN EDUCATIONAL SETTINGS

School-based speech-language pathology and audiology services are generally provided under the authorization of the Individuals with Disabilities Education Improvement Act (IDEA 2004), which is the federal law that authorizes special education in the United States. While most of the paperwork required in schools must comply with IDEA requirements, the IDEA is not the only law that governs or guides what is required, how processes should proceed in school settings, and what documentation is required. Federal laws are identified as public laws (PL), which outline major components of the law. Regulations that implement the laws are set forth in the Code of Federal Regulations (CFR). States are required to enact legislation that aligns state law with federal laws. States can exceed federal law, but they cannot have laws with lower mandates than what exists in federal legislation. State interpretations and provisions may be different from state to state. Additionally, local school board policy and local practice may have specific procedures that are not found in federal or state law but are required for local implementation of state and federal requirements. Parents and staff often become confused about which requirements are federal or state laws, or local practice. Most typically, forms and required paperwork will be designed to comply with legal requirements. Following are the major laws, or "big laws" that pertain to school services and records:

- Family Educational Rights and Privacy Act (FERPA)
- Health Insurance Portability and Accountability Act (HIPAA)
- Individuals with Disabilities Education Improvement Act (IDEA 2004)
- Rehabilitation Act of 1973 and Section 504
- Elementary and Secondary Education Act (ESEA)/No Child Left Behind (NCLB)
- Americans with Disabilities Act (ADA)

This chapter reviews each of these laws and their application to speech-language and hearing services in schools. A summary of these laws, their purpose, and the types of documentation required are provided in Table 20–1.

Laws Regulating Student Records: FERPA and HIPAA

Laws in education are centrally concerned with protecting student confidentiality, specifically related to students with disabilities. These students are considered a protected class of individuals. The Family Educational Rights and Privacy Act (FERPA) is the federal law that addresses student records, including who can access student education records. This law ensures that parents have an opportunity to have the records amended and provides families some control over the disclosure of information from the records. According to FERPA, educational records are records that are (1) directly related to the student and (2) maintained by an educational agency or institution or by a party acting for the agency or institution (20 USC 1232g[a][4][A])(FERPA) (Moore, 2010a). The legislation provides clarification on parents' access to student records, in addition to limiting the transfer of records by requiring consent for record transfers.

An overview of the requirements for access to school records is outlined in Table 20–2. (U.S. Department of Education, 2011). These requirements pertain to all student records, but they set forth the foundation for confidentiality of student records and student information under IDEA. Speech-language pathologists, audiologists, and other educators, including administrators, can sometimes be confused about requests for student records. What if the parents are divorced and do not get along? What if we need to talk to the doctor, but the parent does not agree to the contact? What if the grandmother who takes care of the student is asserting that the student's parents are not making the best choices, and she needs to see the student records? There are a variety of circumstances of records requests or informational releases that might seem in the student's best interest but do not fall within the parameters of allowable provisions. The best advice to school personnel is to always check with administration or legal counsel if you have a question. However, here are some good, quick rules to live by:

- Do not generate letters or records that do not otherwise exist in the student records. This situation may apply if a parent or attorney for the student requests that you generate an opinion regarding which parent is better suited for custody, or if a child's family should be deported when access to services may not be available in another country. Generating documents that render opinions about such issues can pull you into legal battles in which you have no business.
- Be extraordinarily cautious about student information that you put in e-mail or other electronic methods. Increasingly, e-mail may be considered a student record and subject to subpoena.
- Thorough documentation about phone calls, attempts to schedule meetings, and therapy notes are all necessary and important. Some of these documents can be considered student records, so be cautious about ensuring that documentation is professional.

TABLE 20–1 Summary of Federal Laws Pertaining to Documentation in Schools

Federal Law	Original Enactment	Most Recent Authorization	Legal Foundations	Documentation

Individuals with Disabilities Education Improvement Act (IDEA 2004)	November 29, 1975, originally passed as PL 94-142, the Education for All Handicapped Children Act	December 3, 2004	• Individuals with Disabilities Education Improvement Act (IDEA 2004) requires the provision of special education and related services for students identified as children with disabilities (CWD).
			• When students are identified as having a disability, they become members of a protected class; therefore, they secure procedural safeguards, which are realized in the procedural requirements of special education.
			• Foundational concepts in special education:
			  • Free appropriate public education (FAPE)
			  • Least restrictive environment (LRE)
			  • Zero reject
			  • Due process of law for families and children
			    • Time lines
			    • Consent
			    • Appeal procedures
				• **Purposes:**
				  • To show that legal requirements were met, including time lines and regulations
				  • To demonstrate that parents were included in the decision making
				• **Typical documents:**
				  • Individualized Education Program (IEP)
				  • Assessment reports
				  • Parent rights
				  • Consent forms

Rehabilitation Act of 1973; Section 504	September 26, 1973	December 2008	• Section 504 of the Rehabilitation Act of 1973 is a federal civil rights law that prohibits discrimination against individuals with disabilities in programs and activities that receive federal financial assistance. • Section 504 is intended to prohibit discrimination on the basis of disability.	• **Purpose:** To ensure that you document the process. Section 504 has regulations but not the tight time lines and definitive criteria that special education has. • **Typical documents:** • 504 Accommodation Plan

(Continues)

TABLE 20–1 Summary of Federal Laws Pertaining to Documentation in Schools (*Continued*)

			• All IDEA students are also covered by Section 504, but not all 504 students are eligible for services under IDEA. It is not necessary for IDEA-eligible students to have a 504 plan.	• Reports • Consent for data collection
Family Educational Rights and Privacy Act (FERPA)	August 21, 1974, as part of the reauthorization of the Elementary and Secondary Education Act (ESEA), the Education Amendments of 1974	October 26, 2001, as part of the USA Patriot Act of 2001	• FERPA provides student's parents the right to access educational records and also the right to protect transferability of records without their consent.	• **Purpose:** To provide regulations regarding sharing of student records to ensure the protection of privacy rights • **Typical documents:** School records as defined under the law
Elementary and Secondary Education Act (ESEA)/ No Child Left Behind (NCLB)	April 11, 1965	NCLB was the reauthorization of Elementary and Secondary Education Act (ESEA; e.g., Title I); signed into law January 8, 2002, and underwent reauthorization in 2011	• ESEA/NCLB intends to ensure that all children reach proficiency on state content standards and state assessments. • Close the achievement gap between high- and low-performing students, minority and nonminority students, and between advantaged and disadvantaged students. Ensure that students have access to highly qualified teachers.	• **Purpose:** To ensure the academic achievement of all students, including students with disabilities, English learners, students from low socioeconomic homes, and minority students • **Typical documents:** • Testing results • Data • AYP (adequate yearly progress) and other accountability reports
Health Insurance Portability and Accountability Act (HIPAA)	August 21, 1996	April 14, 2003	• HIPAA sets forth simplified health insurance administration by establishing standards and requirements for the electronic transmission of certain health information.	• **Purpose:** Privacy of protected health information

(*Continues*)

(*Continued*)

			• Specifically addresses protected health information (PHI), which includes any physical or mental health information.
			• Education records subject to the protections of FERPA are excluded from HIPAA.
			• HIPAA privacy rule mandates that a "covered entity" may not use or disclose PHI except as permitted by the rule. A school district is considered the "covered entity." The PHI is germane, in most cases, to conducting evaluation and development of the IEP and/or 504.
			• Intent of both HIPAA and FERPA is confidentiality.
			• Some of the agencies that work with school districts (i.e. medical) and want records must abide by HIPAA's PHI rules, so there must be consent in order to exchange information.
				• **Typical documents:** Most school records are covered under FERPA and excluded from HIPAA, including:
				  • IEPs
				  • Evaluations
				  • IEP meeting tapes
				  • Medicaid reimbursement claims
				  • Student health records
				  • Personal notes, when the personal note has become a school record (Shorter, 2004)

Americans with Disabilities Act (ADA)	July 26, 1990	September 26, 2008	ADA (1990) deals with accessibility to public domains (including communication access) and "prohibits discrimination on the basis of disability in employment, programs, and services provided by state and local governments, goods and services provided by private companies, and in commercial facilities" (U.S. Department of Justice, 1999, in Moore & Montgomery, 2008).	• **Purpose:** Prohibits discrimination against people with disabilities; intended to give broad protections by providing physical and communication access
				• **Typical documents:**
				  • Employment records
				  • Facilities records
				  • Some school records
				  • Other records that document provision of accessibility for the public

TABLE 20–2 FERPA Requirements for Access to School Records

FERPA Requires Schools to:

- Provide student with an opportunity to inspect and review his or her education records within 45 days of the receipt of a request;
- Provide a student with copies of education records or otherwise make the records available to the student if the student, for instance, lives outside of commuting distance of the school;
- Redact the names and other personally identifiable information about other students that may be included in the student's education records.

FERPA Does Not Require Schools to:

- Create or maintain education records;
- Provide students with calendars, notices, or other information that does not generally contain information directly related to the student;
- Respond to questions about a student.

Under FERPA a School Must:

- Consider a request from a student to amend inaccurate or misleading information in the student's education records;
- Offer a student a hearing on the matter if it decides not to amend the records in accordance with the request;
- Offer a student a right to place a statement to be kept and disclosed with the record, if as a result of the hearing the school still decides not to amend the record.

A School Is Not Required to Consider Requests for Amendment under FERPA That:

- Seeks to change a grade or disciplinary decision;
- Seeks to change the opinions or reflections of a school official or other person reflected in an education record.

A School Must:

- Have a student's consent prior to the disclosure of education records;
- Ensure that the consent is signed, dated, and states the purpose of the disclosure.
- Ensure the information disclosed has been appropriately designated as directory information by the school.

Adapted from U.S. Department of Education (2011)

Under FERPA, all schools are required to provide an annual notification to parents and the community regarding the rules for access to student records. The means of notification can include student newspaper, calendar, student programs guide, rules handbook, or other means likely to inform students. The notification does not have to be made individually to students. (U.S. Department of Education, 2011). This annual notification spells out the rights of parents and specifies the information that must be provided by the school.

Parents have the right to:

- Inspect and review records
- Seek amendment of inaccurate or misleading information in their education records
- Consent to most disclosures of personally identifiable information from education records

This chapter emphasizes the critical importance of documentation. In schools, the rules pertaining to student records lay the foundation for what information should be documented in addition to the rules for who has access to these records. School personnel should assume that anything that is written has the potential for being accessed or reviewed by the parents and/or their counsel. Further information about assessment reports and Individualized Education Program (IEP) requirements follows later in this chapter.

One final consideration about student records is the requirement for maintaining or destroying these records. Record retention requirements are determined by the type of pupil record it is. School-based practitioners should check with their local district to determine what the policies and procedures are for maintaining and destroying records. Following is a list of three major types of pupil records: mandatory permanent, mandatory interim, and permitted student records.

- *Mandatory permanent pupil records* are required by state law and usually include identifying information about the pupil; when the student attended the schools in the district; and records of subjects taken, grades, immunizations, and date of graduation or exit.
- *Mandatory interim pupil records* are held for a stipulated period of time and include health information, special education information, language training records, progress reports, parental restrictions, parent/pupil challenges to records, parent authorizations/prohibitions for student participation in certain programs, and results of standardized tests.
- *Permitted pupil records* include counselor/teacher rating scales, standardized tests older than three years, routine discipline, behavioral reports, discipline notices, and attendance records. (Moore, 2010a)

The Health Insurance Portability and Accountability Act (HIPAA) is the law that pertains to protected health information (PHI). Originally enacted in 1996, the 2003 amendments addressed electronic transmission of records and increased restrictions on accessibility to health records. Because school personnel are often seeking information from health care providers, there is periodically confusion and questions regarding which HIPAA requirements apply in school settings. The answer is that education records are subject to the protections of FERPA and are excluded from HIPAA. The HIPAA privacy rule mandates that a "covered entity" may not use or disclose PHI except as permitted by the rule. A school district is considered the "covered entity." The PHI is germane, in most cases, to conducting evaluation and development of the Individualized Education Program (IEP) and/or 504 plan. Again, the intent of both HIPAA and FERPA is confidentiality. Speech-language pathologists and audiologists practicing in health care settings will have greater awareness of the influence of HIPAA in their work settings than professionals working in schools. Most school records are covered under FERPA and excluded from HIPAA, including IEPs; evaluations; IEP meeting tapes; Medicaid reimbursement claims; student health records; and personal notes, when the personal note has become a school record (Shorter, 2004).

IDEA 2004 Documentation Requirements

The Individuals with Disabilities Education Improvement Act (IDEA 2004) is the law that authorizes special education in the United States. The IDEA was originally enacted as the Education for All Handicapped Children Act, PL 94-142, in 1975. The foundation of this law is rooted in civil rights, taking its influence of "separate but equal is not equal" from the Supreme Court decision *Brown v. Board of Education* in 1954 (Moore & Montgomery, 2008). Because of these roots in civil rights, students who are identified as children with disabilities (CWD) are considered members of a protected class in this country. Consequently, they engender procedural rights and protections in order to ensure these civil rights. It is for this reason that documentation under the IDEA is critical, as it is the proof that school districts and service providers have followed the foundational components of the rights provided under the law.

Attorneys and school district administrators often tell staff that their work needs to be "legally defensible." Documentation is the vehicle through which personnel create the "legally defensible" record, which, in essence, shows that the process was followed and that the district's IEP team created a program that met the requirements of the law. In special education, processes are extraordinarily important. School-based personnel will participate as members of teams that create documentation that serves to verify that the processes were followed. Records should be able to stand on their own. Through the records created, the story of the student's experience should be told, and the reader should be able to "thread the needle," connecting all components of the student's history. If and when the school district is challenged in a due process hearing, it is the documentation that will provide the evidence that "something took place" (i.e., logs, postal receipts, fax confirmations, and so on). The documentation serves as the historical record, but if we think of it as telling the child's story, we are more inclined to ensure that we are doing our part in demonstrating the reasons why decisions were made and actions were taken.

Special education eligibility is determined through a multidisciplinary assessment. The speech-language pathologist and/or audiologist will need to complete a report documenting the findings of the assessment. Assessment reports and prereferral/response-to-intervention processes and documentation are discussed in another section. The eligibility determination and IEP meeting process are outlined in Figure 20–1.

The main document under IDEA is the Individualized Education Program. The IEP is to be developed either following an assessment or for an annual review. Most IEPs are now electronic or web-based. In many electronic systems, the IEP form reflects all of the federal requirements, designed to ensure that IEP teams meet the required elements. The benefit of electronic systems is that they are developed so that no portion of the IEP can be left blank. However, there is some criticism that electronic systems lend themselves to looking like they are not individualized, specifically with goal development, and/or that they do not allow for parent input. Ensuring and documenting parent input is critical, especially with an electronic system. One of the best ways to do this is within the notes section of the IEP (see Figure 20–2).

While electronic IEPs may seem to make documentation easier, it is the IEP process that is critical. Figure 20–2 illustrates how the IEP process should occur. The IEP document itself should include meaningful interpretation of data by building a bridge, or "threading the needle" between the student's performance (i.e., assessment or other data, student classroom performance, student grades, observational information, input from other teachers and specialists) and the proposed goals. Other texts (Moore & Montgomery, 2008) describe the components of the IEP, and that is not the intention of this chapter. What is important for this chapter is the content of the documents developed, in order to ensure compliance, accuracy, and legal defensibility. The following sections highlight key areas for documentation in the special education process.

Report Writing

The most typical report completed in a school setting is an assessment report. Some school districts require an annual report of student progress, but such reports typically follow a format laid out by the local education agency (LEA). An assessment report must document

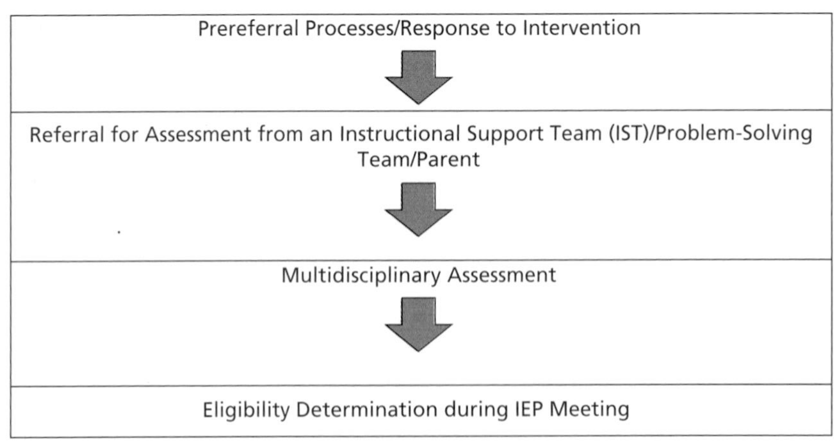

FIGURE 20–1 Special Education Identification Process

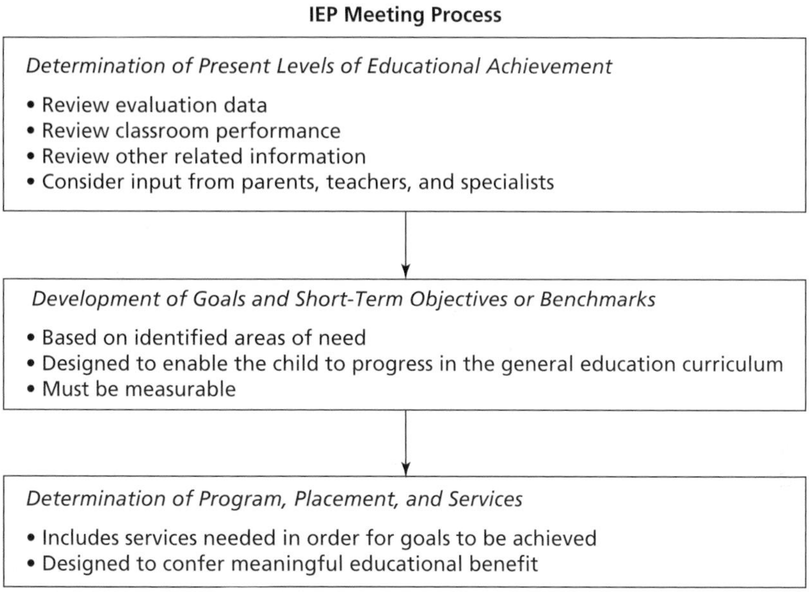

IEP Meeting Process

Determination of Present Levels of Educational Achievement
• Review evaluation data • Review classroom performance • Review other related information • Consider input from parents, teachers, and specialists

↓

Development of Goals and Short-Term Objectives or Benchmarks
• Based on identified areas of need • Designed to enable the child to progress in the general education curriculum • Must be measurable

↓

Determination of Program, Placement, and Services
• Includes services needed in order for goals to be achieved • Designed to confer meaningful educational benefit

FIGURE 20-2 IEP Meeting Process

From *Making a Difference for America's Children: Speech-Language Pathologists in Public Schools*, (2nd ed., p. 160), by B.J. Moore and J. K. Montgomery, 2008, Austin, TX: PRO-ED. Copyright 2008 by PRO-ED. Reprinted with permission.

suspected areas of need; connect to findings in other reports, including both prior speech and language reports, as well as reports from other service providers; document current areas of concern; and be written in a professional manner, using professional terminology. In some school districts, it is becoming increasingly common for the multidisciplinary assessment team (MDAT) to write one comprehensive report to ensure that the connection between the thoughts of the professionals is obvious in the report. While this is a highly recommended practice, it may not be the practice in every district.

Assessment reports generally follow the following format (Moore, 2010a, 2010b):

- Reason for assessment
- Background information
- Assessments:
    - Standardized assessments or tests
    - Observation in natural setting
    - Nonstandardized assessments or methods
    - Activities within natural setting
- Behaviors observed during assessment
- Information on progress in academic or curricular areas
- Information on classroom assessments and statewide assessments
- Information from others (teacher, parent, aide, other MDAT members)
- Input from the student on his/her disabling condition, thoughts, desires, and wishes
- Impressions
- Summary/conclusions
- Recommendations

Pitfalls in assessment reports come when school personnel do not connect their assessment results to the actual daily classroom work in schools. Assessment reports that only provide test results and discussion of clinical findings and do not connect these results to classroom performance do not meet the premise of "threading the needle" among assessments, IEP development, and academic achievement.

The same is true for audiology reports. An audiogram placed in the student file without interpretation connected to the classroom or in concert with findings from other MDAT members does not serve the student well. Both speech-language pathologists and audiologists in schools can assume that their clinical impressions must be directly and overtly connected to the student's classroom performance. Not only is this good practice, it is required by law and is good for the student.

Therapy Notes, Progress Monitoring, Personal Notes, and E-mail

During training in communication sciences and disorders, speech-language pathologists and audiologists are drilled in the requirements of documenting client performance during therapy. Hegde and Davis (2005) instruct clinicians: "You should chart your client's performance in each session" (p. 169). Justice (2006) states: "During every treatment session the experienced clinician probes the client's skills and progress, making adjustments to the treatment process to enhance the effectiveness of the session and the overall treatment plan" (p. 119). Oftentimes, however, when working in educational settings, these habits are prone to slippage. Keeping therapy notes for therapeutic sessions is an expectation in a school setting, just as in any other setting.

As instructed by Hegde and Davis (2005), progress should be charted for each session. Progress monitoring is a "hot topic" in school settings currently, particularly with the advent of response-to-intervention (see Response to Intervention section). Speech-language pathologists and audiologists are trained in these methods and may serve as a resource to educational personnel. Charting and progress monitoring are expectations of our professional work and are required in all work settings for clinical practice, including schools. IEP goals are written with measurable targets. To track phonological production, fluency counts, or grammatical units, charting or progress monitoring will occur and should be part of the therapy notes.

Although it is not a requirement in schools, following a SOAP note format is useful for therapy note documentation in schools as well as medical and private practice settings. See Figure 20-3.

Writing a SOAP note for school settings may seem onerous to school-based clinicians, but this type of documentation will pay off for both Medicaid billing and for any legal challenges. In fact, the therapy note does not have to be onerous. Consider the following example for an in-class session:

S – Student chatting with friends before class began. Attentive to teacher instructions.

O – Applied vocabulary strategies for verbal rehearsal during class activity. Student observed three times using strategy appropriately with history terms *tariff*, *taxation without representation*, and *revolution*.

A – First application of strategy without prompting.

P – Continue per IEP.

Keeping this type of a note is not difficult and not particularly time consuming. Do remember, however, to initial and date each note so that authentication of the author of the note is provided. Writing the note at the end of the session or right after the session is completed ensures both accuracy and completion of the requirement.

- Subjective — Write your opinion or impressions regarding relevant student or client behavior or status in a brief statement
- Objective — Record measurable information or progress monitoring data collected for each task during the therapy session
- Assessment — Describe your analysis and/or interpret data for current session and compare to student's or client's previous level of performance
- Plan — Identify proposed therapy targets for the next session

FIGURE 20-3 SOAP Notes

Information based on Hegde and Davis (2005) and Moore (2010a, 2010b)

Keeping therapy notes is important for many purposes. In addition to therapeutic interactions, school-based practitioners are encouraged and reminded about keeping documentation of all interactions with parents and all issues pertinent to the case. Particularly in challenging or "high-profile" cases, school-based practitioners may feel a need to keep "personal notes" or a "personal file." Sometimes, these notes pertain to challenging interactions with parents or other agencies. Although courts and legislatures have protected the use of personal notes, especially if used for the purpose of serving as a memory aid or reminder of a situation, a personal file may still be subpoenaed. Special education or school personnel may sometimes feel threatened or that they need to document situations for their own personal reasons, separate from the requirements of the law or professional responsibilities. Thus, always be cognizant that someone else may read that file.

School personnel also need to be cautious regarding e-mail. E-mail can be subpoenaed. In most work settings, e-mail is widely used. E-mail can be problematic because it is easily forwarded; it can also end up in a student file, making it part of the student record and, as such, available to the parent. You may, in fact, wish to print and save some e-mail, but do so with the knowledge that it may be considered a student record. In some cases, this may be appropriate. Practitioners should be very careful with what to put in e-mail. As a general rule, if you don't want the child's parent, your boss, your mother, or a judge reading the e-mail, don't send it! (Moore, 2010a, 2010b)

One other caution about electronic communication involves social networking. Facebook, Twitter, YouTube, and the ever-emerging world of social networking are widely accessed. Within these domains, individuals typically feel free to share widely their daily experiences, including their feelings about bosses, coworkers, and other situations in their lives, including, in the case of educators, information about children. Children should be protected at all times, especially by those who are responsible for their well-being. Remember, too, that FERPA and IDEA have confidentiality protections that are easily violated when personally identifiable information is shared. This is true in the lunchroom, the faculty lounge, and also on social networking sites, where anyone can access information. Again, be careful and cognizant of the problems this can present. See Chapter 9 for issues related to e-mail and finding employment.

Some systems for electronic billing of Medicaid also have electronic systems for note taking. Both IDEA and Medicaid require that school districts maintain records for at least three years after the student separates from the educational system. Storing of files is an inefficient system in many school districts, so electronic storage is simple. Additionally, this method ensures that records are not lost. However, for some speech-language pathologists and audiologists, especially those who have been practicing for many years, electronic documentation may not be as comfortable or easy.

One final comment on therapy notes and documentation: As recommended throughout this chapter, in addition to maintaining therapy notes, you should get into the habit of documenting all communications with parents, teachers, and issues pertaining to a student. Many school-based practitioners find it easy to keep all documentation in one file. Many clinicians just keep individual files on each student, maintaining therapy notes on one side and other documentation on the other side of the file. Most local education agencies (LEAs) have a procedure for keeping such records as well as how these records are to be disposed of at the appropriate time.

The following tips summarize this section:

- Yes, it's true: *if it's not documented, it didn't happen!*
- Get yourself into the habit of documenting everything, including conversations with parents, phone calls, intervention notes, and anything else.
- Do not rely on your memory. It will fail you, and it will not be the same as someone else's, especially that of a parent.
- Lack of documentation is lethal. Poor documentation is worse. (Moore, 2010a, 2010b)

IEP and IFSP Components

The IEP and the Individualized Family Service Plan (IFSP), developed for infants and toddlers receiving services under Part C of the IDEA, are the cornerstones of documentation in special education. The documentation requirements provide the foundation for ensuring that the LEA has designed a plan that is individualized to a given child's unique needs. Through the IEP process (see Figure 20–2), a document is developed that, in essence, is the contract whereby the responsible parties develop a program intended to confer educational benefit to the student

(Moore & Montgomery, 2008). These are more than words. The IEP process results in a document that is legally binding and portable, meaning that the family can take this document to any school district in the United States and that district will be required to provide the services identified in the IEP without delay. If you have ever been confused by the lack of clarity in an incoming IEP document, you understand why clear documentation on the IEP is so important to the student. Sometimes this happens even within one's own district. See Chapter 15 for discussion of policies and procedures in educational settings.

IFSPs are developed with a different focus than the IEP. Services to infants and toddlers occur primarily in the home, and issues related to infants and toddlers are addressed through family system support and through direct services to the child. IFSPs are outcome driven, and the documentation of an IFSP is designed accordingly. Providing services in a natural environment, and combining resources of educational and other state and local agencies, is a common way of dealing with these needs of the children and families. Programming for infants and toddlers is very different from state to state and is not addressed here. Early intervention (EI) is a growing area of service under IDEA due to technological advances and increasing awareness of the importance of providing services to children and families as early as possible. The specialization of documentation requirements is highly dependent on state and local regulations. See Chapter 16 for in-depth discussion of early intervention.

Present Levels of Academic Achievement

Special education requirements ensure monitoring of student progress in the general curriculum since the inception of the federal law in 1975. However, mandates for accountability are more recent, with the reauthorizations of IDEA in 1997 and 2004. The 2001 reauthorization of the Elementary and Secondary Education Act (ESEA), known as No Child Left Behind (NCLB), put into place requirements for school districts to demonstrate academic growth in various subgroups, including students with disabilities. These mandates have led to heightened awareness of the need for speech-language pathologists, in particular, to be developing "educationally relevant IEPs" (Brannen et al., 2000) and delivering services through "curriculum-relevant" therapy (Wallach, 2008).

Under IDEA 2004, documentation of a student's present level of performance (PLOP) became a requirement to identify the student's present levels of academic achievement and/or functional performance (IDEA §§ 614[d][A][i][I]). Statements about students' performance should always be positive, never using negative language (Hegde & Davis, 2005; Moore & Montgomery, 2008). The IDEA (2004) regulations require that all IEPs include a statement of the child's present levels of academic achievement and functional performance. Information must include how the child's disability affects involvement and progress in the general curriculum (i.e., the same curriculum as for nondisabled children).

For preschool children, as appropriate, documentation should focus on how the disability affects the child's participation in appropriate activities (34 CFR § 300.320).

This change in language is directive. Previously, PLOP statements were broad and generic. The IDEA 2004 requirement ensures that the IEP team is considering the student's needs in relation to academic achievement. Figure 20–2 illustrates the redundancy that is built into the process. The multidisciplinary assessment team assesses all areas of suspected disability and then identifies the areas of academic need that result from the deficits identified in the assessment. If the IEP meeting is not a review of an initial or triennial assessment, then there will be no assessment upon which to base the present levels. According to Moore and Montgomery (2008, pp. 133, 135):

> Depending on the type of meeting being held, present levels of educational performance are considered by any and all of the following methods:
>
> - Reviewing assessment(s), including statewide, school-wide or classroom, as well as specialist or psycho-educational assessments
> - Reviewing classroom work
> - Reviewing grade reports
> - Reviewing teacher or specialist report (oral or written)
> - Considering parent and student information and interests
> - Reviewing the previous year's goals and the progress made
> - Considering new information brought forth by any member of the team

- Considering reports on student progress and behavior by service providers
- Reviewing discipline and behavioral information
- Considering statewide assessment results

The question for the IEP team, including the speech-language pathologist and/or audiologist, is how the communication disorder affects a student's ability to progress in the curriculum. To know this information, all personnel must be in communication, be familiar with the curricular requirements of the student's grade level and/or program, and address how the student's disability impacts his/her ability to progress in the curriculum. For students with more significant disabilities, functional performance is documented in this area of the IEP.

As a result of this shift in thinking and requirements, the present levels of academic achievement should not include simply rewriting individualized standard test scores or information from previous IEPs. Instead, the link between the areas of need and goals should be evident. For example: "Sara's difficulties in word retrieval and rapid naming adversely affect her reading comprehension abilities. She is able to participate in the classroom activities utilizing the core text with support provided through the Learning Lab program. Her independent reading level is 2.0 according to the Accelerated Reader assessment given on March 3, 2011."

Some students who receive speech and language services for articulation, fluency, voice, or even language-related issues may not have deficits in core academics. In these cases, it is important that their grade-level performance be documented on the IEP. Sometimes, practitioners are tempted to leave blank areas where the student has no needs, but this is not the correct procedure. Another rule of documentation is "Leave nothing blank." On the other hand, functional performance related to the student's communication needs, such as phonology, fluency, or voice, should be documented in the IEP. For example: "Bobby's speech is characterized by multiple disfluencies, most often sound repetitions and prolongations. The focus of his current IEP is learning to utilize fluency shaping techniques across the school environment."

Goals, Objectives, and Benchmarks

IEP goals must be measurable and should be based on common core standards. Electronically based IEP systems often have an expanded base of prewritten goals from which to pick. The ASHA website also has resources for development of IEP goals. A quick guide to writing IEP goals is provided by the Association of California School Administrators (2006):

Who:	the student
Does what:	observable behavior
When:	by reporting date
Given what:	conditions
How much:	mastery or criteria
How will it be measured:	performance data

Benchmarks are no longer required for annual academic goals, but some LEAs still prefer these to be written. What is required is reporting to parents on the progress toward the goal. This reporting must occur on the same schedule as general education updates students' progress. Again, most districts have processes for such reporting, but frequently these quarterly reports are not included in the IEP file, which means there is no evidence that the requirement was followed. The IEP must describe how progress of the pupil toward meeting the annual goals will be measured. Additionally, the IEP must include when the periodic reports will be made. The record needs to reflect that goals have been reported to the parents at the required intervals (Moore, 2010a).

All states currently have state standards that are used for IEP development. As of the writing of this chapter, 45 states have adopted the Common Core State Standards, a joint initiative of the National Governors Association Center for Best Practices and the Council of Chief State School Officers (National Governors Association Center for Best Practices, Council of Chief State School Officers, 2010). The Common Core State Standards are intended to improve the current state standards, which are now more than 10 years old, through integration of skills and also attention to the needs of students with disabilities and English learners. It is expected that in the next few years more states will move in this direction. Consequently, all school-based personnel should pay attention to these standards, as they will reshape all of education.

If a student is failing to make progress on the agreed-upon IEP goals, it is the responsibility of the service provider to reconvene the IEP team to discuss the reasons for the lack of progress. Failure to make progress on IEP goals can be seen as a denial of the student's free appropriate public education (FAPE). It is highly recommended and required to meet whenever students are not making progress, to address the issue (i.e., document it), and to adjust the IEP accordingly. Examples of adjustments include changing or dropping a goal or service. Do not let lack of student progress go undocumented. Lack of progress needs to be addressed for all concerned.

IEP Meeting Notes

Whether to keep IEP meeting notes is often a local district or LEA decision, and some administrators have very strong opinions about how they want the special education personnel in the district to operate. This author is one of those special education directors who has strong opinions about meeting notes and highly recommends the use of meeting notes for several reasons. Meeting notes should document (1) the purpose of the meeting; (2) the offer of parent rights and procedural safeguards; (3) that the IEP team followed the IEP process (Figure 20–2); (4) parental participation, including questions and issues raised by the parent and how those issues were addressed; (5) recommendation of goals and adjustments made, if applicable; (6) discussion of the consideration of continuum of services; and (7) the district's offer of FAPE.

Response-to-Intervention (RtI)

Response-to-Intervention (RtI) models are a hot topic in school-based services. These general education models are widely variable across all school districts. In many cases, speech-language pathologists and audiologists have been involved with the development of the model at their school. In other cases, speech-language pathologists and audiologists are not involved in RtI services at their schools. At the heart of RtI is the belief that early and systematic approaches to assist students who are having academic and behavioral challenges can prevent students from ultimately requiring special education. Many processes are involved in these models of intervention. A problem-solving team analyzes universal screening and progress monitoring data and makes determinations about what will happen if a student does not respond to the intervention program. In consideration of documentation for RtI programs and the participation of speech-language pathologists and audiologists, a key is to look to the processes and programs in existence at a school site or district.

Speech-language pathologists and audiologists may be involved in many different aspects of RtI, including planning and providing services in any of the three tiers of intervention (Moore & Montgomery, 2008). At the core of RtI operations is progress monitoring and data-driven decision making. Rudebusch (2008) provides numerous examples of tracking systems, worksheets, and progress monitoring systems that can be used by clinicians participating in RtI. Similarly, the development and availability of programs such as the San Diego City Schools' *Articulation Differences and Disorders Manual* (San Diego City Schools, 2004–2005) and *START-IN* (Montgomery & Moore-Brown, 2005) and others are increasingly providing the resources that can help school-based personnel participate and document their involvement in RtI.

Documentation under Other Educational Laws: ESEA and Section 504

The final two laws that require data and documentation are the Elementary and Secondary Education Act (ESEA) and Section 504. Although these laws may seem unrelated, both strive to ensure access to equal opportunities in educational programs. Just like IDEA, these laws also address the participation of students with some sort of disadvantage who otherwise may be denied or have limited access to resources designed to support their successful participation in school.

The Elementary and Secondary Education Act (ESEA)

ESEA was enacted in 1965 during the civil rights era, under the administration of Lyndon Baines Johnson. ESEA authorized Title I, which provides local school districts with financial assistance for the education of low-income children. In 2001, the ESEA was reauthorized under then-President George W. Bush and was renamed No Child Left Behind (NCLB). The new law enhanced accountability provisions in American schools. There were many provisions in NCLB, but one of the most noteworthy was the establishment of subgroups for which schools and school districts would be held accountable in terms of academic achievement. These subgroups include students from low socioeconomic status (SES) homes, minority students, students who are English learners, students with disabilities, and all students. Under the requirements of NCLB, all of these subgroups, including the disability subgroup, are to meet grade-level proficiency by the year 2014. The measurement of the progress of these subgroups is known as adequate yearly progress (AYP), and it measures the movement of the subgroups toward the goal (Moore & Montgomery, 2008).

Although NCLB is not without controversy because of its accountability provisions and mandates for proficiency, there is no doubt that educators have changed the way they have instructed students in the various subgroups, including students with disabilities. In addition to NCLB, the emphasis on academic achievement was strengthened when IDEA 2004 was passed, aligning the accountability requirements of general and special education. Special educators, including speech-language pathologists and audiologists, are well aware of NCLB requirements, including the participation of their students in statewide assessment. In the previous section on IDEA and IEP requirements, the concepts of "educationally relevant" IEPs and "curriculum-relevant" services were mentioned. These concepts are necessary realities when serving students in special education, regardless of their disability or area of need. School-based personnel need to attend to the requirements of both general and special education because general and special education are connected through accountability. Table 20–1 cites testing results, data, and AYP reports as being the typical documents that demonstrate compliance with ESEA. In reality, though, the typical documentation will be related to changes to the reading and math programs, the emphasis on preparation for state testing, the analysis of end-of-the-quarter benchmark data for core content courses, and the use of standards in classroom instruction and IEP goal development that will reflect the influence of this law.

ESEA is due to be reauthorized sometime in 2012. The name of the law has already reverted in common vernacular away from the use of the term NCLB. Although it is anticipated that the stringent requirements to have all children grade-level proficient by the year 2014 (just a little more than two years away as of the writing of this chapter) are expected to change, the accountability provisions are expected to remain. Requirements for holding schools, students, and professionals to high expectations are expected to continue through new reauthorizations of ESEA and IDEA. School-based speech-language pathologists and audiologists will need to continue to be vigilant in how they document IDEA and RtI services and how they connect services to academic standards.

Section 504 and the Americans with Disabilities Act (ADA)

Section 504 of the Rehabilitation Act of 1973 is a federal civil rights law that prohibits discrimination against individuals with disabilities in programs and activities that receive federal assistance. The interpretation of who is disabled under Section 504 is broader than under IDEA. Most recently reauthorized in 2008, the provisions of 504 have actually been broadened. Students are deemed eligible as students with a disability under Section 504 if the student is determined to be an individual who:

> Has a physical or mental impairment that substantially limits one or more major life activities, including caring for one's self, performing manual tasks, walking, seeing, hearing, speaking, breathing, sleeping, learning, reading, concentrating, thinking, communicating, and working. (34 CFR 504.3)

Students are found to be eligible following a data collection process or assessment. If a student is eligible, a 504 Accommodation Plan will be developed. While 504 does not have the same time lines as IDEA, there are procedural safeguards, rights, and protections provided under this law. Students who are eligible under 504 may be entitled to receive services available through special education to address their needs. It is necessary to document how assessment and plan development follow prescribed 504 processes. The process often feels unfamiliar to special and general education personnel because of the lack of specific requirements. A good rule of thumb is to follow the well-established time lines of special education.

The Americans with Disabilities Act is not an education law but, like 504, is a law that applies to educational settings in that education receives federal funds. ADA is a law that requires access in public domains, including both physical access to buildings, as well as communication access for individuals with hearing loss and other communication limitations. Through the ADA, physical modifications to public buildings have been realized. These structural changes include creating accessible restrooms, providing accessible audio systems, and putting in ramps so that individuals with mobility challenges are not limited in movement around a building. Issues relating to documentation of accessibility can and do still arise in IEP meetings. Special education generally needs to work with the facilities department of the district to ensure that facilities are accessible to students. Special education personnel may also get involved when members of the public need access, even though the issue is not student related.

Special Issues with Documentation in Schools

Documentation requirements in schools are cumbersome, and failure to comply can bring about liability for the school district. Worse, at times failure to comply can bring about hard feelings between school professionals and parents. In concluding this section on documentation in schools, we consider some special issues.

Request for Records When parents or their representatives request records, all educational records need to be provided. This means health records, cumulative records, discipline reports, teacher records, and the special education file. Be sure to share any request for records with your principal or special education office administrator immediately, as time lines apply. A request for records often indicates that the family is unhappy with some aspect of their child's program.

Request for Copies of Protocols Speech-language pathologists and audiologists are sometimes confused about providing copies of protocols to parents when requested. The confusion comes because we are told that it violates copyright laws to copy protocols. Copying protocols is a violation of copyright laws if an individual copies a blank protocol in order to avoid spending the money to purchase new protocols. Once a protocol has been used during an assessment, the protocol becomes a student record and is permitted to be copied. When this record is copied, be sure to copy all pages of the protocol, including the blank pages.

Providing Parents Copies of Records in Their Primary Language Parent participation is a cornerstone of special education. School districts have a responsibility to ensure that parents can fully participate in the IEP process. Having oral interpretation at an IEP or other school meeting is commonly understood, but parents whose primary language is other than English also have the right to have copies of IEPs and assessment reports provided to them in their primary language. The LEA will have procedures to complete such requests.

Legal Considerations First and foremost, the legal documentation required in special education gives assurance that the required procedures have been followed. In a due process hearing, when a parent's testimony, or the testimony of a witness, contradicts the testimony of the district's witnesses, credence will be given to any documentation the district can provide to support the witness's testimony. In a legal battle, the judge will look for both substantive and procedural violations. The procedural requirements are those that involve the procedures: time lines, notices, IEP meeting documentation, and so on. The question will be "Did the district fail to comply with the procedures mandated under IDEA, and, if so, did the procedural violation rise to the level of a denial of the child's right to a free appropriate public education (FAPE)?" The substantive component of the IEP is the essence of the program. Based on what was delivered, did the student receive an educational benefit? Again, the standard the judge will consider is whether the student received FAPE. IDEA does not allow judges to determine that FAPE was denied simply because some procedural violations occurred. However, if the procedural violation led to a denial of FAPE, the district will lose the case.

A request for a test protocol, like a request for records, can be an indicator that the family is unhappy or feels the need to share the records with someone, such as a legal representative. If the family or representative requests a copy of a test protocol, it may be that person's intention to have someone check your scoring (Moore, 2010a). If someone is launching a challenge to the results and recommendations, a natural place to start for that person could be the test protocol to find any possible scoring error. Such an error might tumble the foundation upon which the recommendations were based. The lesson is to be very careful when scoring assessments. We all make mistakes, but big problems can occur if scoring errors were made and if the incorrect score was relied upon for making recommendations for goals, service, or placement recommendations. The moral of this story is that documentation is not only writing things down but also being careful in ensuring accurate administration and scoring. Legally defensible documentation relies on linking to evidence-based practice and threading the needle between assessment, identification of needs, and IEP goal development. Again, see Chapter 15 for an in-depth discussion of school-related issues.

DOCUMENTATION IN HEALTH CARE SETTINGS

While services in school settings are authorized under the requirements of federal education laws, services in health care settings are authorized under insurance requirements, which primarily are based on the requirements of Medicare. As mentioned earlier in this chapter, unless a client is paying directly for services (e.g., private pay) in a private practice setting, all other speech, language, and audiology services are paid for through third-party payers, all of whom have specific regulations. Health care settings include hospitals, rehabilitation centers, home health care, skilled nursing facilities, or other long-term care settings. In some cases, private practice and university clinic settings may also accept and bill Medicare and other health insurance.

Documentation in health care settings is all about reimbursement and may require a "shift in thinking" for speech-language pathologists and audiologists, who may believe documentation should focus on procedures and performance (Coleman, Majerus, Meska, & Goulding, 2008). According to Hapner (2008), increased scrutiny on the need for skilled services and therapy caps increases the attention that speech-language pathologists and audiologists need to pay to documentation. Additionally, remember that the individuals who are reviewing claims are typically not speech-language pathologists or audiologists. Consequently, clinicians in these settings need to be sure they not only know the requirements but also document so someone outside of the profession can understand the notes (Coleman et al., 2008; Hapner, 2008; Sutherland Cornett, 2006; Swigert, 2003). Reviewers need to be able to determine easily if the services are medically necessary and that criteria are met (Coleman et al., 2008). Hapner (2008) warns, "Poor record keeping poses a threat to evaluation and follow-through with therapy, to insurance reimbursement, and to the development of a clinical record that meets legal standards" (p. 33).

Medicare provides health insurance for individuals who are over 65 years of age and for individuals with certain disabling conditions. Medicare is divided into two programs: Medicare Part A and Medicare Part B. Part A is hospital insurance and covers services provided in hospitals, skilled nursing facilities, home health care services, and hospice. Part B services cover physician services, audiology testing services, outpatient services, and rehabilitation services (ASHA, n.d.-b). Telepractice is also an acceptable way to deliver speech-language and audiology services under Medicare (ASHA, n.d.-d). Documentation requirements are the same.

Billing and documentation under Medicare are extremely complex. This chapter provides general information about documentation issues under the Medicare system; however, specifics about codes, fees, and other related issues are not addressed here. ASHA's website and the website for the Centers for Medicare & Medicaid Services (CMS) have information that is particularly helpful. See Chapters 13 and 14 for further discussion of issues related to health and insurance.

Clinical notes are required under Medicare for purposes of billing and documenting services. These documents include evaluation notes, treatment encounter notes, progress notes, and discharge notes. An important part of documentation in health care settings is the billing codes. There are three types of codes: CPT codes, HCPCS codes, and ICD-9-CM codes (see Table 20–3). The system of codes is regulated by the Centers for Medicare & Medicaid Services, which has established recognized codes under HIPAA (ASHA, n.d.-f).

Although billing codes, their updates, and changes often dominate discussions about documentation in health care settings, Hapner (2008) clarifies the importance of clinical note writing:

- allows documentation of events, findings, and clinical impressions during encounters with patients;
- enhances clinical follow-through with the transfer of information from evaluation to intervention, or from session-to-session to ensure the progression of therapy;
- is used to transfer information from speech-language pathologist to physician; or
- is used to transfer information from one speech-language pathologist to another to continue the clinical process (p. 34).

Medicare requires that services provided need to be "reasonable and necessary." The ASHA document

TABLE 20–3 Billing Code Systems

Code System	Abbreviation	Services Covered	Administrator
Current Procedural Terminology	CPT	Procedures or services	American Medical Association (AMA)
Healthcare Common Procedures Coding System	HCPCS	Devices, supplies, equipment	Centers for Medicare & Medicaid Services (CMS)
International Classification of Diseases-10th Revision-Clinical Modification	ICD-10-CM	Diagnoses and disorders	National Center for Health Statistics

Adapted from ASHA (n.d.-f)/end table/

Speech-Language Pathology Medical Review Guidelines (2011) identifies the threshold components for this standard:

- **Reasonable:** appropriate amount, frequency, and duration of treatment in accordance with accepted standards of practice
- **Necessary:** appropriate treatment for the patient's diagnosis and condition
- **Specific:** targeted to particular treatment goals
- Effective: expected to yield improvement within a reasonable time
- **Skilled:** requiring the knowledge, skills, and judgment of a speech-language pathologist, that is, complex and sophisticated (p. 8)

Types of Clinical Documentation

Creation of a clinical record provides "an overall indicator of clinical service and quality, and serves as a basis for planning care and for service continuity" (Sutherland Cornett, 2006, p. 3). Each of the different types of notes has specific requirements, depending on the purpose of the note.

Evaluation notes require the following:

- Documentation of diagnosis, description of problem, date of onset, current functional status
- Use of standardized measures for objective testing to document patient status
- Statement of prognosis and time frame for therapy
- List of prognostic indicators that will be used to determine progress

Treatment encounter notes require the following:

- Documentation of every treatment day and of every treatment service
- Record of all skilled interventions and justification for billing
- Identifying information, treatment provided, signature of professional providing the service
- Total treatment time
- Comprehensive information so that another clinician could conduct follow-up therapy with a reasonable expectation to progress in the therapeutic process
- Tip: Use SOAP note format (see Figure 20–3).
- Tip: Include ICD-10 and CPT codes in notes to assist the reviewer.

Discharge notes require the following:

- A summary of all treatment provided and a statement that the therapist agrees with discharge

  Allowed is the use of the ASHA National Outcome Measurement System (NOMS) Functional Communication Measures (FCM) for reporting on the Physician Quality Reporting Initiative (PQRI)

Plan of care and progress notes require the following:

- Inclusion in the clinical record
- Documentation of medical necessity and need for ongoing service

- Physician certification and approval of the care and treatment plan every 30 days
- Any changes to long-term and short-term goals, and the plan of care
- Completion after evaluation but before treatment begins; signed by treating physician
- Diagnosis, medical condition that relates to the speech/language diagnosis, long-term goals, frequency, and duration of treatment
- Tip: Be sure to include "PLAN OF CARE" on the note so the reviewer knows that is what it is.

  (ASHA, n.d.-g; Hapner, 2008; Sutherland Cornett, 2006)

Coleman et al. (2008) report that denials of Medicaid claims are typically due to either failure to justify medical necessity (i.e., linking the medical diagnosis to the change in functioning abilities) or failure to justify the use of skilled services (i.e., making a skilled analysis and determining the need for treatment through a review of the objective data gathered from patient performance). For residents in skilled nursing facilities (SNF), goal writing needs to be based on the requirements of the 1990 Omnibus Reconciliation Act, which calls for functional goals and outcomes for the resident. Specialized forms exist for these purposes. Use of SOAP notes, justification of medical necessity for treatment, and the previously stated requirements for progress notes are also suggested by these authors for use in the SNF.

Other resources that are useful on the ASHA website are the article "Clinical Record Keeping in Speech-Language Pathology for Health Care and Third-Party Payers" (Paul & Hasselkus, 2004), as well as the Outpatient Speech-Language Pathology Service Audit Template (Sutherland Cornet, 2006). Individuals working in health care settings should also be aware of the impending development of electronic medical records (EMRs) (ASHA, n.d.-a).

Although information provided here deals primarily with Medicare requirements, private health plans also cover speech-language and audiology services. As stated, many plans match or model Medicare requirements, but individual plans do vary in the amount, type, and conditions covered. Most services provided in hospitals are generally covered, but there are variations among plans (e.g., health maintenance organizations, preferred provider organizations, and individual, indemnity, or fee-for-service). The benefits authorized under any plan should always be researched prior to treatment (ASHA, n.d.-e). The writing guidelines are the same for both Medicaid and Medicare.

DOCUMENTATION IN PRIVATE PRACTICE AND UNIVERSITY CLINICS

Speech-language pathologists and audiologists working in private practice settings may have a variety of different types of clients and payers. Regardless of the type of client or who is funding the service, clinical notes are expected in accordance with the ASHA Code of Ethics (ASHA, 2010), although the type of client and payer may dictate the form of the notes.

Speech-language pathologists in private practice were not able to bill Medicare until July 1, 2009, following the passage of the Medicare Improvements for Patients and Providers Act of 2008 (MIPPA). An advisory on Medicare billing for speech-language pathologists in private practice is available at the CMS website (Centers for Medicare & Medicaid Services [CMS], n.d.-a).

Speech-language pathologists and audiologists in private practice who take private insurance may belong to networks within health maintenance organizations (HMOs) or preferred provider organizations (PPOs). Some private practitioners do not want to deal directly with insurance companies and the paperwork of billing. In these cases, private practitioners may require their patients or their families to pay directly for the service and then provide them with the appropriate forms with codes to bill for reimbursement.

Some speech-language pathologists may serve in other capacities, such as providing contract services to school districts; providing vendor services to early childhood agencies, courts, or other social service agencies; or establishing themselves as nonpublic agencies for specific contracting possibilities with public schools. Other speech-language pathologists may develop a relationship with a private school and take referrals from the private school or work with cases when students need services. In these situations, the private practitioner may be paid by the school or directly by the student's parent. In each of these situations, the type of documentation depends on who is paying for the service and that entity's documentation requirements.

Private practice is the only setting in which direct fee-for-service may be received. In these cases, documentation for service is not established based on a third-party payer's requirements, but a client paying by fee-for-service still requires a billing statement. Therapy notes, including progress notes, should be maintained as part of keeping appropriate clinical records consistent with all of the reasons previously outlined in this chapter.

Services in university clinics may be provided by student clinicians or by university staff. Clients who receive services from students sign a contract indicating that they are aware that a student who is supervised will be providing the services. Universities use these clinics to teach students the art of documentation. If a faculty or staff member is providing services, the university may bill private insurance, Medicare, or Medicaid, or take private pay.

DOCUMENTATION FOR AUDIOLOGICAL SERVICES

Audiologists who work in school settings follow all of the procedures discussed in the section on Documentation in Educational Settings. Audiologists in school settings typically provide testing such as hearing screening, pure-tone testing, otoacoustic emissions, and impedance audiometry. Additionally, audiologists provide consultative services and fitting and oversight of hearing aids, FM systems, and possibly mapping management of cochlear implants. Medically based audiological testing is not part of school-based services. Under Medicare, hearing and balance testing is covered under "other diagnostic tests," but Medicare has no provision to pay for routine hearing testing or audiological therapeutic services (CMS, n.d.-b). Audiology services must come from a physician's referral. Some private insurance providers require prior authorization, especially for certain procedures.

According to ASHA (n.d.-c), requirements include documenting the details of a physician's referral, services performed, and the follow-up provided to the physician. Requirements for documenting audiological testing are included in Chapter 15, section 80.3 of *The Medicare Benefit Manual* (CMS, n.d.-a), which includes the following:

> *Documenting for Audiological Tests.* The reason for the test should be documented either on the order, and/or the audiological evaluation report, and/or in the patient's medical record. Examples of appropriate reasons include, but are not limited to:
>
> - Evaluation of suspected change in hearing, tinnitus, or balance
> - Evaluation of the cause of disorders of hearing, tinnitus, or balance
> - Determination of the effect of medication, surgery or other treatments

Information on CPT codes and other requirements for audiology under Medicare can be found on the ASHA websites provided or from CMS. All of the information provided previously regarding Medicare documentation applies when appropriate to audiology services, but the specifics of documentation are too complex and lengthy for this chapter.

Audiologists who work in private practice or other clinical settings may also be dispensing audiologists. Fitting and selling hearing aids involves documentation related to these activities. ASHA scope of practice documents, guidelines, and state licensure laws have information pertinent to any requirements and necessary documentation.

SUMMARY

Learning to keep clear, concise, and complete documentation is one of the best habits a clinician can form. The benefits of appropriate documentation extend first and foremost to providing appropriate clinical care to the student/client/patient, then to the employer and payer for compliance, and finally to the provider to ensure development of a legal record and to meet mandates for reimbursement. Lack of adequate documentation can lead to numerous types of problems, with time and energy then needed to contest, follow up, and challenge issues related to the lack of documentation.

This chapter attempted to define issues related to documentation in all settings in which speech-language pathologists and audiologists work. While each setting has its own requirements and standards, there is no doubt that conducting high-level professional services includes both the delivery of competent services as well as the documentation of these services because "if it's not documented, it didn't happen."

CRITICAL THINKING

1. What skills do you think are important in writing good clinical evaluation reports versus other types of written documentation?
2. As a student, you are frequently required to write "lengthy" clinical evaluation reports, yet in the real clinical world, you will write much briefer ones. What is the rationale for learning to write long, comprehensive reports?
3. How do technology and the Internet affect documentation in our professions? What are the advantages and disadvantages of using technology for documentation?
4. Suppose you feel pressure from a parent to alter a report so that a child might access clinical services. What does our Code of Ethics say about fraudulent documentation? What would you do in this case?
5. What do you think when you read another clinician's reports that have obvious stylistic errors, numerous acronyms, and typographical errors? How should you ensure that you are using standard American English writing skills in your own documentation?
6. What federal laws guide our documentation in school and medical settings?
7. Ask to review a diagnostic report from your current clinic. What features do you like about the report? What could be improved? What would a professional from another discipline think about the report? Does it make a convincing case in a focused, clear, and succinct manner?
8. You work in the public schools, and a professor who teaches diagnostic methods has asked you to be on a panel and address her class about report writing in the educational setting. What would be five suggestions you would give students to help them write effective reports in the schools?
9. How do you think that electronic report writing will affect our report-writing skills in medical settings? What are the advantages and disadvantages of this style of report writing?

REFERENCES

American Speech-Language-Hearing Association. (2010). *Code of ethics*. Available from http://www.asha.org/policy

American Speech-Language-Hearing Association. (2011). *Speech-language pathology medical review guidelines*. Retrieved from http://www.asha.org/uploadedFiles/SLP-Medical-Review-Guidelines.pdf

American Speech-Language-Hearing Association. (n.d.-a). *Electronic medical records*. Retrieved from http://www.asha.org/slp/healthcare/EMR.htm

American Speech-Language-Hearing Association. (n.d.-b). *Medicare*. Retrieved from http://www.asha.org/public/coverage/medicare.htm

American Speech-Language-Hearing Association. (n.d.-c). *Medicare frequently asked questions: Audiology*. Retrieved from http://www.asha.org/Practice/reimbursement/medicare/audiology-medicare-FAQs/

American Speech-Language-Hearing Association. (n.d.-d). *FAQs on telepractice reimbursement and licensure*. Retrieved from http://www.asha.org/Practice/telepractice/TelepracticeFAQs/

American Speech-Language-Hearing Association. (n.d.-e). *Private health plans: An overview*. Retrieved from http://www.asha.org/practice/reimbursement/private-plans/overview/

American Speech-Language-Hearing Association. (n.d.-f). *Introduction to billing code systems.* Retrieved from http://www.asha.org/practice/reimbursement/coding/code_intro.htm

American Speech-Language-Hearing Association. (n.d.-g). *Speech-language pathology and the Physician Quality Reporting System.* Retrieved from http://www.asha.org/Members/research/NOMS/PQRI/

Americans with Disabilities Act (ADA), 42 U.S.C. §§ 12101 *et seq.* (1990).

Association of California School Administrators. (2006). *Handbook of goals and objectives related to state of California content standards.* Sacramento, CA: Author.

Brannen, S. J., Cooper, E. B., Dellegrotto, J. T., Disney, S. T., Eger, D. L, Ehren, B. J., et al. (2000). *Developing educationally relevant IEPs: A technical assistance document for speech-language pathologists.* Rockville, MD: American Speech-Language-Hearing Association.

Centers for Medicare & Medicaid Services. (n.d.-a). *Medicare billing for speech-language pathologists in private practice.* Retrieved from https://www.cms.gov/MLNProducts/downloads/SpeechLangPathfctsht.pdf

Centers for Medicare & Medicaid Services. (n.d.-b). *Audiology services.* Retrieved from https://www.cms.gov/Medicare/Medicare-Fee-for-Service-Payment/PhysicianFeeSched/Audiology.html

Code of Federal Regulations, Title 34, 504.3. Section 504 of the Rehabilitation Act of 1973.

Code of Federal Regulations, Title 34, 300.320. Individuals with Disabilities Education Improvement Act of 2004.

Coleman, J., Majerus, N. J., Meska, S., & Goulding, B. (2008). *Special challenges of documenting SLP services in the LTC setting.* Retrieved from http://www.asha.org/Events/convention/handouts/2008/2228_Goulding_Bill.htm

Elementary and Secondary Education Act (ESEA), 20 U.S.C. §§ 2701 *et seq.* (1965).

Family Educational Rights and Privacy Act (FERPA), 20 U.S.C. §§ 1232g (1974).

Hapner, E. R. (2008, March). Documentation that works [Abstract]. *Perspectives on Voice and Voice Disorders*, 33–42. Retrieved from http://div3perspectives.asha.org/cgi/content/abstract/18/1/33

Health Insurance Portability and Accountability Act (HIPAA), 45 CFR Parts 160, 162, and 164 (2002).

Hegde, M. N., & Davis, D. (2005). *Clinical methods and practicum in speech-language pathology* (4th ed.). Clifton Park, NY: Delmar Cengage Learning.

Individuals with Disabilities Education Improvement Act of 2004 (IDEA), 20 U.S.C. §§ 1400 *et seq.* (2004).

Justice, L. M. (2006). *Communication sciences and disorders: An introduction.* Upper Saddle River, NJ: Pearson.

Medicare Improvements for Patients and Providers Act of 2008, Pub. L. No. 110-275. Retrieved from http://www.gpo.gov/fdsys/pkg/PLAW-110publ275/pdf/PLAW-110publ275.pdf

Montgomery, J. K., & Moore-Brown, B. J. (2005). *START-IN: A response to intervention (RtI) program for reading.* Greenville, SC: Super Duper Publications.

Moore, B. J. (2010a). *Documentation for SLPs and audiologists in schools* [Audio program]. Rockville, MD: American Speech-Language-Hearing Association.

Moore, B. J. (2010b, October). If it's not documented, it didn't happen. *Perspectives on Administration and Supervision, 20*, 106–110.

Moore, B. J., & Montgomery, J. K. (2008). *Making a difference for America's children: Speech-language pathologists in public schools* (2nd ed.). Austin, TX: PRO-ED.

National Governors Association Center for Best Practices, Council of Chief State School Officers. (2010). *Common core state standards.* Washington, DC: Author. Retrieved from http://www.corestandards.org

No Child Left Behind Act of 2001, 20 U.S.C. §§ 6311 *et seq.* (2002).

Omnibus Reconciliation Act of 1990, Pub. L. No. 101-508. Retrieved from http://www.law.cornell.edu/usc-cgi/get_external.cgi?type=pubL&target=101-508

Paul, D., & Hasselkus, A. (2004). *Clinical record keeping in speech-language pathology for health care and third-party payers*. Retrieved from http://dev2010.asha.org/uploadedFiles/slp/healthcare/CRKSpeechED.pdf

Rehabilitation Act of 1973, Section 504, 29 U.S.C. §§ 794 (1973).

Rudebusch, J. (2008). *The source for RTI*. East Moline, IL: LinguiSystems.

San Diego City Schools. (2004–2005). *Articulation differences and disorders manual*. Retrieved from http://www.csha.org/pdf/CSHAArticulationManual.pdf

Shorter, T. N. (2004). *Understanding HIPAA: A guide to school district privacy obligations*. Horsham, PA: LRP Publications.

Sutherland Cornett, B. (2006, September 5). Clinical documentation in speech-language pathology: Essential information for successful practice. *The ASHA Leader*.

Swigert, N. (2003). Dollars and documentation. *Perspectives on swallowing and swallowing disorders (dysphagia), 12*(2), 32.

U.S. Department of Education. (2011, February). *The Family Educational Rights and Privacy Act: Guidance for eligible students*. Retrieved from http://ed.gov/policy/gen/guid/fpco/ferpa/for-eligible-students.pdf

Wallach, G. P. (2008). *Language intervention for school-age students: Setting goals for academic success*. St. Louis, MO: Mosby Elsevier.

RESOURCES

American Psychological Association. (2010). *Publication manual* (6th ed.). Washington, DC: Author.

American Speech-Language-Hearing Association. (2011). *Coding for reimbursement frequently asked questions: Speech-language pathology*. Retrieved from http://www.asha.org/practice/reimbursement/coding/coding_faqs_slp.htm

Association of California School Administrators http://www.acsa.org/

Goldfarb, R., & Serpanos, Y. (2011). *Professional writing in speech-language pathology and audiology*. San Diego, CA: Plural Publishing.

Hacker, D. (2000). *Rules for writers*. Boston, MA: Bedford/St. Martin's.

Lamar University. *Professional writing*. Retrieved from http://dept.lamar.edu/cofac/deptspeech/files/professional_writing.pdf

NHIC Corp. (2010). *Physical, occupational & speech therapy billing guide*. Retrieved from http://www.medicarenhic.com/providers/pubs/Physical%20and%20Occupational%20therapy%20Guide.pdf

Purdue Online Writing Lab (OWL) http://owl.english.purdue.edu/

Shipley, K., & McAfee, J. (2008.) *Assessment in speech-language pathology* (4th ed.). Clifton Park, NY: Delmar Cengage Learning.

Stein-Rubin, C., & Fabus, R. (2012). *A guide to clinical assessment and professional report writing in speech-language pathology*. Clifton Park, NY: Delmar Cengage Learning.

21

Successful Leadership: Influencing Others to Follow Your Lead

Ann W. Kummer, PhD

SCOPE OF CHAPTER

In the professions of audiology and speech-language pathology, many of us consider ourselves as "clinicians" but not necessarily as "leaders." We evaluate and treat individuals for a variety of communication and swallowing disorders. We counsel families, and we work with physicians, teachers, and other professionals. Most of us are not in what would be classified as a "leadership position." Regardless, leadership skills are important for clinicians and all professionals in the workplace, as well as for those of us who are in management or administration positions.

This chapter discusses the types of leadership roles that all professionals play, regardless of their position in the organization. The common characteristics of effective leaders are described. The chapter outlines the various sources of power and the most effective ways to influence others to follow your lead. Finally, the need for effective communication skills in all leadership roles is emphasized, with a discussion of methods to improve these skills in leadership situations. You will find that there are numerous exciting and realistic ways you can demonstrate leadership both within your professional employment and within the larger profession.

LEADERSHIP AND THE ROLES OF A LEADER

Leadership is the process of influencing or directing others to follow (Yukl, 1981). A leader, therefore, is a person who influences others to act in a certain way in order to achieve certain goals.

Whether they entail leading a large organization or leading a family to follow a treatment plan, leadership roles can be divided into three basic categories—the visionary role, the motivational role (Golper & Brown, 2004), and the coaching and/or mentoring role. The combination of these roles requires the leader to engage in high levels of both task-oriented (visionary) activities and relationship-centered (motivational) activities. These activities all have the primary purpose of accomplishing certain goals through the entire team (leader and followers).

Visionary Role

The visionary role encompasses the way in which leaders define, strategize, and plan to set a path for others to follow. An effective visionary leader attends to four aspects of this role: mission, vision, values, and strategy.

Mission In the visionary role, the leader must first define the mission of the organization (or group, committee, or team) and be sure that this is clear to all within the organization. The *mission* is the organization's primary purpose or function. Even when chairing a small committee, the leader should make the mission of the committee clear so that the members know what is expected and what is outside the realm of responsibility for the committee. A clear mission statement helps to determine the activities of the members of the organization and direct them toward a common focus. Examples of mission statements include the following:

- Hospital X provides a high standard of patient care, research, and education to improve the health care of infants, children, and adolescents in the community, the nation, and the world.
- The dysphagia team improves the quality of life for patients with feeding and swallowing disorders by providing quality care and education to their families.
- The mission of Special Interest Group X is to promote the development of knowledge and skills among affiliates through research and the exchange of information in our specialty area.
- Therapy is done with patient G.K. for the correction of all misarticulated phonemes.

Vision Once the mission is clear, the leader must develop a vision. A *vision* is the long-term goal that reflects what the organization would like to be in the future. Using information at hand, leaders must be able to plan prospectively, process many different kinds of information, and use their perceptions as a basis for judging environmental forces. The vision should always be developed with input from a variety of stakeholders (i.e., patients and families, senior management, referring physicians, third-party payers, staff, and so on). It should be developed with both an analytical and objective perspective, as well as an emotional and subjective view. Examples of vision statements include the following:

- To be a leading resource for the community of scientists and clinicians specializing in XYZ disorders
- To be the leader in improving the outcomes for at-risk infants

Once the vision is developed with input, the leader must be able to bind people together around a common sense of identity and purpose for a shared vision (Senge, 2006).

Values The next aspect of the visionary role is defining values. *Values* involve the principles that are important as a group attempts to carry out the mission and achieve the vision. Values provide the followers with a guideline of acceptable and expected performance and behavior (Dye, 2000). Values also let the followers know what is not acceptable. Knowingly or not, leaders always set the tone for standards of behavior in the group. If the leader allows goals to be accomplished through inappropriate behavior, the followers will either do the same, or leave. So that everyone knows the "rules of the game," it is important for the leader to determine the values of the organization or group. The following are examples of typical value statements:

- We will treat patients and families as partners and members of the health care team.
- We recognize the value and worth of all individuals—regardless of racial, cultural, or personal differences.
- We will provide service to our customers with respect for their time.
- We will treat our coworkers with respect and dignity.
- We will work cooperatively with all team members and acknowledge their contributions to the goals of the team.

Strategic Plan The last aspect of the visionary role involves developing a strategic plan. The *strategic plan* is a detailed document that serves as a guide or road map for achieving the goals of the vision. It usually has specific steps with time lines for accomplishment. Just like the vision, the strategic plan must take into account the interest of all stakeholders. When developing a strategic plan, the leader must also consider what resources will be needed (money, people, time, materials, equipment, space, training, and technology) to accomplish the goals. Once completed, the strategic plan should serve to focus and guide the activities of the organization toward accomplishment of the predefined goals.

A visionary role can be created for an entire organization, a department, a program, or even for clinical activities. Table 21–1 provides an example of how the visionary role can be applied to the role of a clinician.

To implement the strategic plan and work toward the vision, the leader is dependent on other people. A leader may have a great strategy, but all will fail unless he or she has the power to influence others to follow the plan. Therefore, once the visionary tasks have been completed, the leader takes on the motivational role.

Motivational Role

In the motivational role, the leader must be able to clearly communicate the plan and demonstrate the need to implement the plan. After the followers are convinced of the need to implement the plan, the leader must then continuously encourage and energize them to accomplish the predetermined goals. To do that, the leader must be involved in constant communication, training, mentoring, and coaching. Once followers have the knowledge and skills to do the job, it is important to motivate and empower them to do the job independently. Great leaders are able to delegate and empower the followers to take responsibility, be creative, and be successful. In fact, John Quincy Adams said: "If your actions inspire others to dream more, learn more, do more and become more, you are a leader."

TABLE 21–1 Leadership as Applied in the Role of a Clinician

- **Mission:** To work with patients with feeding and swallowing disorders
- **Vision:** To be able to significantly improve or correct the disorder treated and make a positive impact on the life of every patient
- **Values:** To conduct therapy with honesty and integrity; to give the best effort possible for each session; to include the family in the therapeutic process; to respect the wishes and goals of the patient and family; and to treat patients and families with respect and dignity
- **Strategy:** To learn as much as possible about each patient; to develop comprehensive, individualized treatment plans; to seek advice and feedback from others as needed; to coordinate treatment with other caregivers; to train the family to understand the problem and how to work with the patient at home; to provide a home program of therapy and update after each treatment session; and to attend at least one continuing education course on dysphagia each year

When considering what motivates employees, most people think of salary and benefits as the primary motivators. Although these may be the main considerations when a person considers taking a job, they become less important as motivators once the person is in the job, as long as the employee perceives the compensation to be fair. To keep employees in the position and make sure they are productive in working toward the goals and vision of the organization, the employees need different types of motivators. In this regard, the leader's emotional intelligence is important in enhancing the interactions with the employees and in creating a positive and supportive work environment to keep employees motivated and happy.

It can actually be said that in the motivational role, the primary job of the leader is to *make each employee (or team member) happy.* For example, if employees are happy, they will willingly be influenced by the leader to work hard to achieve the goals of the organization. Employees will also be loyal and less likely to leave for another job. To make employees happy, the leader must first ensure that the employees have the necessary support and resources to do the job well. Second, the leader needs to determine what the employees need to receive (in addition to remuneration) in exchange for good work. In many cases, employees just need to feel appreciated by their supervisor. Positive feedback (i.e., I'm proud of you. You did a great job! You are important to this organization and to me!) goes a very long way in making employees happy in their job.

When the leader works to provide the employees all that is needed to do a good job and be happy, including appreciation, positive feedback, and recognition, the leader is practicing a type of "servant leadership" (Frick, Spears, & Senge, 2004; Greenleaf, Spears, & Vaill, 1998; Greenleaf, Beazley, Beggs, & Spears, 2003). Leaders who serve their employees in this way will have much more influence over those employees and will be "paid back" with hard work and loyalty in the future.

Coaching and/or Mentoring Role

An effective leader must often take on the role of a coach or mentor. Although these two roles are similar, there are some subtle differences that have an impact on the outcomes achieved (McLeod, 2003; Whitmore, 2009).

A *coach* is someone who supports, encourages, and provides constant feedback to an individual or group in order to achieve specific goals or improve performance on specific tasks. A coach does not necessarily need to be a specialist or expert in a particular area. Instead, the coach's job is to enable individuals to find answers within themselves as a result of trial and error, feedback, and encouragement. Coaching is an important leadership role because the leader is always dependent on others to accomplish specific tasks.

A *mentor* is someone who is usually older, wiser, and more experienced than those who are being mentored. The mentor's job is to impart knowledge and to help those being mentored to develop specific skills and expertise. Mentoring is an important role for an effective leader because the more knowledge and skill that the followers or employees have, the better they will be able to support the goals of the leader and mission of the organization.

In audiology and speech-language pathology, we are trained to help others to change behaviors. Clients should not be the only beneficiaries of these coaching and mentoring skills; rather, they should be incorporated in other leadership activities with employees, committee members, coworkers, and graduate students.

Certainly, the leader of an organization should foster a culture of continuous learning through coaching and mentoring at all levels. This will help to increase the success of individual employees and the organization as a whole. Truly effective leaders take pride in the successes and accomplishments of those under their leadership. In addition, when continuous learning is part of the culture, outcomes continue to improve and job satisfaction remains high.

Leader Role versus Manager Role: What Is the Difference?

In general, a leader is a person who develops a plan or course of action, while a manager is responsible for seeing that the plan is implemented (Zaleznik, 2004). In this regard, the leader must *communicate* the plan to the manager and *influence* the manager to follow directions related to the plan. In an organization, therefore, a manager typically oversees and controls the day-to-day operations and resources to implement the mission and vision set by the leader (Mintzberg, 1998). In contrast to a leader, a manager usually has a particular position of authority that does not change with the situation.

The roles that the leader and manager play in an organization are very different, although they are

TABLE 21–2 Differences between the Roles of a Leader and Manager

Leader	Manager
Originates ideas	Follows directions
Asks what and why	Asks how and when
Has global perspective	Has a day-to-day perspective
Looks toward the future	Focuses on the present
Watches the horizon	Watches the bottom line
Develops	Implements
Makes the rules	Plays the game
Promotes change	Maintains a steady course
Plans	Does
Takes initiative and risks	Follows a predetermined course
Deals with people	Deals with things
Looks at the forest	Looks at the trees

From *Business Matters: A Guide for Speech-Language Pathologists,* by L. A. C. Golper and J. Brown, 2004, Rockville, MD: American Speech-Language-Hearing Association. Reprinted with permission.

not mutually exclusive, and they can overlap (Kotter, 1998). Table 21–2 shows the contrasting roles of the leader and manager. Since the roles are different, the skills that are required to fulfill these roles are also different. As a result, some individuals are better suited for one role versus the other.

It has been said that most companies are overmanaged and underled. If true, these organizations will remain static and have difficulty dealing with a culture of rapid change. For an organization to be truly successful, it is important to have both effective leaders and effective managers. Having a balance between the two is particularly important for service and health care organizations that have to compete in an increasingly complex and ever-changing environment.

Leadership Roles Are Situational

We usually think of leaders as those who are at the top of an organizational chart or those who are in positions of power or authority. However, opportunities for leadership are not reserved for those who are in administrative positions only. Leadership is not job-specific; instead it is situation-specific. Therefore, anyone can be a leader in certain situations.

We all serve as both leaders and followers, depending on the situation, the group, and the environment. For example, in one day an individual can be a department director (leader), a committee member (follower), a middle manager (leader and follower), a parent (leader), an advocate for legislative change (leader), a clinician (leader), a student supervisor (leader), and a member of a patient care team (leader and follower).

In the professions of speech-language pathology and audiology, many opportunities for leadership roles are available through the American Speech-Language-Hearing Association (ASHA), the American Academy of Audiology (AAA), local and state associations, and other professional organizations. Even in the purely clinical arena, each clinician serves as a leader every day. For example, the speech-language pathologist (SLP) is the leader of his or her client's treatment "team." In this role, the SLP sets the vision and mission for the treatment of the patient and influences the patient, family members, and other treating professionals to take certain actions to achieve the goals. The SLP has the ability to influence others through the demonstration of professional knowledge, expertise, and skill. This builds the trust and confidence in the SLP's ability, which is required for others on the treatment team to follow the SLP's direction. The SLP must have the ability to effectively communicate the plan with good interpersonal skills. Therefore, even when a clinician does not hold a formal position of authority, the person must have good leadership and communication skills to be effective in the workplace.

LEADERSHIP CHARACTERISTICS

Many authors list personality and behavioral characteristics that are typical of great leaders. Great leaders are not always the most visible or most vocal people. In fact, great leaders blend personal humility with strong ambition for the organization (Collins, 2001). These leaders take pride in the accomplishment of others (Clarke, 2005; Maxwell, 1999). They channel their ambition to work for the good of the organization or team, rather than for their personal gain or egos. In fact, when a leader focuses on recognition of others, the productivity of the group will often increase (Clarke, 2005).

Table 21–3 includes a compilation of common leadership characteristics. Covey (2000) surveyed 54,000 people about characteristics of effective leaders. In his survey, the most frequent characteristics named, in order of frequency, were integrity, communication, people(-oriented), visionary, and caring.

It should be noted that the characteristics in Table 21–3 have a common theme and, therefore, are categorized under three main headings: character, relationship orientation, and competence. It soon becomes apparent that the first two categories (character and relationship orientation) are related to the leader's personal power. The last category (competence) is what establishes the leader's expert power. To determine if you have these qualities, see the Assessment of Leadership Qualities in the appendix.

TABLE 21–3 Common Characteristics of Effective Leaders

Character: Demonstrates integrity, honesty and trustworthiness; admits mistakes and apologizes; has extreme humility and modesty; ambition is for the institution rather than just for self; tells the truth; has a personal and organizational code of ethics; is fair to all; doesn't use power for selfish purposes; is a role model of behavior; is genuine and candid; is inspiring; respects others; has self-awareness, self-regulation, and self-discipline; is diplomatic and tactful

Relationship orientation: Listens to others and communicates effectively; shows respect; takes time for people; has strong interpersonal skills; is concerned about the welfare of employees; recognizes others; appreciates the contributions of others; shows confidence in the ability of others; works cooperatively; gives frequent positive feedback; smiles and is courteous; shows compassion; is positive in dealings with others; is emotionally mature; is empathetic and supportive; is respectful, trustworthy, and fair-minded; doesn't take advantage of others; empowers others and delegates; supports and celebrates the successes of others

Competence: Shows the knowledge and skills to get the job done; is ambitious and achievement-oriented; is assertive and decisive; is a problem-solver; is a visionary and is forward-thinking; doesn't get discouraged about setbacks or failures; is tolerant of stress; has strong need to produce results; takes initiative and risks; focuses on results; benchmarks and networks with others; demonstrates a desire to make a difference; is committed; engages in continuous performance and quality improvement; is passionate about the mission and vision

Adapted from *Business Matters: A Guide for Speech-Language Pathologists,* by L. A. C. Golper and J. Brown, 2004, Rockville, MD: American Speech-Language-Hearing Association.

LEADERSHIP POWER

Effective leadership depends as much on the follower accepting direction as it does on the leader giving it. "Followers" include employees, committee members, students, patients, clients, and so on. Because the followers must consent to being influenced by the leader, the leader must obtain the trust and loyalty of the followers in order to influence them to follow a certain path. How the leader obtains this trust and loyalty often depends on the leader's relationship with others and ability to communicate effectively with the followers.

All leaders need *power* to achieve their goals through others (Maxwell, 2002). A leader's power is the ability to influence others to believe or act in a certain way. Although power often has a negative connotation, the use of the right type of power can be very positive and is necessary for effective leadership.

Many authors have described five basic sources of leadership power (Hellriegel, Slocum, & Woodman, 1983; Yukl, 1981):

1. Legitimate power
2. Reward power
3. Punishment power
4. Expert power
5. Personal power

Although they are sometimes labeled differently, the meanings behind the labels for these sources of power are the same.

Legitimate (or Position) Power

The most obvious source of power is called legitimate (or position) power. This is the power that is given to the boss, supervisor, or chairperson by virtue of a particular leadership *position*. The boss is the designated leader of a group and has legitimate authority to tell his or her staff what to do, when to do it, and how to do it. This source of power is solely based on the level of authority that is inherent in the position and is not based on any personal or professional attributes of this leader.

Reward Power

The second source of power is reward power. Reward power is the leader's ability to give the followers something of value in return for their work. If the leader is the boss, then the ability to offer salary, benefits, and promotion is the basis of this type of power. The reward or incentive does not need to be monetary, however. The leader may have the ability to reward with special privileges or assignments. Even the ability to publicly recognize and thank the follower gives the leader reward power.

Punishment (Coercive) Power

Punishment (coercive) power is the opposite of reward power. Punishment power is the ability to take something away from the follower as a result of noncompliance. The things that might be taken away are also things that serve as effective rewards for the employee (i.e., salary, benefits, promotion or job security, and so on). The employee may also be coerced to comply with the demands of the leader due to a fear of reprisal, lack of respect, or embarrassment if there is noncompliance with the leader's demands. Although this type of power is effective in the short term, it leads to employee dissatisfaction in the long run. Unhappy employees can result in poor performance and reduced productivity and ultimately lead to turnover, all of which are costly to the organization. Therefore, effective leaders use punishment power sparingly, if at all.

Expert Power

Expert power is unrelated to the leader's position or legitimate authority. Instead, leaders have expert power when employees or others recognize their special knowledge, skill, and expertise, particularly in difficult situations. An effective leader must have sufficient, maybe even extensive, knowledge in appropriate areas for expert power. With this source of power, employees or followers have confidence in the leader's ability to understand the issues and to lead them competently. In this case, the employees or followers respect the leader and feel they are in good hands. The greater the expertise, the more authority and power the leader will have.

Personal (or Referent) Power

Personal (or referent) power is a source of influence that depends on the leader's personality, likeability, and charisma. For this type of power, leaders' personal characteristics are more important than their position or level of authority. Personal power results in the type of influence that a best friend or admired colleague would have on an individual. To have personal power, the leader must be high in "emotional intelligence," which is the ability to manage relationships effectively and work well with others (Goleman, 1995, 2002, 2004; Heifetz, 2004). Leaders with personal power tend to have excellent communication skills, since effective communication enhances interpersonal relationships. Personal power is also gained when the leader shows a great deal of respect and encouragement for others and displays characteristics of honesty, integrity, and trustworthiness. As a result of these characteristics, followers develop a strong personal identification with the leader and want to please the leader with compliance.

Considering these five sources of power, which is most effective in influencing others? Although the first three sources of power are typically associated with being the "boss," most good leaders would agree that a more effective source of influence is expert power and the *most* effective source of influence is personal power (Hellriegel et al., 1983; Yukl, 1981). These sources of power are necessary for effective leadership, yet they are unrelated to the leader's formal position in an organization. Note that the three categories of common leadership characteristics just noted support the concept that personal power (through character and relationship orientation) and expert power (through competence) are very strong sources of influence. In contrast, a person with authority, but lacking expert or personal power, will have great difficulty influencing others in the long run, especially in situations where the followers do not see personal value in following the person's lead.

LEADERSHIP: A BALANCING ACT

In addition to understanding sources of power, the leader should understand the mutual dependency that is inherent in the leader-follower relationship. Both parties have need for something from the other. As such, there must be a balance in the relationship whereby the leader and follower both receive what they value in exchange for what they give. In the work setting, the boss or supervisor is dependent on the employee for a certain amount and type of work. The chairperson of a committee is dependent on the members to complete their tasks in order to accomplish committee goals. The followers (employees, committee members, and so on) expect certain rewards from the leader in exchange for their efforts. These rewards may be material (such as pay) or psychological (such as appreciation or recognition). The leader must continuously "serve" the followers and satisfy their needs in order to retain the position of leadership and power.

Successful organizations have one thing in common—they realize that employees are the organization's most valuable resource. Leaders who understand the importance of employee satisfaction through appropriate rewards are likely to find that the employees reciprocate with good job performance (quality and quantity) and with loyalty to the organization.

Within the concept of mutual dependency and the need for balance in the relationship, the roles of "boss" and employee should be reconsidered. Contrary to popular belief, the employee does not work "for" the boss. Instead, they both work for each other for the benefit of the organization. In fact, effective bosses or leaders will realize that their job is to make the employee happy because a happy employee is an effective employee. They can achieve this goal by acting as a "servant leader." If employees are happy with the rewards received in exchange for their work and the employees have all the necessary resources for the job, they are likely to provide quality services, be productive, and stay in the position. Since the costs of poor quality, low productivity, and turnover are significant, making the employee happy is an important responsibility for the boss.

DEVELOPMENT OF LEADERSHIP SKILLS: NATURE VERSUS NURTURE

Are good leaders born that way... or are they the result of their training and experience? The answer to this question is that it is probably a combination of both. Leadership skills can be learned and constantly improved, particularly in a model environment (Heller, 1999). Good role models and mentoring relationships are crucial in the development of leadership skills. In addition, an entrepreneurial culture can help the individual learn to take on the responsibilities that are typically given to leaders. In fact, the best way to develop leaders in an organization is to create challenging opportunities for young or inexperienced employees to "step up" and take responsibility and then to provide coaching and mentoring. Successful businesses are those that encourage and reward employees who help to develop leaders within their ranks.

Although many leadership skills can be learned and developed, some individuals have more "leadership potential" than others. This potential has a great deal to do with personality traits and communication abilities. In this way, nature has a role in the making of a good leader. Certainly, great leaders are not all alike and they accomplish their goals through many different methods and approaches. However, research shows that they do share certain personality and behavioral characteristics. In fact, it has been said that "leaders are effective because of who they are inside" (Maxwell, 2002).

LEADERSHIP THROUGH EFFECTIVE COMMUNICATION

Business communication refers to the method in which we exchange information in the workplace in order to convey a plan or direction and influence others to follow. When the people (leaders and staff) in an organization fail to communicate effectively with each other, the accomplishment of goals is very difficult and the organization is at risk.

Communication in the Profession of Communication Disorders

As audiologists and speech-language pathologists, we are very aware of the importance of communication skills in interpersonal relationships. We are experts in communication disorders, and we know what to do to remediate those disorders. However, we often forget that effective communication is more than just hearing clearly, understanding a message, and speaking intelligibly. Effective business communication requires a high level of listening skills and the ability to convey a message in a clear and positive manner.

In our own professional business, we need to be able to communicate effectively with our "customers," including patients or clients, families, physicians, teachers, colleagues, other health care providers, administrators, third-party payers, and so on. It is clear that without effective interpersonal communication skills, quality and productivity will suffer due to the lack of ability to influence, persuade, and negotiate—all necessities for workplace success.

Communication in Leadership Roles

Although most of us can hear and convey our ideas effectively, we are often ineffective when it comes to truly listening to others. The visionary role is dependent on the leader's ability to understand the environment and the needs of the organization in order to craft a plan. This means the leader must listen carefully to others to obtain the necessary information.

The leader's success in performing the motivational role depends on his or her ability to communicate the plan and to engage others to embrace the plan and follow direction. Effective communication is the crux of motivating employees, and employee motivation is critically important to the job's success. Employees are motivated when managers communicate clear expectations, instructions, and time frames. This fosters within the employees a sense of security, respect, power, and control in their jobs. On the other hand, employees are demotivated when they are unsure of the leader's direction, expectations, and priorities.

Furthermore, the leader must recognize the mutual dependency between a leader and followers and understand what motivates the followers. This is important so that there is a balance in the relationship between what is received by the leader and what is received by the followers. As part of this, leaders need to communicate constant encouragement and support, as well as acknowledgment and appreciation for achievement of outcomes.

Leaders need to effectively communicate for a variety of purposes. Some examples of these include the following:

Communication of Mission, Vision, Values, and Strategies

The leader must be able to grasp the "big picture" in order to determine the mission, vision, values, and strategies of the organization. The leader should be knowledgeable about inside and outside forces and activities that have the potential to affect the organization. In addition, the leader must consider and analyze the organization's strength, weaknesses, opportunities, and threats (SWOT) to determine the strategic plan. To accomplish these tasks, the leader must communicate with all stakeholders, including *external customers* (i.e., patients/clients, families, physicians, other professionals, and insurance companies) and *internal customers* (i.e., senior management and staff). The leader must be able to listen carefully to others, gather information, analyze the information, and then determine the plan with input and constant feedback from others. The leader then needs to be able to share the plan with the followers. Throughout all of these activities, the leader must be able to listen carefully and communicate effectively with others.

Communicating Expectations The leader cannot realistically expect followers to perform in a certain way if the followers do not know the expectations of performance. Few of us, if any, can read minds. Unclear expectations can not only result in failure but also cause the follower to feel very insecure and unhappy. The leader will encounter additional problems when it is time to provide feedback on behavior or performance, especially if there are issues with performance or accomplishment. Therefore, the leader must communicate clear expectations of performance. A discussion about expectations is important to be sure the follower has a clear understanding of what is expected and when. This discussion should take place verbally in person, and it should also be documented in writing for further reference.

Providing Constructive Feedback The term *constructive feedback* tends to have a negative connotation. In fact, constructive feedback can be both positive and negative. Positive feedback is news or input to an employee about a good effort or result. Employees or followers should be given generous positive feedback. In addition, they should be continuously encouraged and supported so they have confidence, a positive attitude, and the desire to do the job well.

Negative feedback is news to an employee about inadequate performance, areas of weakness, areas that need improvement, and opportunities for growth. Unfortunately, the word *negative* can stir up feelings of defensiveness and resistance. Therefore, this word should be avoided when talking to the employee. Instead, the focus of this type of feedback should be on change, improvement, and professional growth.

Whenever possible, constructive feedback should be information-specific, issue-focused, and based on observations rather than subjective impressions. Successful leaders develop a routine that includes frequent, in-depth discussions about performance with employees or followers. Bosses should let employees know that the purpose of the feedback is to help them be successful.

Giving honest feedback is very hard for most leaders. As a result, leaders sometimes soften the negative feedback to avoid confrontation or hard feelings. This may hurt employees in the long run, however, especially if they did not get a clear message of what to do differently. A strong leader is one who can give both positive and negative feedback. Open and honest feedback helps employees by giving them guidance as to how to perform, what is expected in the future, and how to be successful. Honest feedback of this type is also good for the ultimate goals of the organization because it helps the employee to contribute appropriately to team goals.

Asking the employee specific questions is a very useful tool in the feedback process. Such questions might include: What have you accomplished this year? What is the reason that this was successful? What were your challenges or disappointments? What could you have done differently or better in retrospect? What would you like to learn to do this year? How can I help? Asking questions is a great way to start a meaningful discussion and unveil unclear expectations that affect performance. It also helps employees to self-evaluate and it encourages them to take responsibility for learning and developing skills.

Giving Rewards and Recognition Effective leaders understand that recognition, praise, and thanks for doing a good job are highly motivating to employees. This may be especially true for those in professional positions, such as audiologists and speech-language pathologists. Recognition signifies that someone noticed the individual's hard work and appreciated it. At the same time, recognition communicates to others what the organization values and rewards.

Recognition is easy to give and inexpensive (usually free). Yet for some leaders, giving praise and recognition is difficult or simply forgotten. Given the studies that indicate the power of recognition in the workplace, it should be a priority for leaders in all positions of leadership! Recognition and praise become particularly important in situations where pay is restricted by regulations, policies, or the organization's budget.

Recognition does not need to be formal. Employees value personalized, spur-of-the-moment recognition for their contributions. They also appreciate public recognition (in a meeting, for example) that is timely and addresses the unique contributions of the individual. Note that frequent recognition of others enhances the leader's personal power.

Sharing Relevant Information The leader should keep employees informed of anything that has the potential to affect them, the work unit, or the organization. When the leader is not proactive in communicating with employees, the employees must rely on rumors and the "grapevine." This form of communication is inefficient and usually inaccurate. In addition, it is often very destructive in that it undermines the leader's effectiveness, and it can cause the leader to constantly correct misinformation and misperceptions (Bartolome, 1999).

Sharing information, whether it is good news or bad news, has a positive effect on the performance of others because it helps to foster a positive atmosphere where there is honesty and trust in the organization. Withholding information can have a negative effect because it can cause fear, insecurity, and distrust (Golper & Brown, 2004). Therefore, an effective leader is one who recognizes the importance of frequent communication with followers and communicates good and bad news openly and honestly. In some organizations, this open environment with honest communication of both the good and the bad is called *transparency*.

Managing Conflict Most leaders know that conflict over issues is natural and often necessary. Conflict helps individuals to consider different options and ultimately to make better choices. By avoiding conflict, some leaders do more harm to the organization. Ignoring conflict and ducking tough issues can ultimately lead to a culture that cannot tolerate honesty and straight talk (Argyris, 1999). Therefore, the leader must encourage team members to speak opening and honestly, argue (in a positive way), and challenge each other. The leader's job is to be sure that discussions and honest disagreements do not become personal.

When conflict does become personal, the leader must deal with it directly and swiftly to maintain a positive work environment. The leader should meet with those in conflict individually or in small groups to allow people the opportunity to vent anger. It is important, however, that everyone knows in advance why these meetings are being held and that they understand that personal attacks and blame are not appropriate in these meetings. The challenge for the leader is to listen carefully to all sides and then arbitrate a resolution. This situation can truly test the leader's communication and negotiation skills.

Developing Relationships, Trust, and Loyalty Establishing effective working relationships with others takes time and effort. However, the best leaders make certain that each person in the group feels connected and valued. (This promotes the balance in the relationship and gives the members their necessary rewards.) When leaders communicate individually with others, clarify expectations, coach and mentor, give employees the opportunity to do their best, recognize and praise them, and encourage individuals to develop their skills, this develops good working relationships and loyalty and builds the leader's personal power to keep the followers productive and task-oriented.

Engaging in Advocacy Advocacy involves taking responsibility to influence others to do certain things. It is a process of marshaling resources and information to bring about a change (Golper & Brown, 2004). Audiology and speech-language pathology offer many opportunities to be involved in advocacy efforts for our clients and the profession as a whole.

Advocacy requires that the leader is knowledgeable (and therefore has expert power) and has good communication skills in order to persuade others. In our professions, advocacy can include working with legislators on issues such as mandating that health care plans offer a benefit option for audiology and speech pathology coverage; repealing the therapy cap under Medicare; determining requirements for state licensure; requiring schools districts to hire only master's-level speech-language pathologists, and so on.

Although we typically think of advocacy as involving the legislative process, it is actually much more extensive and is something leaders must do frequently. For example, a department director may advocate for increased salaries, more space, or additional equipment based on a strong argument using relevant information. A committee leader may advocate for a change in a procedure based on the information that has been gathered and analyzed by the committee. A clinician may advocate for a change in the frequency of therapy based on information gathered regarding the patient's needs, previous response to therapy, and prognosis.

Advocacy involves influencing others. Therefore, the effectiveness of advocacy efforts clearly depends on the leader's power (expert power and even personal power) and the leader's communication skills to convince others of the need for the change.

Barriers to Effective Communication

Although there is little argument that leaders need to have effective communication skills, certain barriers often disrupt the communication process. One common barrier is when the leader does not clearly communicate directions and expectations to the followers. This happens when the leader mistakenly believes that more information is best and, as a result, gives too much extraneous information or writes directions in the style of a term paper. Instead, an effective leader communicates in a way that is clear, succinct, and to the point. This can be done best if the leader thinks of communicating (both verbally and in writing) using a bullet list format (Clarke, 2004).

The leader's inability to listen effectively may pose another communication barrier (Nichols & Stevens, 1999). Hearing is passive and takes no effort. Listening, on the other hand, is active. It requires that we focus on the speaker, maintain attention, and seek to understand. Since listening requires effort, it is no surprise that when we hear others speak, we typically remember only a small portion of what we have heard.

One problem is that people can listen and attend to other things at the same time. Because only a part of our mind is paying attention, it is easy for our minds to drift and think about other things while listening to the speaker. We can also be distracted by issues competing for our attention, like the conversation at the next table. In some cases, we are busy thinking about a response instead of listening to the other person. Our emotions and interpersonal relationship with the speaker also affect our ability to listen and understand. Finally, personal filters, assumptions, judgments, biases, culture, and beliefs can distort what we hear.

Because listening is so difficult and we listen with a personal bias, what we think we heard and understood can be very different from what the speaker actually intended to communicate. To counter these barriers, effective leaders participate in a process called "active listening."

Active Listening

Active listening is a structured form of listening and responding that focuses the attention on the speaker. The goal of active listening is to improve the mutual understanding of both parties through specific techniques. Some of the principles of active listening include the following:

Focus on the Speaker You already know your thoughts. Therefore, spend more time trying to understand the other person's thoughts. Listen about 80 percent of the time and talk about 20 percent of the time.

Empathize Try to "walk in the other person's shoes" and see the other person's perspective. Empathizing does not mean you need to agree with the speaker. It just means that you must ignore your own thoughts and perceptions for the moment and see the issue from the other person's perspective.

Acknowledge Show that you are listening and trying to understand through verbal and nonverbal confirmation. Use nonverbal communication and body position (e.g., leaning forward) to encourage the speaker and signal interest.

Don't Interrupt Let the speaker complete the point without interruption and without rushing him or her.

Ask Questions Ask sincere and relevant questions to clarify a statement or gather more information. A question that begins with "why" (i.e., "Why do you think that?") can put the person on the defensive. Therefore, this type of question should be avoided.

Paraphrase to Confirm Understanding Paraphrasing is a technique that good active listeners use frequently. It is a way to confirm understanding by restating the information that was received. The speaker confirms, clarifies, or explains further based on the listener's restatement. Some common ways to paraphrase or confirm understanding may start with the following: "What I hear you saying is ... Is that what you meant?" or "It seems that you are frustrated when ... Is that correct?"

Effective Methods of Communication In past generations, communication was accomplished by phone, mail, or in person. Also, workers in the majority of professions had predictable work hours, often 9 to 5. Those days have changed. Many people check e-mail messages (or voice mail) before leaving home in the morning and before going to bed at night. Late-night e-mails from workaholics, insomniacs, and all others are now common. Effective leaders are also effective communicators through e-mail. They respect the e-mail recipient's time by writing e-mails that are concise and have more bullet lists than paragraphs (Clarke, 2004).

Although e-mail communication is convenient, it does not replace the need for individual or group meetings. In fact, any communication that involves emotion, problem solving, or differences of opinion is best done with a traditional face-to-face meeting. Meetings are also important because they can make people feel part of the group. Participative meetings help people to feel that their opinion is heard and that it matters. It gives them an opportunity to ask questions and clarify misunderstandings. In addition, meetings allow individuals to communicate more effectively with tone, posture, eye contact, and body language. Thus, an effective leader must determine the most important mode of communication (fast versus personal) for each type of situation.

SUMMARY

There is general agreement that a leader must have power to be effective. Although this chapter discussed five sources of power, most authors agree that expert power and personal power are the most effective in influencing others to achieve maximum performance. These sources of power are important as the leader fulfills the major roles that were discussed in this chapter. For the visionary role, the leader needs knowledge and competence. Therefore, expert power is important. For the motivational role, the leader must interact with the followers. Therefore, personal power is needed.

Communication skills are also extremely important in these leadership roles. For the visionary role, the leader must be able to listen carefully to obtain information in order to develop the plan. For the motivational role, the leader must then communicate the plan clearly in order to influence others to act.

In summary, effective leaders require expertise, strong interpersonal skills, and excellent communication skills. Emotional intelligence contributes to personal power and, therefore, is a key factor in the ability to influence others. Personal power and influence are related to balance in a relationship. If employees feel that they are given positive feedback and are appreciated for their work, they are happier and work harder. If the followers like (personal power) and respect (expert power) the leader, they will *want* to follow the leader's direction. Therefore, although it's a cliché, when a leader needs to influence others to perform, "it pays to be nice!"

CRITICAL THINKING

1. Think of influential people and people of authority in your work setting and in your personal life. Consider each person's primary source of influence or power. Which of these people are most influential and why?
2. Consider your present clinical situation. What situations require leadership there? Who assumes that leadership? How effective are these individuals?
3. What are some ways that audiologists and speech-language pathologists can assume leadership roles in the profession at the national, state, local, and individual practitioner level?
4. What is meant by "servant leader"? Why is it important for the followers to be satisfied with the leadership in their workplaces?
5. Some people think that good leaders "have the biggest mouths." Assess this statement with regard to the relationship between leadership and communication skills.
6. Make up a "leadership evaluation tool" that includes criteria and a rating scale by which you could assess the leadership within your clinical situation. What criteria are most important? Use the tool to evaluate your leadership. What feedback would you give your leadership based on administration of this tool?
7. You have just begun your first professional position. One of your colleagues speaks to you in what you consider a condescending manner. This has happened a number of times, and you feel that the other professional's communication style is demeaning and discouraging for you. What would you do? Would you discuss this with your supervisor? What leadership would you expect from your supervisor to manage this situation?
8. What can undergraduate and graduate programs do to develop the communication and leadership skills among students in audiology and speech-language pathology?

REFERENCES

Argyris, C. (1999). Skilled incompetence. In *Harvard Business Review on effective communication* (pp. 101–118). Boston, MA: Harvard Business School Publishing.

Bartolome, F. (1999). Nobody trusts the boss completely—Now what? In *Harvard Business Review on effective communication* (pp. 79–100). Boston, MA: Harvard Business School Publishing.

Clarke, M. (2004). *Communication land mines: 18 communication catastrophes and how to avoid them.* Raleigh, NC: Martin Productions.

Clarke, M. (2005). *Leadership land mines: 8 management catastrophes and how to avoid them.* Raleigh, NC: Martin Productions.

Collins, J. (2001). *Good to great.* New York, NY: Harper Business.

Covey, S. (2000). Leadership is a choice. In *Lessons in leadership program guide* (4). Lexington, KY: Wyncom.

Dye, C. F. (2000). *Leadership in healthcare: Values at the top.* Chicago, IL: Health Administration Press.

Frick, D. A., Spears, L. C., & Senge, P. M. (2004). *Robert K. Greenleaf: A life of servant leadership.* San Francisco, CA: Berrett-Koehler Publishers.

Goleman, D. (1995). *Emotional intelligence.* New York, NY: Bantam Books.

Goleman, D. (2002). *Primal leadership: Realizing the power of emotional intelligence.* Boston, MA: Harvard Business School Publishing.

Goleman, D. (2004). What makes a leader? *Harvard Business Review, 82*(1), 82–91.

Golper, L., & Brown, J. (2004). *Business matters: A guide for speech-language pathologists.* Rockville, MD: American Speech-Language-Hearing Association.

Greenleaf, R. K., Beazley, H., Beggs, J., & Spears, L. C. (2003). *The servant-leader within: A transformative path.* Mahwah, NJ: Paulist Press.

Greenleaf, R. K., Spears, L. C., & Vaill, P. B. (1998). *The power of servant leadership.* San Francisco, CA: Berrett-Koehler Publishers.

Heifetz, R. A. (2004). Question authority. In S. Clarke (Ed.), Voices: Leading by feel. *Harvard Business Review, 82*(1), 27–37.

Heller, R. (1999). *Learning to lead.* New York, NY: DK Publishing.

Hellriegel, D., Slocum, J. W., Jr., & Woodman, R. W. (1983). *Organizational behavior* (3rd ed.). St. Paul, MN: West Publishing.

Kotter, J. P. (1998). What leaders really do. In *Harvard Business Review on leadership* (pp. 37–60). Boston, MA: Harvard Business School Publishing.

Maxwell, J. C. (1999). *The 21 indispensable qualities of a leader: Becoming the person others want to follow.* Nashville, TN: Maxwell Motivation.

Maxwell, J. C. (2002). *Leadership 101: What every leader needs to know.* Nashville, TN: Maxwell Motivation.

McLeod, A. (2003). *Performance coaching—The handbook for managers, H.R. professionals and coaches.* New York, NY: Crown House.

Mintzberg, H. (1998). The manager's job: Folklore and fact. In *Harvard Business Review on leadership* (pp.1–36). Boston, MA: Harvard Business School Publishing.

Nichols, R. G., & Stevens, L. A. (1999). Listening to people. In *Harvard Business Review on effective communication* (pp. 1–24). Boston, MA: Harvard Business School Publishing.

Senge, P. M. (2006). *The fifth discipline: The art & practice of the learning organization.* New York, NY: Doubleday.

Whitmore, J. (2009). *Coaching for performance: Growing people, performance and purpose* (3rd ed.). London, England: Nicholas Brealey Publishing.

Yukl, G. A. (1981). *Leadership in organizations.* Englewood Cliffs, NJ: Prentice Hall.

Zaleznik, A. (2004). Managers and leaders: Are they different? *Harvard Business Review, 82*(1), 74–81.

RESOURCES

Websites

American Academy of Audiology (AAA)
http://www.audiology.org

American Speech-Language-Hearing Association (ASHA) Member Center
http://www.asha.org/members

Harvard Business Review
http://hbr.org

Appendix 21-A

Assessment of Leadership Qualities

Instructions: Rate your leadership qualities the way you think others would rate you based on their perception. Then ask others to rate you anonymously and compare your perception with theirs. Any rating under 3 is an important area for development.

	1	2	3	4
Character				
Has integrity, honesty, trustworthiness, code of ethics				
Admits mistakes and apologizes; has humility and modesty				
Has ambition for organization, not just for self				
Doesn't use power for selfish purposes				
Is fair to all				
Is a role model of behavior; is inspiring to others				
Has self-awareness, self-regulation, and self-discipline				
Is diplomatic and tactful, respectful, genuine, caring				
Relationship Orientation				
Has strong interpersonal skills				
Is concerned about the welfare of employees				
Listens to others and communicates effectively				
Recognizes and appreciates the contributions of others				
Is empathetic, supportive, respectful, compassionate, and positive				
Gives frequent positive feedback; smiles and is courteous				
Doesn't take advantage of others				
Shows confidence in the ability of others; empowers others				
Supports and celebrates the successes of others				

	1	2	3	4
Competence and Drive				
Shows the knowledge and skills to get the job done				
Is achievement-oriented with a strong need to produce results				
Is assertive, decisive, committed, a problem-solver				
Takes initiative and risks				
Is a visionary and forward-thinker				
Doesn't get discouraged about failures or setbacks				
Is tolerant of stress				
Benchmarks and networks with others				
Engages in continuous performance and quality improvement				
Is passionate about the mission and vision of the organization				

Key:

1. Never
2. Sometimes
3. Usually
4. Always

22

Infection Prevention

Rosemary Lubinski, EdD

SCOPE OF CHAPTER

Little did you know upon entering the profession of audiology or speech-language pathology that, in addition to your professional knowledge base and clinical skills, you would need to know about such topics as communicable diseases and universal precautions. Whether you practice in a health care institution; educational setting; private practice; or community speech, language, or hearing clinic, it is essential to know procedures to protect yourself, your family, and your clients from the spread of infectious diseases. Although infectious diseases are not new or unique to the populations with which we work, changing demographics of our society, mainstreaming into educational settings, increased service to high-risk populations, and increases in certain communicable diseases are a few of the factors that prompt serious attention to risk management. Therefore, this chapter provides a rationale for protecting yourself and others, presents a basic discussion of infection pathways and types, and outlines ways of incorporating a hygiene plan into your clinical practice with all clients. Finally, we discuss some special situations related to the topic of infection prevention. This chapter encourages you to use a commonsense approach to creating a hygienic environment that minimizes the potential of infection transmission.

IMPORTANCE OF INFECTION PREVENTION TO SPEECH-LANGUAGE PATHOLOGISTS AND AUDIOLOGISTS

Although those of you who practice in health care facilities are likely to be aware of clean practices or risk management, this subject is often "ignored" by professionals working in other settings such as schools or private practice (McMillan & Willette, 1988). This is most unfortunate because clients with infectious diseases can range from toddlers in early intervention programs to elderly people seeking a hearing aid from a dispensing audiologist. The reasons for an increase in infections are complex but include changing and increased population growth, increased poverty, expansion of populations into remote areas, environmental degradation, improved transportation providing easier spread of disease, and inadequate public health infrastructure (Engender Health, 2005). Changing demographics of our client population suggest that you are likely to work with individuals who may be at high risk for contracting or transmitting an infection, including inpatients who are acutely ill and those with communicable diseases such as hepatitis B, HIV (the virus that causes acquired immune deficiency syndrome, or AIDS), tuberculosis, influenza, staphylococcus, and cytomegalovirus. All of these individuals are high-risk populations, usually because of their repressed immune systems, complicated medical conditions, and poverty.

In addition, speech-language pathologists have created new roles within shock trauma centers, high-risk neonatal programs, and AIDS programs and have become responsible for swallowing management programs in which the focus may be on working with critically ill patients. Audiologists, too, have created special hearing health programs for high-risk populations. For example, immitance procedures require the use of probe tips, vestibular testing may result in vomiting, cerumen management may result in blood transmission, and intraoperative monitoring for cochlear implants places the audiologist in operating rooms.

Federal legislation (i.e., PL 94-142, Section 504 of the Rehabilitation Act, and PL 99-457) and various state laws focus on the right of disabled individuals to a free appropriate public education in the least restrictive environment (American Speech-Language-Hearing Association, 1991). This means that children with compromised health resistance may be attending public schools and may be in need of communication services. Thus, speech-language pathologists and audiologists in educational settings need to be as vigilant as colleagues in health care institutions of risk-management procedures.

The increase in the prevalence of diseases also necessitates such awareness. Although AIDS may be the best-known infectious disease, in actuality, other diseases are more prevalent, such as herpes simplex and hepatitis B. Contact with individuals with certain infectious diseases such as cytomegalovirus may have health implications for professional women who work during pregnancy.

The nature of our hands-on contact with clients during speech mechanism examinations, respiratory and laryngeal assessments, inspections of the outer ear, hearing aid fittings, swallowing assessments and treatments, fittings of surgically implanted hearing devices, and care of clients with a laryngectomy or tracheotomy also increases the risk for infection transmission. Any procedure that brings you in direct contact with body fluids necessitates precautions.

Lest we forget, speech-language pathologists and audiologists themselves may be sources of infections that can be transmitted to clients. The state of low resistance to illness of many of our clients already mentioned makes them more susceptible to the infections we might transmit to them. For example, what may appear to be a "common cold" to you may result in bronchitis or pneumonia for frail elderly residents of a nursing facility. These illnesses, in turn, may result in increased nursing care, additional medications, relocation to an acute care hospital, prolonged illness, or death. You may also have a more serious communicable disease that requires the use of precautions to protect your clients.

McMillan and Willette (1988) remind us of the ethical responsibility we have to protect our patients from all health and safety dangers. The most basic ethical responsibility you have regarding spread of infection is to reduce the probability of its occurrence to its lowest possible level in your interactions with clients. When a patient suffers an infection, "progress is slowed, revenue may be decreased due to absence, and the risk of malpractice accusation may increase" (p. 37).

Nosocomial infections are infections inadvertently contracted in a health care facility. Health care workers today are highly aware of the fact that hospitals and other facilities are unhealthy environments, in that the risk for exposure to a staphylococcal virus or other infectious agents is much higher in a health care facility than it is at home. Nosocomial infections affect approximately 1 in 10 hospitalized patients, with an estimated annual cost of $6.7 billion per year in the United States (Graves, 2004). This is an increase of more than $2.2 billion from 1992 data provided by the Centers for Disease Control and Prevention (CDC) (1992). Direct cost increases are related to need for more care and extended stays. Dixon (1987) added that indirect costs such as loss of income are incalculable, though likely high. In addition, nosocomial infections add substantially to health care costs. Various hospital and rehabilitation program accrediting bodies, such as The Joint Commission, require that facilities have ongoing, comprehensive infection control procedures in place as part of their patient safety program to maintain their accreditation. Finally, in an era of cost containment, the importance of surveillance of nosocomial infections is critical in providing quality, cost-efficient care. The Centers for Disease Control (CDC) (1992) estimates that preventing just 6 percent of nosocomial infections would offset the cost of infection control programs in hospitals. Keep in mind, too, that nosocomial infections divert costly hospital resources, and infection prevention is expensive in itself (Graves, 2004).

According to the ASHA Code of Ethics, any certified professional must not discriminate in the delivery of professional services on the basis of disability. Thus, certified professionals are required to provide services to high-risk individuals, including those with HIV. ASHA's Legislative Council passed the following resolution in 1988 (ASHA, 1989):

> RESOLVED, That it is the position of the American-Speech-Language-Hearing Association that persons with HIV disease (including individuals with AIDS, ARC, and individuals who are seropositive) and those who are regarded by others as having the disease, should be entitled to civil rights protections under Section 504 of the Rehabilitation Act of 1973, as amended (LC-29-88).

INFECTION AND ITS PATHWAY

Infections are caused by microorganisms that are found on your skin, in the air and water, and/or in plants, animals, soil, and people. Some of these are *normal flora,* and others are *pathogens*. Both kinds can cause infections, particularly in people who are at high risk (Engender Health, 2005).

The transmission of an infection follows a predictable pathway. There must be a source of infection, a means of transmission, and a susceptible host. This is referred to as the *chain of infection* (Castle & Ajemian, 1987; Interorganizational Group for Speech-Language Pathology and Audiology, 2010). The source of infection may be a person, for example, the client or clinician, or it can be an inanimate object such as equipment that has been contaminated by an infected person. Thus, clinicians and clients may infect each other, or one client can infect a second client through indirect contamination of inanimate objects such as toys, a microphone, or a speculum (McMillan & Willette, 1988). Clients can also infect themselves (autoinfection). Remember that you can infect others while being unaware that you are infected. This is called being an asymptomatic carrier.

An infection can be transmitted in many ways, including (1) touching another person, particularly with your hands during assessment, intervention, or daily care; (2) touching one infected client and then using the same hand to touch the oral area of yourself or another client; (3) touching an inanimate object that has been contaminated; (4) coughing or sneezing (airborne transmission); (5) ingestion of contaminated food or water; and (6) contact or a bite from an animal or insect such as mosquitoes or fleas.

The final link in the chain of infection is the availability of a susceptible host. It is known that individuals become more vulnerable to contracting an infection when they have reduced immunological defense systems because of their illness(es) and/or malnourishment. Therapies received, such as radiation therapy and insertion of medical equipment (e.g., catheters or intravenous tubes), may also increase their susceptibility. Infants, the elderly, and those with chronic debilitating diseases are more susceptible to infection by the very nature of their frailty.

EXAMPLES OF COMMUNICABLE DISEASES

Examples of infections are so numerous that a complete discussion of all agents is beyond the scope of this chapter. Here, we consider eight common chronic communicable diseases: staphylococcal infections, hepatitis B, HIV/AIDS, cytomegalovirus, herpes, tuberculosis, scabies, and influenza.

Staphylococcal Infections

Staphylococcal infections, often called "staph," comprise a group of infections that are common in hospitals and other medical settings. Staph infections range from simple and localized skin infections, such as pimples and boils, to serious wounds, urinary and bloodstream infections, and pneumonia. Newborns, nursing mothers, and patients who have compromised immune systems are at high risk for contracting staph infections (Merck, 2005). Staph infections that become resistant to antibiotics are called *methicillin-resistant staphylococcus aureus* (MRSA). While MRSA is more common in hospitals, 12 percent of the cases involve people in community settings (CDC, 2005b).

Hepatitis B Virus (HBV)

According to statistics compiled for 2003, hepatitis B virus (HBV) is a common, potentially life-threatening infection. It affects about 73,000 people in the United States per year (CDC, 2005e). About 5,000 people die from the disease each year (CDC, 2005e). Further, the prevalence of hepatitis B is estimated to be at least 1 million people in the United States, with costs estimated to be at least $700 million per year. HBV incubation is 120 days on average, and the onset of acute disease is insidious. HBV is transmitted via blood, during sexual activity, and perinatally (CDC, 1999a, 1999b, 1999c). Symptoms include loss of appetite or anorexia, malaise, nausea, vomiting, abdominal pain, itching all over the body, joint pain, dark urine, pale-colored stools, and jaundice (EmedicineHealth, 2012). Such symptoms, which occur in about 70 percent of patients with HBV, usually occur 9 to 12 weeks after exposure to the hepatitis B virus (CDC, 2005d, 2005e). Individuals at high risk for harboring or contracting hepatitis B include sexually active individuals, intravenous drug users, patients of hemodialysis units, hemophiliacs, residents of some institutions for the developmentally disabled and prisons, infants born to infected mothers, and immigrants from areas of high endemicity, including east Asia, Africa, most Pacific Islands, parts of the Middle East, and the Amazon basin Centers for Disease Control and Prevention, 1999c). Health care workers who come in contact with blood or patient secretions containing blood are potentially among the high-risk groups for contracting HBV. It should be remembered that the risk of contracting hepatitis B is much greater than that for HIV. A preventive vaccine is available for HBV; its immunological effect remains intact for about 15 years (CDC, 2005d, 2005e).

HIV/AIDS

Human immunodeficiency virus (HIV) is generally well known by the public. Acquired immune deficiency syndrome (AIDS) is the fifth leading cause of death in the United States among people ages 25 to 44 (National Center for Health Statistics, 1999). HIV precedes AIDS, and the disease may be nonsymptomatic for 10 years before AIDS diagnosis. HIV is found in blood, semen, saliva, tears, nervous system tissue, breast milk, and female genital tract secretions, though not all have been found to transmit infection to others. HIV attacks the immune system and increases susceptibility to life-threatening illnesses.

The CDC (2011) estimates that in 2006 nearly 1.2 million people were living with HIV in the United States. About one-quarter of those were unaware of their infection. The majority of these are individuals between 25 and 44 years of age, and the states with the highest cumulative number of cases include New York, California, Florida, and Texas. The most common causes of transmission are male-to-male sexual contact and injection drug use (CDC, 2005a). In 2008, there were about 489,696 people living with AIDS in the United States, three-quarters of whom were men (Kaiser Family Foundation, 2010). To date, there is no cure for AIDS, although there is active research to develop drug treatments and prevention vaccines.

The many symptoms of HIV/AIDS are listed in Table 22–1. Of particular interest to speech-language pathologists and audiologists are changes in speech and language, impaired cognitive functioning, and hearing loss. Communication difficulties include voice disorders related to Kaposi's sarcoma in the larynx, motor speech disorders, language disorders, and general withdrawal from socialization. In addition, if the patient is intubated, an assistive communication device may be necessary (Flower & Sooy, 1987). Conductive and sensorineural hearing impairments are also common and may necessitate the use of a hearing aid or other assistive listening device (Flower, 1991). For a more in-depth discussion of HIV/AIDS and communication disorders, see Flower (1991) and Swanepoel and Louw (2010).

TABLE 22–1 Symptoms of HIV/AIDS

Common Symptoms	Additional Symptoms
Prolonged, unexplained fatigue	Speech and language difficulties
Prolonged fever	Hearing loss
Chills	Cognitive/memory impairment
Swollen glands/lymph nodes	Visual impairments
Joint swelling and bone pain	Generalized itching
Mouth lesions	Chest pain
Sore throat	Muscle pain
Shortness of breath	Genital sores
Constipation and/or diarrhea	Numbness and tingling
Tumor (Kaposi sarcoma)	Cold intolerance
Skin rashes	
Seizures	
Weight loss	
Malaise	
Headache	

Cytomegalovirus (CMV)

Cytomegalovirus is a common infection affecting between 50 and 85 percent of adults in the United States by age 40 (New York State Department of Health, 2011) but is most widespread in less developed areas of the world. At high risk are unborn babies of mothers infected with CMV during pregnancy, those who work with children, and those with compromised immune systems such as transplant recipients and those with HIV (ASHA, 1991; CDC, 2002). CMV is a member of the herpes virus group (cold sores, chickenpox, shingles, and mononucleosis) and the Epstein-Barr virus, which causes infectious mononucleosis (CDC, 2002; Crawford & Studebaker, 1990). Transmission is primarily through contact with body fluids such as urine, genital secretions, and eye and nose secretions. CMV is the primary cause of congenital viral infection in the United States and creates a variety of problems with hearing, vision, mental abilities, and motor coordination (CDC, 2002). Once an individual is infected, the virus remains alive but dormant for life, and recurrence is rare unless the individual's immune system is compromised. There is no current cure for CMV.

Cytomegalovirus is of concern for women of childbearing age if they contract the disease during pregnancy (ASHA, 1991). The affected individual may appear asymptomatic or have a protracted mononucleosis-like illness. Any employed woman who is pregnant and who works with young children should be educated concerning CMV and its transmission. Women of childbearing age may wish to be tested to determine susceptibility to CMV infection. In general, frequent hand washing and appropriate disposal of diapers help to minimize the spread of infection.

Herpes Simplex Virus (HSV)

Herpes simplex virus (HSV) may take two forms: Type 1 and Type 2. Type 1 (herpes labialis) usually manifests itself by infections of the lips, mouth, and face. Frequent signs include cold sores or fever blisters in the orofacial region. Most people have been infected with Type 1 virus by the age of 20. Type 1 is precipitated by overexposure to sunlight, fever, stress, and certain foods and drugs (University of Maryland Medical Center, 2011). It may also cause infections in the cornea. Type 2 is usually associated with genital infection. Both forms of the infection may be recurrent. The virus is contagious during the blister and wet ulcer stages and can be transmitted through saliva, urine, genital secretions, or contact with broken skin or mucous membranes. Individuals with herpes labialis should refrain from working with infants, burn patients, or immunocompromised patients (Valenti, 1992). Type 2 genital herpes can be spread during vaginal delivery or sexual activity. Infected individuals should seek medical help if herpes symptoms do not resolve within a week or if there are frequent recurrences.

Tuberculosis (TB)

Tuberculosis (TB) is a contagious bacterial infection primarily of the lungs and is caused by mycobacterium tuberculosis (CDC, 2005f). In the mid-1980s, a resurgence of TB became evident in the United States after 30 years of decline. The resurgence is attributed to the increase in antibiotic-resistant strains of the disease, the HIV epidemic, an increase in the number of homeless individuals, an increase in immigration from Asian countries, physician nonadherence in prescribing the recommended drug regimen, and few resources for prevention and care. Although TB can affect anyone of any age, it is seen more often in older people who have been exposed to tuberculosis and immunocompromised individuals. Fortunately, in the United States, the estimated rate of TB cases has seen a steady drop from the late 1990s and to the early years of the twenty-first century (National Center for Health Statistics, 2004).

Populations most at risk for contracting tuberculosis are those living with the consequences of poverty, such as poor nutrition, poor ventilation, crowding, and poor hygiene. Other individuals with weakened immune systems and who are at high risk include substance abusers; those with diabetes, silicosis, cancer of the head or neck, or leukemia; and those on specialized treatments for rheumatoid arthritis or Crohn's disease (CDC, 2005f). Of particular concern is that the tuberculosis rate of nursing facility patients is four times higher than that of age-matched community residents (Boscia, 1986).

According to the CDC (2005f), TB bacteria can attack any part of the body, including the kidney, spine, brain, and lungs. People in the latent stage of the disease do not usually become sick. In the active stage, however, TB is spread via airborne droplets from sneezes or coughs. Once in the lungs, the bacteria travel to other parts of the body. The primary symptoms of pulmonary tuberculosis are coughing, which spreads the mycobacterium tuberculosis through the air; fatigue; night sweats; chills; coughing up blood; low-grade fever; and weight loss (CDC, 2005f). If you work in a hospital or nursing home, an annual tuberculosis screening may be mandatory. This may include one or more of the following tests: chest X-ray, sputum cultures, blood tests, and the tuberculin skin test (Mantoux tuberculin skin test) (CDC, 2012). Individuals with latent TB infection will have a positive skin test but a normal chest X-ray and sputum test. Those with active TB can spread the disease to others; they will have a positive skin test and an abnormal chest X-ray or positive sputum test (CDC, 2005f). Treatment for the infection includes a program of medications. Compliance with the medication program is essential because noncompliance leading to treatment failure may result in drug resistance, relapse, increasing disability, and death (Hellman & Gram, 1993). Symptoms often improve within two to three weeks, although the prescribed medication program must be followed for a lengthy period of time.

Scabies

Scabies is an infectious skin rash caused by infestation with the mite *Sarcoptes scabiei*. Transmission is through prolonged skin-to-skin contact with an infected individual and may be spread by sharing clothing, towels, and bedding. A quick handshake is unlikely to spread the infestation. Scabies spreads quickly in crowded settings such as hospitals, nursing homes, and child care centers. Again, those with compromised immune systems and the elderly are at risk. Symptoms include pimplelike irritations; burrows or rash on the skin, especially between the fingers and in skin folds throughout the body; intense itching, especially at night; and sores caused by scratching (CDC, 2005c). It may take four to six weeks for symptoms to appear for those who have never been infected and only a few days for those with previous infestation. Control measures include mass cleaning of patient bedding, clothing, and food trays and skin application of a pesticide, usually lindane, for all employees or others who have come in contact with the infected individual (Sherertz & Hampton, 1987). Universal precautions include adequate hand washing, gloving, and gowning, which are essential when working with an infected client (Polder, Tablan, & Williams, 1992).

Influenza Viruses

Influenza, or the "flu," is a highly contagious infection of the respiratory tract. It usually occurs from late fall to early spring. Flu affects all age groups, and its severity can range from mild to severe illness. Each year 20,000 Americans, most of them elderly, die from influenza or secondary complications. Symptoms include some combination of fever, chills, muscle aches and pain, sweating, dry cough, nasal congestion, runny nose, diarrhea, sore throat, headache, malaise, and fatigue (CDC, 2004). Flu spreads in the respiratory droplets of an infected individual who may or may not show active flu symptoms. It is especially important to prevent transmission of type A and type B influenza viruses to high-risk groups such as the elderly and patients of all ages with chronic cardiac, pulmonary, renal, or metabolic diseases. Outbreaks of influenza in acute care and chronic care hospitals as well as nursing homes can have serious health care and morbidity implications. Prevention includes yearly vaccine immunization and measures to limit the spread of the disease, including universal precautions such as frequent hand washing, covering your mouth and nose with a tissue when you cough or sneeze, appropriate disposal of tissues, restrictive admission to a facility, separation of infected patients, and prohibition of individuals with respiratory symptoms from visiting high-risk patients (CDC, 2004; Fedson, 1987). If you contract influenza, it is critical that you check with your employer's infection control personnel for guidelines regarding client contact. Some physicians may prescribe antiviral medications, and all will recommend rest and plenty of liquids.

PROGRAM FOR INFECTION PREVENTION

All settings in which you practice as a speech-language pathologist or audiologist should have an infection prevention program in place. The general purpose of such programs is to minimize the potential of infection transmission to clients and staff members and hopefully stop the cycle of transmission. Although plans differ according to settings, certain commonalities exist across infection prevention programs. Staff need to (1) be aware of potential risks associated with their settings and professional procedures; (2) know their institutional and departmental infection prevention management plans for minimizing infection spread; (3) know how to implement the infection prevention management plan; (4) know how to modify the plan to meet individual situations; and (5) know when and to whom to report incidents. Common barriers to implementing prevention programs include staff underestimating the risks involved; lack of knowledge of appropriate infection prevention practices and their role in implementing this program; and inadequate supplies, equipment, and space in low-resource settings (Engender Health, 2005).

If you work in a health care institution such as a hospital or nursing home, there will be a multidisciplinary Infection Control Committee (ICC) responsible for reducing the occurrence of infections through the establishment and monitoring of general policies and procedures for infection control. These rules usually emanate from standards established by federal and state governments and agencies, professional organizations, and accreditation agencies such as The Joint Commission. The ICC is charged with approving programs of prevention and investigating, reporting, and monitoring infections (Castle & Ajemian, 1987). Each facility will have a plan that details the exposure classification of each employee, a record of employee vaccinations, a plan for infection control training, universal precautions implementation plans, and postexposure plans and records (Interorganizational Group for Speech-Language Pathology and Audiology, 2010).

In addition to complying with general infection prevention procedures established for the entire institution, individual departments such as speech-language pathology or audiology will be required to state in writing specific policies and procedures for ensuring infection prevention during their contact with clients. See Chapter 19, Policies and Procedures.

Settings other than hospitals should also have infection prevention programs. For example, home health care programs; educational settings; private practices; and community speech, language, or hearing clinics should each have and implement a systematic written program for ensuring to the highest extent possible the prevention of infection transmission between staff and clients or among clients. Committees similar to the ICC implement and monitor the infection prevention program and provide orientation and continuing education on this topic for all staff.

Pre-employment Screening and Follow-Up

A pre-employment medical evaluation is one of the requirements of employment in most organizations and certainly in all health care institutions. The purpose of this examination is to identify individuals who may serve as sources of an infectious agent and, therefore, compromise clients, staff, or families with whom they would come in contact. The most important aspects of the screening focus on identification of rubella, hepatitis B, and tuberculosis (Castle & Ajemian, 1987). The pre-employment evaluation usually includes a communicable disease history, a history of immunization, and a physical examination. Most organizations also have established policies for immunizations, yearly medical reevaluations, protocols for documentation of employees exposed to communicable diseases, and guidelines for a return to work for these individuals. Information regarding such protocols can be found in your employee handbook or your department's policy and procedure manual or can be obtained from your institution's infection prevention committee.

Prior to employment and periodically thereafter, you will likely need to show evidence of a negative response to the Mantoux skin test for tuberculosis. You may know this test by the acronym PPD (purified protein derivative) for the type of tuberculin used in the test. Two to three days after the injection, your arm will be examined and the reaction area measured. In some health care settings, you may be required to take the two-step Mantoux test, which involves testing of the opposite arm one to three weeks later. In both cases, if there is a positive response, you must check with your primary care physician for a chest X-ray. Some health care agencies may also require vaccinations for hepatitis B, influenza, measles, mumps and rubella, tetanus, diphtheria, pertussis, meningitis, and varicella. Keep a record of all vaccinations and reports and provide one for your employer.

Orientation and Training in Infection Prevention

One of the first tasks you will be required to complete upon employment in most institutions is to participate in a general orientation. Part of this orientation will be devoted to understanding infection prevention needs and protocols along with other protocols aimed at ensuring a healthy and safe work environment. During this orientation, you will become familiar with the management or hygiene plan designed for your department, its rationale, and specific ways to implement the plan into daily practice. In-service education programs to update an existing hygiene plan will also occur as needs arise.

Hygiene Plan

The hygiene plan designed for your department will focus on creating an environment with every reasonable effort made to limit exposure to infectious agents. Potential infectious agents include all body fluids: blood, semen, drainage from scrapes and cuts, feces, urine, vomitus, respiratory secretions, and saliva, along with anything that has come in contact with body fluids (e.g., bandages, prostheses, and instruments). In general, hygiene plans will have as their cornerstone the adoption of *universal precautions.* The underlying premise of universal precautions is that one adopts practices that minimize and, if possible, eliminate the risk of transmitting any infection, whether potential or actual. Thus, every clinician, including trainees, assistants, and volunteers, working with every client in every setting must assume a preventive approach to reducing infection transmission. A universal approach to clients ensures that all are treated equally, without discrimination, and with confidentiality regarding their medical status.

Hygiene Plan Techniques

The hygiene plan techniques presented here focus on what you can do to help prevent the transmission of an infectious disease. The first technique discussed, hand washing, is considered the most basic approach to infection prevention. The other basic techniques focus on respiratory etiquette. Both of these should be considered routine client care. Other techniques include barrier techniques such as the use of gloves, masks, gowns, and lab coats. Finally, sterilization and disinfection are discussed as additional priority methods.

Hand Washing There is no substitute for hand washing in the prevention of infection transmission. Although this is a simple and cost-effective means of preventing

TABLE 22–2 Guidelines on When to Wash Hands

- Upon arrival at work
- Immediately, if they are potentially contaminated with blood or body fluids
- Between patients
- After removing gloves
- Before and after handling inpatient care devices
- Before preparing or serving food
- Before and after performing any personal body function
- When hands are obviously soiled, such as after sneezing, blowing one's nose, or using the bathroom
- After changing diapers
- Before leaving your work setting
- For isolation patients, before removing gown and mask and after removing gown and mask

Source: American Speech-Language-Hearing Association. (1989). AIDS/HIV: Report: Implications for speech-language pathologists and audiologists. *ASHA*, 29, 33–37. Reprinted with permission.

the spread of infectious agents to noncontaminated areas and personnel, it is estimated that health care workers wash their hands only about half the time they should (Engender Health, 2005). The goal of hand washing is to reduce as much as possible the presence of contaminating organisms on hands that touch clients or objects in the environment that might be contaminated. Simply, you should wash your hands thoroughly with plain or antiseptic soap and running water before and after contact with each client, even when gloves are worn. The use of liquid soaps is preferred over bar soap. A general minimum guideline for hand washing is 10 seconds, or the amount of time it takes to sing one stanza of "Happy Birthday." Wearing gloves does not negate the need for hand washing. Table 22–2 lists guidelines for when to wash hands, and Table 22–3 lists the recommended steps in washing hands. If water conservation is an issue in your geographical area, adaptations in the continuous flow of water will be needed. If you do not have access to a water source, you can use disposable antiseptic wipes or alcohol-based hand rubs or gels. Any wipes should be disposed of properly. Be sure to use an emollient lotion after the use of alcohol-based rubs to balance their drying effect.

The two most common hand-drying techniques recommended are the use of disposable paper towels and hand dryers. Towels should be disposed of properly and not reused.

Respiratory Etiquette Another important risk-reduction technique clinicians should use is respiratory etiquette. This involves procedures that contain respiratory secretions from people with signs or symptoms of respiratory infection (Interorganizational Group for Speech-Language Pathology and Audiology, 2010). Practitioners should have signs in appropriate languages at the entrance to their clinical environments about the need to alert clinicians to any possible respiratory infections. Keep in mind that influenza and other serious respiratory illnesses are spread by coughing, sneezing, and unclean hands. Specific strategies to reduce the spread of germs include (1) covering your mouth and nose with a tissue when you cough or sneeze, (2) disposing of the tissue in an appropriate receptacle immediately, (3) coughing or sneezing into your upper sleeve or elbow but not your hands if a tissue is unavailable, (4) washing your hands or using an alcohol-based hand rub if you have contact with respiratory secretions, and (5) if necessary, wearing a face mask to protect others. The CDC provides printable fliers and posters titled "Cover Your Cough." These are available in a variety of languages and can be

TABLE 22–3 Hand-Washing Steps

- Remove all jewelry, except for plain wedding bands.
- Obtain paper towel from dispenser.
- Slightly lean forward over sink and avoid touching sink.
- Turn on water to comfortably warm level.
- Wet hands and forearms.
- Apply liquid hospital-grade antiseptic soap.
- Vigorously wash hands, wrists, and forearms, weaving fingers and thumbs together for 30 to 60 seconds.
- Thoroughly rinse forearms, wrists, and hands.
- Dry hands, then wrist and forearm using a paper towel.
- Avoid rubbing hands too hard to prevent chapping.
- Use clean paper towel to turn off the faucet and turn the doorknobs if foot or electronic controls are not available.
- Dispose of all paper towels in an appropriate container.
- Use emollient to decrease the risk of skin cracking.

Information compiled from Kemp, R., & Bankaitis, A. (2000). *Infection control in audiology.* Retrieved from http://www.audiologyonline.com/articles/article_detail.asp?article_id=214 and *Infection Control: A Policy and Procedure Manual* by M. Palmer, 1984, Philadelphia: W.B. Saunders.

found at the CDC's website, provided in the Resources section of this chapter.

Personal Protective Equipment Gloves, masks, face shields, goggles, gowns, hats or bonnets, and lab coats, otherwise known as *personal protective equipment (PPE),* are used to prevent the possibility of transmitting airborne or spattered infectious agents such as droplets of blood or other body fluids onto your skin or clothes. Most of these PPEs are disposable, used only once, and thrown away according to agency and manufacturer directions.

Gloves provide a barrier, though not an impermeable one, to microorganisms that may be transmitted between client and clinician. Wearing gloves becomes particularly important during an oral-facial examination, during middle ear testing, when handling or fabricating ear molds and other prostheses, during swallowing assessments and therapies, and during assessments of respiratory and laryngeal functioning. Gloves should be worn during each of these tasks. Speech-language pathologists and audiologists are most likely to use single-use (disposable), nonsterile gloves. Palmer (1984) suggests that the method for putting on disposable, nonsterile gloves should be as consistent as the methods for sterile gloves. If nonsterile gloves are used, hands should be washed before and after gloving. All gloves should be changed before each new client contact. Finally, gloves should be discarded in a properly marked container after each use or when torn during contact with a client.

Palmer (1984) recommends an acceptable method for putting on nonsterile gloves when no gown is used. Remember not to touch any surface with a contaminated glove that you will later touch without gloves, such as doorknobs, telephones, and pens. Failure to take this precaution may result in harmful exposure of disease to you and your coworkers and clients. Palmer (1984) provides the following guidelines for gloving:

- Wash and dry hands first.
- Grasp the inside of the right glove with left hand.
- Insert the right hand into glove and pull glove on.

- Place the left hand into the left glove and pull glove on.
- Remove gloves by pulling the contaminated outer side in onto itself.
- Discard gloves in appropriate place.
- Wash and dry hands after gloves are removed.

Remember that masks should be worn only once, donned prior to gown or gloves, and discarded when they become moist. Palmer (1984) suggests the strings must be tied securely for a snug fit. "If you wear glasses, the mask should fit snugly over your nose and under the edge of your glasses to prevent fogging" (p. 57). Your hands should be washed before and after removing the mask. Isolation gowns must be worn when working with an infected patient or when a patient is in protective isolation. In donning a gown, touch only the inside of the gown. Shoe covers also may be required in isolation areas. All of these protective clothing items should be disposed of in proper containers. Finally, if washable lab coats are used, they should be changed daily or as needed throughout a day, if contaminated. Otherwise, you should use disposable gowns and, after use, dispose of them properly. The Occupational Safety and Health Administration (OSHA) (1992) mandates that any clothing worn as personal protective equipment should be laundered, maintained, or disposed of by the employer and not sent home with the employee for cleaning.

Decontamination: Cleaning, Disinfection, and Sterilization
There are three levels of decontamination in infection control. The lowest level of decontamination includes alcohol wipes, mild detergent soap, or agents such as hydrogen peroxide. This type of decontamination is not sufficient for cleaning instruments or contaminated services in a clinical setting (Golper, 1998). Contaminated surfaces need at least moderate decontamination, requiring disinfecting agents. Disinfection and sterilization typically begin with cleaning the surface to remove any obvious foreign material from objects through washing. This step normally precedes both disinfection and sterilization (Rutala, 1987).

Sterilization is considered to be the highest level of decontamination. Sterilization entails a complete destruction of microorganisms and their spores through physical or chemical processes (Rutala, 1987). Sterilization is necessary for any surgical instrument or device or any object that will be used from one patient to another and potentially carries body fluids. Sterilization can be accomplished by use of a steam autoclave, dry heat oven, chemical vapor sterilization, or immersion in a chemical agent (such as Cidex) for 10 hours. Items such as impedance probe tips, otoscopic specula, and other heat-sensitive instruments must be cleansed of debris prior to being sterilized in a chemical agent. Be sure to check the manufacturer's instructions regarding proper sterilization procedures for all equipment prior to sterilization.

Disinfection is a lower level of decontamination than sterilization but will sufficiently destroy most organisms on clinical surfaces. Disinfection involves cleaning objects and the surfaces of materials and furniture touched by a client and staff. Materials include all therapy materials, toys, games, and other items used in assessment or therapy. All surfaces of tabletops, chairs, and chair arms should be disinfected after each use. All equipment or materials used during an evaluation that are not inserted in the oral cavity should be disinfected after each use. Metal surfaces should be cleaned by using a registered germicide, and nonmetal surfaces can be disinfected with a solution of household bleach at a 1:10 dilution with water. The items should be sprayed, vigorously washed, lightly misted again, and left moist (McMillan & Willette, 1988). Any used paper towels should be disposed in proper containers. The use of any cleaning, or disinfection agents, or sterilization of materials or equipment should adhere to the manufacturers' instructions. Additionally, you should note that cleaning agents or other chemical products can pose a hazard to employee health through skin or aerosol exposure; thus, organizations are required to tell all employees what chemicals are present in their environment. Your facility will have a Material Safety Data Sheet (MSDS) notebook containing a chemical fact sheet on all chemicals in your work area (everything from correction fluid to disinfecting agents), and you will be asked to verify that you have reviewed the MSDS notebook in your area and are aware of the appropriate steps to take if you have a reaction to these agents.

Toys Toys are such a common part of our interaction with pediatric clients that special mention should be made about their place in infection prevention. Whenever possible, use toys that have washable surfaces, especially when working with children in diapers. If possible, each group of children should have its own toys. Avoid furry or fabric dolls and stuffed animals. All toys, game boards and pieces, materials, and furniture should be washed and disinfected after each assessment or therapy session. Toys that have been mouthed by a child should be isolated immediately from other children and then properly washed and disinfected before continued use with other children. In general, it is best not to include toys in waiting room areas as daily disinfection is impractical.

Regulated Waste Containers Your setting will have specific guidelines for what is considered "regulated waste" in that agency. OSHA (1992) defines regulated waste as liquid or semiliquid blood or other potentially infectious material (OPIM), items contaminated with blood or OPIM, contaminated sharp objects (sharps), and pathological and microbiological wastes containing blood or OPIM. Individual containers for such regulated waste must be closable, suitable to contain the type of materials enclosed to prevent leakage, and labeled with the biohazard symbol or color coded (usually red) to warn employees of the potential hazards within. Local and state laws govern where and how regulated wastes will be disposed. Check with your department's policy and procedure manual section on infection prevention as to appropriate disposal methods for items you use.

Separation of People with Infectious Diseases Speech-language pathologists may need to provide clinical services to patients who are in isolation in a hospital, home, or other health care facility. Isolation is defined as the separation of individuals who have a specific infectious illness from those who are healthy (CDC, 2004). This is done to stop the spread of the illness. Examples of infectious diseases that may require isolation include tuberculosis and severe acute respiratory syndrome. If it is known that a person has been exposed to an infectious agent but is not symptomatic, this individual may be placed in quarantine to prevent possible spread. Clinicians working with individuals in isolation or quarantine should follow all hand-washing, personal protective equipment, and equipment disinfectant procedures mandated by your hospital or health care agency.

ISSUES OF SPECIAL CONCERN

You should be aware of four special issues regarding infection control. First, a medical history of your patients may be helpful in reducing potential exposure. Second, the settings in which we work pose particular infection prevention challenges. The third issue addresses the special needs of female speech-language pathologists or audiologists who work during childbearing years. These professionals should be aware of the relationship of infection prevention and pregnancy. The final issue to be addressed is how to report a possible infection exposure incident.

Medical Case History

Clinicians should take or review a patient's medical history when possible. While this appears an obvious step in preparing to work with a client, review of the medical history has direct implications for infection prevention. For example, a patient who takes an anticoagulant may be at greater risk for bleeding. Another patient who had a bone marrow transplant may be in an immunocompromised state. Medical history review will help clinicians determine a risk assessment that involves identifying hazards and those at risk, evaluating risks, taking preventive actions, and monitoring outcomes (Interorganizational Group for Speech-Language Pathology and Audiology, 2010). Other factors that might be reviewed include recent history of infectious diseases, travel history, history of drug abuse or sexually transmitted diseases, and congregate living.

Educational Settings

A practical issue that arises in an educational setting such as a public school is how to apply universal precautions. Keep in mind that there are more students attending schools with compromised health than ever before. Hand washing between your sessions with students may not be easily available or possible because of the location of a therapy room or inability to leave a child or children unsupervised in a room while you go to another room for washing. When possible, the speech-language pathologist or audiologist in this setting should seek a room with or very near hand-washing facilities. A possible alternative to hand washing is to cleanse hands with disposable antiseptic wipes or no-rinse hand sanitizers (for example, Purell). Hand washing with soap and water should be done as soon as possible thereafter. Professionals in education settings should be acutely aware of the need to disinfect tables, chairs, and clinical materials between use and appropriate disposal of gloves, tongue blades, or any other potentially infected clinical materials. It is also important that any cleaning materials be kept out of the reach of children at all times.

Long-Term Care Facilities

Although less attention has been paid to nosocomial infections in long-term care facilities (LTCF) compared with acute care hospitals, the population of 1.6 million residents in this setting is considered a high-risk group. The increased risk for nosocomial infections among this population is related to living in close quarters, participation in numerous group activities, malnutrition and dehydration, underlying systemic diseases, use of indwelling devices such as catheters, immobility, fecal incontinence, impaired cognitive skills, decreased ability to maintain personal hygiene, and frequent use of multiple medications, including sedatives and tranquilizers (Garibaldi & Nurse, 1992). Ambulatory residents who may be incontinent or coughing also serve as a possible means for spreading infections. Risk also increases because of decreased staffing and staff who may be unaware of infection prevention procedures. The prevalence of infections acquired in nursing homes varies from a low of 6.7 percent (Eikelenboom-Boskammp, Cox-Claessens, Boom-Poels, Drabbe, Koopmans, & Voss, 2011) to a reported high of 16.2 percent (Garibaldi, Brodine, & Matsumiya, 1981). This variation may be due to difficulty in diagnosing infections within the elderly population. The most common types of infections found in this population include respiratory, urinary tract, skin and soft tissue, and gastrointestinal infections (Mathei, Niclaes, Suetens, Jans, & Buntinx, 2007). It should be noted that the mortality rate for pneumonia among LTCF residents is significantly higher than that of community-based elders.

The high prevalence of nosocomial infections among LTCF residents may be due to the low turnover rate of residents, the high ratio of patients to staff, lack of compensation to staff for sick leave, inadequate immunization requirements, and frequent turnover of nonprofessional employees. Infections that occur at epidemic rates in LTCFs include respiratory tract infections, gastroenteritis, and urinary tract infections (Garibaldi & Nurse, 1992; Infections in Long-Term Care, 1999). Thus, if you work in this setting, consider the higher possibility of transmitting an infection to or contracting one from the population of the institution.

Day Care Centers

Children attending day care centers or nursery programs are at increased risk for contracting and transmitting a variety of diseases (Sherertz & Hampton, 1987). The reasons why infections may spread so easily in this setting are similar to those discussed for nursing home settings. Professionals who work in these settings or whose own children attend them should be aware of the increased potential for contracting and transmitting infections. Toys belonging to the day care center or to children themselves should be disinfected on a daily basis. Of particular concern in day care centers is the issue of proper diapering techniques. The Fountain Valley School District, Fountain Valley, California, provides the following guidelines for diapering and suggests that similar guidelines be used with children who use potty chairs. Be sure to wear gloves during this procedure and dispose of them and the diaper in accordance with your setting's guidelines.

- The professional puts on disposable gloves.
- The child lies on a disposable towel.
- The soiled diaper touches only your hands.
- The diaper is disposed of in a plastic bag to be taken home or to an appropriate receptacle.
- There is proper cleansing of the child's bottom.
- There is proper disposal of the washcloth or towelette.
- The child's hands are washed.
- The diapering area and equipment are cleaned and disinfected.
- The caregiver's gloves are disposed of properly.
- The caregiver's hands are washed thoroughly.

A second concern in day care centers is how to identify a child who is too ill to remain at the center or in need of immediate medical attention. An in-depth discussion of this topic is beyond the scope of this chapter. The reader is referred to an excellent resource, *What You Can Do to Stop Disease in the Child Day Care Centers* (CDC, 1984).

Staff Who Are Pregnant

Staff members who are pregnant may be concerned about contracting an infection that may affect their unborn child. Infections that have the greatest potential for affecting a fetus include those due to rubella, enterovirus, hepatitis B, syphilis, toxoplasma, cytomegalovirus, and varicella. Women who are pregnant should discuss their potential risk for contracting infections in their workplace with their personal physician and the infection prevention personnel in their facilities.

Reporting Exposure Incidents

According to OSHA (1992), you should immediately report any situation in which you have been exposed to a potentially infectious agent. Early reporting will help you receive the medical care you may need, help prevent the spread of the infection to others, and assist your employer in assessing the situation surrounding the exposure incident in an effort to prevent further occurrences. Your employer must provide you with a free medical evaluation and treatment if the exposure occurred during your employment. Again, if you are exposed to a potentially infectious agent, check with your departmental policy and procedure manual for specific guidelines for how, when, and to whom to report the incident.

SUMMARY

An important aspect of risk management in any work setting is to prevent the transmission of infectious disease. It is your responsibility to understand the risks involved and know and implement universal precautions. The source of an infection can be people, objects, or surfaces (toys, doorknobs, keyboards, phones). Infections are spread through direct contact with the body fluids of another person, through cross-contamination involving the clinician as the means of transmission, from one client to another, through airborne transmission of agents, or through indirect contact with contaminated surfaces of objects. The best precaution to prevent infection transmission is to adhere to universal precautions with all clients, regardless of known or unknown pathology. Universal precautions include routine, vigorous hand washing before and after client contact; appropriate use and disposal of gloves, masks, and gowns; application of barrier techniques; and proper disinfection/sterilization of clinical tools and materials. The Codes of Ethics of both ASHA and the American Academy of Audiology require their members to provide appropriate services to individuals with known infectious disease and to use universal and reasonable precautions in working with all clients. Confidentiality regarding protected health information must always be maintained. Remember that infection prevention is a necessary component of quality service delivery.

CRITICAL THINKING

1. Consider your current employment or training setting. What routine precautions do you take to prevent the transmission of infections? How did you learn about these precautions?
2. Why is hand washing one of the best ways to prevent transmission of infections? Practice proper hand-washing techniques.
3. Suppose you worked with a colleague who had a severe cold and cold sores around the lip area. You notice that the coworker does not observe any special precautions to prevent the transmission of her infections to pediatric clients. What would you do?
4. You work in a hospital at which you frequently get referrals to assess patients with AIDS. What ethical and legal issues should you consider in working with these patients?
5. What are some populations and settings that are high risk for infection transmission? Why is the risk higher with these populations?
6. Suppose one of your clients who has a cold coughs and sneezes repeatedly during a session in your presence. What should you do?
7. What infection precautions should you take if you work in early intervention and provide services in children's homes? How would you explain the rationale for your procedures to the family?

REFERENCES

American Speech-Language-Hearing Association. (1989). AIDS/HIV: Report: Implications for speech-language pathologists and audiologists. *ASHA, 29,* 33–37.

American Speech-Language-Hearing Association. (1991). Chronic communicable diseases and risk management in the schools. *Language, Speech, and Hearing Services in Schools, 22,* 345–352.

Boscia, J. (1986). Epidemiology of bacteriuria in an elderly ambulatory population. *American Journal of Medicine, 80,* 208–212.

Castle, M., & Ajemian, E. (1987). *Hospital infection control: Principles and practice.* New York, NY: John Wiley and Sons.

Centers for Disease Control and Prevention. (1984). *What you can do to stop disease in child day care centers.* Washington, DC: Author.

Centers for Disease Control and Prevention. (1992). Public health focus: Surveillance, prevention and control of nosocomial infections. *Morbidity and Mortality Weekly Report, 41,* 783–787.

Centers for Disease Control and Prevention. (1999a). *AIDS/HIV.* Available from http://www.cdc.gov/nchs/fastats/aids-hiv.htm/

Centers for Disease Control and Prevention. (1999b). *HIV/AIDS surveillance report 1999, 11*(1), 1–44.

Centers for Disease Control and Prevention. (1999c). *Viral hepatitis B—fact sheet.* Available from http://www.cdc.gov/ncidod/diseases/hepatitis/b/fact/htm

Centers for Disease Control and Prevention. (2002). *Cytomegalovirus (CMV) infection.* Available from http://www.cdc.gov/cmv/

Centers for Disease Control and Prevention. (2004). *Key facts about the flu: How to prevent the flu and what to do if you get sick.* Washington, DC: Department of Health and Human Services.

Centers for Disease Control and Prevention. (2005a). *Basic statistics: HIV/AIDS.* Retrieved from http://www.cdc.gov/hiv/stats.htm

Centers for Disease Control and Prevention. (2005b). *CA-MRSA Information for the public.* Retrieved from http://clearviewregional.edu/docs/hs/nurse/CA-MRSA%20Public%20FAQs%20%20CDC%20Infection%20Control%20in%20Healthcare.htm

Centers for Disease Control and Prevention. (2005c). *Parasites-Scabies.* Retrieved from http://www.cdc.gov/parasites/scabies/

Centers for Disease Control and Prevention. (2005d). *Hepatitis B fact sheet.* Available from http://www.cdc.gov/hepatitis

Centers for Disease Control and Prevention. (2005e). *Hepatitis B frequently asked questions.* Available from http://www.cdc.gov/ncidod/diseases/hepatitis.b/faqb.htm

Centers for Disease Control and Prevention. (2005f). *Questions and answers about TB 2005.* Available from http://www.cdc.gov/nchstp/tb/faqs/qa_introduction.htm

Centers for Disease Control and Prevention. (2011). *Basic statistics.* Retrieved from http://www.cdc.gov/hiv/topics/surveillance/basic.htm#hivest

Centers for Disease Control and Prevention. (2012). *Tuberculosis.* Retrieved from http://www.cdc.gov/tb/topic/testing/default.htm

Crawford, M., & Studebaker, G. (1990). Cytomegalovirus: A disease of hearing. *The Hearing Journal, 43,* 25–30.

Dixon, R. (1987). Costs of nosocomial infections and benefits of infection control programs. In R. Wenzel (Ed.), *Prevention and control of nosocomial infections* (pp. 19–25). Baltimore, MD: Williams & Wilkins.

Eikelenboom-Boskamp, A., Cox-Claessens, J., Boom-Poels, P., Drabbe, M., Koopmans, R., & Voss, A. (2011). Three-year prevalence of healthcare-associated infections in Dutch nursing homes. *Journal Hospital Infections, 78,* 59-82.

EmedicineHealth. (2012). *Hepatitis B.* Retrieved from http://www.emedicinehealth.com/hepatitis_b/article_em.htm

Engender Health. (2005). *Infection prevention.* Retrieved from http://www.engenderhealth.info/pubs/quality/infection-prevention.php

Fedson, D. (1987). Immunizations for health care workers and patients in hospitals. In R. Wenzel (Ed.), *Prevention and control of nosocomial infections* (pp. 116–174). Baltimore, MD: Williams & Wilkins.

Flower, W. (1991). Communication problems in patients with AIDS. In J. Mukand (Ed.), *Rehabilitation for patients with HIV disease.* New York, NY: McGraw-Hill.

Flower, W., & Sooy, C. (1987). AIDS: An introduction for speech-language pathologists and audiologists. *ASHA, 27,* 25–30.

Garibaldi, R., Brodine, S., & Matsumiya, S. (1981). Infections among patients in nursing homes: Policies, prevalence, problems. *New England Journal of Medicine, 305*, 731-5.

Garibaldi, R. L., & Nurse, B. (1992). Infections in nursing homes. In J. Bennett & P. Brachman (Eds.), *Hospital infections* (pp. 491–532). Boston, MA: Little, Brown.

Golper, L. A. C. (1998). *Sourcebook for medical speech pathology* (2nd ed.). Clifton Park, NY: Delmar Cengage Learning.

Graves, J. (2004). Economics and preventing hospital-acquired infection. *Emerging Infectious Diseases, 10*, 561–566. Available from http://www.cdc.gov/eid

Hellman, S., & Gram, M. (1993). The resurgence of tuberculosis. *American Association of Occupational Health Nurses Journal, 41,* 66–71.

Interorganizational Group for Speech-Language Pathology and Audiology. (2010). *Infection prevention and control guidelines for speech-language pathology*. Retrieved from http://www.caslpa.ca/PDF/infection_prevention_control_guidelines/Infection_Prevention_control_Guidelines_SLP.pdf

Kaiser Family Foundation. *HIV/AIDS*. Available from http://www.statehealthfacts.org

Mathei, C., Niclaes, L., Suetens, C., Jans, B., & Buntinx, F. (2007). Infections in residents of nursing homes. *Infections Disease Clinics of North America, 21,* 761–772.

McMillan, M., & Willette, S. (1988). Aseptic technique: A procedure for preventing disease transmission in the practice environment. *ASHA, 31,* 35–37.

Merck. (2005). Staphylococcal infections. *The Merck Manual.* Retrieved from http://www.merckmanuals.com/professional/index/ind_st.html

National Center for Health Statistics. (1999). *National vital statistics reports* (v. 27). Hyattsville, MD: Author.

National Center for Health Statistics. (2004). *National vital statistics reports* (v. 52). Hyattsville, MD: Author.

New York State Department of Health. (2011). *Cytomegalovirus*. Retrieved from http://www.health.ny.gov/diseases/communicable/cytomegalovirus/fact_sheet.htm

Palmer, M. (1984). *Infection control: A policy and procedure manual.* Philadelphia, PA: W.B. Saunders.

Polder, J., Tablan, O., & Williams, W. (1992). Personnel health services. In J. Bennett & P. Brachman (Eds.), *Hospital infections.* Boston, MA: Little, Brown.

Rutala, W. (1987). Disinfection, sterilization, and waste disposal. In R. Wenzel (Ed.), *Prevention and control of nosocomial infections* (pp. 257–282). Baltimore, MD: Williams & Wilkins.

Sherertz, R., & Hampton, A. (1987). Infection control aspects of hospital employee health. In R. Wenzel (Ed.), *Prevention and control of nosocomial infections* (pp. 116–174). Baltimore, MD: Williams & Wilkins.

Swanepoel, D., & Louw, B. (2010). (Eds.). *HIV/AIDS: A clinical resource for communication, hearing and swallowing disorders.* San Diego, CA: Plural Publishing.

University of Maryland Medical Center. (2011). *Herpes simplex virus*. Retrieved from http://www.umm.edu/altmed/articles/herpes-simplex-000079.htm

Valenti, P. (1992). Selected viruses of nosocomial importance. In J. Bennett & P. Brachman (Eds.), *Hospital infections* (pp. 789–822). Boston, MA: Little, Brown.

RESOURCES

American Academy of Audiology (AAA)

AAA has an Infection Control Task Force that has published the document *Infection Control in Audiological Practice.* This publication outlines the importance of infection control in audiology practice, general housekeeping and environmental infection control practices, and ways to control human sources of infection. Retrieved from http:www.audiology.org/resources/documentlibrary/Pages/InfectionControl.aspx?PF=1.

American Speech-Language-Hearing Association (ASHA)

ASHA provides a number of resources for speech-language pathologists including ASHA policy documents, information on infection control basics and disease prevention in health care, resources for school-based SLPs, practice guidelines, articles, and links. SLPs should access http://www.asha.org/slp/infectioncontrol.htm. Audiologists should access http://www.asha.org/aud/infection-control.htm.

Centers for Disease Control and Prevention (CDC)

1600 Clifton Road
Atlanta, GA 30333
Telephone: 800-232-4636
Website: http://www.cdc.gov

Originally established in 1946 as the Communicable Disease Center in Atlanta, Georgia, the Centers for Disease Control and Prevention is a federal agency within the Department of Health and Human Services. The CDC is responsible for national programs aimed at prevention and control of communicable and airborne diseases and other preventable conditions. The agency is composed of nine major divisions that consult with related state and local health programs; develop programs for chronic disease prevention, environmental health, and occupational safety and health; and focus on research, education, information, and epidemiological data collection and analysis. The agency also provides international consultation on these topics.

Commission on Accreditation of Rehabilitation Facilities (CARF)

6951 E. Southpoint Road
Tucson, AZ 85756
Telephone: 502-325-1044
Website: http://www.carf.org

This accreditation agency includes standards based on universal precautions in its survey and review of rehabilitation agencies.

Interorganizational Group for Speech-Language Pathology and Audiology

This is a group of Canadian organizations devoted to collaboration of regulatory groups, professional associations, and university programs in developing practice standards and guidelines. One of its projects was the development of guidelines for infection prevention and control guidelines for speech-language pathology. Its in-depth manual describes a rationale for infection prevention techniques and standard and routine precautions. Find information on infection prevention at the following web address: http://www.caslpa.ca/english/resources/infection_prevention_control_guidelines.asp

Occupational Safety and Health Administration (OSHA), U.S. Labor Department

200 Constitution Avenue, N.W.
Washington, DC 20210
Website: http://www.osha.gov/

Part of the U.S. Labor Department, the Occupational Safety and Health Administration develops policies, disseminates information, and enforces occupational safety and health standards. This agency also determines compliance with occupational safety and health standards through inspections and determines and enforces penalties for noncompliance. It was established in 1971 following enactment of the Occupational Safety and Health Act of 1970.

23

Child Abuse and Elder Mistreatment

Rosemary Lubinski, EdD

SCOPE OF CHAPTER

Sometime during your employment as an audiologist or speech-language pathologist, you may suspect that a child or elder client is a victim of abuse or neglect. Depending on the state in which you are employed, you will have either a professional and/or a mandated obligation to report incidences of suspected abuse. This chapter presents broad definitions and characteristics of various types of child abuse, possible causes for such mistreatment, the scope of the problem, and suggestions for what to do when indicators may be present. Similarly, various types of elder abuse and neglect are discussed. This chapter is intended to supplement and not replace individual state definitions, procedures, or requirements for coursework or certification on these topics.

CHILD ABUSE AND NEGLECT

Clinicians must be able to identify the signs and symptoms of child abuse and neglect. In addition, you need to be aware of the potential causes and factors that put a child at risk for these forms of maltreatment. Finally, you need to know who may act as an abuser and how common child abuse and neglect are in our society.

Child Abuse

Broadly defined, child abuse occurs when children under 18 years of age are physically or mentally harmed by a parent or other person legally responsible for their care. This may involve physical injury by other than accidental means, sexual offense against the child, or allowing the child to engage in such acts. Physical abuse involves the use of force, such as striking, beating, pushing, shoving, shaking, slapping, kicking, pinching, or burning, that results in injury, pain, or impairment. The abuse may or may not be executed with an object. The unjustifiable use of drugs and physical restraints may also be considered physical abuse.

Child abuse may also include other forms of neglect such as malnutrition, dehydration, psychological mistreatment, and failure to treat mental or physical ills that may impair growth and development. Emotional abuse, also called *mental cruelty*, *emotional neglect*, or *emotional maltreatment*, occurs when there is some type of nonphysical actions toward a child that result in psychological stress and may lead to physical or psychological illness. Emotional abuse may entail threatening a child verbally or nonverbally, terrorizing, isolating or placing the child in a closed confinement, withholding nurturance and affection, and knowingly permitting the child's maladaptive behavior. Table 23–1 describes potential types and indicators of child abuse and neglect.

Maltreatment and Neglect

Maltreatment occurs when children under 18 years of age are neglected or have serious physical injury inflicted on them by other than accidental means. The parent or other person legally responsible for care fails to provide a minimum degree of care and the child's physical, mental, emotional, or educational well-being has been or is in danger of being impaired. Neglect is considered an act of omission. According to the U.S. Department of Department of Health and Human Services (2006), neglect can be categorized as physical, medical, inadequate supervision, environmental, emotional, and educational. Specific examples of neglect include when a responsible adult has not provided a child with adequate nutrition, clothing, shelter, protection from safety hazards, personal hygiene, nurturing or affection, or education although financially able to do so or offered means to do so. Neglect also occurs when the responsible adult has not provided the child with proper supervision or guardianship. This may occur when this individual inflicts or allows harm to be inflicted, places the child at risk of harm, uses excessive corporal punishment, or uses substances that impair self-control.

A child who has been abandoned by his or her parents or other legally responsible person is also considered neglected. Emotional neglect occurs when there is a "state of substantially diminished psychological or intellectual functioning in relation to, but not limited to such factors as failure to thrive, control of aggression or self-destructive impulses, ability to think and reason, or acting out and misbehavior" (Center for Development of Human Services at Buffalo State College, n.d., p. 17). Such neglect may cause children to be permanently damaged or may be responsible for more deaths per year than abuse.

Continuum of Abuse and Neglect

Abuse and neglect range in severity from mild to moderate to severe (U.S. Department of Health and Human Services, 2006). Severity is determined by such factors as degree of harm or risk and the chronicity of the problem. Keep in mind that one occurrence of abuse or neglect may be serious and warrant identification and intervention.

Causes and Risks

There are numerous, interrelated possible causes of and risk factors for child abuse and neglect. Table 23–2 lists four major categories, including parent/caretaker characteristics, parent-child relationship characteristics, child characteristics, and environmental factors. It should be noted that these are *potential* risk factors, and the presence of any one is not an absolute predictor of child abuse or neglect. Further, it is likely these factors are not mutually exclusive and do not all arise within the parent/caregiver. Finally, causes and risk factors must be considered within a framework of a cultural background of child-rearing practices and economic and political values. The origins of abuse and neglect should also be considered from a socio-ecological perspective. For example, poverty may contribute to a parent abusing a child, and

TABLE 23–1 Types and Potential Indicators of Child Abuse and Neglect

Possible Signs of Physical Abuse

- Unexplained bruises or welts in different places, in clusters, in various stages of healing, and/or in shape of instrument used
- Unexplained burns
- Unexplained lacerations or abrasions
- Unexplained skeletal injuries, for example, bites, fracture, bald spots, detached retina
  - Inappropriate clothing for weather to conceal injuries
- Extremes in behavior—aggressive to withdrawn
- Easily frightened or fearful—for example, of parents, adults, physical contact, going home, or when other children cry
- Self-destructive
- Hurts others
- Poor social relationships—craves attention, poor relationships with peers, manipulates adults
- Reports fear of parents, injuries, unbelievable reasons for injuries
- Poor academic performance
- Short attention span
- Language delays
- Runaway
- Truancy and or delinquency

Possible Signs of Sexual Abuse

- Difficulty walking
- Abnormalities in genital/anal areas—itching, pain, swelling, bruises, frequent infections, discharge, poor sphincter control
- Venereal disease
- Pregnancy
- Report of abuse
- Drop in academic performance
- Poor peer relationships
- Unwillingness to change, for example, gym clothing
- Unusually sophisticated sexual knowledge and behavior
- Depressed, apathetic
- Suicidal
- Sexually aggressive
- Regression to earlier developmental stages

Possible Signs of Emotional Maltreatment

- Failure to thrive in infancy
- Poor appearance
- Infantile or regressive behavior
- Developmental lags
- Extremes in behavior
- Poor self-concept
- Depressed, apathetic
- Suicidal

Possible Signs of Neglect

- Hunger and malnutrition, begs for or steals food
- Poor hygiene, lice, body odor
- Inappropriate clothing for weather and context
- Unattended physical problems or medical needs
- Lack of supervision especially in dangerous activities or contexts
- Constant fatigue
- Developmental lags
- Extremes in behavior
- Depressed, apathetic
- Seeks attention or affection
- Truancy or delinquency

TABLE 23–2 Possible Causes of and Risks for Child Abuse and Neglect

Parent/Caretaker Characteristics

- Personal history of abuse
- History of family violence
- Single parenthood or absence of parent
- Social isolation and lack of emotional support
- Parental/caregiver immaturity or lack of parenting knowledge
- Marital problems of parents
- Physical or mental health problems
- Life crises such as financial problems, unemployment or underemployment, death of spouse
- Substance abuse
- Adolescent parents
- Lack of knowledge in areas of housekeeping, nutrition, and medical care
- Expectation that child act like an adult (e.g., leaves young child alone or to care for other younger children)
- Has low frustration tolerance and poor judgment; cannot delay gratification
- Lack of motivation to learn productive child-raising practices
- Does not believe there is a problem, is unconcerned, or refuses to cooperate

Child Characteristics

- Infant
- Child with special needs (e.g., mental retardation, health problems, sensory impairments, learning difficulties, communication difficulties)
- Twins or multiple births
- Premature baby
- Baby born during time of family trauma
- Baby or young child who cries excessively (colicky), has feeding difficulties, resists being held
- Stepchild
- Child of unplanned or unwanted pregnancy
- Adolescence, teenager's striving for independence, teenager's dependency on teenage culture

Parent-Child Relationship Characteristics

- Parent's unrealistic expectations for development, achievement, or responsibility
- Lack of nurturing child-rearing skills
- Use of violence as an accepted means of personal interaction
- Inadequate bonding between parent and child
- Delay or failure to seek needed health care
- Perception that child is evil or different

Environmental Factors

- Lack of social support
- Homelessness
- Poor or inadequate housing
- Large family in crowded housing
- Poverty
- Withdrawal of governmental social, housing, and economic support

thus, intervention would need to focus on both the parent and remediation of poverty (U.S. Department of Health and Human Services, 2006).

Several of these etiological factors bear more discussion. First, 40 percent of physical abuse of children is caused by people who themselves were abused as children (Check, 1989). These adults were inadequately parented during their own childhood and have carried over this negative child-rearing style to their own interactions with children.

Second, younger parents, particularly teenagers, appear more at risk for committing child abuse. Teenagers may be emotionally immature to take on the responsibilities of parenting and have limited parenting, coping, and homemaking skills. Teen mothers may be at greater risk for not completing their education, have limited work options, and face financial stress (U.S. Department of Health and Human Services, 2006).

Third, substance abuse contributes to drug-exposed newborns and inappropriate parenting styles. Substance abuse frequently co-occurs with other problems. For example, young parents may also be involved with substance abuse. Substance abuse is also a major contributor to criminal activity.

Fourth, parents under stress because of unmet internal needs, lack of support, unemployment, financial or familial crises, and their own health and emotional problems are more vulnerable to committing child abuse and neglecting their children.

Fifth, children who have challenging needs may be more susceptible to abuse and neglect. Children with a myriad complex of chronic needs may stress parents/caregivers beyond their limits, particularly when parents or caregivers have limited education, support, and respite and possibly face financial concerns. Parents may not know how to deal with challenging behavioral characteristics such as noncompliance and resort to inappropriate measures to gain control. Children with communication disabilities pose double challenges. Parents may become frustrated by lack of meaningful intelligible communication. Further, children with communication problems may not be able to report their own abuse to parents or other caregivers/educators.

Statistics vary on the prevalence of child abuse among children with disabilities, but evidence does indicate that it may be at least 1.8 times greater than for children without disabilities (Hibbard & Desch, 2007; Sullivan & Knutson, 2000). There is some indication that children with behavior disorders are at greater risk for physical abuse and those with speech/language disorders are at risk for neglect (Sullivan & Knutson, 2000).

Finally, very young children are at the highest risk for abuse and death from abuse. According to the National Center on Child Abuse and Neglect, children less than 1 year old were more likely to be neglected than at any other time of their lives (U.S. Department of Health and Human Services, 1994). The demands of infant care may tax parents or caregivers, particularly those with limited parenting skills, support, or patience.

Munchausen by Proxy

Munchausen syndrome is a disorder in which an individual deliberately creates fictitious physical and/or mental health symptoms to gain attention and sympathy, particularly from medical personnel. When this pattern of exaggeration, fabrication, and inducement is applied to the symptoms of others (usually children), it is called Munchausen by proxy (MBP). This is considered a recognized type of maltreatment that may involve physical, sexual, or emotional abuse; neglect; or a combination (Lasher, 2004). MBP perpetrators are usually mothers who appear to be good caretakers, may have extensive health care knowledge and experience, and are convincing in their concern. Some may change health care providers frequently to avoid suspicion and subject their child to unneeded medical tests and procedures. Some may inflict injury to magnify the symptomatology. Most will deny the maltreatment even when confronted with evidence.

Possible indicators of MBP include some combination of the following: frequent emergency room admissions, recurrent episodes of the same complaint, treatment that does not produce expected results, a pattern of the problem arising in the perpetrator's presence and disappearing in his or her absence, and recurrences when the child goes home after treatment. The parent exhibits characteristics commensurate with the pattern described (Lasher, 2004). Confirmation of this diagnosis is difficult but necessary because of the potential for serious harm to a child. SLPs and audiologists who work in medical settings should be alert to this category of child abuse.

Who Is an Abuser?

Child abuse spans all ethnic, social, economic, and racial lines. Abusers may be parents, guardians, relatives, or friends. Eighty percent of abusers are parents, and women (53.8 percent) comprise the majority of abusers (U.S. Department of Health and Human Services Bureau, 2009). A typical profile of an abuser is a young adult in his or her mid-20s, with limited education, living at or below the poverty level, and depressed. Nearly all child abusers were inadequately parented in their own childhood, and most were abused as children (Andrews University, 1999). It should be noted that child-child abuse also occurs, such as adolescent-child sexual abuse, sibling incest, and cousin-cousin incest.

Extent of the Problem

Each year the U.S. Department of Health and Human Services Children's Bureau (2009) publishes data on child maltreatment that are collected and analyzed by the National Child Abuse and Neglect Data System (NCANDS). Note that these data are aggregate as a child may be reported as a victim of one or more types of abuse or neglect. In 2009 there were about 3.3 million referrals to Child Protective Services (CPS) in the United States involving the alledged maltreatment of 6.0 million children. About one-quarter of these were found to be victims with substantiated cases. Children from birth to 1 year had the highest rate of victimization. Boys presented as 48.2 percent of the victims and girls 51.1 percent. Whites accounted for 44 percent of the cases; African Americans, 22.3 percent; and Hispanics, 20.7 percent. Neglect accounted for the highest percent of maltreatment (78.3 percent), followed by physical abuse (17.8 percent), sexual abuse (9.5 percent), and psychological maltreatment (7.6 percent). Eighty-one percent of abuse cases were committed by parents, and women constituted 53.8 percent of perpetrators as compared with 44.4 percent male. Four-fifths of perpetrators were between the ages of 20 and 49 years. The national data estimate that 1770 children died from abuse or neglect. Most of these child fatalities involved children younger than four, boys, and were attributable to neglect or multiple maltreatments.

Effects of Child Abuse and Neglect

Child abuse and neglect have numerous negative effects that may be obvious immediately or may be more covert and manifest themselves later in life. There may be some combination of social, emotional, behavioral, academic, and physical consequences. Each of these negative effects may in some way influence communicative and cognitive development. For example, child neglect has been associated with the failure of the brain to develop and impoverished cognitive and social skills (U.S. Department of Health and Human Services, Children's Bureau, 2010). The Children's Bureau states: "Children who are neglected early in life may remain in a state of 'hyperarousal' in which they are constantly anticipating threats, or they may experience dissociation with a decreased ability to benefit from social, emotional, and cognitive experiences. To be able to learn, a child's brain needs to be in a state of 'attentive calm,' which is rare for maltreated children" (p. 22). The brain of abused or neglected children may be as much as 20 percent smaller than that of nonabused children. Abuse particularly affects the development of language skills. Effects in the education realm include lower IQ; poorer scores on reading, language, and math skills; and overall lower academic performance. Children who are abused or neglected may be diagnosed with oppositional defiant disorder, conduct disorder, post-traumatic stress disorder, depression, anxiety, and sexual abuse of others.

The estimated annual financial costs are extremely high, totaling more than $103.8 billion (Wang and Holton, 2007). Direct costs are estimated to be at least $33 billion and include costs for hospitalization, chronic health problems, mental health services, child welfare, and law enforcement and judiciary. The remaining indirect costs are related to special education, mental health, juvenile delinquency, lost productivity to society, and adult criminality.

Societal consequences go beyond the financial. Indirect effects include increased child and adult criminal activity, mental illness, substance abuse, and domestic violence. The fact that one-third of neglected children are likely to maltreat their own children creates a vicious cycle that affects generations (U.S. Department of Health and Human Services, Children's Bureau, 2010).

What to Do If You Suspect Abuse

You cannot ignore signs of abuse. First, you must know if you are a mandated reporter of abuse in your state. You must also know what constitutes abuse in your state, what reasonable cause is, and what to do when you suspect abuse. Your confidentiality will be protected if you have made the report in good faith. If you work in a larger organization, policies and procedures will be in place to guide you in the steps to take when reporting abuse. You are advised to inform your supervisor of your suspicions.

Who Is a Mandated Reporter of Abuse?

Each state has specific people who are required by law to report suspected child abuse or neglect. For example, according to New York State Law Chapter 544, Identification and Reporting of Child Abuse and

Maltreatment—Explaining Reporting Requirements—Study Requirements for Licensing (1989), speech-language pathologists and audiologists are not specifically named in this category. They may, however, be considered under some other mandated personnel category such as a school official; a day care center worker; or a member of hospital personnel engaged in the admission, examination, care, or treatment of patients. It is best to review your school, hospital, or agency's policy and procedure manual for precise guidelines in your facility, locality, and state. Note that if you are a mandated reporter, you can face criminal and civil liability for not reporting suspected abuse (U.S. Department of Health and Human Services, 2006). Even if you are not a mandated reporter, you have an ethical responsibility to document in writing possible signs of abuse or neglect and report these to your supervisor immediately.

What Is Reasonable Cause?

If you suspect a child has *possibly* incurred abuse or neglect, you have reasonable cause to report a possible problem. Reasonable cause is based on personally observed physical and behavioral evidence and/or a report from the child and your own professional training and experience. According to the Center for Development of Human Services at Buffalo State College (n.d.), "the reporter should only be *able to entertain the possibility that it could have been neglect or nonaccidental* in order to possess the necessary reasonable cause."

When and to Whom to Report

Suspected child abuse or neglect should be reported immediately by telephone, at any time of day, seven days a week. Depending on the state, a written report may be required within a specified time limit. For example, New York State requires that a written report be filed within 48 hours of the oral report. Where to report cases of child abuse depends on whether you are a mandated reporter. For example, in New York State, mandated reporters and concerned members of the general public call different numbers of the New York State Child Abuse Hotline. Each state will have similar child abuse hotlines listed in the local telephone book. In addition, national phone numbers are listed in the Resources section at the end of this chapter. Again, your agency, hospital, or school will have specific guidelines for policies and procedures regarding reporting of possible child abuse.

Immunity and Confidentiality

You have immunity from any civil or criminal liability if you or your agency has reported a suspected case of child abuse or neglect in *good faith*. Your name will be kept confidential unless you provide written permission for its release.

Consequences for Failing to Report

If you are a mandated reporter and willfully fail to report a case of suspected child abuse or maltreatment, you may be guilty of a misdemeanor and have a civil liability for damages caused by such failure. Remember that failure to report your suspicion may result in continued and more severe harm to a child.

ELDER ABUSE, NEGLECT, AND EXPLOITATION

Elders are among the most vulnerable members of our society. Their ability to protect themselves may be hampered by physical, cognitive, and communication problems. As with child abuse, you need to be aware of the signs and symptoms of elder abuse and what to do if you suspect such maltreatment. Remember that elder abuse or neglect can take place in the home or in formal care settings.

Elder Abuse

Elder abuse is a general term that describes intentional and neglectful actions by a person(s) in trust or a caregiver who causes harm to an elder (National Center on Elder Abuse, 2010). For an action to be classified as elder abuse, a person either does something or fails to do something that harms an elder. Elder abuse may occur in the home or in institutional settings, or it may be self-imposed (Administration on Aging, 1998). The seven most common forms of elder abuse include physical abuse, sexual abuse, emotional or psychological abuse, neglect, abandonment, financial or material exploitation, and self-neglect. Table 23–3 provides a summary of the seven major types of elder abuse and potential signs or symptoms of each type.

TABLE 23–3 Types and Potential Indicators of Elder Abuse, Neglect, and Exploitation

Possible Signs of Physical Abuse

- Cuts, wounds, punctures, choke marks
- Unexplained fractures, broken bones, skull fractures
- Bruises, welts, discolorations on face or body
- Bedsores or significant skin problems
- Detached retina, hematomas
- Injuries left untreated or improperly cared for
- Poor skin hygiene or condition
- Dehydration without illness-based cause
- Malnourishment without illness-based cause
- Loss of weight
- Cigarette or rope burns
- Soiled clothing or bed
- Broken eyeglasses, hearing aids, other assistive devices
- Signs of being restrained
- Sudden change in elder behavior
- Elder report of physical abuse
- Death or murder

Possible Signs of Sexual Abuse

- Bruises around breasts or genital area
- Unexplained sexually transmitted diseases
- Unexplained vaginal or anal bleeding
- Torn, stained, or bloody underclothing
- Inappropriate display of affection by caregiver
- Elder report of sexual abuse

Possible Signs of Psychological/Emotional Abuse

- Hesitancy to express feelings in public
- Ambivalence, deference to others, passivity, cowering
- Lack of eye contact
- Clinging, trembling
- Depression
- Confusion or disorientation
- Fear
- Withdrawal
- Denial
- Helplessness, hopelessness
- Severe anxiety or agitation
- Anger
- Confabulations
- Elder report of verbal or emotional mistreatment
- Extreme withdrawal
- Elder becomes noncommunicative, especially in presence of caregiver
- Attempted suicide

Possible Signs of Financial or Material Exploitation

- Improper signatures on financial documents or unusual activity in bank accounts
- Identity theft
- Financial statements do not come to elder's home without explanation
- Power of attorney given or changed without explanation
- Change(s) in will or other documents without explanation
- Financial mismanagement of funds, including unpaid bills
- Elder states that he or she has been signing papers without understanding their content
- Missing personal items
- Heightened concern by elder regarding financial management
- Lack of amenities, including appropriate clothing, entertainment, and so on that elder could afford
- Promises of care by caregiver or family
- Provision of unnecessary services or purchase of items

(*Continues*)

(Continued)

- Unauthorized withdrawal of funds using an ATM or credit card
- Elder receives eviction notice from house he or she owned
- Elder report of financial or property mismanagement
- Caregiver concerned that too much money is spent on the elder

Possible Signs of Abandonment

- Desertion of an elder at a hospital, nursing home, or other institution
- Desertion of an elder at a public location
- Report by elder of being abandoned

Possible Signs of Neglect

- Dirty environment
- Fecal or urine smell
- Environmental safety hazards
- Rashes, sores, lice, or other infestation
- Untreated medical condition
- Malnourishment or dehydration
- Inappropriate or inadequate clothing and grooming

Possible Signs of Self-Neglect

- Inability to handle activities of daily living, including personal care and meal preparation
- Suicide attempts
- Inadequate financial management
- Dirty, unsafe living environment
- Homelessness
- Refusing medical or personal care
- Willful isolation
- Alcohol or other drug abuse
- Slovenly appearance
- Malnourishment or dehydration
- Not keeping medical or other important personal appointments

Specific Types of Elder Abuse

Many types of elder abuse are similar to those of child abuse, including physical abuse involving injury, pain, or impairment and sexual abuse whereby individuals receive inappropriate and unwanted sexual activities imposed on them. Several other types of abuse are particular to elders or have different characteristics and are described in the following sections.

Physical Abuse This type of abuse involves the nonaccidental use of force that results in pain, injury, or impairment (Helpguide, 2010). Physical abuse may also include the inappropriate use of drugs, restraints, or confinement.

Emotional or Psychological Abuse Elders who experience undue emotional pain or distress are said to be emotionally abused. A common type of emotional abuse is administered verbally through verbal attacks, insults, threats, intimidation, humiliation, or harassment or by giving the elder the "silent treatment." Nonverbal abuse involves ignoring or terrorizing the older person. Other forms of emotional abuse include infantilization of the elder and isolation from people and activities of choice.

Neglect Elder neglect is defined as "an act of omission, of not doing something, of withholding goods or services" (Quinn & Tomita, 1986, p. 34). Neglect involves deliberately ignoring the needs of an elder and may take the form of financial neglect, by failing to attend to financial obligations, and physical neglect, when the elder receives inadequate food, water, clothing, shelter, personal hygiene, medicine, comfort, or personal safety (Administration on Aging, 1998). Neglect can be intentional (active), characterized by a conscious effort to inflict harm, or unintentional (passive), which is associated with laziness or lack of knowledge (Cicirelli, 1986).

Self-Neglect Self-neglect occurs when elders harm themselves. For example, elders may improperly or inadequately care for their own health, safety, clothing, nutrition, hygiene, or shelter. Potential factors that lead to self-neglect include long-term chronic self-neglect through adulthood, dementia, illness, malnutrition, overmedication, depression, substance abuse, poverty, and isolation (Woolf, 1998).

Abandonment Abandonment is the deliberate desertion of an elder by a person who has responsibility for that elder. Abandoned elders are left alone frequently and for extended time periods in their home or other setting by caregivers. This is particularly dangerous for those elders who cannot provide for their own daily needs such as food, personal care, and medications. In addition, the loss of socialization opportunities may have a deleterious effect on the elder and contribute to cognitive and emotional decline.

Financial or Material Exploitation This type of abuse occurs when an elder's funds, property, or material assets are illegally or improperly used, usually without authorization or permission. Examples of financial or material exploitation include fraudulent check cashing or use of a credit card; forgery of a signature; misuse or theft of money, property, or other possessions; coercion into signing a document (e.g., a will); identity theft; or the improper use of conservatorship, guardianship, or power of attorney (Administration on Aging, 1998; Helpguide, 2010).

Who Is Abused?

According to the National Center on Elder Abuse (2010), the majority of elder abuse victims are female (67.3 percent). The median age of elders abused by others is 77.9 years and 77.4 years for elders who neglected themselves. Two-thirds of the victims of domestic abuse are white, 18.7 percent are African American, and 10 percent are Hispanic.

Who Is at Risk?

Any elder is at risk for abuse, although those who have mental or physical disabilities are at the greatest risk. Recent data indicate that about 67 percent of elders with substantiated reports of abuse were female, 43 percent were over age 80, and 77 percent were Caucasian; 89 percent of incidents occurred in the home (National Center on Elder Abuse, 2010). Elders are at risk when their caregivers over- or underestimate their abilities and thus have unreasonable expectations for performance. Elders are also at risk if there is a history of domestic abuse in their family or in that of a professional caregiver. The likelihood of abuse increases when caregivers have difficulty with temper control; physical, mental, or substance abuse problems; and immature personalities. Elders themselves may increase their risk for abuse if they verbally insult or psychologically taunt their caregivers, especially with threats of withholding inheritances (Quinn & Tomita, 1986). Other factors that place elders at risk include dependency and isolation, family conflict, and financial stress. Those elders with dementia and mental disorders are at significant risk for abuse as care for these individuals is particularly stressful and time consuming (National Center on Elder Abuse, 2011).

Who Is an Abuser?

Those who abuse elders come from all racial, economic, educational, and socioeconomic strata (Quinn & Tomita, 1986). In 2004, the National Center on Elder Abuse (2010) reported that 52.7 percent of alleged perpetrators of abuse were female and three-quarters were under the age of 60. It also found that adult children are the most frequent abusers of the elderly (34.6 percent) and other family members (21.5 percent). Formal caregivers who have poor working conditions, low salary, and limited education are at higher risk for becoming an abuser.

Extent of the Problem

Reliable statistics on elder abuse and neglect are difficult to find. According to the National Center on Elder Abuse (2010), about 1 in 10 elders may be a victim of elder abuse, but few of these cases are reported. National data indicate that there may be between one million and two million older Americans who have been abused or neglected. These data are considered gross underestimations of the true number of cases. It is predicted that for every reported incident of elder abuse, five go unreported.

The most common types of elder maltreatment are, in decreasing order of frequency, neglect (49 percent), emotional/psychological abuse (35 percent), financial/

material exploitation (30 percent), physical abuse (27 percent), abandonment (4 percent), sexual abuse (3 percent), and other (1.4 percent). These frequency data are not mutually exclusive, as more than one type of abuse may be reported for an incident.

Why Does Elder Abuse Occur?

Elder abuse and neglect are generally attributed to the following factors:

- Physical and mental impairment of the elder
- Caregiver stress
- Violence as a problem-solving strategy
- Individual problems of the abuser
- Society's negative portrayal of the elderly
- Greed (Quinn & Tomita, 1986)

It is likely these hypothesized causes work in tandem rather than individually. Meeting the needs of frail, physically and/or mentally challenged elders is a time- and effort-consuming task, especially for caregivers with limited personal resources and reduced or immature psychological stamina. In some cases, a "triggering crisis" may instigate an incident of abuse. In other cases, long-term, unrelieved stress and physical fatigue may result in an explosion of violence. Some families may routinely use abuse as a problem-solving strategy. Some elders may purposely antagonize their caregivers, whereas others with reduced cognitive abilities may not understand or appreciate the care received. Finally, society stigmatizes the disabled and their caregivers. Limited financial or social incentives are available for caregivers who may sacrifice career and social lives for their elder family member. Some caregivers may deliberately hasten the progression of decline because it will result in a greater or earlier financial inheritance. Reinharz (1986) commented that elder abuse is not a modern problem and represents "twin cultural themes of honor and contempt" toward the elderly.

Certain caregiving contexts appear to trigger abuse, and many of these are related to the stress involved. For example, feeding, incontinence, interrupted sleep, and incessant vocalizations are all extremely stressful for caregivers, especially when they occur repeatedly and without respite. These situations become even more problematic if the caregiver is an alcohol or drug abuser or has a history of being abused or abusive.

Elders may be afraid to report abuse because of their fear of what will happen to them if their caregiver is removed. Many elders greatly fear they will be forced to leave their home and relocate to an institutional setting where there will be less independence, loss of control, and loss of familiar surroundings and property. Thus, many elders refrain from mentioning incidents of abuse because they perceive the alternative of institutionalization to be worse than the abuse they receive in their home.

Elder Abuse in Long-Term Care Facilities

Working with elders in long-term care facilities can be a challenging job, particularly when residents have demanding physical and psychological needs, salary and societal regard are low, and training is minimal. Pillemer and Moore (1990) state that possible risk factors for staff abuse of elders in long-term care settings include patient aggression and provocation, staff burnout, staff age, and conflict regarding daily routines. In their confidential interviews of 577 nurses and aides, Pillemer and Moore found that more than 75 percent of staff had observed psychological abuse, 41 percent admitted to committing such abuse, about 33 percent had observed physical abuse, and 10 percent had committed physical abuse. Physical abuse is the most commonly reported abuse against elders in nursing homes, followed by sexual abuse, neglect, and monetary abuse. Male nursing aides committed two-thirds of the reported cases of abuse. Prevention undoubtedly lies in higher qualifications for staff, more staff training, and enforcement of mandatory abuse reporting (Quinn & Tomita, 1997).

WHAT TO DO?

Each state determines whether audiologists and speech-language pathologists are mandated to report child or elder abuse. If you suspect elder abuse, it is best to document in writing the indicators and discuss the policy and procedure of your setting for reporting these potential signs of elder abuse.

In most states, the Adult Protective Services agency (APS) is the major site responsible for both investigation of reported cases of elder abuse and for providing help to victims and their families. This agency is often contained within the county department of social services. Other organizations that have primary roles in investigation and follow-up of elder abuse referrals include the Area Agency on Aging, county departments of social services, the local law enforcement agency, the medical examiner/coroner's office, hospitals, the state long-term care ombudsman's office, mental health agencies, and facility licensing or certification organizations. Investigations may lead to provision of community supportive services, financial or legal assistance, counseling referrals, or guardianship. Alleged perpetrators may face criminal investigations and prosecution.

SUMMARY

When providing intervention services in home, community, or institutional settings, audiologists and speech-language pathologists need to be vigilant for signs of abuse. Young children and elders with communication problems and other disorders are particularly vulnerable to abuse because of their high-intensity needs. Abuse can take a variety of forms, including physical, psychological, sexual, financial, or neglect. Abuse or neglect can occur in any age, ethnic, or economic group; in urban, suburban, or rural settings; and in any type of setting by paid caregivers, family members, or others. Speech-language pathologists and audiologists need to know their individual state regulations regarding mandated reporting of child or elder abuse and should know their agency's particular guidelines for reporting suspected cases of child abuse. Identification of abuse against those with whom we work may help prevent further abuse and provide abusers with the help they need to refrain from this type of dangerous and humiliating behavior.

CRITICAL THINKING

1. What steps would you take if you suspected child or elder abuse?
2. How would you consider cultural differences in child-raising practices in deciding if a child had possibly been abused?
3. What might be the effects if you do not report a suspected case of child or elder abuse?
4. Should speech-language pathologists and audiologists be legally described as "mandated" reporters of child abuse in every state? Why or why not?
5. When visiting a home for an early intervention evaluation, you notice that the children in the home are dirty, dressed inappropriately for the heating conditions in the home, and frequently scratch themselves. The physical environment of the home is also filthy. The mother, however, is an excellent informant and greatly interested in the speech and language development of her children. The mother and children appear to have a warm relationship. What would you do?
6. You are hired by a private practice on an hourly wage to provide clinical services in a long-term care facility. You notice some signs of resident neglect in the facility but are reluctant to say anything because it may jeopardize your position in the facility. What would you do? What would the Code of Ethics of the American Speech-Language-Hearing Association or American Board of Audiology say about this issue?
7. Create scenarios that might be indicative of child or elder abuse. Consider what you should do in each situation.

REFERENCES

Administration on Aging. (1998). *The national elder abuse incidence study: Final report September 1998.* Retrieved from http://www.aoa.gov/AoARoot/AoA_Programs/Elder_Rights/Elder_Abuse/docs/ABuseReport_Full.pdf

Andrews University. (1999). *Child abuse.* Available from http://www.andrews.edu/

Center for Development of Human Services at Buffalo State College. (n.d.). *Identification and report of child abuse and maltreatment: A course for mandated reporters.* Buffalo, NY: Author.

Check, W. (1989). *Child abuse.* New York, NY: Chelsea House Publishers.

Cicirelli, V. (1986). The helping relationship and family neglect in later life. In K. Pillemer & R. Wolf (Eds.), *Elder abuse conflict in the family* (pp. 49–66). Dover, MA: Auburn House Publishing.

Helpguide. (2010). *Elder abuse and neglect.* Retrieved from http://www.helpguide.org/mental/elder_abuse_physical_emotional_sexual_neglect.htm

Hibbard, R., & Desch, L. (2007). Maltreatment of children with disabilities. *Pediatrics, 119,* 1018–1025.

Lasher, L. (2004). *MBP overview and definitions.* Available from http://www.mbpexpert.com/

National Center on Elder Abuse. (2010). *Why should I care about elder abuse*? Newark, DE: Author.

National Center on Elder Abuse. (2011). *Risk factors for elder abuse.* Retrieved from http://www.ncea.aoa.gov/NCEAroot/Main_Site/FAQ/Basics/Risk_Factors.aspx

New York State Law Chapter 544, Identification and Reporting of Child Abuse and Maltreatment—Explaining Reporting Requirements—Study Requirements for Licensing. (1989).

Pillemer, K., & Moore, D. (1990). Highlights from a study of abuse of patients in nursing homes. *Journal of Elder Abuse and Neglect, 2,* 5–29.

Quinn, M. J., & Tomita, S. (1986). *Elder abuse and neglect.* New York, NY: Springer Publishing.

Quinn, M. J., & Tomita, S. (1997). *Elder abuse and neglect* (2nd ed.). New York, NY: Springer Publishing.

Reinharz, S. (1986). Loving and hating one's elders: Twin themes in legend and literature. In K. Pillemer & R. Wolf (Eds.), *Elder abuse conflict in the family* (pp. 25–48). Dover, MA: Auburn House Publishing.

Sullivan, P., & Knutson, J. (2000). Maltreatment and disabilities: A population-based epidemiological study. *Child Abuse and Neglect,* 24, 1257–1273.

U.S. Department of Health and Human Services, Administration for Children and Families. (2006). *Child neglect: A guide for prevention, assessment, and intervention.* Washington, DC: U.S. Government Printing Office.

U.S. Department of Health and Human Services, Children's Bureau. (2009). *Child maltreatment 2009.* Available from http://www.acf.hhs.gov/programs/cb/stats_research/index.htm#can

U.S. Department of Health and Human Services, Children's Bureau. (2010). *Child maltreatment 2008.* Available from www.acf.hhs.gov/programs/cb/pubs/cm08/index.htm

U.S. Department of Health and Human Services, National Center on Child Abuse and Neglect. (1994). *Child maltreatment 1992: Reports from the states to the National Center on Child Abuse and Neglect.* Washington, DC: U.S. Government Printing Office.

Wang, C., & Holton, J. (2007). *Total estimated cost of child abuse and neglect in the United States.* Chicago, Illinois: Prevent Child Abuse America. Retrieved from http://www.preventchildabuse.org/about_us/media_releases/pcaa_pew_economic_impact_study_final.pdf

Woolf, L. (1998). *Elder abuse and neglect.* Retrieved from http://www.webster.edu/~woolflm/abuse.html

RESOURCES

NOTE: The web addresses and phone numbers of these resources are fluid and should be checked for currency at time of use.

Administration on Aging
U.S. Department of Health and Human Services
330 Independence Avenue, SW
Washington, DC 20201
Telephone: 202-619-0724
Website: http://www.aoa.gov

Adult Protective Service (APS)
Call directory assistance and request the number for the department of social services or aging services in your county.

American Academy of Pediatrics
Check this website for information on what to know about child abuse developed by the American Academy of Pediatrics: http://www.aap.org/en-us/search/pages/results.aspx?k=child%20abuse

Area Agency on Aging
Look in the government section of your telephone directory under the terms *aging* or *elderly services*. This agency can provide the phone number for the local ombudsman for long-term care in your area.

Child Help USA Hotline
Telephone: 800-422-4453 (24 hours)
Website: http://www.childhelp.org

Elder Abuse Resources
Website: http://www.vachss.com

Eldercare Locator
For those who want to identify aging services in specific communities, call this Administration on Aging agency.
Telephone: 800-677-1116

Medicaid Fraud Control Units (MFCU)
Every State Attorney General's Office has an MFCU to prosecute Medicaid provider fraud and patient abuse in long-term care or home health care settings.

Mental Help Net
Provides information and referral numbers for numerous national hotlines. Website: http://mentalhelp.net/

National Center for Missing and Exploited Children
Helps families and professionals.
Telephone: 800-843-5678

National Center on Child Abuse and Neglect. (1993). *A report on the maltreatment of children with disabilities.* Washington, DC: U.S. Department of Health and Human Services.

National Center on Elder Abuse
State directory of help lines, hotlines, and elder abuse prevention resources. Website: http://www.ncea.aoa.gov/NCEAroot/Main_Site/Find_Help/Resources/Elders_Families.aspx

National Committee to Prevent Child Abuse
Website: http://www.healthline.com/galecontent/national-committee-to-prevent-child-abuse

National Domestic Violence Hotline
Helps children, parents, friends, and offenders of family violence.
Telephone: 800-799-7233

National Parent Hotline
Call for support from trained persons. Part of Parents Anonymous.
Telephone: 855-4APARENT
Website: http://www.nationalparenthelpline.org

National Respite Locator Service
Helps parents, caregivers, and professionals caring for children with disabilities, terminal illnesses, or those at risk of abuse.
Telephone: 800-677-1116

Youth Crisis Hotline
Helps individuals reporting child abuse of children ages 12 to 18.
Telephone: 800-448-4663

24

Service Delivery for Culturally and Linguistically Diverse Populations

Hortencia Kayser, PhD

SCOPE OF CHAPTER

During the past 40 years, speech-language pathologists and audiologists have become increasingly aware of the needs of culturally and linguistically diverse populations through the efforts of the American Speech-Language-Hearing Association (ASHA), state associations, and professional caucuses. Professionals are faced daily with the challenges of providing appropriate assessment and treatment to populations that historically have received little attention. The immigration pattern into the United States has also increased awareness that evidence-based practice is not available to these diverse populations (Scheffner Hammer, 2011). This chapter provides an overview of issues you will confront as a speech-language pathologist or audiologist in working with culturally and linguistically diverse populations.

The chapter begins with a demographic profile of culturally and linguistically diverse individuals in the United States. You are then introduced to factors that define and affect professional and clinical practice such as ASHA's position statements concerning individuals who are culturally and linguistically diverse, training needs in our professions, and specific issues affecting assessment and treatment of communication disorders in these populations.

DEMOGRAPHICS AND DESCRIPTIONS

Culturally and linguistically diverse (CLD) populations historically include Native, Hispanic, African, and Asian Americans. ASHA (2005) expanded the definition to encompass issues related to age, experience, ability, gender, race, ethnicity, language, religion, politics, physical challenges, sexual orientation, and socioeconomic status. This chapter focuses only on culturally and linguistically diverse populations, but you should be aware that diversity encompasses a broad range of characteristics. You will need to learn to work sensitively and competently with clients and colleagues who represent a variety of diverse backgrounds and attributes.

The U.S. Census Bureau (2008) predicts significant growth in CLD populations over the next 25 years. By 2042, minorities will constitute a majority in the United States. The Hispanic and African American populations are the two largest minority groups in the United States, 16.3 percent and 12.6 percent, respectively. The Asian population comprises about 5 percent of the U.S. population. The Hispanic population has become the largest ethnic group in the United States and will nearly triple to 133 million by 2050. The African American population will increase to 15 percent, and Asians will grow from 5.1 percent to 9.2 percent during this period (U.S. Census Bureau, 2010). The Hispanic population can be described as an explosion of newcomers for all parts of the nation. Table 24–1 provides demographics for the major groups in the United States as reported by the U.S. Census Bureau (2010).

TABLE 24–1 United States Population, 2010

Group	Estimate	Percentage*
Total	308,745,538	100.0
White	223,553,265	72.4
Hispanic	50,477,594	16.3
African American	38,929,319	12.6
Asian	14,674,252	4.8
Two or more races	9,009,073	2.9
American Indian and Alaska Native	2,932,249	0.9
Native Hawaiian/ Pacific Islander	540,013	0.2

From *Overview of Race and Hispanic Origin: 2010*, U.S. Census Bureau, 2010, Washington, DC: Author.

* Percentages do not add up to 100% because Hispanics can be of one or more races.

The increasing numbers of immigrant populations that have entered the United States are becoming an important factor in the nation's sociocultural, economic, and educational planning. The American Community Survey (U.S. Census Bureau, 2009) reported that about 12.5 percent of the population is foreign born. The largest contributors to this number come from Mexico (30 percent) and South and East Asia (about 23 percent).

An important factor in the description of new immigrants is their ability to speak English. In 2009, 21 percent of students in schools spoke a language other than English at home (National Center for Education Statistics, 2009). The 5.5 million English language learners (ELLs) in the public schools speak more than 276 languages. The American Community Survey (U.S. Census Bureau, 2008) reported that the children of immigrant families between the ages of 5 and 18 are perceived to speak English very well for all groups. Families from Mexico (54.3 percent), South America (66.8 percent), and the Middle East (55.5 percent) reported that their children spoke English very well (Pew Research Center, 2010). In contrast, families from the Caribbean (43.1 percent), Central America (45.5 percent), and South/East Asia (48 percent) had fewer children who spoke English very well.

The parents of immigrant children present a different language profile. Individuals older than 18 years are less likely to speak English very well. South and East Asian (41.6 percent) and Middle Eastern (47.2 percent) adults reported that they speak English very well. The adult populations from Mexico (20.4 percent), the Caribbean (24 percent), Central America (24.3 percent), and South

America (34.5 percent) had fewer people reporting that they spoke English very well. The younger the immigrant population group, the more likely the children will speak English well.

According to the 2006 American Community Survey (Brault, 2008), about 15 percent of the noninstitutionalized U.S. population over the age of five has a disability. This translates to more than 54 million people. The prevalence of disabilities among minority populations in the United States, however, appears higher, with Hispanics at about 17 percent and African Americans at 21 percent. The prevalence of disability among all races and ethnic groups for those receiving public assistance rises to 62 percent. Further, African American and Hispanic children live disproportionately in low-income and single-parent homes (Fujiura, Yamaki, & Czechowicz, 1998).

In 2009, of the 6.6 million students 3 to 21 years of age served through the Individuals with Disabilities Education Act (IDEA, 2004), about 22 percent had speech or language impairments, and 1 percent had hearing impairments (National Center for Education Statistics, 2011). Note, too, that many of the students in other disability categories also had speech, language, and/or hearing impairments.

Preschool and school caseloads reflect the growing diversity among students. According to the National Center for Education Statistics in 2010, 6 percent of children aged 3 to 5 and 9 percent of students 6 to 21 years of age were served under IDEA. Interestingly, the prevalence of American Indian/Alaska Native preschoolers receiving services was higher than any of the minority groups (9 percent). The percentage of minorities receiving these services during school age was higher for African Americans (12 percent), Hispanics (9 percent), and American Indians/Alaska Natives (14 percent) than for whites and Asians.

In 2009, the prevalence of poverty in the United States was estimated to be about 14.3 percent of the population (U.S. Census Bureau, 2009). The number of people in poverty in 2009 (43.6 million) is the largest number in the 51 years for which poverty estimates have been published (U.S. Census, 2010). The poverty rate for African Americans was 25.8 percent and for Hispanics, 25.3 percent. The poverty rate for children of all races and ethnic groups was 20 percent. Poverty was also associated with being foreign born, living in principal cities, residing in the South, and being in a household headed by a single female.

Poverty also affects individuals' ability to access health insurance and hence health care. In 2009, about 10 percent of children under 18 years of age had no health insurance. Nineteen percent of African Americans were uninsured, as were 32.1 percent of Hispanics (U.S. Census Bureau, 2009). Swartz (2009) in her analysis of health care and poverty states, "As we have come to appreciate how poor health can affect learning, which in turn is related to a person's productivity and earnings, awareness has grown that investing in ways to improve access to health care pays off in areas beyond health outcomes" (p. 69). Access to diagnostic and intervention programs for communication disorders, either in educational or health care settings, is also an important priority for all racial and ethnic groups in poverty.

Speech-Language Pathologists and Audiologists from Diverse Backgrounds

ASHA represents more than 150,000 speech-language pathologists; audiologists; and speech, language, and hearing scientists. In 2010, approximately 7.1 percent of certified members identified themselves as belonging to a racial, ethnic, or multiracial group. Table 24–2 provides a description of ASHA's membership by ethnicity or race (American Speech-Language-Hearing Association [ASHA], 2010a, 2010b). The largest groups are Hispanics (2.8 percent) and African Americans (2.2 percent).

Approximately 7,401 speech-language pathologists and audiologists, or 5.3 percent of the ASHA membership, have identified themselves as bilingual. The most common bilingual speaker can speak English and Spanish (2.1 percent). The majority of these professionals are located in the states of New York, California, Texas, Florida, Illinois, New Jersey, Massachusetts, and Pennsylvania. Thus, there appears to be a dearth of professionals who are from culturally and linguistically diverse backgrounds to meet the growing needs of these populations. We need professionals who understand cultural differences and who speak languages other than English (Scheffner Hammer, 2011).

Preparation of Communication Disorders Professionals from Diverse Backgrounds

Recruiting bicultural and bilingual students, educators, clinicians, and scientists has become an important priority for ASHA (2004). Recruitment begins

TABLE 24–2 American Speech-Language-Hearing Association Certified Membership by Ethnicity or Race, 2010

Race/Ethnicity	Total Number of Certified Speech-Language Pathologists and Audiologists
White	90,089
Race not specified	46,204
Hispanic	4,050
African American	3,093
Asian	1,960
Multiracial	1,276
American Indian/ Alaska Native	315
Native Hawaiian/ Pacific Islander	145
Total	143,081

From *Membership and Affiliation Profile: Highlights and Trends*, American Speech-Language-Hearing Association. (2010b). Adapted with permission. Available from http://www.asha.org/research/memberdata

in the elementary schools, through participation of audiologists and speech-language pathologists in recruitment fairs, parent programs, health fairs, and other community events that will introduce students to our professions. High school recruitment fairs are excellent avenues for young adults to hear about these professions. Universities can also promote recruitment programs that target culturally diverse students during recruitment trips, career fairs, and university events.

An important group to recruit is speech assistants. Professional assistants may need help in identifying college programs and financial assistance programs to support their education. A partnership between school districts and universities that provide online graduate courses could be developed to promote recruitment and graduation of CLD students in assistant programs. These individuals should then be encouraged to continue their education at the graduate level to become fully certified and licensed professionals.

Retention of students from CLD groups requires a commitment from college or university administrations for scholarships, tuition waivers, graduate assistantships, and financial aid packages. Academic assistance in the form of writing centers, tutoring sessions, and support groups from other CLD students all serve to support student success. Professionals who are culturally proficient and bilingual are of utmost importance for the professions to provide effective services for an increasingly culturally and linguistically diverse nation.

Preparation in Cultural Competence

Preparation in cultural competence begins at the undergraduate and graduate levels. ASHA includes cultural and linguistic diversity in a number of its standards for obtaining the Certificate of Clinical Competence (CCC) in speech-language pathology or audiology. Thus, college and university programs are expected to demonstrate that students have knowledge and skills in working with clients from diverse backgrounds. Some programs infuse these topics across coursework and clinical practicum and others also have specific coursework devoted to this topic.

To help prepare more professionals who are linguistically and culturally competent, a number of colleges and universities are creating innovative programs. The following are examples, but undoubtedly not a complete listing, of such programs. A certificate in bilingual speech-language pathology is available at the University of El Paso (Texas), San Diego State University, and Marquette University. Teachers College, Columbia University offers a bilingual/bicultural program focus to its master's program in speech-language pathology. The Department of Speech and Hearing Sciences at Arizona State University has a bilingual training track to prepare SLPs to work with bilingual populations. Texas Christian University also has an optional emphasis in bilingual speech-language pathology. Penn State University offers a program titled Multiplying Opportunities for Services and Access to Immigrant Children (MOSAIC) to train SLPs to work with English language learners. Students interested in developing skills to work with these populations should query their colleges, universities, and even potential employers about such opportunities.

Preparation in becoming more culturally competent begins but does not end at the graduate level.

Continuing education is an excellent opportunity to learn about various cultural groups and improve assessment, intervention, and counseling approaches for these clients and their caregivers. Educational opportunities are offered at national, state, and local conferences and through information provided by ASHA's Office of Multicultural Affairs. Lubinski and Matteliano (2008) prepared a *Guide to Cultural Competence in the Curriculum: Speech-Language Pathology* that provides a framework for developing multicultural knowledge and skills. ASHA's Special Interest Group 14, Culturally and Linguistically Diverse Populations, devotes its *Perspectives* publication to this topic and sponsors programs at the annual national convention.

ASHA DOCUMENTS

ASHA has been proactive in educating its membership concerning multicultural issues. A number of ASHA documents have made a tremendous impact on service delivery to culturally and linguistically diverse populations with communication disorders. These statements embody decades of discussion among speech-language pathologists, audiologists, and university researchers concerning best practices and the ethical responsibility of clinicians and researchers. As the decades have passed, the issues have become clearer and the commitment to resolve these concerns has become greater among CLD professionals and the association. Reading the complete position statements is the responsibility of the professional in clinical practice or in research. The following is a summary of each of these important position statements.

Social Dialects

The purpose of the position paper on social dialects (ASHA, 1983a) was to clarify ASHA's view of social dialects. The policy document makes it clear that dialectal variation of English is not a communication disorder. According to the position, all social dialects are adequate, functional, and effective varieties of English. Thus, children and adults are not to be admitted to treatment programs or identified as disordered solely on the basis of their dialect. However, individuals who speak a nonstandard English dialect may elect to have speech and language services to develop Standard American English. If a speech-language pathologist provides this service, the practitioner must work to preserve the integrity of the client's dialect. The speech-language pathologist must also have the clinical competency to provide this service by knowing the linguistic characteristics of the client's native dialect.

This position statement addressed an important issue. Children in the public schools were identified as speech and language disordered because of their use of African American English (AAE), Spanish Influenced English, or another social dialect that is viewed as nonstandard use of English. Individuals with these speech and language characteristics are not communicatively disordered. Recognition of these dialects as complete forms of a community's language becomes important in the scope of practice of speech-language pathologists and audiologists.

Clinical Management of Communicatively Handicapped Minority Language Populations

The clinical management position statement (ASHA, 1985) recommended those clinical competencies necessary to assess and treat communication disorders in culturally and linguistically diverse populations and to describe alternative strategies when these competencies are not met. Five competency areas were identified for bilingual speech-language pathologists and audiologists: (1) language proficiency (native or near-native fluency in both the minority language and the English language), (2) normative processes (ability to describe the process of normal speech and language acquisition for both bilingual and monolingual individuals, and how those processes are manifested in oral and written language), (3) assessment (the ability to administer and interpret formal and informal assessment procedures to distinguish between communication difference and communication disorders), (4) intervention (the ability to apply intervention strategies for treatment of communicative disorders in the native language), and (5) cultural sensitivity (the ability to recognize cultural factors that affect the delivery of speech-language pathology and audiology services to non-English-speaking communities).

The position statement acknowledged the difficulty in acquiring bilingual speech-language pathologists and audiologists; therefore, five alternative strategies for acquiring bilingual personnel were included: (1) establish contacts (e.g., find consultants who can provide the service); (2) establish cooperatives (e.g., a group of agencies or school districts could share one bilingual speech-language pathologist or audiologist); (3) establish networks (e.g., ties could be developed between agencies and university programs that might have bilingual graduate students, and these students can then be recruited by the agencies); (4) establish Clinical Fellowship and graduate practicum sites (e.g., bilingual graduate students could be used to assist personnel in schools and other facilities); (5) establish interdisciplinary teams (e.g., a team approach could be developed among the monolingual speech-language-pathologist or audiologist and bilingual professionals such as teachers, psychologists, and nurses who are knowledgeable of nonbiased assessment procedures and development of the client's language).

The final recommendation in the position statement listed those individuals who may serve as interpreters or translators. It is important to know the difference between these two terms. Interpreters communicate one language into the other orally. Translators communicate one language into the other by written form. Interpreters can be recruited from language banks, bilingual professional staff, family members, or friends of the client. Note that use of the family or friend is the last resort because interpreters must have training and knowledge of clinical procedures. Family members may not interpret accurately because of cultural roles, protection of the family member, or not understanding the professionals' statements (Kayser, 1989).

This position statement was of particular importance because it served as the basis in curriculum development for many minority-emphasis graduate programs in speech-language pathology and audiology. The majority of the competencies for clinicians who serve CLD clients are stated clearly, but the language proficiency competency for speech-language pathologists and audiologists was not well defined and has been revisited by several ASHA committees several times with no clear resolution. Since the acceptance of this paper by ASHA's Executive Board and Legislative Council, research and best practices with English language learners have advanced our understanding of assessment and treatment practices with diverse populations. The clinical management paper is in the process of revision by the Multicultural Issues Board to address current evidence-based practice in assessment and intervention.

Bilingual Speech-Language Pathologists and Audiologists

The primary purpose of this ASHA position paper was to define the term *bilingual*, to protect the public from clinicians who claim to have bilingual abilities, and to serve as a model for clinicians who aspire to become bilingual (ASHA, 1989). The definition stated that speech-language pathologists or audiologists who identify themselves as bilingual must be able to speak their primary language and speak (or sign) at least one other language with native or near-native proficiency in semantics, phonology, morphology/syntax, and pragmatics during clinical management. Many bilingual professionals have attempted to meet the intent of this definition and, through continuing education, have met the academic competencies as outlined in the 1985 clinical management position statement (ASHA, 1985). Language proficiency in the second language can be evaluated through testing services in university language programs or by state education agencies that certify teachers. Regardless of the method chosen by clinicians to document academic competencies and language proficiency, they are bound by the ASHA Code of Ethics to provide quality services to all clients (ASHA, 1994). ASHA does not provide a mechanism to determine the language proficiency of bilingual professionals and depends upon self-identification through the Office of Multicultural Affairs. ASHA keeps a registry of bilingual professionals.

The Speech-Language Pathologist and English as a Second Language

The growing number of children in schools from culturally and linguistically diverse populations has increased the likelihood of professionals serving as instructors of English as a Second Language (ESL). School districts may not have ESL instructors and thus view the speech-language pathologist as the alternative language service provider for a child who does not speak English. This position statement on provision of ESL instruction by speech-language pathologists in school settings (ASHA, 1998) states that ESL instructors require specialized academic preparation in areas such as second language acquisition, comparative linguistics, and ESL pedagogy. Speech-language pathologists typically do not have this academic preparation in their graduate studies program. Speech-language pathologists must therefore examine their education and experience relative to their state's credentialing for ESL teachers. The clinician who does not have this specialized background should not provide direct instruction in ESL but should collaborate with ESL instructors to provide preassessment, assessment, and intervention with children who are English language learners.

This is an important statement because it defines for school speech-language pathologists ASHA's position on our scope of practice, how we can enhance service delivery systems, how to appropriately identify and serve students from culturally and linguistically diverse groups, and how important it is to comply with the ASHA Code of Ethics (ASHA, 1994), state and federal mandates, and school district policy.

Students and Professionals Who Speak English with Accents and Nonstandard Dialects: Issues and Recommendations

This paper was a combined position statement and technical report (ASHA, 1997). The technical report was developed to describe the inequities and discrimination reported to the National Office concerning employment practices, clinical training, and selection of CLD graduate students into graduate programs in communication sciences and disorders. The technical paper provided guidelines and suggestions for clinical and graduate faculty to improve circumstances for graduate students with accents or dialects viewed as nonstandard English. ASHA's position is that students and professionals in communication sciences and disorders who speak with accents and/or dialects can effectively provide speech, language, and audiology services to individuals with communication disorders as long as they have the expected knowledge. No research indicates that individuals who speak with accents are less likely to perform well in clinical situations than a Standard American English speaker. Additionally, ASHA members must not discriminate against people who speak with an accent or dialect in educational programs, employment, or service delivery. This paper was a critical turning point in the fair treatment of professionals and graduate students in communication sciences and disorders. The recruitment and retention of CLD students in speech-language pathology and audiology are important outcomes of this paper.

Knowledge and Skills Needed by Speech-Language Pathologists and Audiologists to Provide Culturally and Linguistically Appropriate Services

This competency paper was written to encourage clinicians to continue lifelong learning to develop the knowledge and skills required to provide culturally and linguistically appropriate services, and it specifies the knowledge and skills needed (ASHA, 2004). It also serves as a guide to identify those weaknesses and strengths in our knowledge in serving CLD populations. The seven topics addressed in this paper expanded our scope of practice in the following areas: (1) cultural competence, (2) language competencies of the clinician, (3) language, (4) articulation and phonology, (5) resonance/voice/fluency, (6) swallowing, and (7) hearing/balance. Each section identifies specific areas of knowledge and skills necessary to appropriately serve culturally and linguistically diverse populations. Professionals who work in different clinical settings may view the whole document as daunting, but its purpose is to identify those sections that are of critical importance for an individual's clinical practice.

Cultural Competence

The ASHA Board of Ethics (2005) provided a definition of cultural competence with the purpose of promoting sensitivity and increasing awareness of cultural diversity. The board used specific sections of the Code of Ethics and related these to cultural diversity. For example, Principle of Ethics I, Rule C speaks directly to the issue of clinical and research activities by prohibiting discrimination in the delivery of services or the conduct of research and scholarly activities on the basis of race, ethnicity, gender, age, religion, national origin, sexual orientation, or disability. Rules A and B direct members to provide services competently and to use every resource, including referral when appropriate. Referral is necessary when cultural or linguistic differences negatively influence outcomes. Principle of Ethics II, Rule C states that members shall continue professional development throughout their careers. This means that clinicians should develop the knowledge and skills required to provide culturally and linguistically appropriate services. Principle of Ethics I, Rule E prohibits delegation of tasks that are beyond the competence of a bilingual assistant or interpreter without adequate supervision from a certified clinician. This is particularly important when the clinician does not speak the language that the assistant is using in treatment. The final principle, Ethics IV, Rule H, provides guidance in our interactions with colleagues and students, prohibiting discrimination against these individuals for any reason.

These documents have provided guidance and proactive commitment to diversity within the fields of speech-language pathology and audiology. As the association has grown, the professions have become aware of the ethical responsibility to cultural competence and appropriate services to culturally and linguistically diverse populations. See Chapter 5 on ethics for further discussion.

CLINICAL ISSUES AFFECTING CULTURALLY AND LINGUISTICALLY DIVERSE POPULATIONS

Three major clinical issues confront speech-language pathologists and audiologists when providing services to CLD populations. The first is an understanding of bilingualism and second language acquisition and its impact on decisions made by professionals in the areas of assessment and treatment. The second is the use of evidence-based practice with culturally and linguistically diverse populations and the recognition that research among white children does not generalize to CLD groups. The third issue is the appropriate assessment and treatment of children and adults using interpreters and/or professionals. The remainder of this chapter briefly discusses these issues.

Bilingualism and Second Language Acquisition

Baetens-Beardsmore (1986) stated that the term *bilingualism* has different meanings for different individuals. For some, it may be equal abilities in two languages, for others, it may be the functional use of a second language. Bilingualism has been defined with varying degrees of strictness, depending on how proficient or competent a speaker must be to be considered bilingual. Valdes and Figueroa (1995) defined bilingualism as knowledge of "more than one" language. Their framework for bilingualism is described as a continuum of proficiencies. Children may be fluent in Spanish, L1, but have limited proficiency in English, L2. Some children are fluent in English but may have limited fluency in Spanish. Between these points, there is individual variation in the proficiency for each language.

Societal and individual variables affect the individual differences in children's bilingualism and proficiency in the two languages. Societal factors include urban or rural habitation, distance from the native tongue country, frequency of visits to the homeland, number of speakers of the language in the community, length of residence in the United States, native literacy in the community, native language education, and church or community centers that serve as a gathering place for use of the native language. In addition, individual variables that influence bilingualism include ethnic identity, emotional attachment to the native language, emphasis on family ties, language attrition (loss), motivation to use the home language, attitude toward the mainstream community, and need for use of the native language and English (Baetens-Beardsmore, 1986).

Internationally Adopted Children

Recently, internationally adopted children have become an important population for service delivery. In the past 30 years, more than 265,000 children have been internationally adopted. In 2009 alone, more than 12,700 international adoptions took place in the United States (U.S. Department of State, 2009). The majority have come from Asia and Eastern European countries. The speech and language reports on these children have been mixed. For example, Glennon and Masters (2002) reported few delays in language development 21 to 36 months postadoption for children from Eastern Europe and China. Yet, Glennon (2002) reported that children adopted from Eastern Europe are at risk of developing language and learning problems if scaled scores were below 75 on the Communication and Symbolic Behavior Scales-Developmental Profile and/or if the child had significant delays in symbolic play. Glennon (2007) suggests that early assessment can be useful in making early intervention decisions with these children.

Research continues at more than 60 agencies across the country. The majority of these centers are located in medical centers and focus on the health, growth, and well-being of internationally adopted children. Centers for speech and language development are still in development across the country. The majority of these children come from different environmental backgrounds that either have supported or not supported these children's growth and development, including speech and language. Hearing health and sensitivity may not have been addressed while the children were in orphanages. Losing their first language will likely be inevitable unless the adopting parents insist on supporting the language through involvement in a native language community or educational programming.

How children progress in their development of English while they lose their native language is still unknown. It is likely that the majority of these children, if adopted before the age of one year and placed in rich language environments and homes, will learn English and become academically successful in American schools. Older children may have more difficulty. Research is needed for clinicians to appropriately respond to the needs of internationally adopted children and their families. For more information on international adoptions and speech-language development, see Hwa-Froelich (2011) and Pollock (n.d.) in the Resources section of the chapter.

Evidence-Based Practice in Assessment and Treatment

Professionals do their best to correctly identify speech, language, and hearing disorders in individuals. This includes the assessment of individuals who are second language learners and culturally and linguistically diverse. It is difficult to provide service to a population when you do not speak the language of the client and are unfamiliar with the cultural norms. Assessing individuals only in English does not provide an appropriate or equitable evaluation. Kohnert (2008) succinctly describes the problem. She states: "Surface similarities between typically developing children learning a second language and monolingual children with language disorders lie at the heart of difference or disordered diagnostic challenge faced by SLPs and special educators" (p. 98).

Assessment and treatment of culturally and linguistically diverse clients should include practices that rely on evidence-based research. The literature has focused on recommendations for clinical practice with CLD populations. There is a growing awareness among professionals of the limitations of expert opinion as the basis for clinical decision making. ASHA (2005) recommended that professionals incorporate the principles of evidence-based practice in clinical decision making to provide high-quality clinical care. Evidence-based practice refers to current high-quality research evidence that is integrated with practitioner expertise and client preferences and values into the process of making clinical decisions (ASHA, 2005). The four recommended steps toward the implementation of a treatment program include (1) framing the clinical question, (2) finding the evidence, (3) assessing the evidence, and (4) making the clinical decision. For professionals working with CLD populations, finding and assessing the evidence are the most difficult steps to complete because of the lack of evidence. When professionals have limited evidence, ASHA (2005) recommends that they evaluate individual studies based on the type of study design and whether the study was implemented appropriately. Ultimately, the treatment provided to clients should consider patient preference, cost-effectiveness, potential harm, and availability of alternative treatments.

The profession recognizes that many speech-language pathologists and audiologists lack the knowledge to serve CLD populations (Roseberry-McKibben, 2002), but we are bound by the ASHA Code of Ethics to do all that we can to serve and learn about CLD populations in our clinical practice (ASHA, 2005).

Assessment The first step toward appropriate services is to recognize that test instruments are to serve us in identifying the strengths and weaknesses of these clients' English capabilities, which includes their perception of English sounds. The test instruments alone do not tell us whether a speech, language, or hearing disorder exists in the client, which means we use resources beyond the test instrument to help identify communication disorders in CLD clients.

Test instruments are important for accurate and objective assessment of individuals with communication disorders in monolingual English-speaking populations. They help determine the client's communication abilities by comparing the performance to a "typically developing" population. Norms are usually developed from primarily middle-class, English-speaking subjects of European background. Some test instruments include a small percentage of CLD populations in their test development statistics, but once the means are calculated, this only serves to lower the norms and not appropriately assess the CLD groups.

When speech-language pathologists assess individuals who do not fit normative data provided for test instruments, accurate assessment becomes problematic for a number of reasons. First, it is inappropriate to administer tests in a language different from that given to the test instrument normative group. If a test instrument is translated, this compromises test validity and reliability. In addition, cultural and linguistic differences may affect the interactions between the client and clinician and thus compromise testing results.

Culture must play a dominant role in the development of any diagnostic or behavioral test. When tested, clients may perform differently because of their cultural background (Kayser, 1989; Kummerer, Lopez-Reyna, & Tejero-Hughes, 2007). Because of a client's linguistic differences, belief systems, and cultural background, results in levels of communicative competence may vary from those of the mainstream population. Test instruments typically reflect the culture of the test developer and present speech and language stimuli thought to be familiar to all individuals. A CLD client may not, however, have had the same cultural and language experiences as the majority population. A limited number of test instruments have been developed for CLD populations. Unfortunately, variations of the language and the cultural expectations of children may change with assimilation into the mainstream culture. In addition to test instruments, the professionals should be alerted to other means of assessment of children and adults from another culture. Typically, nonstandard procedures or modified procedures are used for assessment.

The use of nonstandard or modified procedures in the assessment of linguistically diverse clients is a common practice among clinicians (Erickson & Iglesias, 1986; Kayser, 1989a, 1995a,b). The clinician initially administers a test using standardized procedures. The clinician readministers the test by altering the procedures to allow more response time or to allow for dialectal variations in the client's responses. Other modified procedures include rewording instructions, providing more examples, having the child explain the "error" response, administering items beyond the test ceiling, and allowing other similar test responses. The purpose of these modified procedures is to obtain as much information as possible about a client's strengths and weaknesses in communication and not rely on the final test score and how the client compares to a mainstream English-speaking population.

Another suggestion is to adapt a test instrument so that it becomes culturally appropriate for the target population (Kayser, 1995a). The test instrument is adapted so that the content and/or tasks become culturally familiar to the client. For example, the vocabulary may be adapted to words used in the community. The task used to elicit a response may be unfamiliar or unnatural to the individual; therefore, a change is made so that the area of speech and language tested can be assessed using a more culturally acceptable task. Once tests are adapted, the original test no longer exists. The norms are now invalid and inappropriate for comparisons. The adaptation of a standardized test results in the loss of standardization, thus reducing validity and reliability. The professional must describe the performance of the client and compare this performance to known developmental norms for a particular population.

An alternative approach to testing is to use systematic observations of the target individual, ethnographic interviewing of the family concerning the client's use of language and communicative competence, published questionnaires for parents and teachers, review of supporting documents from other agencies, and dynamic assessment.

Dynamic assessment includes a test-teach-retest protocol for observing and evaluating the learning process of a child or adult from a CLD background (Gutierrez-Clellen, Peña, & Quinn, 1995; Peña & Gillam, 2000; Peña, Iglesias, & Lidz, 2001). The clinician begins by assessing children's abilities in areas such as vocabulary or narratives. The teach session, also called *mediation,* requires the clinician to attempt to teach the child something about what is expected in the assessment phase. The retest phase is repeated to assess the outcomes of the learning process. Dynamic assessment allows the clinician to make inferences about the child's learning potential and what strengths the child has in learning. Significant research supports dynamic assessment in distinguishing children who are language impaired from children with typical language skills.

Testing does not provide speech-language pathologists and audiologists all of the answers to our questions about clients from CLD backgrounds. Available test instruments will provide a limited view of the client's abilities. Clinicians must explore new methods of assessment to distinguish language differences from disorders in these populations. See the ASHA website for a variety of resources for assessing CLD populations.

Treatment Culturally diverse communities may have their own traditional ways of caring for individuals with disabilities. When families hold beliefs that are different from the mainstream, they may be unlikely to seek out educational, medical, or other health care services (Rodriguez, & Olswang, 2003; Saenz & Huer, 2003; Salas-Provance, Erickson, & Reed, 2002). Intervention requires that a client's communication needs are met through an understanding of what the family needs, values, and considers appropriate intervention services. Treatment programs for CLD clients should consider language of instruction, content of therapy that is culturally sensitive and facilitates learning, and appropriate collaboration with interpreters for optimum outcomes.

Language of Instruction English has been the language of choice for interventions for the majority of CLD clients, whether or not the client speaks English. Choice may not exist if intervention in the home language is not possible. Research supports the use of the native language in therapy. Perozzi (1985), Perozzi and Chavez-Sanchez (1992), and Kiernan and Swisher (1990) began the investigation of language of instruction with Spanish-English-speaking and Native American children. Their work with single-subject designs supported native language instruction. They concluded that it may be instrumental in helping CLD children with language impairments to develop skills in both the native language and the majority language. Both research groups suggested that a bilingual curriculum is better than teaching only in English. Gutierrez-Clellen (1999) reviewed the literature concerning language choice in intervention with bilingual children and presented evidence from bilingual education in Canada and the United States that concluded that instruction in the native language is beneficial to learning the English language. Gutierrez-Clellen (1999) and Kohnert, Yim, Nett, Kan, and Duran (2005) recommend the use of the native language for instruction because of an additive effect that occurs for those children who maintain the use of the native language while learning English. Additive bilingualism occurs in children, and the results are higher performance in academic achievement as well as higher proficiency in two languages than if children were instructed only in English.

Treatment Content Cultural sensitivity has been a theme among advocates for culturally and linguistically diverse individuals with communication disorders (Kayser, 1993; Saville-Troike, 1986). Cultural sensitivity may then affect the content of the therapy. Kayser (1993) states that background research about a culture may be necessary to plan appropriate culturally sensitive therapy. Preparation may include observations of the community and discussion with bilingual professionals and families to understand those aspects of culture that may be unfamiliar, offensive, and inappropriate within the therapy session. Recognizing the values and community activities also will provide clinicians with a wealth of content and materials for speech and language treatment as well as aural stimuli for the audiologist. For example, one clinician learned about an Easter custom among Mexican American families. Children and adults cracked colorful dried eggshells filled with confetti over each other's heads. These eggshells are called *cascarones*. Although the clinician had worked with Hispanic children for 20 years, she had never heard of this custom. She introduced the topic in therapy with groups of Hispanic children on her caseload and was surprised that the children could explain, describe, and sequence the making of these cascarones (Kayser, 1995b).

Lynch and Hanson (2004) recommend four effective ways to begin to gather information about other cultures: (1) learning through books, the arts, and technology; (2) talking and working with individuals from the culture who can act as cultural guides and mediators; (3) participating in the daily life of another culture; and (4) learning the language of another culture. Working with clients from other cultures will take an investment of time, effort, reading, and recognizing when to ask more questions to fully understand what else you need to know.

Paraprofessionals, Interpreters, and Translators

Using a nonprofessional as an interpreter may appear to be an adequate solution to an immediate need, but the process of interpretation can be problematic. Interpreting for another individual is a learned skill and not an ability that comes naturally. Langdon (1988) reports that interpreters may omit, add information, use the wrong word, or transpose information. Interpreters must be trained carefully before they are used for client-family conferences, assessment, and treatment.

Paraprofessionals and interpreters provide two separate clinical roles that require different training. A *paraprofessional,* as defined by ASHA (1983b, 1993), is any person who, after receiving on-the-job or academic training, provides clinical services that are prescribed and directed by a certified speech-language pathologist or audiologist. An *interpreter* is one who conveys information from one language to the other in the oral modality. A *translator* conveys information in the written modality (Langdon, 1992). Paraprofessionals, interpreters, and translators should have a minimum of a high school diploma with communication skills that are adequate for the tasks assigned by the clinician. Interpreters and translators should have oral and written abilities in English and the minority language. All bilingual individuals are not capable of acquiring these skills. Professional interpreting and translation require training and advanced linguistic skills in two languages (Kayser, 1989, 1995a).

Langdon (1992) suggests that the roles of the interpreter and translator require an ability to stay emotionally uninvolved with the discussions or content of the material. Both must maintain confidentiality and neutrality, accept the clinician's authority, and be able to work with other professional staff (Kayser, 1989, 1995a). When a family member or friend becomes the interpreter, information relayed to the family may be omitted or misunderstood (Kayser, 1989, 1995a). Interpreters are increasingly part of the practice of speech-language pathologists and audiologists. Training for both the professional and the interpreter/translator will produce valid and reliable interactions with the client who does not speak or read English.

The paraprofessional/interpreter's role may include screening of speech, language, and/or hearing; treatment activities that do not require clinical decision making; chart recording; clinical record maintenance; preparation of clinical materials; and testing of hearing aids. The paraprofessional and/or interpreter should not be responsible for interpreting data, determining caseloads, transmitting clinical information to other professionals, preparing reports, referring clients to other professionals, or using a title other than that assigned by the professional (ASHA, 1993). See Chapter 12 for more on the topic of paraprofessionals.

AUDIOLOGY AND MULTICULTURAL POPULATIONS

The American Speech-Language-Hearing Association (2010a) reported that there are approximately 711 audiologists in the association that are from culturally and linguistically diverse populations. The number of bilingual audiologists in clinical settings is limited, and therefore alternatives must be adopted to ensure that CLD populations are served appropriately (Newman-Ryan, DeLeon-Northrup, & Villarreal-Emery, 2005). Language barriers and cultural differences do influence the audiometric evaluation of non-English-speaking populations (Hodgson & Montgomery, 1994). Clients who do not understand English can have a frustrating experience when they are uncertain of what is expected of them for a response and what exactly the audiologist will be administering during the evaluation. It becomes especially frustrating for both the clinician and client when questions arise during the protocols. Hodgson and Montgomery (1994) recommend answering three questions during an evaluation: (1) How great is the loss of hearing sensitivity? (2) What type of hearing loss is present? (3) How good is word recognition ability as a function of clarity of hearing? The first two questions can be answered with little to no ability of the audiologist to speak the client's language. The third question must be answered with the use of speech. Perception of another language with the confounding variable of hearing loss makes the evaluation less likely to be valid. Testing with words that are familiar makes the evaluation much more reliable and valid.

Northrup (1985) provided additional guidelines for audiologists who are not proficient in the client's native language:

1. Use gestures with clear and simple instructions.
2. Use translated written cards for literate clients.
3. Be aware of limitations in using a case history with clients.
4. Be cautious in interpreting the data.
5. Inform the client that test procedures are not harmful.
6. All consent documents should be in the client's native language, or an interpreter must be available to explain the forms.
7. Before testing, determine language preference.

The audiologist should also consider that CLD groups may have a different prevalence of hearing disorders and ear infections. For example, Native Americans have persistent ear infections, presumed to be caused by an anatomical difference in the angle of the eustachian tube. Many cultures have specific beliefs about the appropriate interactions of opposite genders, such as the audiologist touching the patient's head or ears. Sensitivity to these possibilities is important. The reporting of the test results becomes problematic when there is no interpreter who can relay the information to an individual who does not understand English. Sensitive information such as a progressive hearing loss or the effects of sickle cell anemia on a hearing mechanism should be provided with cultural sensitivity (Scott, 2002). The use of interpreters who understand audiometric terminology becomes extremely important to the audiologist in explaining the procedures and results with sensitivity to the client's cultural background. Similarly, translators must have proficiency in both languages as well as a knowledge base of hearing loss terminology.

Audiologists have an important role in educating CLD populations of all ages. Identifying children through neonatal screenings, relaying information to parents in the native language, and providing follow-up services through medical professionals and speech-language pathologists who can provide ongoing services for these children become paramount. Exposure of children to unsafe noise levels, such as at arcades and sporting events, is a concern. The American Academy of Audiology (2010) reports that as many as 12 percent of children between the ages of six and nine have noise-induced hearing loss. Children from all populations are at risk of acquiring noise-induced hearing loss, and audiologists need to inform parents from all backgrounds of the consequences of prolonged exposure to noisy environments.

CLD groups have other areas of need. Audiologists may work with clients and families regarding aural rehabilitation, hearing aid use, assistive listening and alerting devices, and acoustic needs in the classroom or workplace. In addition, cochlear implants should be available to individuals from other cultures. Auditory processing disorders may be related to learning disabilities, and thus, it is imperative that audiologists accurately diagnose this type of problem in all children. Keep in mind Kenneth Wolf's (2004) comment, "Audiologists should approach cultural competence as they do clinical competence: with a commitment to lifelong learning. Although the body of literature in audiology and the number of courses available have not been vast, they are growing. We need to seek and apply new knowledge so that we can successfully meet the hearing health care challenges presented by the rapidly changing demographics of the United States."

WHAT IS THE NEXT STEP IN DEVELOPING CULTURAL COMPETENCE?

ASHA (2011) suggests that you might develop your cultural competence through a variety of activities. For example, you might volunteer for a multicultural constituency group or join Special Interest Group 14. You can also mentor students from minority backgrounds; participate in local, state, and national advocacy and lobbying programs; and encourage at the grassroots level a greater awareness of multicultural issues in your own workplaces. Identifying and solving a particular unmet communication need in your own community may be the best action. Further, mobilizing your clients from diverse backgrounds to become self-advocates encourages them to assume responsibility for their communication needs. Some professionals may choose to learn another language or visit another country to become more familiar with cultural differences. Finally, our research agenda in both speech-language pathology and audiology should encourage focused study of the communication characteristics, needs, and intervention approaches for multicultural groups of all kinds.

SUMMARY

This chapter introduced a variety of issues that confront speech-language pathologists and audiologists working with culturally and linguistically diverse populations with communication disorders. ASHA position statements were briefly described concerning culturally and linguistically diverse populations. Each of these issues has an impact on the quality of service provided to multicultural populations. Issues discussed included demographics; communication disorders in culturally and linguistically diverse populations; testing; treatment; and paraprofessionals, interpreters, and translators. ASHA has been a leader among professional associations in providing its membership with information concerning culturally and linguistically diverse people and continues to provide information to the public and its members. Advocacy at the grassroots or state and national levels is critical to bringing quality services to these growing populations.

CRITICAL THINKING

1. The ASHA position statements concerning culturally and linguistically diverse populations have made a tremendous impact on the clinical practice in our fields of speech-language pathology and audiology. Describe your perceptions of these position statements and how you might approach cultural competency in service provision to CLD populations.
2. Standardized testing is only one part of the diagnostic evaluation of CLD populations. How would you describe the inadequacies of tests to another professional? To the client? To parents? What nonstandardized assessment procedures are useful for CLD populations? How would you report these results in your documentation?
3. Providing treatment to children and adults who speak a language different from yours is a challenge to most professionals. How would you approach this challenge and whom would you ask for assistance? What are the advantages and disadvantages of using family versus professional interpreters?
4. Everyone has a culture. How would you describe your own culture? How do you think your own cultural background affects your provision of clinical services?
5. What are some ways you could increase your understanding of another culture that is near you at home, work, or school? Suppose you take a clinical position that serves a CLD population. How would you upgrade your knowledge base and skills to work effectively in this position?
6. What ethical issues might you face in working with individuals from different cultural and linguistic backgrounds? Review the ASHA or AAA Code of Ethics for issues that affect service to CLD populations.
7. How can we attract more individuals from diverse backgrounds into speech-language pathology and audiology? What would you recommend to your school district to recruit individuals from diverse backgrounds to become speech-language pathologists and audiologists?

REFERENCES

American Academy of Audiology (2010). *Hearing loss in children*. Retrieved from http://www.howsyourhearing.com/hearinglossinchildren.html

American Speech-Language-Hearing Association. (1983a). Position paper: Social dialects and implications of the position on social dialects. *ASHA, 25,* 23–27.

American Speech-Language-Hearing Association. (1983b). *Guidelines for the employment and utilization of supportive personnel.* Rockville, MD: Author.

American Speech-Language-Hearing Association. (1985). Clinical management of communicatively handicapped minority language populations. *ASHA, 27,* 29–32.

American Speech-Language-Hearing Association. (1989). Bilingual speech-language pathologists and audiologists. *ASHA, 31,* 93.

American Speech-Language-Hearing Association. (1993). *Position statement and guidelines for the education/training, use, and supervision of support personnel in speech-language pathology and audiology.* Rockville, MD: Author.

American Speech-Language-Hearing Association. (1994). Code of ethics. *ASHA, 36* (Suppl. 13), 1–2.

American Speech-Language-Hearing Association. (1998). Provision of English as-a-second-language instruction by speech-language pathologists in school settings. *ASHA, 40* (Suppl. 18).

American Speech-Language-Hearing Association. (2004). Knowledge and skills needed by speech-language pathologists and audiologists to provide culturally and linguistically appropriate services. *ASHA Supplement, 24*.

American Speech-Language-Hearing Association. (2005). Cultural competence. *ASHA Supplement, 25*.

American Speech-Language-Hearing Association. (2010a). *Demographic profile of ASHA members providing bilingual and Spanish-language services*. Rockville, MD: Author.

American Speech-Language-Hearing Association. (2010b). *Highlights and trends: ASHA counts for year end 2010*. Rockville, MD: Author.

American Speech-Language-Hearing Association. (2011). *The ABC's of empowerment through volunteering in ASHA*. Available from http://www.asha.org/practice/multicultural/opportunities/ABC/

American Speech-Language-Hearing Association Joint Subcommittee of the Executive Board on English Language Proficiency. (1997). Students and professionals who speak English with accents and nonstandard dialects: Issues and recommendations. *ASHA, 40* (Suppl. 18).

Baetens-Beardsmore, H. (1986). *Bilingualism: Basic principles*. San Diego, CA: College-Hill Press.

Brault, M. (2008). *Disability status and the characteristics of people in group quarters: A brief analysis of disability prevalence among the cilivlian noninstitutionalized and total populations in the American Community Survey*. Retrieved from http://www.census.gov/hhes/www/disability/GQdisability.pdf

Erickson, J., & Iglesias, A. (1986). Assessment of communication disorders in non-English proficient children. In O. Taylor (Ed.), *Nature of communication disorders in culturally and linguistically diverse populations* (pp. 181–218). San Diego, CA: College-Hill Press.

Fujiura, G., Yamaki, K., & Czechowicz, S. (1998). Disability among ethnic and racial minorities in the United States. *Journal of Disability Policy Studies. 9*, 111–130.

Glennon, S. (2002). Language development and delay in internationally adopted infants and toddlers: A review. *American Journal of Speech-Language Pathology, 11*(4), 333–339.

Glennon, S. (2007). Predicting language outcomes for internationally adopted children. *Journal of Speech, Language, and Hearing Research, 50*, 529–548.

Glennon, S., & Masters, M. G. (2002). Typical and atypical language development in infants and toddlers adopted from Eastern Europe. *American Journal of Speech-Language Pathology, 11*(4), 417–433.

Gutiérrez-Clellen, V. F. (1999). Language choice in intervention with bilingual children. *American Journal of Speech-Language Pathology, 8*, 291–302.

Gutierrez-Clellen, V. F., Peña, E., & Quinn, R. (1995). Accommodating cultural differences in narrative style: A multicultural perspective. *Topics in Language Disorders, 15*, 54–67.

Hodgson, W. R., & Montgomery, P. (1994). Hearing impairment and bilingual children: Considerations in assessment and intervention. *Seminars in Speech and Language, 15*(2), 174–182.

Individuals with Disabilities Education Improvement Act of 2004, Pub. L. No. 108-446 (2004).

Kayser, H. (1989). Speech and language assessment of Spanish-English speaking children. *Language, Speech, and Hearing Services in Schools, 30*, 226–244.

Kayser, H. (1993). Hispanic cultures. In D. Battle (Ed.), *Communication disorders in multicultural populations* (pp. 114–157). Boston, MA: Andover Medical Publishers.

Kayser, H. (1995a). *Bilingual speech-language pathology: An Hispanic focus*. Clifton Park, NY: Delmar Cengage Learning.

Kayser, H. (1995b). Intervention with children from linguistically and culturally diverse backgrounds. In M. E. Fey, J. Windsor, & S. F. Warren (Eds.), *Language intervention: Preschool through the elementary years* (pp. 315–332). Baltimore, MD: Paul H. Brookes.

Kiernan, B., & Swisher, L. (1990). The initial learning of novel English words: Two single-subject experiments with minority-language children. *Journal of Speech and Hearing Research, 33*, 707–716.

Kohnert, K. (2008). *Language disorders in bilingual children and adults.* San Diego, CA: Plural Publishing.

Kohnert, K., Yim, D., Nett, K., Kan, P. F., & Duran, L. (2005). Intervention with linguistically diverse preschool children: A focus on developing home language(s). *Language, Speech, and Hearing Services in Schools, 36,* 251–263.

Kummerer, S. E., Lopez-Reyna, N. A., & Tejero-Hughes, M. (2007). Mexican immigrant mothers' perceptions of their children's communication disabilities, emergent literacy development, and speech-language therapy program. *American Journal of Speech-Language Pathology, 16,* 271–282.

Langdon, H. (1988). *Working with an interpreter/translator in the school setting. Dimensions of appropriate assessment for minority handicapped students: Recommended practices.* Presented at the State Conference for School Superintendents, Tucson, AZ.

Langdon, H. (1992). Speech and language assessment of LEP/bilingual Hispanic students. In H. Langdon & L. R. L. Cheng (Eds.), *Hispanic children and adults with communication disorders* (pp. 201–271). Gaithersburg, MD: Aspen Publishers.

Lubinski, R., & Matteliano, M. (2008). *A guide to cultural competence in the curriculum speech-language pathology.* Buffalo, NY: Center for International Rehabilitation Research Information and Exchange.

Lynch, E. W., & Hanson, M. J. (2004). *Developing cross-cultural competence* (3rd ed.). Baltimore, MD: Paul H. Brookes.

National Center for Education Statistics. (2009). *The condition of education.* Available from http://nces.ed.gov/programs/coe/.figures.figure-lsm-1.asp

National Center for Education Statistics. (2010). Status and trends in the education of racial and ethnic groups. Available from http://nces.ed.gov/pubsearch/pubsinfo.asp?pubid=2010015

National Center for Education Statistics. (2011). *The condition of education 2011. Children and youth with disabilities.* Available from http://nces.ed.gov/programs/coe/indicator_cwd.asp

Newman-Ryan, J., DeLeon-Northrup, B., & Villarreal-Emery, C. (2005). Testing balance function in Spanish-speaking patients: Guidelines for non-Spanish-speaking clinicians. *American Journal of Audiology, 4*(2), 15–23.

Northrup, B. D. (1985). Audiologic assessment and multicultural populations. In *Communication disorders in multicultural populations* (pp. 1–22). Rockville, MD: American Speech-Language-Hearing Association.

Peña, E. D., & Gillam, R. B. (2000). Dynamic assessment of children referred for speech and language evaluations. In C. Lidz & J. Elliott (Eds.), *Dynamic assessment: Prevailing models and applications* (Vol. 6, pp. 543–575). Oxford, England: Elsevier Science.

Peña, E. D., Iglesias, A., & Lidz, C. (2001). Reducing test bias through dynamic assessment of children's word learning ability. *American Journal of Speech-Language Pathology, 10,* 138–154.

Perozzi, J. A. (1985). A pilot study of language facilitation for bilingual, language handicapped children: Theoretical and intervention implications. *Journal of Speech and Hearing Disorders, 50,* 403–406.

Perozzi, J. A., & Chavez-Sanchez, M. L. (1992, October). The effect of instruction in L1 on receptive acquisition of L2 for bilingual children with language delay. *Language, Speech, and Hearing Services in Schools, 23,* 348–352.

Pew Research Center. (2010). Statistical portrait of Hispanics in the United States, 2008. Available from http://www.pewhispanic.org/2010/01/21/statistical-portrait-of-hispanics-in-the-united-states-2008/

Rodriguez, B. L., & Olswang, L. B. (2003). Mexican-American and Anglo-American mothers' beliefs and values about child rearing, education, and language impairment. *American Journal of Speech-Language Pathology, 12,* 462–492.

Roseberry-McKibbin, C. (2002). *Multicultural students with special language needs.* Oceanside, CA: Academic Communication Associates.

Saenz, T. I., & Huer, M. B. (2003). Testing strategies involving least biased language assessment of bilingual children. *Communication Disorders Quarterly, 24*(4), 184–193.

Salas-Provance, M. B., Erickson, J. G., & Reed, J. (2002). Disabilities as viewed by four generations of one Hispanic family. *American Journal of Speech-Language Pathology, 11,* 151–162.

Saville-Troike, M. (1986). Anthropological considerations in the study of communication. In O. Taylor (Ed.), *Nature of communication disorders in culturally and linguistically diverse populations* (pp. 1–19). San Diego, CA: College-Hill Press.

Scheffner Hammer, C. (2011, May). Broadening our knowledge about diverse populations. *American Journal of Speech-Language Pathology, 20*, 71–72.

Scott, D. M. (2002). Multicultural aspects of hearing disorders and audiology. In D. E. Battle (Ed.), *Communication disorders in multicultural populations* (3rd ed.). Boston, MA: Butterworth-Heinemann.

Swartz, K. (2009). Health care for the poor: For whom, what care, and whose responsibility? *Focus, 2,* 69–74.

U.S. Census Bureau. (2008). *An older and more diverse nation by midcentury.* Washington, DC: Author.

U.S. Census Bureau. (2009). *Income, poverty, and health insurance in the United States: 2009–Highlights.* Washington, DC: Author.

U.S. Census Bureau. (2010). *Overview of race and Hispanic origin: 2010.* Washington, DC: Author.

U.S. Department of State. (2009). *Adoption annual report.* Available from www.adoption.state.gov

Valdes, G., & Figueroa, R. (1995). *Bilingualism and testing: A special case of bias.* Norwood, NJ: Ablex Publishing.

Wolf, K. E. (2004, April 13). Cultural competence in audiology. *The ASHA Leader, 26*, 9–13.

RESOURCES

American Speech-Language-Hearing Association. (2001). *Guide to speech-language pathology assessment for multicultural and bilingual populations.* Rockville, MD: Author.

Battle, D. (2001). *Communciation disorders in multicultural populations.* Boston, MA: Butterworth-Heinemann.

Bialystok, E. (2001). *Bilingualism in development: Language, literacy, & cognition.* Cambridge, England: University of Cambridge.

Crowley, C. (2003). *Diagnosing communication disorders in culturally and linguistically diverse students* (ERIC Digest; Eric Identifier ED482343). Retrieved from http://www.ericdigests.org/2005-1/diverse.htm

Genesee, F., Paradis, J., & Crago, M. B. (2004). *Dual language development & disorders: A handbook on bilingualism & second language learning.* Baltimore, MD: Paul H. Brookes.

Goldstein, B. A. (2004). *Bilingual language development & disorders in Spanish-English speakers.* Baltimore, MD: Paul H. Brookes.

Hwa-Froelich, D. (2011). *Supporting development in internationally adopted children.* Baltimore, MD: Paul H. Brookes Publishing Company.

Hwa-Froelich, D., & Westby, C. (2003). Frameworks of education: Perspectives of Southeast Asian parents and Head Start staff. *Language, Speech, and Hearing Services in Schools, 34,* 299–319.

Kayser, H. (2002). Hispanic cultures and language. In D. Battle (Ed.), *Communication disorders in multicultural populations* (2nd ed., pp. 157–196). Boston, MA: Butterworth-Heinemann.

Kayser, H. (2008). *Educating Latino preschool children.* San Diego, CA: Plural Publishing.

Kohnert, K. (2008). *Language disorders in bilingual children and adults.* San Diego, CA: Plural Publishing.

Langdon, H. W. (2008). *Assessment & intervention for communication disorders in culturally & linguistically diverse populations.* Clifton Park, NY: Delmar Cengage Learning.

Pollock, K. (n.d.). Speech-language development in children adopted internationally. Available from http://www.rehabmed.ualberta.ca/spa/phonology/Completged.htm

Stone, J. H. (2005). *Culture and disability.* Thousand Oaks, CA: Sage.

Taylor, O. (1986). Historical perspectives and conceptual framework. In O. Taylor (Ed.), *Nature of communication disorders in culturally and linguistically diverse populations* (pp. 1–19). San Diego, CA: College-Hill Press.

U.S. Department of Health and Human Services. (1985). *Report of the Secretary's Task Force on Black and Minority Health* (Vol. 1, Executive Summary, Publication 491-313/44706). Washington, DC: U.S. Government Printing Office.

U.S. Department of Health and Human Services. (2004). *National healthcare disparities report. Priority populations: Racial and ethnic minorities* (pp. 87–100). Washington, DC: Author.

Internet Sources

Adoption Institute
http://www.adoptioninstitute.org/

American Speech-Language-Hearing Association Multicultural Affairs and Resources
http://www.asha.org/practice/multicultural

Audiology in Multicultural Populations
http://www.asha.org/practice/multicultural/aud.htm

Bilingual Therapies (bilingual speech pathologist resources)
http://www.bilingualtherapies.com/bilingual-speech-pathologist-resources/websites/

Center for Capacity Building for Minorities with Disabilities Research
http://www.uic.edu/orgs/empower/Center%20web%20page/ccbmdr.htm

Center for International Rehabilitation Research Information & Exchange
http://cirrie.buffalo.edu

Diversity RX
http://www.diversityrx.org

Multicultural Constituency Groups
http://www.asha.org/practice/multicultural/opportunities/constituency.htm

Special Interest Group 14, Communication Disorders and Sciences in Culturally and Linguistically Diverse (CLD) Populations
http://www.asha.org/SIG/14/

U.S. Department of Health and Human Services, Office of Minority Health, Think Cultural Health
https://www.thinkculturalhealth.hhs.gov

U.S. Department of Health and Human Services, Office of Minority Health, National Standards on Culturally and Linguistically Appropriate Services
http://minorityhealth.hhs.gov/templates/browse.aspx?lvl=2&lvlID=15

25

Supervision and Mentoring

Melanie W. Hudson, MA

SCOPE OF CHAPTER

This chapter is written by a supervisor for both supervisees and beginning supervisors. The information in this chapter is based on both the literature and personal experiences in supervising and in training supervisors in a variety of professional contexts. Good sources for more in-depth discussion of supervision in general and in speech-language pathology and audiology in particular include Anderson (1988), McCrea and Brasseur (2003), and Carozza (2011). The chapter begins with an overview of the foundations of the supervisory process including a description of the Dreyfus Model of Skill Acquisition (1980) and Anderson's Continuum Model (1988). It includes a model of supervision that can be applied across all levels of experience and settings, and moves to practical issues discussions. Specific discussion is directed to current issues such as the Clinical Fellowship experience and the AuD externship; ethics; cultural, linguistic, and generational differences; technology; training; accountability; and research needs.

A BRIEF HISTORY OF SUPERVISION AND MENTORING

An appreciation of the history of supervision and mentoring is as important to the preprofessional as it is to the seasoned clinician. Supervision and mentoring have been integral parts of both professions from their early beginnings. It is safe to state that each member of the professions of speech-language pathology and audiology has participated in the supervisory process during the course of his or her clinical training, certainly as a supervisee and perhaps also as a supervisor. In her recently published book, *Science of Successful Supervision and Mentorship*, Carozza (2011) explains the importance of knowledge of the history of supervisory education and research and how such knowledge relates to providing effective supervision. As interest in supervision and mentoring increases, and as they continue to play such a significant role in professional growth and development, it is helpful to understand the evolutionary progress of this distinct area of practice.

It was not until the last quarter of the twentieth century that a true understanding of supervision as a process in clinical education was established. Anderson (1988), Farmer and Farmer (1989), and Ulrich (1985) provide informative summaries of the early development of the supervisory process when the professions of speech pathology and audiology were in their infancy. During the 1960s and 1970s, conferences and publications devoted exclusively to issues pertaining to supervision began to appear on the professional horizon (Anderson, 1970; Kleffner, 1964; Halfond, 1964). In 1970 the Council of College and University Supervisors was established, expanding in 1974 into the Council of University Supervisors in Speech-Language Pathology and Audiology (CSSPA). In 1975 the American Speech and Hearing Association (ASHA) Committee on Supervision was established and some communication sciences and disorders (CSD) programs began course offerings in supervision. In 1985 the American Speech-Language-Hearing Association (ASHA) adopted a position statement describing competencies associated with appropriate supervision, with an emphasis on supervision of students (ASHA, 1985). As interest continued to grow, there were several national conferences devoted to the topic, resulting in more publications, along with major books that continue to define the knowledge base (Anderson, 1988; Casey, Smith, & Ulrich, 1988; Crago & Pickering, 1987; Farmer & Farmer, 1989). During the 1990s, there was a move toward combining theory and practice in supervision, and the *ASHA Certification and Membership Handbook* was revised to document the requirements for the Clinical Fellowship Year (CFY) (ASHA, 1997).

At the beginning of the new millennium, there was more emphasis placed on quality clinical education for audiologists and speech-language pathologists. ASHA developed new standards for students' courses of study that required documentation of knowledge and skills, including both formative and summative assessment in addition to new standards for academic program accreditation and certification of personnel (ASHA, 2000). Further research on the topic of merging theory and practice in supervision led to the publication of two major books (Dowling, 2001; McCrea & Brasseur, 2003). With the publication of these books, supervisors have a better understanding of how to implement effective supervisory practices that are supported by evidence and research.

Several factors during the preceding decade stimulated interest in supervision, including expanded scope of practice, personnel shortages, and sustained influx of new professionals (O'Connor, 2008). For example, supervisors may find themselves in situations in which they do not feel qualified to provide supervision because an individual case is out of their scope of practice. Or, due to a shortage of qualified clinicians in a facility, a supervisor does not have the appropriate amount of time to provide the required supervision and mentoring thus jeopardizing the supervisee's ability to meet certification and/or licensure requirements. These and other types of similar situations may also present ethical dilemmas for both the supervisor and the supervisee.

In keeping with some of these variables, ASHA revised its certification guidelines for the Clinical Fellowship (CF) experience (Council for Clinical Certification, 2005). You will note that this revision includes discontinuing the "Y" designation for "year" to denote the adjustment in the length of time to complete requirements. These revised guidelines also include replacing the term *supervisor* with *mentor* to reflect the higher degree of autonomy now placed on the clinical fellow or extern. Policy documents regarding CF mentoring (ASHA, 2007) and ethical issues pertaining to supervision of student clinicians (ASHA, 2010c), a technical report (2008b), and a document addressing knowledge and skills for clinical supervision (ASHA, 2008c) were also published. The American Board of Audiology (ABA) and almost all states now have specific supervision requirements in place to ensure appropriate levels of supervision and/or mentoring for the beginning clinician. Individuals entering into a supervisory or mentoring relationship need to become familiar with regulations and guidelines applicable to their specific circumstances. Whether you are a supervisor, mentor, preceptor, clinical fellow, AuD extern, or hold a provisional certificate or license, the success of the experience depends on assuming this responsibility. Regulations, standards, and guidelines are covered in more detail later in this chapter.

Supervision and mentoring have played significant roles in the development of speech-language pathology and audiology since the early history of both professions. Over the years, research and evidence have demonstrated how effective supervision and mentoring support service delivery and positive outcomes. As a result, university programs, professional organizations, and government agencies have learned to recognize the value of effective supervision and mentoring of the new clinician. Their attempts to address this need by establishing regulations and guidelines for clinical supervisors and mentors are evidence of this belief.

THE SUPERVISORY PROCESS

Supervision as a process is more easily understood when presented in the context of learning or acquiring clinical skills and knowledge in audiology and speech-language pathology. The insightful student of supervision will be able to draw a parallel between supervisee performance and supervisor expectations when such a process is taken into consideration.

The Dreyfus Model of Skill Acquisition

The Dreyfus Model of Skill Acquisition (1986) describes a learning process consisting of five stages: *novice, advanced beginner, competent, proficient,* and *expert.* It is used as a means of assessing and supporting progress in the development of skills. It also provides a definition of acceptable level for the assessment of competence. Similar in its design to a developmental continuum, the learner, or supervisee, progresses from one stage to the next as the level of clinical knowledge and skills increases.

At the *novice* stage, the learner has minimal knowledge connected to practice. Because supervisees at this stage have no experience in the application of rules, behavior is predictably inflexible. The novice needs to be closely supervised and cannot be expected to use discretionary judgment. The supervisor would naturally need to incorporate a more direct style of supervision, such as modeling behaviors for supervisees.

At the *advanced beginner* stage, supervisees are able to demonstrate marginally acceptable performance, but with limited situational perception. They are beginning to treat knowledge in context but still treat attributes and aspects separately and with equal importance. For example, they may not perceive the relationship between a hypernasal vocal quality and restricted movement of the mandible thus viewing them as distinct areas for treatment.

At the *competent* stage, supervisees are able to plan with more independence, deliberately using analytical assessment to treat problems in context. Competent supervisees can view actions in terms of long-term goals and are able to incorporate conscious, deliberate planning to achieve those goals. These supervisees are also able to use standardized and routine procedures while recognizing their relevance to a given situation. For example, after conducting a pure-tone audiometric screening, supervisees would be able to assess the necessity of impedance testing or the use of a bone oscillator to help determine type of hearing loss.

At the *proficient* stage, supervisees are able to see the situation as a whole in terms of long-term goals. This holistic understanding improves decision making as maxims are used for guidance, and supervisees are now able to modify plans in terms of what should be expected. Proficient supervisees perceive deviations from what is typical and, as a result, are able to make clinical judgments more easily. These supervisees are also able to see what is most important in a situation and to take responsibility for their own decisions. If working with a nonverbal child with autism, for instance, these supervisees would recognize the value of joint attention training before attempting to initiate a system of picture exchange for communication.

At the *expert* stage, clinicians are able to make decisions based not only on a set of rules but also using their experience to manipulate these rules to achieve the end goal. Expert clinicians have an intuitive grasp of situations and rely on an analytical approach to problem solving only when unfamiliar situations occur. Expert clinicians are able to see the end goal and know just how to achieve it. They see the big picture and are able to consider various alternatives, possibly going beyond existing standards to achieve the end result.

The goal of a supervisor is to ensure that the supervisee progresses from one stage to the next while employing effective strategies that promote increasing levels of independence. Implementation of models of the supervisory process that utilize such strategies help achieve this goal.

Anderson's Continuum of Supervision

Jean Anderson's book *The Supervisory Process in Speech-Language Pathology and Audiology* (1988) had a major impact in the area of supervision. The profound influence of her work is reflected in the fact that her approach to the supervisory process is reflected in the current accreditation standards for academic programs in communication sciences and disorders (ASHA, 2000). Anderson (1988) defines supervision as "a process that consists of a variety of patterns of behavior, the appropriateness of which depends on the needs, competencies, expectations and philosophies of the supervisor and supervisee and the specifics of the situation (tasks, client, setting, and other variables)" (p. 12). This definition supports flexibility, self-evaluation, and critical thinking. It also promotes collaboration, a key component of the process. Prior to the publication of this book, supervisory style was characterized by stricter control and higher levels of direction on the part of the supervisor. Very little, if any, collaboration existed between the supervisor and the supervisee.

Anderson's Continuum of Supervision (1988) is the most widely recognized supervision model in speech-language pathology and audiology (Dowling, 2001). This continuum model was influenced by the theoretical framework of Cogan (1973), whose ongoing cycle of supervision was designed to improve the performance of teachers. Anderson employs different strategies and styles that may be incorporated at different stages of the supervisory process, depending on the situation. The continuum model allows for the eventual competent independence of the supervisee while the degree of involvement of both the supervisor and supervisee shifts as they move along the continuum.

The continuum consists of three stages, *evaluation-feedback, transitional,* and *self-supervision* (see Figure 25–1). It is important to understand that the stages are not time-bound, but allow for the supervisee to be at any given stage, or point along the continuum, depending on circumstances, including knowledge and skills. An important feature of this model is that it also promotes the

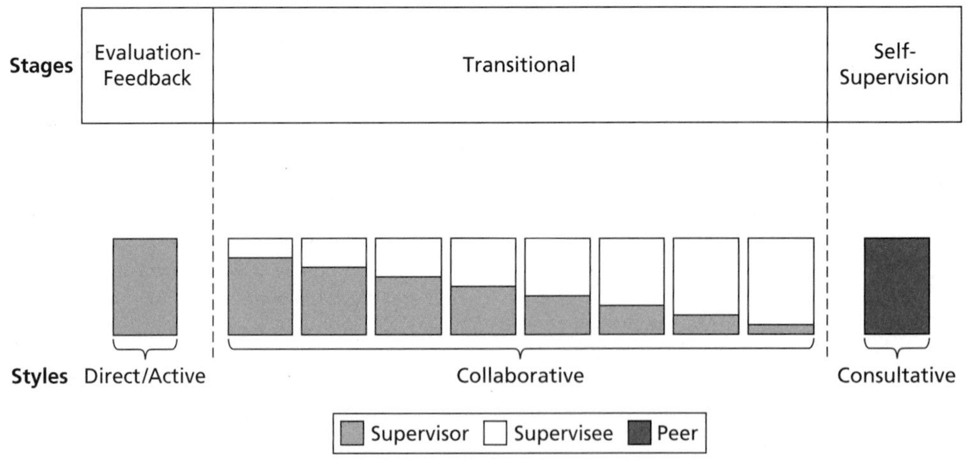

FIGURE 25–1 Anderson's Continuum of Supervision

From *The Supervisory Process in Speech-Language Pathology and Audiology* (p. 27), by E. S. McCrea and J. A. Brasseur, 2003, Boston, MA: Allyn & Bacon. Copyright © 2003 by Pearson Education. Reprinted with permission.

professional growth of the supervisor. As supervisees progress along the continuum, supervisors learn to adjust their supervisory style according to the needs of the supervisees. The supervisor may choose to become more or less directive as appropriate, according to the knowledge and skills of the supervisee.

Students and entry-level clinicians with minimal knowledge and skill work closely with their supervisors at the *evaluation-feedback* stage of the continuum. The supervisee who is a marginal student or who is working in a new setting would be most likely seen in this stage, with the supervisor having a dominant role and employing a more direct style of supervision. The goal at this initial stage is for the supervisee to move as quickly as possible from a level of dependence on the supervisor to one that is more consultative in nature (McCrea & Brasseur, 2003). As the student or new clinician begins to demonstrate the ability to employ critical thinking skills and principles of reflective practice (self-evaluation), then movement to the *transitional* stage is appropriate.

At the *transitional* stage, supervision is a shared process and the supervisee is moving toward more independence. Supervisors now use a less direct style of supervision and employ methods that include the supervisee as an active participant in the supervisory process. Supervisors encourage the development of problem-solving skills, critical thinking, and reflective practice to guide the supervisee to higher levels of independence and competence. Individual circumstances and situations will necessitate a fluidity of movement within this stage as dictated by experience, comfort level, and skill of the supervisee (McCrea & Brasseur, 2003).

The *self-supervision* stage is attained when supervisees no longer rely upon the feedback of their supervisors to analyze their work but are able to self-analyze their clinical behavior. The relationship between supervisor and supervisee becomes more of a peer interaction. At this stage, supervisees are truly competent, independent clinicians, having assumed complete responsibility for their own professional development, although they still desire peer interaction (McCrea & Brasseur, 2003).

Key Elements of the Supervisory Process

We learn from Anderson's continuum (1988) that an effective supervisory model should have a framework for systematic development of the process of supervision. The key components of such a framework should include collaborative planning, observation and data collection, analysis of data, and evaluation and feedback. Each of these elements should support principles of reflective practice that lead to self-supervision. Although professional demands and responsibilities may vary from setting to setting, these key elements are universal and not specific to any particular setting or profession.

Planning Supervisors need to consider more than just the relationship with the supervisee as part of the planning process. McCrea and Brasseur (2003) describe the concept of "fourfold planning" (p. 106) for all participants, including the client, the clinician, the supervisee, and the supervisor, as the foundation of the ongoing supervisory process. The needs of each of these participants should be considered and addressed appropriately when setting goals. Thus, supervisors must balance helping supervisees plan for their clients and for their own clinical and professional growth. In all cases, goals should be measurable, serve as a guide for action, and serve as a source of motivation. The supervisee will more likely achieve specified goals if the supervisor offers continued support and recognizes effort and success.

Observation and Data Collection The purpose of observation is to collect data on some aspect(s) of the clinical work being done. Anderson (1988) described observation as the point at which supervision changes from being solely an art to more of a science and stressed that it must be an active process if it is to be of value. She also stated that "observation without data is a waste of time" (p. 123). Objectivity in the supervisory process is achieved through clinical observation and data collection.

A supervisor may want to gather information about the supervisee's communication skills, or monitor a specific clinical activity to assess quality of service delivery. Data may also be collected by the supervisees themselves, depending on the objectives set as part of the planning process. These data would typically be centered on client or patient behavior and organized in such a way that they can be related to actions of the supervisee. In any case, data collection should correspond to the goals established in relation to expected clinical activities and professional growth.

A variety of tools can be used to observe and collect data in audiology and speech-language pathology.

Casey et al. (1988) identified seven types of data collection, including verbatim recording, selective verbatim, rating scales, tally, interaction analysis, nonverbal analysis, and those that are individually designed. To facilitate self-supervision, or reflective practice, the Kansas Inventory of Self-Supervision (Mawdsley, 1987) is an excellent example of an individually designed system for collecting specific data. New clinicians should become familiar with several data collection tools to diversify their clinical skills. Whichever methods are employed, the resulting data are analyzed so that they become logical and meaningful and have a specific purpose.

Analysis Analysis of collected data allows supervisees to observe the relationship of their behavior to that of the client. It also affords an opportunity for supervisors to observe how their actions may influence the behavior and performance of their supervisees. As cited in McCrea & Brasseur (2003, p. 193), Cogan (1973) listed the purposes of analyzing data:

- Determining if objectives from the planning stage were met
- Identifying salient patterns in the teacher's (supervisee's) behavior
- Identifying unanticipated learning by the student (client/patient)
- Identifying critical incidents in the interaction (behavior that significantly affects the learning or relationship between teacher and student)
- Organizing the data to determine what was learned
- Determining if what was planned was carried out
- Developing a database for the rest of the supervision program

The results of analyzed data may yield information that provides an opportunity for supervisors to improve their interactions and become more effective at their job. The results may also yield information that informs the clinician whether or not certain clinical procedures are effective. Objective data must be collected so that events can be reconstructed for accurate analysis (Goldhammer, Anderson, & Krajewski, 1980). The reconstruction of the collected data also promotes accountability and thus maintains compliance with codes of ethics for both professions. Before an objective evaluation of performance or effectiveness can occur, data must be carefully examined and interpreted. The process of analysis also provides supervisors with an opportunity to examine and interpret their own behavior to see how it influences the supervisory relationship. For instance, if the supervisor has been employing a more direct style of supervision, the supervisee may not have demonstrated sufficient confidence in determining if a certain clinical procedure would be appropriate in treatment for the client. In this situation, the supervisor would need to move from a direct style of supervision to a more flexible one that affords the supervisee with more input in the decision-making process.

Evaluation The importance of collection of objective data is underscored when an evaluation component is being considered. Current literature on supervisor accountability discounts the acceptability of a totally subjective evaluation on the part of the supervisor (Anderson, 1988). When the supervisory relationship is based on a collaborative and consultative model, the effective supervisor relies on the results of analysis of objective data as part of the evaluation process. Objective data support the observations that the supervisor shares with the supervisee. Dowling (2001) states that "if supervisees are truly self-evaluating, they are aware of their levels of performance and assessment becomes a joint sharing of known information" (p. 227). The process of evaluation is ongoing in nature, and supervisees always have an understanding of their strengths and weaknesses. The effective supervisor assists supervisees in describing and measuring their own progress and achievement as part of this ongoing process (ASHA, 2008c). In other words, there would be no surprises at a prescribed evaluation conference with the supervisor using a collaborative model that employs tools for self-assessment.

Principles of active learning support engaging students in written self-analysis of their discrete and nonverbal clinical behaviors (Gillam, Roussos, & Anderson, 1990). Many university CSD programs have developed their own tools for self-assessment of clinical knowledge and skills to support these principles. Weltsch and Crowe (2006) studied the effectiveness of a supervisory approach designed to facilitate self-analysis by graduate clinicians. They concluded that having student clinicians complete written self-analyses of recorded target intervention behaviors may lead to greater clinical competency. The Supervisee Performance Assessment Instrument (SPAI) (Fall & Sutton, 2004) is an example of an instrument used for self-assessment by the supervisee. Its design supports collaboration by allowing the supervisor and supervisee to target specific areas for evaluation that can be tailored to certain individuals or groups. The format uses a nonhierarchical type of scaling and a large number of evaluation criteria.

Professionals in both educational and health care settings have developed a variety of self-assessment tools, including rating scales and performance checklists. Many of these may be adapted for use by audiologists and speech-language pathologists. Dowling (2001) discusses the importance of evaluation but states that overemphasis on this component of the process may be destructive to the supervisory relationship. The use of self-assessment tools may serve to place the evaluation component of the supervisory process in the proper context to support a collaborative supervisory relationship.

CORE Model of Supervision and Mentoring

Hudson (2010) describes the CORE Model of Supervision and Mentoring incorporating these key elements of the supervisory process. Based on the combined works of individuals who have made significant contributions to the knowledge base of the supervisory process, including Anderson (1988), Brasseur and McCrea (2003), Cogan (1973), and Dowling (2001), the model comprises a cycle with four major components: *collaboration, observation, reflection,* and *evaluation.*

The goal of the first component of this model, *collaboration*, is to establish an effective and trusting working relationship between supervisor and supervisee, emphasizing the joint nature of the supervisory relationship. ASHA (2008b) describes supervision as a collaborative process, with shared responsibility for many of the activities throughout the supervisory experience. This is where the supervisor sets the stage for growth in relation to the supervisory process by explaining policies and procedures; performance expectations; and assessment procedures, including data collection. In addition, the supervisor guides the supervisee in establishing performance goals and objectives to promote clinical knowledge, personal improvement, productivity, and self-directed learning.

The *observation* component allows the supervisor to record data that will be used during the processes of analysis and evaluation. McCrea and Brasseur (2003) state that observation is the place where real objectivity begins in the supervisory process. The observation and data collection are based on the goals and objectives that were established during the collaboration component of the model. The supervisor should specify the purpose for each observation and what supervisee behavior data will be collected. For instance, the supervisor may be collecting data on the number of times the supervisee uses the phrase "good job" when the goal was to use appropriate positive reinforcement consistent with client performance of targeted skills.

The *reflection* component is where evidence-supported strategies to promote reflective practice are specifically identified to promote self-supervision and independence. These strategies may include the use of journals, portfolios, and self-evaluation checklists (Hudson, 2010). As in Anderson's model, the ultimate goal of this component is for the supervisee to engage in critical thinking for solving professional problems as an independent, competent clinician (McCrea & Brasseur, 2003). The supervisor plays an important role in supporting guided reflection as the supervisee implements predetermined goals, tackles new situations, embraces challenges, and meets expectations.

The purpose of the *evaluation* component is to provide the supervisee with feedback that is objective, data-based, verifiable, and systematic. This feedback should be designed to motivate and enhance performance. Dowling (2001) states that managing feedback is a fundamental issue in building constructive supervisory relationships. Self-assessment tools that support principles of reflective practice are an important ingredient of this component. As specific skills in need of improvement are identified, or as new situations occur as part of this process, they are addressed by rotating to the *collaboration* component and then proceeding through the remaining components of the cycle.

SUPERVISORY STYLE AND COMMUNICATION SKILLS

What do you think of when you hear the word *style*? In the context of supervision, definitions that have been offered include "a distinctive manner of responding to supervisees" (Ladany, Walker, & Melincoff, 2001, p. 263) and "the way in which the personality and convictions of the supervisor are demonstrated in the supervisory relationship" (Leighton, 1991; Long, Lawless, & Dotson, 1996, p. 589). Anderson (1988) discusses the influence of personal characteristics and interpersonal style on the type of supervisory style chosen by the supervisor. She also refers to supervisory style as it applies to stages of her continuum model: direct-active style at the evaluation-feedback stage, collaborative style at the transitional stage, and consultative style at the self-supervision stage. A study of supervisory styles in nursing revealed two styles used by clinical nurse supervisors: emotional style and cognitive style (Severinsson, 1996; Severinsson & Hallberg, 1996). Research tells us that supervisors tend to use one style even when they think they do not (McCrea & Brasseur, 2003). Experience tells us that certain styles are more effective in some situations than in others. Supervisors should be aware of the supervisory style that they choose and develop an appreciation of how various styles affect the supervisory relationship.

Most of us recognize the role that communication style can play in our interpersonal relationships. The influence of interpersonal communication skills on the supervisory process has been widely studied, and research demonstrates that the communication skills of the supervisor play a key role in the clinical performance of the supervisee and the overall success of the supervisory relationship (McCrea & Brasseur, 2003). Essential components of effective communication may include active listening, asking purposeful questions, and responding appropriately to questions when asked. Each of these has both verbal and nonverbal aspects. Verbal behaviors that support active listening include saying "fine," "I see," "good," "mmm," or "uh-huh" (Shipley, 1997).

Nonverbal behaviors that support active listening include facing the listener, maintaining eye contact, and using appropriate facial expressions and head movements. Purposeful questions are well thought out and are formulated to encourage the supervisee to think creatively and develop problem-solving skills. In a study on questioning behaviors of supervisors, Smith (1979) found that when supervisors dominated the questioning process by asking for factual information, they deprived supervisees of the opportunity to problem-solve, self-analyze, and self-direct their own behavior. This type of communication style on the part of the supervisor would certainly present a challenge for the new clinician who is striving for independence.

The effective supervisor promotes self-supervision as the supervisee grows toward competence and independence. Strategies that encourage critical thinking on the part of the supervisee are an important part of this growth, and knowing how to *ask* questions is an essential communication skill for the supervisor when facilitating critical thinking. Cunningham (1971) developed a category system for questioning by dividing questions into broad and narrow categories. The narrow category includes cognitive memory questions (recall, identify/observe, yes/no, define, name, designate) and convergent questions (explain, state relationships, compare, and contrast). The broad category includes divergent questions (predict, hypothesize, infer, reconstruct) and evaluative questions (judge, value, defend, justify, choice). Supervisors need to consider the types of questions they employ when facilitating critical thinking as part of the supervisory process.

The manner in which the supervisor *responds* to questions also plays an important role in interpersonal communication style and has an effect on the supervisory relationship. Carin and Sund (1971) stress the importance of a diplomatic reply to questions that are answered incorrectly by redirecting, helping the respondent move closer to a better answer, and not blocking communication by responding negatively. In a study of classroom teacher behavior, they reported that when wait time was extended for students to reply to questions, it resulted in longer responses, fewer "I don't know" answers, more whole sentences, and increased speculative thinking. Supervisors should learn to adjust their wait time when asking questions to afford the supervisee the opportunity to reflect and formulate considered responses.

Providing feedback is a key element of supervision and mentoring, typically linked to the evaluation component of the supervisory process. Supervisors and supervisees alike may even consider "supervising" and "providing feedback" as synonymous. But no matter how much of a role feedback may play, it is a fundamental expectation of both parties in the supervisory relationship. In a traditional supervisory model, feedback is usually provided in written form, or it may be spontaneous or unscheduled verbal interaction (Anderson, 1988). Feedback may also be provided at a scheduled conference, either in person or by telephone or other real-time electronic method. These sessions typically consist of the supervisor giving suggestions, reviewing expectations, and discussing overall performance while the supervisee listens and perhaps provides clarification and asks questions. In a collaborative/consultative model, feedback is part of an ongoing process, and formal feedback sessions are less likely to take place. The communication styles of the supervisor and the supervisee can determine how receptive the supervisee is to feedback, so both need to tread carefully when in this territory.

The supervisee is more likely to be receptive to feedback if it is constructive. Pfeiffer and Jones (1987, p. 121) list 10 characteristics of constructive feedback:

1. It is descriptive rather than evaluative.
2. It is specific rather than general.
3. It is focused on the behavior rather than the person.
4. It takes into account the needs of both the receiver and the giver of the feedback.
5. It is directed toward performance rather than personal characteristics.
6. It is well timed.
7. It involves sharing of information rather than giving advice.
8. It involves the amount of information the receiver can use, rather than the amount of information we would like to give.
9. It is checked to ensure clear communication.
10. It is checked to determine the degree of agreement of the receiver.

To be effective, feedback should be part of an ongoing process, supported by careful analysis of data and related to the goals developed as part of the initial collaborative planning phase of the supervisory process. Feedback should always serve to promote critical reflection on the parts of both the supervisor and the supervisee. It should enable both parties to explore why some strategies worked and others did not. This will naturally lead to the collaboration involved in outlining specific, measurable, action-oriented, realistic, and time-bound goals for improvement.

Both supervisors and supervisees need to recognize how their individual communication styles affect the supervisory relationship. A great deal of literature is available pertaining to communication style among the realms of counseling, education, self-improvement, career development, and management, to name a few. Professional conferences also offer courses on this topic, sometimes with an emphasis on the influence of cultural, linguistic, and generational issues on communication skills in the professional setting. Taking advantage of professional development opportunities in this area will enhance not only the supervisory relationship but also any other professional relationships that occur in the work setting.

TRANSITION: SUPERVISOR TO MENTOR/PRECEPTOR

As students, you have come to expect a certain degree of dependency on your clinical supervisor for most, if not all, aspects of your clinical activities. Your supervisor reads your reports, reviews your audiograms, observes you counseling family members, watches how you fit a hearing aid, sees you perform an oral-peripheral examination, helps you introduce a new therapy activity to a client, and so on. Very little you have done as a student clinician has not been observed and/or evaluated by a supervisor. It is no wonder that as your knowledge and skills develop, and your supervisor naturally becomes less directly involved in your clinical activities, that you may, on occasion, develop a sense of panic. As you approach graduation, and your first professional employment, you are told that you will have a mentor or preceptor instead of a supervisor. Now, the sense of panic may really begin to set in. So, just what is the difference between a supervisor and a mentor/preceptor?

Consider this fact: as a paid professional, your employer has rightfully assumed that your clinical knowledge and skills are worth whatever you are being paid. If that is the assumption, why would the employer feel the need to assign someone to work closely beside you, watching you perform daily tasks that your resumé indicates you know how to do independently? On the other hand, you just graduated and are new to the job, so it is understandable that some sort of coaching or even some direction on occasion would be in order. Hence, the mentor or preceptor is put in place, and you are now entering into a special relationship that will assist you in your quest for growth through learning.

Shea (1997) describes the mentor as someone whose role is to gently guide the new clinician by offering knowledge, insight, perspective, or wisdom. ASHA (2008a) describes mentoring as a collaborative process of shared responsibility. This concept of shared responsibility sets the stage for a relationship that offers more give and take, more exchange of ideas, and more working as a team than was the case in the student-supervisor relationship. If your previous supervisory relationships were truly collaborative, and you were guided in the art of reflective practice, the transition from supervisor to mentor/preceptor will feel quite natural. Mentors/preceptors are expected to lead by example. As role models, they will demonstrate ethical conduct, responsibility, and perspective taking and have knowledge of strategies that foster self-evaluation. They will appreciate learning styles, personality types, and consider how race, culture, gender, and age may influence personal interactions. Your mentor/preceptor will guide you to proficiency, where you will obtain a greater understanding and appreciation of the big picture, the holistic view of a situation. You and your mentor/preceptor will discuss why some strategies worked and some did not as you continue to develop confidence to take the initiative and try new strategies on your own. In this strategic partnership, you will feel empowered to explore new territory and stretch your skills with the knowledge that you have a foundation of support, your mentor/preceptor.

REGULATIONS, STANDARDS, AND GUIDELINES

At the preprofessional level, the Council on Academic Accreditation (CAA) states that academic programs are required to demonstrate that "Clinical supervision is commensurate with the clinical knowledge and skills of each student..." (Standard 3.5B; CAA, 2004). Before providing direct services in any setting, supervisors, mentors, preceptors, student clinicians, clinical fellows, AuD externs, and audiologists with provisional board certification need to be aware of professional association standards for certification, state licensure laws, and federal/state reimbursement programs such as Medicaid and Medicare. State licensure boards and state boards of education have their own regulations and requirements, and supervision requirements may not match those of professional associations such as ASHA and the ABA. Thus, it is important to refer to all applicable sources. Each state has information that is readily available on requirements for certification and licensure and is easily obtainable on their Internet websites. ASHA has information on its website on the certification process for speech-language pathologists and audiologists. The ABA also has information available on its website regarding provisional board certification and becoming a member of the American Academy of Audiology (AAA).

Supervisors and mentors/preceptors are fully responsible for the behavior, clinical services, and documentation of their supervisees. This means that supervisors and mentors/preceptors must be aware of the professional competence of the supervisee in specific areas/scopes of practice, to protect not only themselves but also the welfare of the clients and to foster the growth of the supervisee (ASHA, 2008b). If you find yourself in a situation in which you do not feel qualified, competent, or physically or emotionally safe, or if you are in a situation that involves an ethical dilemma, it is absolutely imperative that you inform your supervisor or mentor/preceptor of the situation. If it is the supervisor or mentor/preceptor who has placed you in this situation, you should contact your university program or professional association, such as ASHA or ABA, for direction and guidance.

Clinical Fellowship Experience and AuD Clinical Practicum

Upon completion of the required academic coursework and clinical practicum experiences and after the graduate degree has been conferred, speech-language pathologists and audiologists advance to the next stages of their professional career development. Speech-language pathologists are now ready to begin their Clinical Fellowship (CF) experience in accordance with the ASHA standards for certification for speech-language pathology, and audiologists begin their fourth-year AuD clinical practicum in accordance with the ASHA (2010a) or ABA standards for certification for audiology. The ASHA standards are established by audiologists and speech-language pathologists, respectively, who are members of ASHA's Council for Clinical Certification in Audiology and Speech-Language Pathology (CFCC). The ABA also establishes standards for audiology credentials. Because the two professions diverge at this point, they will be addressed separately in this chapter.

Speech-Language Pathology Clinical Fellowship (SLPCF)

ASHA (n.d.) describes the Clinical Fellowship experience as a transition between being a student and being an independent provider of clinical services and involving a mentored professional experience. The purposes of the CF experience include the following:

1. Integration and application of the theoretical knowledge from academic training
2. Evaluation of strengths and identification of limitations
3. Development and refinement of clinical skills consistent with the scope of practice
4. Advancement from constant supervision to independent practitioner

It is the responsibility of the clinical fellow (CF) to identify a mentor who holds a current Certificate of Clinical Competence (CCC) and, if applicable, state licensure. Some states do not require the completion of a CF experience but have their own provisional licensure requirements that include supervision by a licensed speech-language pathologist who may or may not be required to hold a CCC. In those instances, the CF will need to determine if the supervisor can also serve as a CF mentor. If not, the ASHA website has information on how to find a CF mentor. CFs should determine what the requirements are for the state in which they are going to be working and verify this information before the start of the CF experience. This may be done by contacting the ASHA National Office and by checking with state licensure boards, as appropriate.

It is important that both the CF and the CF mentor are familiar with the ASHA Code of Ethics, the *ASHA Certification and Membership Handbook*, both of which are available on the ASHA website, and any and all applicable state licensure/certification requirements in order not to jeopardize the certification or licensure status of the CF. The CF and the CF mentor need to discuss at the very beginning of the CF experience how the monitoring activities will be completed, including frequency and method of documentation, and how the CF's performance will be evaluated. Both parties should maintain copies of all written feedback and other documentation, including the required forms submitted to ASHA and the state. The specific requirements for completion of the CF experience are provided in Chapter 10.

Finally, the CF and the mentor need to be aware of possible ethical misconduct on the part of the CF mentor. Although these events are not typical, they may include arbitrary termination of the mentoring relationship, failure to complete and sign the required paperwork in a timely manner, failure to provide the required amount and type of mentoring, or recruitment of the CF as an independent practitioner. If any of these or other unfortunate situations occur, the CF should consult with a certification manager at the ASHA National Office immediately.

AuD Clinical Practicum

There have been important developments in recent years in the profession of audiology regarding credentialing. Two professional organizations, ASHA and ABA, both offer a path to certification and membership. Currently, membership and certification in ASHA can be accomplished through the same application process, whereas the ABA credential and membership in AAA are separate (2011). In addition, individual states continue to have their own requirements for licensure, which may or may not mirror either of the professional association standards for certification. As a student approaching completion of graduate studies in audiology, you should consider how you want to be credentialed, and by which (or both) professional associations while pursuing the doctoral degree. More information about requirements for ASHA certification and ABA board certification is provided in Chapter 10.

SUPERVISION AFTER CERTIFICATION

Now that you have earned your Certificate of Clinical Competence, or Board Certification, what can you expect in the way of supervision? The answer to that question will depend on your individual circumstances, including your work setting and the nature of your assigned duties. You should expect to have someone to whom you report directly, perhaps a rehabilitation director, clinic or private practice owner, service coordinator, school principal, or regional supervisor. This individual may or may not share your professional credentials. This supervisor's main goal is to ensure the well-being of the patients, clients, or students whom you serve and to ensure the quality of the services you provide in that setting. As such, you can expect to have some type of supervision and receive an evaluation of your performance by someone in a supervisory capacity. Chapter 10 includes a more detailed discussion of the employee evaluation process, but it bears some mention in this chapter as you will most likely continue to be in a supervisory or mentoring/preceptor type of relationship. The fundamental principles of supervision and mentoring still apply, so you may want to review those principles at this next stage of your career. You may also be asked to provide supervision to a graduate student or an assistant. Now you become the supervisor.

Supervision of Students and Assistants

Graduate programs require students to accrue clinical practicum hours in a variety of settings to prepare them for the professional work environment. You may be asked very early in your post-certification career to supervise a student in your work setting. If that is the case, remember above all other considerations that you are a role model to this individual. You need to keep in mind that your opinions and impressions may carry a great deal of weight and that the student will look to you for guidance and direction in many areas, including clinical skills, ethical behavior, interpersonal skills, and work habits. Typically, the student's university program director or clinic director will have made the necessary arrangements between the university and your worksite for the student placement. You should determine who your contact at the university will be and what type of documentation is expected of you as the student's supervisor. You should also discuss your professional liability with your worksite supervisor and verify that your current licensure and certification will meet the needs of the university.

It is both a responsibility and a privilege to play a part in the early professional growth of a student clinician. The rewards of creating the professional climate in which a student can thrive are well worth the challenges that this unique supervisory relationship will present to you. The opportunity that this relationship will provide will also make a significant contribution to your own professional growth and development.

Supervision of assistants, including speech-language pathology assistants (SLPAs) and support personnel in audiology, presents a unique challenge, particularly for new clinicians who may just be learning how to do their first job. One of the most important issues involves the amount of supervision that is required and the documentation associated with that supervision. Typically, the more complex cases will necessitate increased levels of supervision. As in any supervisory relationship, the basic principles apply to the supervisor of the SLPA or support personnel in audiology, particularly in the areas of ethical behavior, communication, and documentation.

ASHA (1996) has established guidelines for the training, credentialing, use, and supervision of assistants that define the parameters of work for both SLPAs and their supervisors. In addition, beginning in 2011, ASHA began offering an affiliation category for individuals who work in speech-language pathology and audiology. They are required to have the necessary skills to work in a support position, and their duties are performed under direct supervision of an ASHA-certified speech-language pathologist or audiologist. The topic of support personnel in speech-language pathology and audiology is covered extensively in Chapter 12.

Ethical Issues

Professional codes of ethics are established to provide the standards of conduct that guide the behavior of members of the professions of speech-language pathology and audiology. Both ASHA and ABA have codes of ethics that serve this purpose, and supervisors have the responsibility to ensure that their supervisees adhere to ethical principles in every aspect of their clinical activities.

The ASHA Code of Ethics (2010b) specifies compliance with certification and licensure for members and certificate holders as required by their employers, their states, governmental agencies, and by ASHA in the area of their clinical or supervisory work, regardless of the work setting. Several sections pertain to the supervision of student clinicians:

- **Principle of Ethics I:** Individuals shall honor their responsibility to hold paramount the welfare of persons they serve professionally or who are participants in research and scholarly activities and they shall treat animals involved in research in a humane manner.
- **Principle of Ethics I, Rule A:** Individuals shall provide all services competently.
- **Principle of Ethics I, Rule D:** Individuals shall not misrepresent the credentials of assistants, technicians, support personnel, students, Clinical Fellows, or any others under their supervision, and they shall inform those they serve professionally of

the name and professional credentials of persons providing services.

- **Principle of Ethics I, Rule G:** Individuals who hold the Certificates of Clinical Competence may delegate tasks related to provision of clinical services that require the unique skills, knowledge, and judgment that are within the scope of their profession to students only if those services are appropriately supervised. The responsibility for client welfare remains with the certified individual.
- **Principle of Ethics II, Rule A:** Individuals shall engage in the provision of clinical services only when they hold the appropriate Certificate of Clinical Competence or when they are in the certification process and are supervised by an individual who holds the appropriate Certificate of Clinical Competence.
- **Principle of Ethics II, Rule B:** Individuals shall engage in only those aspects of the professions that are within the scope of their professional practice and competence, considering their level of education, training, and experience.
- **Principle of Ethics IV, Rule B:** Individuals shall prohibit anyone under their supervision from engaging in any practice that violates the Code of Ethics.

Supervisors also need to be aware of the issue of *vicarious liability* that describes the supervisor's responsibility concerning the behavior of the supervisee (Newman, 2001). For example, supervisors must consider the welfare of the patient, including confidentiality and privacy, and documentation in keeping with principles of ethical practice. In addition, both inter-professional and intra-professional relationships are areas that have ethical implications and may need to be considered by both the supervisor and the supervisee.

Supervisors also need to be aware of the dual relationship that can develop between the supervisor and the supervisee (Newman, Victor, & Zylla-Jones, 2009). When the relationship between the supervisor and the supervisee becomes more personal than professional, it can compromise the integrity of the supervisory relationship. For example, if a supervisor uses the supervisee as a babysitter, the supervisor now has an additional relationship with the supervisee as an employer. Suppose the supervisee forgets to show up at the supervisor's home one evening when the supervisor and her husband have purchased costly tickets for the symphony? Will the supervisor be able to maintain objectivity when evaluating the supervisee's ability to assume responsibility? This new relationship now presents its own set of problems that can adversely affect the supervisory relationship. Supervisors assume responsibility for maintaining the proper balance in the relationship and for setting and maintaining appropriate boundaries as needed.

Situations involving ethical misconduct, including abuse of power, may also occur on the part of the supervisor. For example, a supervisor may fail to provide a sufficient amount of supervision based on the performance of the supervisee, fail to monitor the supervisee's protection of patient confidentiality, fail to verify appropriate competencies before delegating tasks to supervisees, fail to demonstrate benefit to the patient based on outcomes, and fail to provide self-assessment tools and opportunities to supervisees (King, 2003). The astute supervisee will learn to recognize possible ethical misconduct on the part of the supervisor and should seek appropriate consultation. A good source of reference is ASHA's (2007) Issues in Ethics technical report on *Responsibilities of Individuals Who Mentor Clinical Fellows.*

Adherence to principles of ethical conduct transcends all aspects of clinical practice and professional behavior. The supervisory relationship provides the supervisor with the opportunity to model behaviors necessary for lifelong ethical practice. See Chapter 5 for a more in-depth discussion of ethical issues.

Cultural, Linguistic, and Generational Issues

As we become more diverse as a nation, supervisors will have more and more opportunities to work with individuals from backgrounds different from their own. Because values, behaviors, and beliefs may differ from culture to culture and from one generation to another, supervisors will need to learn to appreciate the effect that these factors have on communication, behavior, and learning styles (ASHA, 2008c). As supervisors and mentors, we should also encourage an understanding of linguistic differences and are obligated to prevent discrimination against people who speak with an accent and/or dialect in educational programs, employment, or service delivery (ASHA, 1998).

Coleman (2000) noted that differences in cultural values have an impact on the nature and effectiveness of all aspects of clinical interventions, including supervisee relationships. He added that in order for interactions with supervisees to be successful, supervisors must consider learning styles and culturally based behaviors of their supervisees. Researchers who have studied clinical intervention strategies related to cultural issues (Anderson, 1992; Battle, 1993; Langdon & Cheng, 1992) promote the use of self-inventory of cultural competence awareness and sensitivity. Munoz, Watson, Yarbrough, and Flahive (2011) state that the roles and responsibilities of the supervisor can still be met even when observing sessions in a language one doesn't speak, while ASHA (2008c) recommends that supervisors provide culturally appropriate feedback to supervisees. It is also important to know when it may be appropriate to use a cultural mediator or advisor concerning effective strategies for interactions with individuals (clients and supervisees) from specific backgrounds. Development of self-awareness on the part of the supervisor sets the stage for increased sensitivity and understanding of situations that may occur during the supervisory process that are solely related to cultural differences. Carozza (2011) offers a cogent discussion of cross-cultural issues in supervision.

McCready (2007) reviewed the research on generational differences in the workforce and noted that the disparities among generations are more complex today than in the past. The experiences of each generation shape the values, beliefs, attitudes, and behaviors that may have a significant effect on the supervisory relationship. For example, a 22-year-old AuD student is in a meeting with his 56-year-old clinical supervisor to discuss a patient with unilateral Meniere's disease. The student begins replying to a text message sent by a fellow audiologist while the supervisor is describing a peaked audiometric configuration. The supervisor is rather offended, believing that the student is not listening, and decides to stop speaking until the student has finished looking at his phone. The student looks up suddenly and asks the supervisor to continue the discussion, quite surprised that she appeared to be offended. The supervisor believes that the student should give her his undivided attention, assuming he can only focus on one thing at a time, while the student believes that multitasking is typical behavior and that his texting while listening should be no reason for the supervisor to take offense.

To bridge this type of generation gap, McCready suggests the formation of smaller study groups within the work setting to investigate the research in this area that can then be presented to the larger group as a whole. She also suggests that the supervisor engage in discussions about generational differences pertaining to a particular work setting or situation and how those differences may or may not apply to that specific setting. In the scenario provided, the supervisor could use the situation to explain the philosophical differences between her generation and that of the AuD student regarding perceptions of multitasking. Where cultural, linguistic, and generational issues are considered, supervisors have a responsibility for their own professional development in order to increase their knowledge and sensitivity. Demonstration of this desire to learn may also motivate supervisees to develop a plan for their own growth in this area.

Supervision of Challenging Supervisees

In graduate CSD programs, some students may present special challenges during the supervisory process (Shapiro, Ogletree, & Brotherton, 2002) and are often referred to as "marginal" students. Dowling (1985, as cited in Dowling, 2001) described marginal students as individuals who "cannot work independently, are unable to formulate goals and procedures, have basic gaps in conceptual understanding, and cannot follow through with suggestions" (p. 162). Understanding how to work effectively with marginal students deserves serious and systematic consideration (Shapiro et al., 2002). By the time these "marginal" students have graduated, they have completed the necessary requirements in their academic courses and clinical work to begin employment. However, new clinicians who experienced some of these challenges as students may need to be carefully monitored by their supervisors once they are in the work setting. In particular, these new clinicians may have difficulty evaluating their skill level accurately (Kruger & Dunning, 1999, as cited in McCrea & Brasseur, 2003). The initial collaborative planning phase of the supervisory process should address this and any other potential areas of concern, and goals should be developed to target those areas specifically. Schober-Peterson and O'Rourke (2008) describe using a formative assessment when working with the "at-risk" student and describe how this type of ongoing assessment encouraged students to take responsibility for their learning and be active participants in the assessment of their knowledge and skills.

This type of ongoing assessment, including providing specific feedback based on objective data collection, can support these new clinicians as they achieve the ultimate goal of self-supervision.

Technology and Supervision

The use of technology in supervision is not necessarily a new concept although the variety of forms to support the supervisory process has expanded significantly over the past several years. The Internet has made it possible for supervisors to use e-mail, instant messaging, social networks, and videoconferencing to communicate with supervisees in real time. Webinars, blogs, and podcasts can store information for access at a later time and may be shared with a large number of individuals. The use of audiotapes and videotapes will likely reveal behaviors that supervisors and supervisees may use for the development of goals for improvement (McCrea & Brasseur, 2003). For example, the supervisor and supervisee may view a videotaped treatment session to verify data, review and discuss subtle behaviors that were not easily observable in real time, or evaluate the success of a treatment technique. The ability to self-analyze behaviors after they have occurred is an extremely effective tool in promoting reflective practice.

Although many universities use videoconferencing routinely for course delivery, it is also an effective technology to support required supervisory visits that may be challenged by time factors and/or geographical distance. Distance supervision, or e-supervision, was described by Dudding (2002) as the use of two-way interactive videoconferencing technology for supervision of graduate students. Dudding (2006) reports that in a later study she found that there was no significant difference in graduate student perceptions of the effectiveness of the traditional versus distance supervision models. She reports that the graduate students "indicated that they felt more in charge of the session and less distracted than when the supervisor was physically in the therapy room" (p. 17).

Tellis, Cimino, and Alberti (2010) described a novel video-capture technology, the Landro Play Analyzer, to supervise clinical sessions and to train students to improve their clinical skills. They were able to observe four clinical sessions simultaneously from a central observation center. In addition, speech samples were analyzed in real time; saved on a CD, DVD, or flash/jump drive; viewed in slow motion; paused; and analyzed with Microsoft Excel. The use of this technology for clinical supervision allowed the authors to monitor multiple sessions as well as provide their student clinicians with specific feedback. Students indicated that they improved their clinical skills because they had the opportunity to review their sessions. Clinicians also reported using this technology successfully with their clients.

Advances in technology have played an important role in the area of supervision and are likely to continue to do so. The opportunities, as well as the challenges, that technology presents and the role that it will continue to play are important issues for supervisors and supervisees alike. ASHA (2008b) stresses the importance of following regulatory guidelines involving confidentiality when using technology in supervision (e.g., videoconferencing). The integral concerns related to ethics, etiquette, access to technical support, licensure regulations, and capital resources should also be considered in any discussion of technology and its application to the supervisory process. See Chapter 26 for a more in-depth discussion of technology.

Training in Supervision

All too often, clinicians are placed in a supervisory role with limited or no supervisory experience. They may be clinically experienced and available, but they do not necessarily have an interest in supervision. Achieving clinical competence does not necessarily mean one has the ability to be an effective supervisor. Therefore, it is important to learn about differing supervisory styles and to develop competence in supervision (ASHA, 2008c). Anderson (1998), Dowling (2001), and McCrea and Brasseur (2003) note that many professionals assume the role of supervisor without adequate training or preparation. Increasingly, data support that supervisors who have had training are more effective than those who have not (O'Connor, 2008). McCrea and Brasseur (2003) note that specific preparation of supervisors is highly recommended.

The ASHA (2008c, pp. 2–8) document *Knowledge and Skills Needed by Speech-Language Pathologists Providing Clinical Supervision* lists 11 items representing core areas that should be acquired by the supervisor:

1. Preparation for the Supervisory Experience
2. Interpersonal Communication and the Supervisor-Supervisee Relationship

3. Development of the Supervisee's Critical Thinking and Problem-Solving Skills
4. Development of the Supervisee's Clinical Competence in Assessment
5. Development of the Supervisee's Clinical Competence in Intervention
6. Supervisory Conferences or Meetings of Clinical Teaching teams
7. Evaluating the Growth of the Supervisee Both as a Clinician and as a Professional
8. Diversity (Ability, Race, Ethnicity, Gender, Age, Culture, Language, Class, Experience, and Education)
9. The Development and Maintenance of Clinical and Supervisory Documentation
10. Ethical, Regulatory, and Legal Requirements
11. Principles of Mentoring

Currently, ASHA (2008c) does not have specific training or continuing education requirements for those seeking to serve as a supervisor or CF mentor, but they must hold a current CCC and the required state licensure. The ABA requires only that mentors for students in an AuD program hold a state license and/or be a certified ABA audiologist. However, some states (e.g., California) or settings may require specific coursework or credentials before granting supervisory status. Although the availability of training in the form of coursework and continuing education (CE) in supervision may not always meet the demand, opportunities are available for continuing education in supervision. ASHA provides CE sessions at its annual convention as well as webinars and teleconferences on supervision. Many state associations also provide CE sessions on supervision. Special Interest Group 11, Administration and Supervision, publishes *Perspectives* three times per year and affords opportunities to earn CE credit. Several recent noteworthy books are also available to those who have an interest in learning more about supervision (Carozza, 2010; Dowling, 2001; McCrea & Brasseur, 2003).

Supervisor Accountability

The evaluation of a supervisor should be based on the demonstration of skills and competencies associated with the supervisory process. Supervisees are often asked to participate in the evaluation process of their supervisors. Do most supervisees have the knowledge required to know what to expect from a supervisor if asked to provide feedback? Even if they did, would they provide feedback that is honest and objective? The answers to these questions support self-evaluation by the supervisor relative to the supervisory process (ASHA, 2008a). However, there are no validated guidelines for the outcomes achieved by supervisors, thus making it necessary for supervisors to use informal measures to evaluate their own supervisory skills and competencies (McCrea & Brasseur, 2003).

Supervisors may consider using items from a self-assessment guide developed by Casey et al. (1988) to assist their effectiveness in acquiring the 13 tasks and 81 associated competencies contained in the ASHA position statement (ASHA, 1985b). Supervisors may also consider using the more recent ASHA (2008c) knowledge and skills document as the basis for their own self-evaluation tool. Analysis of the data from such a self-assessment allows the supervisor to identify supervisory objectives, select procedures, and measure goal outcomes (ASHA, 2008c). A performance appraisal that employs multiple sources of input is referred to as a *360-Degree Assessment* (U.S. Office of Personnel Management, 1997). This appraisal includes self-assessment, and some aspects of a supervisor's performance may also be evaluated by a professional peer, support staff, and an administrator to whom the individual reports. This type of performance appraisal focuses on subjective impressions of global aspects of supervisor behavior and will not necessarily provide insight into the efficiency and effectiveness of an individual supervisor's practice (McCrea & Brasseur, 2003).

The results of a successful evaluation of one's own behavior present an opportunity for quality assurance to ensure accountability. Making a decision to improve as a supervisor promotes job satisfaction, self-fulfillment, and ethical behavior and prevents burnout (Dowling, 2001). Self-assessment is a key ingredient of reflective practice, and the supervisor who uses this tool is also providing the supervisee an effective role model.

FUTURE NEEDS IN SUPERVISION AND MENTORING

Supervision and mentoring are required components of clinical training and credentialing for professional organizations in speech-language pathology and audiology. Because of its pervasive nature in the professions, ASHA (2008a) recognizes supervision as a distinct area of practice. What research is needed to ensure evidence-based practices in the distinct area of supervision? Data collection and analysis as part of the supervisory process provide the foundation for research and evidence to support effective supervisory practice. Anderson (1988) stated, "When the clinical supervision process proceeds as inquiry, personal discoveries have the potential for becoming collective discoveries" (p. 298). These discoveries are made after careful examination of the effects of certain supervisory practices, forming the basis of research. Emphasizing the need for further research, ASHA (2008b) states, "Systematic study and investigation of the supervisory process is necessary to expand the evidence base from which increased knowledge about supervision and the supervisory process will emerge." Following are the possible topics for further research included in this document:

- Exploring different supervisory approaches that promote problem solving, self-analysis, and self-evaluation to develop clinical effectiveness
- Identifying essential components of training effective supervisors
- Examining the efficacy of supervisory training on supervisor/supervisee satisfaction and competence
- Identifying the basic behaviors/skills that supervisors should use in their interactions with supervisees that are essential to an effective working relationship
- Examining how supervisory style affects the development of clinical competence
- Examining different methods to develop more efficient models of supervision
- Examining supervisor behaviors that enhance supervisee growth (e.g., examining the process for negotiating and mutually agreeing on targets for change and measuring the impact that supervisor change has on the supervisee's professional growth) or training supervisors to use specific interpersonal skills (e.g., empathy, active listening) and then measuring how such skills enhance supervisee growth (McCrea & Brasseur, 2003)
- Examining the effectiveness and efficiency of technology in delivering supervision
- Examining the impact of supervision on client outcomes
- Examining supervisory approaches and communication styles with supervisees in consideration of gender, age, and cultural and linguistic diversity
- Examining aspects of the supervisory process (i.e., understanding, planning, observing, analyzing, and integrating) and the relationship of each to the success of the supervisory experience (McCrea & Brasseur, 2003)

In her article, O'Connor (2008) suggests actions that professionals and/or the professions still need to take to ensure quality supervision and more effective clinical education. These actions include consideration of a theoretically based protocol to train individuals for supervision and development of a tool to measure a supervisor's effectiveness that is based on the skills or competencies associated with the responsibilities involved in the supervisory process.

In 2010, ASHA's Special Interest Group 11, Administration and Supervision, conducted a survey of its affiliates to determine if there was an interest in voluntary supervisory training that would lead to a credential in supervision. Ninety-six percent of the respondents rated formal training in supervision as very important or somewhat important. More than 90 percent stated that new supervisors, current supervisors with no formal training, and current supervisors interested in additional training would benefit from supervisory training. The majority of the respondents stated that they had received their training through self-study, on-the-job training, conferences and workshops, and informal networking (Victor, 2010). The results of this survey lend support for the development of a theoretically based protocol to train individuals for supervision.

As noted earlier in this chapter, Casey (1985; Casey et al., 1988) developed a tool to measure a supervisor's effectiveness that was based on the competencies associated with the responsibilities involved in the supervisory process listed in the 1985 ASHA position statement. The more recently revised ASHA (2008a) position statement could serve as the basis for recommendation of a new tool for self-evaluation as supervisors continue their efforts to provide state-of-the-art clinical services.

Both supervisors and supervisees alike have the responsibility to learn about issues in clinical supervision. The most effective supervisors will approach the supervisory relationship with the understanding that supervisees bring not only certain skills, knowledge, and clinical experience to a situation but also their own individual talents, perceptions, and life experiences. They will also appreciate how each of these factors can influence both the supervisory relationship and the overall clinical experience itself. For supervisees to develop critical knowledge and skills leading to competency, they must also learn to analyze their own behaviors to see how their actions influence the supervisory relationship and their clinical experiences. This shared responsibility for supporting the principles of reflective practice will lead to self-supervision of the independent clinician who is committed to lifelong learning and professional growth.

SUMMARY

Supervision plays a major role in the professions of speech-language pathology and audiology because of its pervasive nature. This chapter presented a model of skill acquisition that forms the basis of successful models of supervision including a continuum model and a model comprising four key components of the supervisory process. It also provided an overview of regulations and guidelines leading to professional certification in both speech-language pathology and audiology. Current issues in supervision that are relevant across settings, including professional ethics, cultural differences, technology, training, and accountability, were also discussed. Finally, it set the stage for further exploration of research in this essential area of the professions.

CRITICAL THINKING

1. What are some of the dynamic differences you should anticipate as you move from working with a clinical supervisor in a university setting to a mentor in your professional workplace? What role do interpersonal communication skills play in this relationship?
2. You are a clinical fellow in an elementary school and have just been asked to supervise an SLPA. Is this appropriate? What responsibilities do you plan to assign her? How will you evaluate her performance?
3. Suppose your supervisor during an externship gave you more clinical responsibility than you thought you were prepared to implement. How would you approach your supervisor about this issue?
4. How would videotaping a treatment session assist the supervisor in promoting self-assessment? What other forms of technology do you think facilitate supervision? Why?
5. One of the difficult issues university programs face is when a student has excellent academic ability but clinical skills that are poor or very slow in developing. What evidence should a supervisor present to document clinical skill achievement in such a situation?
6. You work for a large community speech and hearing center and are about to hire a clinical supervisor who can both mentor those in their clinical fellowship and also manage the preschool program for children who are hearing impaired. What qualities would you look for in this professional? What are some questions you might pose to the professional during an interview for this position?
7. Suppose your supervisor abruptly ended the supervisory relationship before you had met the requirements for certification and/or licensure. What would you do?
8. Do you think supervisors should be required to have training before they can become supervisors? If so, what should the training include?
9. You just started your first clinical position and feel that the person assigned to you as a mentor does not provide you with sufficient information and feedback. The individual is "very nice" to you but does not provide the support you need as you start this position. What would you do?
10. In contrast, you are the mentor for a first-year professional who is highly confident but does not listen carefully to your suggestions and information. You feel that she dismisses what you have to offer. What would you do?

REFERENCES

American Board of Audiology. (2011). *Board certification in audiology*. Available from http://www.americanboardofaudiology.org/faq/faqs_board_certification.html

American Speech-Language-Hearing Association. (n.d.). *Clinical fellowship*. Available from http://www.asha.org/Certification/Clinical_Fellowship

American Speech-Language-Hearing Association. (1985). Committee on Supervision in Speech-Language Pathology and Audiology: Clinical supervision in speech-language pathology and audiology. A position statement. *ASHA, 27*, 57–60.

American Speech-Language-Hearing Association. (1996, Spring). Guidelines for the training, credentialing, use, and supervision of speech-language pathology assistants. *ASHA, 38* (Suppl. 16), 21–34.

American Speech-Language-Hearing Association. (1997). *ASHA certification and membership handbook*. Rockville, MD: Author.

American Speech-Language-Hearing Association. (1998). *Students and professionals who speak English with accents and nonstandard dialects: Issues and recommendations*. Available from http://www.asha.org/policy

American Speech-Language-Hearing Association. (2000). *Background information and standards for implementation for the certificate of clinical competence in speech-language pathology*. Rockville, MD: ASHA, Council on Professional Standards in Speech-Language Pathology and Audiology.

American Speech-Language-Hearing Association. (2007). *Responsibilities of individuals who mentor clinical fellows*. Available from http://www.asha.org/policy

American Speech-Language-Hearing Association. (2008a). *Clinical supervision in speech-language pathology* [Position statement]. Available from http://www.asha.org/policy

American Speech-Language-Hearing Association. (2008b). *Clinical supervision in speech-language pathology* [Technical report]. Available from http://www.asha.org/policy

American Speech-Language-Hearing Association. (2008c). *Knowledge and skills needed by speech-language pathologists providing clinical supervision*. Available from http://www.asha.org/policy

American Speech-Language-Hearing Association. (2010a). *Certification*. Available from http://www.asha.org/about/membership-certification/

American Speech-Language-Hearing Association. (2010b). *Code of ethics*. Available from http://www.asha.org/policy

American Speech-Language-Hearing Association. (2010c). *Supervision of student clinicians* [Issues in Ethics]. Available from http://www.asha.org/policy

Anderson, J. (Ed.). (1970). *Proceedings of Conference on Supervision of Speech and Hearing Programs in the Schools*. Bloomington, IN: Indiana University.

Anderson, J. L. (1988). *The supervisory process in speech-language pathology and audiology*. Austin, TX: PRO-ED.

Anderson, N. B. (1992). Understanding cultural diversity. *American Journal of Speech-Language Pathology, 1*, 11–12.

Battle, D. (1993). *Communication disorders in multicultural populations*. Boston, MA: Butterworth-Heinemann.

Carin, A., & Sund, R. (1971). *Developing questioning techniques*. Columbus, OH: Charles E. Merrill.

Carozza, L. (2011). *Science of successful supervision and mentorship*. San Diego, CA: Plural Publishing.

Casey, P. (1985). *Supervisory skills self-assessment*. Whitewater, WI: University of Wisconsin.

Casey, P., Smith, K., & Ulrich, S. (1988). *Self-supervision: A career tool for audiologists and speech-language pathologists* (Clinical Series No. 10). Rockville, MD: National Student Speech Language Hearing Association.

Cogan, M. (1973). *Clinical supervision*. Boston, MA: Houghton Mifflin.

Coleman, T. J. (2000). *Clinical management of communication disorders in culturally diverse children*. Needham Heights, MA: Allyn & Bacon.

Council for Clinical Certification in Audiology and Speech-Language Pathology. (2005). *Membership and certification handbook of the American Speech-Language-Hearing Association.* Available from http://www.asha.org/about/membership-certification/handbooks/slp/slp_standards.htm

Council on Academic Accreditation in Audiology and Speech-Language Pathology. (2004). *Standards for accreditation of graduate education programs in audiology and speech-language pathology programs.* Available from http://www.asha.org/policy

Crago, M., & Pickering, M. (Eds.). (1987). *Supervision in human communication disorders: Perspectives on a process.* San Diego, CA: Little Brown-College Hill Press.

Cunningham, R. (1971). Developing question-asking skills. In J. Weigand (Ed.), *Developing teacher competencies.* Englewood Cliffs, NJ: Prentice Hall.

Dowling, S. (2001). *Supervision: Strategies for successful outcomes and productivity.* Boston, MA: Allyn & Bacon.

Dreyfus, H. I., & Dreyfus S. E. (1986). Five steps from novice to expert. In *Mind over machine.* New York, NY: Free Press.

Dudding, C. C. (2002). The use of videoconferencing in supervision of graduate clinicians. *Perspectives on Administration and Supervision, 12*(1), 8–12.

Dudding, C. C. (2006). Distance supervision: An update. *Perspectives on Administration and Supervision, 16*(1), 16–18.

Fall, M., & Sutton, J. M. (2004). *Clinical supervision: A handbook for practitioners.* Auckland, New Zealand: Pearson Education New Zealand.

Farmer S., & Farmer, J. (1989). *Supervision in communication disorders.* Columbus, OH: Merrill.

Gillam, R. B., Roussos, C. S., & Anderson, J. L. (1990). Facilitating changes in supervisees' clinical behaviors: An experimental investigation of supervisory effectiveness. *Journal of Speech and Hearing Disorders, 55*(4), 729–739.

Goldhammer, R., Anderson, R., & Krajewski, R. (1980). *Clinical supervision* (2nd ed.). New York, NY: Holt, Rinehart, and Winston.

Halfond, M. (1964). Clinical supervision-stepchild in training. *ASHA, 6,* 441–444.

Hudson, M. W. (2010). Supervision to mentoring: Practical considerations. *Perspectives on Administration and Supervision, 20,* 71–75.

Hudson, M. W. (2010). *Supporting professional performance in the clinical workplace.* Short course held at convention of the American Speech-Language-Hearing Association, Philadelphia.

King, D. (2003, May 27). Supervision of student clinicians: Modeling ethical practice for future professionals. *The ASHA Leader, 8,* 26.

Kleffner, F. (Ed.). (1964). *Seminar on guidelines for the internship year.* Washington, DC: American Speech and Hearing Association.

Ladany, N., Walker, J. A., & Melincoff, D. S. (2001). Supervisory style: Its relation to the supervisory working alliance and supervisory self-disclosure. *Counselor Education and Supervision, 40,* 263–275.

Langdon, H. W., & Cheng, L. (1992). *Hispanic children and adults with communication disorders.* Gaithersburg, MD: Aspen Publishers.

Leighton, J. (1991). Gender stereotyping in supervisory styles. *Psychoanalytic Review, 78,* 347–363.

Long, J., Lawless, J., & Dotson, D. (1996). Supervisory Styles Index: Examining supervisees' perceptions of supervisory style. *Contemporary Family Therapy, 18*(4), 589–606.

Mawdsley, B. (1987). Kansas Inventory of Self-Supervision. In S. Farmer, (Ed.), *Clinical supervision: A coming of age.* Proceedings of a national conference on supervision held at Las Cruces, New Mexico State University.

McCrea, E., & Brasseur, J. (2003). *The supervisory process in speech-language pathology and audiology.* Boston, MA: Allyn & Bacon.

McCready, V. (2007). Generational differences: Do they make a difference in supervisory and administrative relationships? *Perspectives in Administration and Supervision, 17*(3), 6–9.

Munoz, M. L., Watson, J. B., Yarbrough, L., & Flahive, L. K. (2011). Monolingual supervision of bilingual student clinicians: Challenges and opportunities. *The ASHA Leader, 16,* 5.

Newman, W. (2001, June/July). The ethical and legal aspects of clinical supervision. *California Speech-Language-Hearing Association Magazine, 30*(1), 10–11, 27.

Newman, W., Victor, S., & Zylla-Jones, E. (2009). *Tools for the first-time supervisor.* Proceedings of session at national convention of the American Speech-Language-Hearing Association, New Orleans, LA.

O'Connor, L. (2008). A new focus on supervision: Looking to the future. *Perspectives on Administration and Supervision, 18*, 17–23.

Pfeiffer, J. W., & Jones, J. E. (1987). *A handbook of structured experiences for human relations training.* San Diego, CA: University Associates.

Schober-Peterson, D., & O'Rourke, C. (2008). Identifying and assisting at-risk graduate students: Process and outcome factors. *Perspectives on Administration and Supervision, 18*, 94–98.

Severinsson, E. (1996). Nurse supervisors' views of their supervisory styles in clinical supervision: A hermeneutical approach. *Journal of Nursing Management, 4*, 191–199.

Severinsson, E., & Hallberg, I. (1996). Clinical supervisors' views of their leadership role in the clinical supervision process with nursing care. *Journal of Advanced Nursing, 24*, 151–161.

Shapiro, D. A., Ogletree, B. T., & Brotherton, W. D. (2002). Graduate students with marginal abilities in communication sciences and disorders: Prevalence, profiles, and solutions. *Journal of Communication Disorders, 35*, 421–451.

Shea, G. F. (1997). *Mentoring: A practical guide* (2nd ed.). Lanham, MD: Crisp Publications.

Shipley, K. (1997). *Interviewing and counseling in communicative disorders—Principles and procedures* (2nd ed.). Boston, MA: Allyn & Bacon.

Smith, K. (1979). *Supervisory conferences questions: Who asks them and who answers them.* Paper presented at the annual convention of the American Speech and Hearing Association, Atlanta, GA.

Tellis, G., Cimino, L., & Alberti, J. (2010). Advanced digital technology for supervising graduate clinicians. *Perspectives on Administration and Supervision, 20*, 9–13.

Ulrich, S. (1985). Continuing education model of training. In K. Smith (Moderator), *Preparation and training models for the supervisory process.* Short course presented at the annual convention of the American Speech-Language-Hearing Association, Washington, DC.

U.S. Department of Personnel Management. (1997). *360-Degree assessment: An overview.* Retrieved from http://www.opm.gov/perform/wppdf/360asess.pdf

Victor, S. (2010). Coordinator's column. *Perspectives on Administration and Supervision, 20*(3), 83–84.

Weltsch, B. R., & Crowe, L. K. (2006). Effectiveness of mediated analysis in improving student clinical competency. *Perspectives on Administration and Supervision, 16*, 21–22.

RESOURCES

Bartlett, S., (2003). Bartlett's action plan. In E. McCrea & J. Brasseur (Eds.), *The supervisory process in speech-language pathology and audiology* (pp. 154–156). Boston, MA: Allyn & Bacon.

Hurst, B., Wilson, C., & Cramer, G. (1998). Professional teaching portfolios. *Phi Delta Kappan, 79*(8), 578–582.

Knowles, M. (1975). *Self-directed learning: A guide for learners and teachers.* New York, NY: Association Press.

McCarthy, M. P. (2009). *Promoting independence through self-evaluation and formative assessment in clinical education.* Presentation at national convention of the American Speech-Language-Hearing Association, New Orleans, LA.

Plutorak, E. G. (1993). Facilitating reflective thought in novice teachers. *Journal of Teacher Education, 44*(4), 288–295.

Rahim, M. A. (1989). Relationships of leader power to compliance and satisfaction with supervision: Evidence from a national sample of managers. *Journal of Management, 15*, 495–516.

Schon, D. A. (1996). *Educating the reflective practitioner: Toward a new design for teaching and learning in the professions.* San Francisco, CA: Jossey-Bass.

26

Technology in the Digital Age

Carol C. Dudding, PhD

SCOPE OF CHAPTER

This chapter provides you with an introduction to the emerging use of technologies in the research, education, and practice of audiology and speech-language pathology. It offers insights into not only the technologies available but also the current and potential applications likely to change how we as professionals diagnose, treat, and interact with the patients we serve. This chapter will explore web-based tools and digital videoconferencing technologies that offer collaboration among professionals and researchers, applications for e-learning and e-supervision, virtual simulations, and service delivery via telepractice.

THE DIGITAL AGE

Digital Natives

If you are a student reading this chapter and were born after the early 1980s, you are considered a digital native or millennial (Jones, Ramanau, Cross, & Healing, 2010; Prensky, 2001b); you are someone who grew up with computers and Internet technologies. You are thought to be fluent in your use of technologies, impatient with linear thinking, and possess the ability to multitask (Jones et al., 2010). You have expectations for how you receive and share information, acquire knowledge, and interact with other people. You view learning as best achieved through action and exploration within a given context (Brown, n.d.). This is in contrast to many of your instructors, supervisors, and employers who are known as digital immigrants. Digital immigrants were exposed to digital technologies later in life. This distinction is important as our professions continue to move forward in research, education, and service delivery. It is a key factor to remember as we continue to develop these new forms of technology.

Impact on Practice Settings

Practicing speech-language pathologists and audiologists are employed in a number of work settings including health care, educational settings, and/or private practice. These practice settings are greatly influenced by technology trends. The health care arena is seeing a surge in health information technologies, such as electronic medical records, electronic billing, and clinical point of care technologies. Health information technologies are projected to increase by 11 percent in coming years ("Health Care Technology Today," 2010). Clinical decision support systems (CDSSs) that aid in assessment and diagnosis will likely "have a profound impact on clinical diagnostics and therapeutics" ("Health Care Technology Today," 2010, p. 41).

Emerging professionals can expect to be involved either professionally or personally in telehealth. *Telehealth* is a term used to describe the delivery of health care services through telecommunication technologies. It is sometimes used interchangeably with the terms *telemedicine* and *telepractice*. The growth and development of telehealth technologies are supported by a federal stimulus package—the American Recovery and Reinvestment Act of 2009—which allocated $2.5 billion for investment in the broadband infrastructure needed to grow these programs. A growing part of the telehealth movement includes the development of patient sensor systems that allow for remote monitoring of patients in long-term care and home health settings. These remote monitoring devices give hope of improving quality of care and reducing health care costs (Rantz et al., 2010). Remote monitoring devices use wireless and Internet technologies to monitor heart rate, oxygen levels, and body temperature and allow for interaction between the patient and medical personnel. These remote monitoring systems and telehealth technologies, in addition to the instrumentation and assistive technologies, will impact all aspects of service delivery in the professions of audiology and speech-language pathology. A more in-depth discussion of the specific technologies follows.

The education arena has certainly been influenced by technologies in the form of educational technologies used in teaching; data management systems that assist tracking student progress; online and web-based therapy portals; computerized assessments and analysis programs; various assistive technologies including augmentative alternative communication (AAC) systems; hearing aids and cochlear implants; and service delivery through telepractice. Once considered an adjunct to teaching, computers are ubiquitous in public school classrooms. Entire organizations, such as the Society for Information Technology & Teacher Education (SITE), have emerged to support research and scholarship in the integration of technology in the classroom. Today's teachers readily employ computer and Internet applications across the curriculum. The National Center for Educational Statistics (2005) reports that nearly 100 percent of public schools in the United States had Internet access, with a growing number employing broadband wireless connections. It was reported that there was one computer for every 3.8 students (National Center for Educational Statistics, 2005). An increasing number of schools are providing teachers and students with handheld computers and tablet-based systems, 17 percent and 8.1 percent, respectively (National Center for Educational Statistics, 2005). Data management systems within the public schools allow tracking of student progress across disciplines, including speech-language services. Through a number of commercially available programs, speech-language pathologists and audiologists based in public schools can access scheduling calendars and student records. They can share information with family members and other professionals and track and report progress toward goals. Many public school systems use dedicated online programs such as IEPOnline to create, track, and share students' Individualized Education Programs (IEPs), thereby streamlining the cumbersome documentation process.

Observe a college campus to see the extent and types of mobile and wireless technologies employed by students in higher education. The emergence of cellular "smart phones" and tablet computers allows students to access the Internet, search databases, connect with others through web conferencing, read books electronically, and communicate via texting from the palm of their hand at a time and location of their choosing. The smart phones and tablets have also yielded an explosion in the development and implementation of application programs known as "apps," many of which support learning.

The remainder of this chapter will focus on some of the specific applications of technology employed in audiology and speech-language pathology, along with the benefits and limitations of each application. When applicable, examples of programs and technologies are provided. These examples are not meant to be an exhaustive list of available products, nor are they meant to serve as an endorsement of a product. Considering the rapid development of digital technologies, it is certain that the technologies discussed in this chapter will soon be outdated. Yet, you are encouraged to consider the technologies and current applications as a starting point in moving forward in the professions of audiology and speech-language pathology. This chapter will help you to think critically about the types and uses of technologies now and in the future.

COMMUNICATION AND COLLABORATION

The emergence of e-mail, text messaging, social networks, and cellular phones has changed the way individuals choose to communicate and share information. These same technologies, along with other VoIP (Voice over Internet Protocol) protocols, offer opportunities for collaboration, consultation, mentoring, and research (Dudding, 2009).

Web Conferencing

Consider the use of web-conferencing software programs such as Skype, Elluminate, and Microsoft Office Live Meeting for collaborating on a research project or discussing a challenging case. These applications, and others like them, allow for real-time communication through use of text, voice, and/or video communication. Desktop sharing allows all participants to view and modify shared documents and applications in real time. Consider a practitioner working with a client with a rare or complex condition. With the use of the aforementioned technologies, practitioners are able to consult with an expert located across the country or indeed across the world. They can virtually meet in real time to discuss a client, view videos of a client's performance, and/or share test results. Now imagine that the same expert is researching a rare or complex condition but has access to a limited number of clients. Once again, through the use of the web-conferencing technologies, the professionals can now collaborate and share information to advance research in this area. No doubt you can imagine any number of scenarios in which the sharing of information among professionals would be beneficial not only to the clients but to the advancement of the professions.

Many of the web-conferencing technologies are inexpensive or free and require an Internet connection, computer, and web camera. These technologies allow participants to communicate in real time, using voice, text, and/or video over the Internet. Participants can either download the required software (e.g., Skype) or log on to an electronic meeting system (e.g., Microsoft Live Meeting).

Users need to be aware of the limitations of this application in terms of quality of audio-video transmission and security of information. The quality of transmission of information during a web conference relies heavily on the Internet speed and bandwidth availability for all participants. Factors such as type of information shared and number of participants can also influence quality. In limited-bandwidth situations, restricting the number of participants and avoiding use of video can improve the quality of the transmission. Another important consideration is that some Internet networking systems and web-conferencing applications lack the security that would allow users to adequately protect the privacy and confidentiality of client information. Features such as firewalls, password-protected applications, and data encryption can improve overall security. Participants should consult with network support personnel and software vendors to determine security levels before sharing client-specific information. A discussion of the Health Insurance Portability and Accountability Act of 1996 (HIPAA) and the

Family Educational Rights and Privacy Act (FERPA) appears at the end of this chapter.

In determining the appropriate web-conferencing technology, users should consider the following questions:

- How many people will be involved? (point-to-point or multipoint)
- When are people available to meet? (synchronous or asynchronous)
- What types of information will be shared? (documents, images, videos, audio, Internet sites)
- What are the security needs and concerns? (client specific, protected information)
- What resources are available? (licensing fees, software, hardware, network access, technology support)

Peer-to-Peer File Sharing and Document Sharing

Another way that professionals and students can collaborate and share information is through peer-to-peer (P2P) file-sharing programs and document-sharing websites such as BitTorrent and GoogleDocs, respectively. These applications allow enrolled users to post, edit, and share documents, music, and a variety of multimedia files. Some applications, such as GoogleDocs, Microsoft Skydive, and Dropbox, allow for storage and retrieval using "cloud computing." Cloud computing is a hosted Internet service that allows users to access the applications through browsers, without housing software or files on a computer, allowing access to your information from any computer at any time. This would be particularly helpful for students and professionals working as a team to create a research paper, procedure manual, or other text-based project. The documents can be either protected or shared with specified users to ensure security of the information. Be aware that P2P applications pose a risk for illegal pirating of music, video, and software. They are also a source for a large number of spyware and viruses. Other helpful web-based collaboration tools include project management sites such as Basecamp and Projectmanager.com. In addition to document sharing, project management sites allow users to assign tasks to specific individuals and track completion of those tasks. Some sites have meeting schedulers, shared calendars, and web-conferencing capabilities for members to discuss the project. These technologies, used individually or together, support and enhance collaboration and research for practicing professionals, students, and researchers in speech-language pathology, audiology, and the speech-hearing sciences.

INSTRUCTION AND TRAINING

Online Learning

Higher education has witnessed an undeniable proliferation of online technologies, especially in the area of distance learning. The Sloan-C Report by Allen and Seaman, *Learning on Demand: Online Education in the United States, 2009,* reveals that more than 4.6 million students were enrolled in at least one online course in the fall of 2008, indicating a 17 percent increase from the previous year. This increase far exceeds the 1.2 percent increase in overall enrollment in higher education (Allen & Seaman, 2010).

There are a number of reported reasons for the increase in online learning in America's universities, including a downturn in the economy, the promise of increased student access, and outreach to students outside of their geographic area. Additionally, some university administrators view online learning as a means to "growth in continuing/professional education, increasing degree completion rates, enhancing the institution's brand value, and providing pedagogic improvements" (Allen & Seaman, 2010, p. 17).

The disciplines of speech-language pathology and audiology are experiencing similar growth rates in the use of distance education technologies in the academic and clinical training of future professionals. A search using the American Speech-Language-Hearing Association's (ASHA) EdFind revealed that 4 percent of speech-language master's degree programs offer complete programs through distance education, and 17 percent offer at least some online courses. Of the 79 doctoral programs in audiology listed within EdFind, 20 percent reported offering at least some courses through distance education. These numbers do not account for the number of graduate courses that are offered as hybrid or blended, that is, courses that employ both face-to-face and online delivery methods.

Instruction through distance learning takes many forms and involves a wide range of technologies. The types of interactions that occur in distance education can be categorized as either synchronous (all participants interacting at the same time) or asynchronous (participants interacting at different times). Many online courses are a blending of these two formats. Technologies that allow for synchronous interaction in online learning include web conferencing, chat rooms, virtual meeting spaces, and conference calls. These technologies allow students and instructors to interact in real time and can incorporate text, video, or audio information. Instructors are able to hold "virtual office hours" during which they interact with students in ways similar to traditional on-campus interactions.

When meeting in real time is not practical or desired, asynchronous interactions and instruction may occur through viewing of recorded presentations, lectures, and videos posted by the instructor, text-based postings on discussion boards, and independent readings and assignments. Often, online learning is delivered through a course management system that allows for user-friendly integration of many of the technologies used in online learning. A popular course management system known as Blackboard allows instructors to post documents, presentations, and video or audio files; set up discussion boards and chat rooms; organize students for collaborative assignments; create and administer online exams and quizzes; view student work; and enter grades into an electronic grade book. Students are able to access the materials posted by the instructor, submit papers and projects, interact with other students and the instructor, and view grades online. Other course management systems are available, some at no cost, to integrate technologies within a user-friendly environment. It is anticipated that the next generation of course management systems used in online learning will look very different from what we have available today, perhaps occurring within virtual classrooms.

In addition to the education and training of future professionals, the technologies discussed have impacted professional development and training in both audiology and speech-language pathology. Beginning in 2003 for audiology and 2005 for speech-language pathology, ASHA-certified professionals are required to obtain 30 hours of continuing education activities within each three-year period. The American Board of Audiology (ABA) and various state licensing agencies also require professional development for recertification and/or licensure. These requirements have created a great need for quality professional development offerings at reasonable costs and convenience. Once again, technology has played a significant role in this area of professional development. FIRST Y*EARS* is an example of a certificate program in auditory learning for children with hearing loss offered through distance learning. In addition to online courses, *webinars* and *webcasts* have emerged, allowing professionals to obtain continuing education while seated at a computer. A webinar (web-based seminar) is a lecture or workshop delivered over the World Wide Web. When the transmission of information is one-way, with no participant interaction, it is referred to as a *webcast.* These methods have proved to be a popular, efficient, and cost-effective way of obtaining required professional development.

A discussion of online learning would be remiss to focus solely on the technologies and not mention the pedagogical aspects. A large amount of research over the years has supported the contention that online learning is as effective or more effective than traditional learning environments (Allen & Seaman, 2007; Lou, Bernard, & Abrami, 2006; Seaman, 2009; Senior, 2010; Williams, 2006). Researchers are exploring pedagogical considerations such as online communities, computer-mediated communication, and interactivity as they contribute to learning in the online environment (Belderrain, 2006; Cox, Carr, & Hall, 2004; Davidson-Shivers, Muilenburg, & Tanner, 2001; Garrison & Cleveland-Innes, 2005; Hmelo-Silver & Barrows, 2008). In 1999, Heinch, Molenda, Russell, and Smaldino developed the ASSURE model to assist in designing courses that involve media technologies. Table 26–1 outlines the components of the ASSURE model.

A number of resources are available for those interested in the design and evaluation of online teaching and technologies. Students and instructors are encouraged to seek out these resources when developing or participating in online learning.

E-supervision

The ABA, ASHA's Council for Clinical Certification, and state licensing and credentialing agencies require student clinicians to complete practicum requirements under the supervision of accredited and/or licensed professionals. Graduate programs in speech-language pathology and audiology recognize the significance of supervision as a means of producing quality clinicians. Bernard and Goodyear (1992) state the importance

TABLE 26–1 The ASSURE Model

A	Analyze learners	• Identify general character • Specify entry competencies • Determine learning style
S	State objectives	• Clearly construct learning outcomes • State desired behaviors • State conditions and degree of performance
S	Select methods, media, and materials	• Select instructional methods • Select media best suited for needs • Modify existing and design new materials as needed
U	Utilize media and materials	• Become familiar with the materials • Prepare the materials, environment • Provide the learning experience
R	Require learner participation	• Prepare in-class and follow-up activities so learner can process the information
E	Evaluate and revise	• Assess before, during, and after instruction • Evaluate the learner, media methods

Based on Heinich, Molenda, Russell, and Smaldino, 1999

of supervision as a "means of transmitting the skills, knowledge, and attitudes of a particular profession. It also is an essential means of ensuring that the clients receive a certain minimum of quality of care while trainees work with them to gain their skills" (p. 2).

As institutions of higher education see a rise in the number of nontraditional applicants pursuing graduate training, along with the increase in distance learning opportunities, fulfilling the supervisory requirements for all students becomes challenging. Students often seek to complete clinical training at sites that are geographically remote from the college campus that may not have access to certified professionals to provide supervision. The time and financial resources required to provide supervision to students at remote locations are substantial (Dudding & Justice, 2004).

E-supervision, the use of digital videoconferencing for supervision, provides a means for students at geographically distant sites to be supervised by clinical instructors located at a college campus or selected base site. E-supervision offers many benefits, including cost-effectiveness and productivity of clinical instruction (Dudding & Justice, 2004). ASHA's recent technical report on supervision expressively permits the use of technology for real-time supervision (American Speech-Language-Hearing Association, 2008).

In establishing an e-supervision program, it is necessary to have a basic understanding of videoconferencing equipment, transmission protocols, and technology support issues. Videoconferencing can be characterized broadly into three categories: (1) desktop/personal conferencing, (2) small group or midlevel conferencing, and (3) telepresence. A program needs to be aware of the level or category of videoconferencing that can be supported by both the on-site and remote location. Table 26–2 describes various categories of videoconferencing available.

An early program of e-supervision for providing live supervision to graduate clinicians using videoconferencing was established at the University of Virginia. Dedicated videoconferencing units were placed within treatment rooms in a number of public schools across

TABLE 26–2 Categories of Videoconferencing

Category	Equipment Requirements	Approximate Costs*	Uses
Desktop/ personal	Computer, webcam, Internet connection, desktop collaboration software	$800 and up	Person-to-person connection, collaboration and sharing of documents and applications
Small group/ midlevel	Dedicated videoconferencing system, monitor, microphone; high-definition video camera	$5,000 and up	Person-to-person, may have option for multipoint; allows for control of remote camera; option of HD video
Telepresence	Fully integrated system, professionally designed and installed, interactive technologies	$300,000 and up	Immersive, "same room" experience; multipoint option; HD video

*For discussion only; does not include IP connection and conferencing fees. Reminder: a minimum of two systems is required.

Virginia with an additional videoconferencing unit set up in the university supervisor's office. The videoconferencing units allowed for real-time, two-way interactions between the supervisor and the graduate student. The supervisor could remotely control the view at the far site employing a pan, tilt, zoom (PTZ) feature. This e-supervision model allowed the university supervisor to supervise several students per day without the travel time between locations (Dudding & Justice, 2004).

Research conducted by Dudding (2004) indicated no significant difference in graduate student perceptions of the effectiveness of the traditional versus distance supervision models. In-depth interviews with graduate students revealed that they perceived the e-supervision model to be an effective means of supervision. One participant reported that videoconferencing was "a terrific tool for supervision when practically speaking, you know, your supervisor cannot be onsite with you. Then you get the same level of supervision" (Dudding, 2006, p. 51). Participants identified additional benefits as increased feelings of autonomy, flexibility, and support from the administration. The distance supervision model was limited in its ability to observe the graduate student while providing services within classrooms, during meetings, and while engaged in interactions with other professionals (Dudding, 2004).

As web camera technologies and high-speed Internet access have developed, other models of e-supervision have emerged employing the web-conferencing technologies as discussed earlier. These technologies are less expensive and require less bandwidth than dedicated videoconferencing systems. However, users should be aware of limitations in audio-video quality and the ability to control the view of the far camera.

Table 26–3 lists additional considerations in selecting a digital videoconferencing system.

E-mentoring

Another application of web conferencing and other communication technologies (e.g., cell phone and e-mail) is in the area of e-mentoring. E-mentoring refers to the use of technology to facilitate and support a mentoring relationship. In the article "The Power of Passionate Mentoring" (Battle, 2007), the author describes the mentoring relationship as a lifelong journey in which "mentors pass along their wisdom, guidance, insight, and understanding of life's experiences to facilitate the education of the mentees and to encourage them to grow and reach their own goals" (p. 1). Mentoring programs can enhance morale, increase productivity, and promote career development

TABLE 26–3 Considerations in Selecting Digital Videoconferencing System

Portability	Can the system be readily moved from location to location within a building or district? Is there an Internet connection available in the desired location?
Ease of use	What type of user setup is required? Is the user interface intuitive and navigable? Can novices readily use the system? What type of user support is available?
Compatibility	Is the system compatible with other systems currently in use? Can the unit interface with a Multipoint Control Unit or bridge to allow for expansion of use?
Connectivity	Does the system conform to the transmission protocols used by the program sites? Can it be used for conferencing with multiple sites? Can it be used with units utilizing a different protocol? What are the system's minimum bandwidth requirements? Does it have wireless capabilities? Can it interface with wireless technologies?
Support	Does the system's manufacturer provide accessible and ongoing technological support for end users and network personnel?
Versatility	What other uses can be served by the videoconferencing system (e.g., course delivery, professional development, collaboration, research)?
Costs	Does the cost of the system outweigh current expenditures for on-site supervision (e.g., mileage)? Is there an option to upgrade equipment at a reduced cost? Does the system's manufacturer provide a discount for institutions of higher education? Is there a discount for purchase of multiple units? What are the costs of any required maintenance agreements? What existing technologies (i.e., computers, web cameras, and so on) can be used?

Adapted from Dudding and Justice, 2004

and retention of employees (U.S. Office of Personnel Management, 2008).

The mentoring process is recognized by the professional organizations governing the professions of audiology and speech-language pathology. The mentoring process is an integral part of ABA requirements for certification in that a minimum of 2,000 hours of mentored professional practice as an audiologist must be completed after required coursework and practicum experiences. ASHA has established two formal mentoring programs to promote career development for students and new researchers: STEP (The Student to Empowered Professional) and MARC (Mentoring Academic Research Careers).

Whether formal or informal, mentoring relationships are based on successful communication. E-mentoring incorporates use of collaboration and conferencing technologies such as e-mail, cell phone, and the web-conferencing technologies discussed previously to support communication in a manner and time convenient to the individuals. Many of the same considerations in the selection of equipment for e-supervision apply to e-mentoring. See Chapter 25 in this text for an in-depth discussion of supervision and mentoring.

Game-Based Learning and Virtual Simulations for Instruction and Learning

Innovators such as Aldrich (2006), Gee (2003), and Prensky (2001a) challenge educators to take hold of twenty-first-century literacy skills to ensure that students are prepared for the new global age of innovation. These skills go beyond print literacy and include "critical thinking, complex-problem solving, and media literacy" (Gee & Levine, 2009, p. 50). Consider the statistics that by the time they are 21 years old, today's youth will have spent 10,000 hours playing computer and video games. Although somewhat controversial, some researchers supply evidence that the brains of these youth are actually changing to accommodate these technologies (Prensky, 2001b, 2001c). Given this information, Prensky and others invoke educators to consider the enormous potential for learning within game-based activities and educational virtual simulations for digital natives.

Game-based learning and simulation technologies have long been used in defense programs, law enforcement, sports training, and the medical field. The U.S. military has a history of extensive use of gaming and virtual simulations in training pilots, medical personnel, commanders, and combat troops. The applications range from war games to teach combat strategy, simulators to train pilots to land on aircraft carriers, and simulated field experiences to prepare troops for the sights, sounds, and smells of the combat field.

The medical field has embraced simulation technologies to create standardized patients and high-tech manikins to train nurses and physicians without the risk of injury to patients. Prestigious medical centers such as Yale, Stanford University, and Johns Hopkins University have developed medical simulation programs. Virtual medical and community health libraries, such as HealthInfo Island, have been established to provide consumer information, training programs, outreach to virtual medical communities, consumer health resources, and one-on-one support (Boulos, Hetherington, & Wheeler, 2007). The Virtual Neurological Education Centre allows participants to experience the symptoms of a neurological disability in an immersive, virtual world environment.

It is realistic to consider the application of serious gaming and virtual simulations in the training of future and in-service professionals in the fields of speech-language pathology and audiology. Currently, audiology students can use virtual audiometers to conduct hearing assessments on virtual clients. A project currently in development, called SimuCase, is an innovative approach to case-based learning. SimuCase is an online simulated case study program in which speech-language pathology students and professionals interact with 3D animated characters to gather relevant information, select and administer tests, and make clinical diagnoses within a virtual learning environment, with no risk of harm to the client. Brundage (2007) explored the use of virtual simulation for the assessment and treatment of stuttering. Researchers in New Zealand are working on similar applications for audiology students.

Second Life is an example of a virtual world application that allows students and instructors to meet as avatars (representations of people) in real time and conduct what appears to be a traditional class meeting in a designated virtual space. Williams (2008), a speech-language pathologist and researcher, explored the use of immersive environments and Second Life for training speech-language pathology graduate students to interact with clients. Results indicated that students consider virtual experiences as similar to real-world interactions with clients. A number of educators predict that avatars and virtual environments are indeed the next generation of online learning.

SERVICE DELIVERY

Technology is incorporated into the diagnosis and treatment of communication disorders in myriad ways. Professionals have access to a number of instrumentation and imaging technologies for use in diagnostics. In the area of intervention, web-based applications and software programs allow for the creation of individualized therapy materials. Game-based activities and virtual simulations can be incorporated into treatment sessions. Assistive technology devices benefit those with communication disorders. Web-conferencing technologies allow for the provision of services through telepractice. It is beyond the scope of this chapter to discuss all of the technologies in detail, but an effort is made to provide an overview of the current applications with an eye toward future development and trends.

Therapy Materials

Many digital immigrants recall days when "dittos" and "Xeroxing" were the mainstays of speech-language intervention programs. In this earlier time, worksheets and clinician-created activities required considerable time and planning. Today, a number of web-based commercially available applications exist, such as BoardMaker and Therasimplicity, that allow clinicians to create customized materials in little time. These technologies are ideal for generating "take-home" activities for clients and families.

An extensive number of computer and video games are available for use in therapy intervention. Some programs have been designed for individuals with a speech-language impairment, while others can be adapted for this purpose. The better examples of these commercially available programs allow for interactivity, provide specific feedback, and are motivating to the user. Williams (2008) proposes that the use of digital games in speech-language intervention introduces the concepts of conflict, cooperation, rules, and constraints while targeting specific communication skill development. Several popular blogs and websites offer a listing of available games, along with suggestions on how to incorporate them into intervention programs. See the Resources section for information on these Internet sites.

Children are not the only population that can benefit from the use of computer and video games. An Internet search reveals several applications intended for brain-injured adults, including those who have aphasia, dementia, or a head injury. Some of these digital applications focus on rehabilitation of skills and encompass the areas of cognitive retraining, word retrieval, and memory drill and practice. Other applications, such as planners, organizers, and altering systems, serve as external memory aids. Research is being conducted on the use of virtual gaming systems for remediation of vestibular and balance problems.

Through the development of apps, nondedicated touch-screen technologies such as the iPhone and iPad have made their way into intervention services in communication sciences and disorders as AAC devices, drill and practice activities, and external memory aids. A search of the Internet yields several websites that offer the top 50 iPhone apps for educators, including applications for note taking, generating task lists, and vocabulary building; calculators; translators; and databases. A similar list has been compiled of applications for use with people with special needs.

As mentioned, consideration should be given to the design, quality, and appropriate application of any technology employed. Following are questions to consider before incorporating a game or simulation into therapy:

- Is the game's cognitive load appropriate for your students or clients?
- Is the game easily modifiable?
- Does the game align with your standards (local, state, and national)?
- Can the game present useful outcomes within a short time period?
- Does the game train or teach?
- Does the game track player progress?
- Are the graphics and gaming quality on par with contemporary entertainment titles? (Rice, 2005)

While digital games offer benefits to both clinicians and clients, you are cautioned to carefully evaluate the claims of any program employed in treatment. It is important to consider the population that the program was designed to address (i.e., age, diagnosis, prerequisite skills, motor, and intellectual ability). Just as one treatment approach does not apply to all types of clients, a single digital game or program cannot address the needs of all clients. The professional should be guided by evidence-based practice in assessing the efficacy of a program employed in intervention. Highly interactive, visually appealing video games do not replace the skills of a highly trained communication disorders professional.

Another application of technology is the use of virtual simulations for intervention. Virtual simulations involve role-play within an environment developed to imitate or estimate how events might occur in real situations. Advantages of simulations within the context of intervention include opportunities for meaningful contextual learning and exposure to real-life challenges. Simulations encourage repeated practice within a safe environment that is challenging and motivating and promotes generalization of skills (Williams, 2008). Proposed ways that virtual simulation environments could be used in the area of language and literacy intervention include the following:

- Immersion of students in a variety of learning environments to explore and practice curricular content such as space, lost civilizations, and historic moments
- Reading skill development with virtual characters and settings
- Animation of stories written by students
- Demonstration of appropriate types of speaking in virtual environments (e.g., negotiation, persuasion, public speaking) (Williams, 2008)

Virtual worlds take simulations one step further in that virtual worlds are an interactive environment accessed by multiple users through an online interface.

Virtual worlds, or "digital worlds," once seemed futuristic but are now part of our youths' culture. McDonald's, Disney, and Coca-Cola have virtual worlds targeted at young children and teens. Second Life is a popular virtual world environment designed for adults. We are challenged to consider ways in which Second Life could be incorporated into clinical service delivery.

Limitations of virtual simulations and virtual worlds are that they are costly to create, they are difficult to modify to specific needs, and few are currently available. Without guidance from an instructor or clinician, virtual simulations and virtual worlds may restrict collaboration, provide limited reflection, and offer limited guided practice on the part of the user (Rogers, 2008).

Instrumentation: Diagnostics and Intervention

Technological advancements have aided in the accurate diagnosis and treatment of communication disorders. Consider some of the tools used by health care professionals that are important to audiologists, speech-language pathologists, and communication scientists. For example, imaging technologies such as magnetic resonance imaging (MRI), functional magnetic resonance imaging (fMRI), diffusion tensor imaging (DTI), and near-infrared spectroscopy (NIRS) have greatly advanced the understanding of brain functioning and aid in the diagnosis and treatment of communication disorders.

Practitioners and researchers within speech-language pathology and audiology use instrumentation technologies to assess the acoustic and aerodynamic aspects of speech production, visualize vocal fold movement through stroboscopy, provide biofeedback, evaluate and remediate the swallowing mechanism, and assess the status of all levels of the auditory and vestibular system through use of immitance measures, otoacoustic emissions (OAEs), auditory evoked potentials (e.g., auditory brainstem response), vestibular evoked myogenic potentials, caloric irrigations, posturography, videonystagmography (VNG), and electronystagmography (ENG).

Graduate students and practicing speech-language pathologists may find relief in software programs capable of performing time-consuming language sample analysis and scoring of tests. Systematic Analysis of Language (SALT) is one example of a computer-assisted language sample analysis software package that will calculate a number of standard measures and compare performance to age-matched peers. A Spanish/English version is also available. A number of popular standardized measures in speech-language testing offer computerized scoring, including Developmental Scoring System, Expressive One Word Picture Vocabulary Test, Functional Communication Profiles-R, Oral and Written Language Scales, Receptive One Word Picture Vocabulary Test, the Stuttering Severity Instrument, and the Test of Language Development.

Low-cost software programs that conduct voice and sound analysis are invaluable to the clinician in both diagnosis and treatment of a variety of speech disorders. Programs such as Waveforms Annotations Spectrograms and Pitch (WASP), WaveSurfer, and PRATT provide basic spectral analysis of the speech signal and in some cases may be used to provide feedback to the speaker.

Assistive Technologies

Assistive technology (AT) refers to technologies that are used to improve or enhance the functioning of an individual with a disability. AT is a specialized area shared with many other professionals such as occupational therapists, physical therapists, and rehabilitation engineers. People with speech, language, or hearing disorders have benefited greatly from AT devices such as programmable digital hearing aids, cochlear implants, voice generators, speech-recognizing software, and the advancement in augmentative and alternative communication (AAC) devices.

The audiology profession has experienced rapid growth in hearing aid technologies since 1987 when the first digital hearing aids were manufactured. Modern digital aids offer advantages in terms of greater user satisfaction through improved fitting measures, noise reduction, feedback reduction, and digital speech enhancement (Ricketts, n.d.). The ASHA 2004 Audiology Survey in Practice Trends (2005a) reported on the types of assistive technology devices dispensed by audiologists. The types of devices included alerting devices, FM systems, assistive listening devices, and technologies meant to assist with telephone communication such as cell phone interfaces, telephone coils, phone amplifiers, and adapters. TTY/TDD (text telephone/telecommunications device for the deaf) systems are another set of telecommunication devices intended to aid people with significant hearing and/or speech impairment in using the telephone. People with TTY/TDD devices can communicate directly with one another through speech and/or text, or they may communicate via a live relay operator who conveys the messages between the users.

Perhaps no technology has impacted the profoundly deaf and hearing-impaired community more than the development of the cochlear implant. A cochlear implant is a device that is surgically implanted in the individual with profound sensorineural hearing loss and provides direct electrical stimulation to the auditory nerve. A cochlear implant is not a cure for deafness, but it does provide people who cannot benefit from hearing aids the perception of the sensation of sound.

Another major area of assistive technologies is the use of augmentative and alternative communication systems to supplement or replace natural speech and/or writing (ASHA, 2002). ASHA defines AAC as a comprehensive system that includes a set of procedures and processes to maximize functional and effective communication through use of aided symbols (e.g., picture communication symbols, line drawings, Blissymbols, and tangible objects) and/or unaided symbols (e.g., manual signs, gestures, and finger spelling) (ASHA, 2002). AAC systems are sometimes classified as either low- or high-technology systems. Low-technology communication systems include symbol boards, books, and object boards that may be made commercially or by a clinician or family member. These systems also include devices operated by electromechanical switches. High-technology communication systems use microcomputers and specialized software. These have the capacity to provide printed and/or voice output. A device that has voice output is referred to as a speech generating device (SGD). The speech may be digitized (recorded human voice) or synthesized (produced from stored digital data).

AAC devices have evolved from expensive and cumbersome devices that required special mounting on wheelchairs, to small, compact, and powerful communication aids. Apple's iPad technology is increasingly popular as an AAC device due to its affordability, cultural acceptance, and the emerging number of apps that are being developed for this specific purpose.

Assistive technology devices will undoubtedly play a larger role as the U.S. population ages. Visual impairment is the most commonly reported disability in the elderly population. Assistive technologies for the visually impaired include magnifying devices, high-intensity reading lamps, recorded books, and high-tech reading machines (Orr, 1997). Elderly people with cognitive and language disabilities may benefit from signaling devices to alert others of their needs; identification aids to convey biographical information; voice amplifiers to increase speech loudness; alphabet and pacing boards to clarify speech communication; and alerts, environmental organizers, and memory books to serve as external memory aids.

Assistive technology for cognition (ATC) is a term referring to devices that help individuals compensate for cognitive impairments. Research has shown that use of ATC devices can help people with acquired brain injury regain independence (LoPresti, Mihailidis, & Kirsch, 2004). Sohlberg (2011) recommends that ATC device selection be team-based and comprehensive with consideration of user's preferences. To ensure long-term success, Sohlberg recommends that the clinician design an individualized training plan to include an acquisition phase, a mastery and generalization phase, and a maintenance phase (2011). Refer to the Resources section for tools to assist in the selection process.

Telepractice

In 2001, ASHA adopted the term *telepractice* to "encompass a range of services provided through telecommunications technology that are not exclusively health related, including clinical services for communication enhancement, and education and supervision" (ASHA, 2005b, p. 1). At that time, a Telepractice Working Group was formed to create guiding documents and position statements for the provision of telepractice in speech-language pathology and audiology. *SLP Services in the Schools: Guidelines for Best Practices* was created to ensure that the provision of services through telepractice meets the same standards as those provided in face-to-face service delivery. The guidelines delineate responsibilities of professionals in terms of confidentiality, ethics, and clinical competencies. A benefit of telepractice is the improved access to services that may not otherwise be available due to geographic limitations, mobility of the client, and/or accessibility to a qualified professional (ASHA, 2005b). Some studies suggest that telepractice results in outcomes equal to or better than those of traditional delivery models (Brennan, Georgeadis, Baron, & Barker, 2004; Farmer & Muhlenbruck, 2001; Karp et al., 2000; Marcin et al., 2004).

Telepractice is being used in communication sciences and disorders in a number of ways. The ASHA website hosts a number of articles supporting telepractice as a way to address the shortage of speech-language pathologists in the public schools, especially in rural areas (Forducey, 2006). Several state departments of education and institutions of higher education are pursuing projects exploring the use of telepractice to provide services to children within the public schools. Other professionals are offering services to treat survivors of combat-related brain injury (Mashima, 2010); providing audiological services and assisting in early hearing detection and intervention (Houston & Muñoz, 2010; Krumm, 2005; Krumm, Ribera, & Froelich, 2002); and diagnosing and treating adults with speech-language and swallowing disorders (Georges, Belz, & Potter, 2006; Houn & Trottier, 2006).

In considering the use of telepractice, it is essential to ensure that the services provided are cost-effective, are in compliance with state and national standards, meet regulatory requirements for reimbursement and licensure, and do not violate interstate licensure laws. It is important that delivery of services through telepractice is acceptable to the clients and families and yields outcomes at least equal to those of face-to-face delivery methods. ASHA has created a new special interest group (SIG18 Telepractice) in the area of telepractice to encourage ongoing discussion, development, and research in this rapidly developing area of service delivery.

Reimbursement for services provided through telepractice varies by state and reimbursement agency. At the time of this writing, the Centers for Medicare & Medicaid Services (CMS) does not allow for reimbursement of telepractice services by audiologists and speech-language pathologists. However, ASHA is supporting federal legislation that would recognize telepractice as an appropriate model of service delivery for audiologists and speech-language pathologists under Medicare. A number of Medicaid offices at the state level have approved or are considering reimbursement for telepractice services for audiology and speech-language pathology. You are encouraged to consult the reimbursement agencies in your state for an updated status.

Telepractice Models and Equipment There are various models of telepractice and types of equipment employed in telepractice delivery areas. One model is known as "store and forward" in which information, such as test results and images, obtained at one site is electronically forwarded to a practitioner at a distant site for consultation. This model is currently not eligible for reimbursement by many insurance carriers. "Face to face" provision of services refers to the use of digital videoconferencing technologies (using web-based or digital videoconferencing units) to provide services in real time, with interaction between the client and the practitioner. This model is gaining acceptance with a number of insurance carriers and regulatory agencies for reimbursement of services. Telepractice may also involve remote monitoring devices and the use of distance learning technologies. Considerations for selection of technology for telepractice are similar to those discussed in the section on e-supervision and e-mentoring.

When employing alternate service delivery models, clients and caregivers should be given a clear and concise explanation of the technologies employed, along with the mention of benefits, limitations, and risks. They should be given an opportunity to ask questions and opt out of services. In the event that the speech-language-hearing professional is dispensing a technology, such as a hearing aid or AT device, the client should be provided with information regarding the full cost, along with a description of the return policy.

COST CONSIDERATIONS

A genuine consideration and concern in the use of any technology is the cost associated with its purchase and use. It is important to consider the actual cost of the technology as going beyond the initial purchase of the equipment or software. In determining the true cost of the technology, it is important to consider the following costs:

- Technology support personnel
- Equipment and software upgrades
- Licensing and maintenance agreements
- Required training
- Peripherals
- Dedicated transmission protocols if IP (Internet Protocol) is not available or adequate

Prior to investing in any technology, it is important to have a clear understanding of the goals, objectives, and needs of the project to guide your purchasing decisions. Avoid being enticed by the "bells and whistles" only to end up with an overpriced technology, or, worse yet, one that is unused because it does not meet your needs.

The costs of technology can be offset by gains in efficiency and effectiveness. For example, e-supervision has benefits of reducing the supervisor's travel costs and time spent traveling. Online learning provides access to students who may not otherwise enroll in a program of study. Web-conferencing technologies reduce the time and expense related to attending meetings. Another cost-saving factor is to consider ways to use the equipment for multiple purposes. Web-conferencing technologies can be used for e-supervision, e-mentoring, distance learning, and professional collaboration, thereby making them more cost-effective.

ETHICAL CONSIDERATIONS

As we integrate existing and emerging technologies into audiology and speech-language pathology, whether it is through collaboration, training, and/or provision of services, it is critical to our professions and to the clients we serve that we maintain the integrity and quality of the services provided. As new technologies continue to emerge, speech-language-hearing practitioners are charged with gaining requisite knowledge for proper and ethical application of these technologies. As professionals engaged in the use of technology in research, training, and service delivery, we must conduct and publish research. This knowledge should be used to update policy documents to reflect best practices.

ASHA's Code of Ethics, Principle II, Rule F directly addresses the use of technology by stating, "Individuals shall ensure that all equipment used in the provision of services or to conduct research and scholarly activities is in proper working order and is properly calibrated" (ASHA, 2010, p. 3). This principle directly addresses use of instrumentation and other clinical equipment. Ethical responsibilities are an inherent part of clinical practice and research regardless of the use of technology. While not specifically aimed at technology, other rules of the ASHA Code of Ethics can be applied when it comes to the use of technology: Principle 1, Rule A, states, "Individuals shall provide all services competently," and Principle 1, Rule B is "Individuals shall use every resource, including referral when appropriate, to ensure that high-quality service is provided" (ASHA, 2010).

In addition to ASHA's Code of Ethics, practitioners are bound by the directives of other agencies such as state licensing boards, federal agencies, insurance carriers, and employers. For example, the federal regulation known as the Health Insurance Portability and Accountability Act (HIPAA) of 1996 requires practitioners to meet stringent privacy and confidentiality requirements that apply to use of many of the technologies discussed in this chapter, including document-sharing technologies. The Family Educational Rights and Privacy Act (FERPA) of 1974 is a federal act that provides protection of educational records. FERPA regulations must be addressed when serving students in K–12 and higher using telepractice. Reimbursement agencies may also have guidelines for use of technologies. In addition to HIPAA regulations, the Centers for Medicare & Medicaid Services provides guidelines for reimbursement for the use of technology in service delivery. Read Chapter 5 for a more in-depth discussion of professional ethics.

SUMMARY

This chapter offers an introduction to the application of technologies in communication sciences and disorders within the digital age. It includes a description of various technologies including videoconferencing, web-based applications and software, computer games, virtual simulations, and digital worlds. In addition, it offers information about current application in the areas of collaboration, research, learning, and service delivery. Attention was given to the benefits and limitations along with guidelines for evaluating each technology. The chapter included information on service delivery models with consideration of the technologies, security, and ethical considerations.

More important, this chapter encourages students and professionals in audiology and speech-language pathology to embrace emerging technologies as opportunities to enhance collaboration, research, education, assessment, and intervention. Jonas Salk, the inventor of the polio vaccine that saved millions of lives, is credited as saying, "This is perhaps the most beautiful time in human history; it is really pregnant with all kinds of creative possibilities made possible by science and technology which now constitutes the slave of man—if man is not enslaved by it." Explore the potential of new and emerging technologies to help better the lives of those that we serve, but do so with an understanding and appreciation of their strengths and limitations so as not to become enslaved by them.

CRITICAL THINKING

1. What are the challenges to existing copyright and intellectual property laws in light of emerging technologies?
2. How might the development of communication technologies (text messaging, IM, video chats, e-mail) and social networks (Facebook and LinkedIn) either assist or hinder people with language and literacy disorders?
3. Consider the learning, social, and cultural characteristics of today's digital youth. What are the implications for the future speech-language pathology and audiology clinical workforce?
4. How does the experienced practitioner best keep informed about the latest technological developments in the field? What role might professional organizations play? What conflicts might arise?
5. What kinds of opportunities does telepractice open to audiology?
6. How could learning based on video games and virtual simulations be incorporated into the training of audiologists and their clinical practice?
7. After reading this chapter, what factors would you consider before enrolling in a professional development and/or educational opportunity offered online?
8. What measures would you put in place to ensure security and confidentiality of client information when utilizing the various technologies discussed in this chapter?
9. How might the high prevalence of digital technologies in our society assist those with communication disorders in reducing perceived handicaps/impairments?
10. How might digital technologies assist audiologists and speech-language pathologists in areas related to prevention?

REFERENCES

Aldrich, C. (2006). 9 Paradoxes of educational simulations. *Training & Development, 60*(5), 49–52.

Allen, E. I., & Seaman, J. (2007). *Online nation: Five years of growth in online learning.* Retrieved from http://www.sloan-c.org/publications/survey/pdf/online_nation.pdf

Allen, E. I., & Seaman, J. (2010). *Learning on demand: Online education in the United States, 2009.* Retrieved from http://sloanconsortium.org/publications/survey/learning_on_demand_sr2010

American Speech-Language-Hearing Association. (2002). *Augmentative and alternative communication: Knowledge and skills for service delivery.* Available from http://www.asha.org/policy

American Speech-Language-Hearing Association. (2005a). *2004 Audiology Survey report: Practice trends in audiology.* Retrieved from http://www.asha.org/uploadedFiles/04AudSurveyPracticeTrends.pdf

American Speech-Language-Hearing Association. (2005b). *Speech-language pathologists providing clinical services via telepractice: Technical report.* Available from http://www.asha.org/policy

American Speech-Language-Hearing Association. (2008). *Clinical supervision in speech-language pathology.* Available from http://www.asha.org/policy

American Speech-Language-Hearing Association. (2010). *Code of ethics.* Retrieved from http://www.asha.org/docs/html/ET2010-00309.html

Battle, D. (2007, February 13). The power of passionate mentoring. Mentoring: The cycle of caring. *The ASHA Leader.* Retrieved from http://www.asha.org/Publications/leader/2007/070213/070213g.htm

Belderrain, Y. (2006). Distance education trends: Integrating new technologies to foster student interaction and collaboration. *Distance Education, 27*(2), 139–153.

Bernard, J. M., & Goodyear, R. K. (1992). *Fundamentals of clinical supervision.* Boston, MA: Allyn & Bacon.

Boulos, M. N., Hetherington, L., & Wheeler, S. (2007). Second Life in medical and health education. *Health Information and Libraries Journal, 24,* 233–245.

Brennan, D. M., Georgeadis, A. C., Baron, C. R., & Barker, L. M. (2004). The effect of videoconferencing-based telerehabilitation on story retelling performance by brain-injured subjects and its implications for remote speech-language therapy. *Telemedicine Journal and e-Health, 10,* 147–154.

Brown, J. S. (n.d.). *Learning in the digital age.* Retrieved from http://net.educause.edu/ir/library/pdf/ffpiu015.pdf

Brundage, S. (2007). Virtual reality augmentation for functional assessment and treatment of stuttering. *Topics in Language Disorders, 27,* 254–271.

Cox, G., Carr, T., & Hall, M. (2004). Evaluating the use of synchronous communication in two blended courses. *Journal of Computer Assisted Learning, 20,* 183–193.

Davidson-Shivers, G. V., Muilenburg, L. Y., & Tanner, E. J. (2001). How do students participate in synchronous and asynchronous online discussions? *Journal of Educational Computing Research, 25*(4), 341–366.

Dudding, C. C. (2004). *Perceptions of the use of videoconferencing for supervision: Differences among graduate clinicians* (Doctoral dissertation, University of Virginia, 2004). Digital Dissertations, AAT 3108759.

Dudding, C. C. (2006). Distance supervision: An update. *ASHA Division 11 Perspectives, 16*(1), 16–18.

Dudding, C. C. (2009). Digital videoconferencing: Applications across the disciplines. *Communication Disorders Quarterly, 30,* 178–182.

Dudding, C. C., & Justice, L. (2004). A model for e-supervision: Videoconferencing as a clinical training tool. *Communication Disorders Quarterly, 25*(3), 145–151.

Farmer, J. E., & Muhlenbruck, L. (2001). Telehealth for children with special health care needs: Promoting comprehensive systems of care. *Clinical Pediatrics, 40,* 93–98.

Forducey, P. (2006). Speech telepractice program expands options for rural Oklahoma schools. *The ASHA Leader, 11*(10), 12–13.

Garrison, D. R., & Cleveland-Innes, M. (2005). Facilitating cognitive presence in online learning: Interaction is not enough. *American Journal of Distance Education, 19*(3), 133–148.

Gee, J. P. (2003). *What video games have to teach us about learning and literacy.* New York, NY: Palgrave Macmillan.

Gee, J. P., & Levine, M. H. (2009). Welcome to our virtual worlds. *Educational Leadership, 66*(6), 48–52.

Georges, J., Belz, N., & Potter, K. (2006, February 7). Telepractice program for dysphagia: Urban and rural perspectives from Kansas. *The ASHA Leader.* Retrieved from http://www.asha.org/Publications/leader/2006/061107/061107d.htm

Health care technology today. (2010, February). *PT in Motion, 2*(1), 41–43.

Heinich, R., Molenda, M., Russell, J. D., & Smaldino, S. E. (1999). *Instructional media and technologies for learning.* Upper Saddle River, NJ: Prentice Hall.

Hmelo-Silver, C. E., & Barrows, H. S. (2008). Facilitating collaborative knowledge building. *Cognition and Instruction, 26,* 48–94.

Houn, B., & Trottier, K. (2006, November 28). Telepractice brings treatment to rural North Dakota. *The ASHA Leader.* Retrieved from http://www.asha.org/Publications/leader/2006/061128/061128f/

Houston, K. T., & Muñoz, K. (2010, May 18). Workshop features telepractice programs for EHDI. *The ASHA Leader.* Retrieved from http://www.asha.org/Publications/leader/2010/100518/Telepractice-Programs-EHDI.htm

Jones, C., Ramanau, R., Cross, S., & Healing, G. (2010). Net generation or digital natives: Is there a distinct new generation entering university? *Computers & Education, 54*(3), 722–732.

Karp, W., Grigsby, R., McSwiggan-Hardin, M., Pursely-Crotteau, S., Adams, L., & Bell, W. (2000). Use of telemedicine for children with special health care needs. *Pediatrics, 105*(4), 843–847.

Krumm, M. (2005, November 8). Audiology telepractice moves from theory to treatment. *The ASHA Leader*. Retrieved from http://www.asha.org/Publications/leader/2005/051108/051108f/

Krumm, M., Ribera, J., & Froelich, T. (2002, June 11). Bridging the service gap through audiology telepractice. *The ASHA Leader*. Retrieved from http://www.asha.org/Publications/leader/2002/020611/f020611_2a/

LoPresti, E. F., Mihailidis, A., & Kirsch, N. L. (2004). Assistive technology for cognitive rehabilitation: State of the art. *Neuropsychological Rehabilitation, 14,* 5–39.

Lou, Y., Bernard, R. M., & Abrami, P. C. (2006). Media and pedagogy in undergraduate distance education: A theory-based meta-analysis of empirical literature. *Educational Technology Research and Development, 54*(2), 141–176.

Marcin, J., Ellis, J., Mawis, R., Nagrampa, E., Nesbitt, T., & Dimand, R. (2004). Using telemedicine to provide pediatric subspecialty care to children with special health care needs in an underserved rural community. *Pediatrics, 113*(1), 1–6.

Mashima, P. A. (2010, November 2). Using telehealth to treat combat-related traumatic brain injury. *The ASHA Leader.* Retrieved from http://www.asha.org/Publications/leader/2010/101102/Using-Telehealth-to-Treat-Combat-Related-Traumatic-Brain-Injury.htm

National Center for Educational Statistics. (2005). *Internet access in U.S. public schools and classrooms: 1994–2003*. Retrieved from http://nces.ed.gov/surveys/frss/publications/2005015/index.asp

Orr, A. (1997). Assistive technologies for older persons who are visually impaired. In R. Lubinski & J. Higginbotham (Eds.), *Communication technologies for the elderly* (pp. 71–102). Clifton Park, NY: Delmar Cengage Learning.

Prensky, M. (2001a). *Digital game-based learning*. New York, NY: McGraw-Hill.

Prensky, M. (2001b). Digital natives, digital immigrants. *On the Horizon, 9*(5). Retrieved from http://www.marcprensky.com/writing/prensky%20-%20digital%20natives,%20digital%20immigrants%20-%20part1.pdf

Prensky, M. (2001c). Digital natives, digital immigrants, part 2. Do they really *think* differently? *On the Horizon, 9*(6). Retrieved from http://www.marcprensky.com/writing/prensky%20-%20digital%20natives,%20digital%20immigrants%20-%20part2.pdf

Rantz, M. J., Skubic, M., Alexander, G., Popescu, M., Aud, M. A., Wakefield, B. J., et al. (2010). Developing a comprehensive electronic health record to enhance nursing care coordination, use of technology, and research. *Journal of Gerontological Nursing, 36*(1), 13–17.

Rice, J. (2005). *Evaluating the suitability of video games for K-12 instruction.* Paper presented at the Association for Educational Communications and Technology 2005 International Convention, Orlando, FL.

Ricketts, T. S. (n.d.). *Digital hearing aids: Current state-of-the-art.* Retrieved from http://www.asha.org/public/hearing/treatment/digital_aid.htm

Rogers, L. (2008). *Virtual worlds: A new window to healthcare education.* Paper presented at the ascilite Melbourne 2008, Melbourne, Australia.

Seaman, J. (2009). *Online learning as a strategic asset: Vol. II: The paradox of faculty voices.* Retrieved from http://www.aplu.org/NetCommunity/Document.Doc?id=1879

Senior, R. (2010). Connectivity: A framework for understanding effective language teaching in face-to-face and online learning communities. *RELC: A Journal of Language Teaching and Research, 41*(2), 137–147.

Sohlberg, M. M. (2011, February 15). Assistive technology for cognition. *The ASHA Leader.* Retrieved from http://www.asha.org/Publications/leader/2011/110215/Assistive-Technology-for-Cognition.htm

U.S. Office of Personnel Management. (2008). *Best practices: Mentoring.* Retrieved from http://www.opm.gov/hrd/lead/BestPractices-Mentoring.pdf

Williams, S. (2008, November 19). *WIRED for success: Digital games, simulations and virtual worlds for language and literacy instruction.* Paper presented at the American Speech-Language-Hearing Association Convention, Chicago.

Williams, S. L. (2006). The effectiveness of distance education in allied health science programs: A meta-analysis of outcomes. *American Journal of Distance Education, 20*(3), 127–141.

RESOURCES

20 Great project management tools. (2010, February 10). Retrieved from http://www.webdesignbooth.com/project-management-tools/

Advancing crisis management training in health care. (2011). Retrieved from http://med.stanford.edu/VAsimulator/

American Speech-Language-Hearing Association. (n.d.). *Special Interest Group 18, Telepractice.* Retrieved from http://www.asha.org/SIG/18/

American Speech-Language-Hearing Association. (n.d.). *Telepractice for SLPs and audiologists.* Retrieved from http://www.asha.org/practice/telepractice/

Boersma, P., & Weenink, D. (n.d.). *Praat: Doing phonetics by computer.* Retrieved from http://www.fon.hum.uva.nl/praat/

Cognitive Training Software. (2011). *BrainTrain.* Available from http://www.braintrain.com

Cohn, E., and Watzlaf, V. (2011). Privacy and Internet-Based Telepractice. *Perspectives on Telepractice,* 1:26–37.

Copyright Clearance Center, Inc. (2005). *The TEACH Act New Roles, Rules and Responsibilities for Academic Institutions.* Retrieved from http://www.copyright.com/media/pdfs/CR-Teach-Act.pdf

David Newmonic Language Resources. (2011). *Speech-language resources.com.* Available from http://www.speechlanguage-resources.com/

The George Lucas Educational Foundation. (2011). *K-12 education & learning innovations with proven strategies that work Edutopia.* Available from http://www.edutopia.org

HITLab. (2008). Available from http://www.hitlabnz.org/

The Johns Hopkins Medicine Simulation Center. (n.d.). Available from http://www.hopkinsmedicine.org/simulation_center/index.html

Kuster, J. (2010, November 27). *Net connections for communication disorders and sciences.* Available from http://www.mnsu.edu/comdis/kuster2/welcome.html

Linden Research, Inc. (2009). *Second Life education—Providers listing.* Available from http://edudirectory.secondlife.com/

Lubinski, R., & Higginbotham, D. J. (Eds.). (1997). *Communication technologies for the elderly: Vision, hearing, and speech.* Clifton Park, NY: Delmar Cengage Learning.

METI. (2010). *Medical education and simulation.* Available from http://www.meti.com

Online Education Database. (2008, December 1). *Top 50 iPhone apps for educators.* Available from http://oedb.org/library/features/top_50_iphones_for_educators

Pannbacker, M., & Lass, N. (2003). Telepractice in speech-language pathology and audiology. *Texas Journal of Audiology and Speech Pathology, 27,* 27–33.

Parrot Software. (2009). *Parrot Software for clinical treatment of speech and memory disorders.* Available from http://www.parrotsoftware.com/parrot_software_for_brain_injury_patients.html

Route 21. (2007). Available from http://route21.p21.org/

Scherer, M., Jutai, J., Fuhrer, M., Demers, L., & DeRuyter, F. (2007). A framework for modeling the selection of assistive technology devices. *Disability and Rehabilitation: Assistive Technology, 2*(1), 1–8.

Scribd Inc. (2011). *IPad apps and accessories for special needs.* Available from http://www.scribd.com/doc/39018411/iPad-Apps-and-Accessories-for-Special-Needs

SimuCase. (2011). SpeechPathology.com. Available from http://www.speechpathology.com/simucase

Society for Information Technology & Teacher Education. (2010). Available from http://site.aace.org/

Speaking of Speech.com. (2008). Available from http://www.speakingofspeech.com/Home_Page.html

TechMatch. (n.d.). Available from https://www.coglink.com:8080/TechMatch/

TMH, Speech, Music and Hearing. (2010, November 23). *WaveSurfer.* Available from http://www.speech.kth.se/wavesurfer/

UCL Division of Psychology and Language Sciences. (2009). *Speech, hearing & phonetic sciences resources.* Available from http://www.phon.ucl.ac.uk/resource/software.html

Virtual Neurological Education Centre. (n.d.). Available from http://healthinfoisland.blogspot.com/2007/03/virtual-neurological-education-centre.html

WordPress. (n.d.). *Community virtual library.* Available from http://infoisland.org/about/

Yale School of Medicine. (2009, October 15). *Simulation medicine emergency.* Available from http://medicine.yale.edu/emergencymed/education/simmedicine.aspx

27

Stress, Conflict, and Coping in the Workplace

Rosemary Lubinski, EdD

SCOPE OF CHAPTER

Most, if not all, professionals will experience stress and conflict at some time in their professional lives. Statistics indicate that three out of four American workers perceive their work as stressful (Maxon, 1999). In fact, some of you may consider this a natural by-product related to a variety of uncontrollable workplace issues. In addition, personal stresses are difficult to isolate from professional life and may complicate how some professionals cope with employment problems. In a time of unprecedented national economic difficulties, it is difficult for many of you to detach professional and personal stresses. Some of you may feel anxious about financial difficulties or an impending loss of your job or that of a spouse.

Your personal and professional lives may be in jeopardy because of a variety of internal and external factors. While some of you may have a strong personal network to help you cope, others may opt to leave the profession or change jobs. Most just carry on despite feelings of chronic stress. As the best treatment for stress and burnout is prevention, this chapter introduces you to these potential problems, provides strategies for self-identification, and suggests prevention and management through positive coping. Maslach (1982) says, "The risk of burnout is less likely to become reality if you get a head start on it" (p. 131). Academic programs, professional organizations, and workplaces have a responsibility to help professionals become and remain "totally healthy" professionals. Keep in mind that not only is workplace stress common, but it has negative personal, service delivery, family, and societal ramifications.

DEFINITIONS AND SYMPTOMS

The first step in dealing effectively with stress and burnout is to know their characteristics. Identification and remediation strategies follow logically from this identification.

Workplace Stress

Employment stress is defined as the detrimental physical and emotional responses that occur when an employee feels there is a conflict between job demands and the control the employee has over meeting demands (Canadian Centre for Occupational Health and Safety, 2008). Stress happens when you do not have sufficient adaptive resources to meet demands (Monat & Lazarus, 1977).

Workplace stress has numerous sources. Some of these are related to our own personal characteristics. Interestingly, younger professionals who are perfectionistic and overachieving may be more at risk than older professionals who have "survived" (Alexander, 2009). Stress may also emanate from the clients with whom we work and the complicated problems they pose. A variety of professional situation factors also may contribute to workplace stress. Some of these are related to the work we do while others derive from interpersonal relationships, the physical environment, external demands, and economic factors. In a study of school-based speech-language pathologists, the top five stressors included too much paperwork, inadequate salary, no time to relax, easily over-committed, and lack of time to complete work (Poche, Tassin, Oliver, & Fellow, 2003). Keep in mind that what may be stressful for one professional may be perceived differently by others. See Table 27–1 for an extended list of sources of stress.

Bullying

One source of burnout that deserves special mention is the presence of coworkers who exhibit bullying behavior. Known as "toxic coworkers" (Cavaiola & Lavender, 2000), these individuals tend to be convincing, charming, and manipulative individuals who have excellent verbal ability but a decided need to criticize and humiliate others. Their goals include attaining their personal self-interests and self-esteem by degrading others, usually those they perceive as a threat. It is estimated that one in six workers is bullied each year, most targets are women, and more than half of the bullies are women (Mezger, 2004). This is interesting since women are supposed to be nurturing and protective of each other. Note that toxic coworkers are often in superior positions but may also be peers (Downs, 2005). Table 27–2 lists other signs of bullying that a coworker may exhibit.

The insidious nature of these individuals may take a serious toll including depression, post-traumatic stress disorder, other physical and psychological stresses, absenteeism, lost productivity, and financial loss to the targets and their employers. Some targets of bullying experience panic attacks and have difficulty concentrating and making decisions. Unfortunately, it is more common that the targets often feel so stressed that they leave their positions while the bully remains in a position of power. Some employers, however, do take action against employees who they can prove have committed psychological harassment. An excellent resource for information on workplace bullies is *The Bully at Work: What You Can Do to Stop the Hurt and Reclaim Your Dignity on the Job*, by Namie and Namie (2003), or go to the Workplace Bullying Institute website (http://www.workplacebullying.org).

Bad Bosses

A particularly difficult workplace stressor is that of the "bad boss." While most supervisors have attained their positions because of their excellent work and desire to lead, some are promoted because of longevity, politics, or the fact that no one wants the position. It is difficult to work with such bosses because they do not view their work with you as a partnership. Their manipulation, mood swings, and lack of support undermine the development of good staff members. For other bosses,

TABLE 27–1 Potential Sources of Stress or Burnout

Client Factors

- Overly demanding clients and/or families
- Complicated, serious problems of clients and/or families
- Lack of client/family responsiveness
- Lack of client/family appreciation

Professional Situation Factors

- Size of caseload—overload or underload
- Too many or lack of clarity regarding responsibilities
- Lack of autonomy
- Little opportunity for self-actualization
- Low pay; few salary increases
- Job insecurity or job loss
- Little opportunity for continuing education
- Tedium
- Excessive paperwork and inadequate time to complete it
- Inadequate working conditions and/or resources
- Under or over promotion
- Discrimination: sexism, ageism, racism
- Inadequate supervision
- Unclear criteria for professional evaluation
- Evaluation based on negative factors only
- Coworker competition or incompetence
- Lack of coworker support
- Bullying behavior by coworkers
- Interdisciplinary conflict or competition
- Unprofessional attitudes on part of supervisor or coworkers
- Lack of positive reinforcement from supervisor
- Rigid or unrealistic institutional policies
- Poor communication between employees and supervisor
- Isolation in the workplace

Personal Factors

- Younger age
- Earlier in career
- Lack of life partner or children
- Higher level of education
- Unrealistic expectations; perfectionism; need for control and to "do it all"
- Impatience or intolerance
- Inability to say "no"
- Inability to delegate work to others
- Lack of confidence
- Need for approval from others
- Hostility
- Impatience
- Personal and/or family health problems
- Family pressures
- Competing demands of job and family

it may be that they have not had any supervisory skills training (VanZant-Stern, 2011). Table 27–3 provides a sampling of the myriad characteristics of bad bosses. Remember that the majority of these bad bosses are not mentally unstable but are bullies at the management level. You are not the cause of their actions.

Effects of Stress

Chronic stress takes an insidious and vicious physical and psychological toll on an individual. Physical effects of stress can range from mild to extreme. Such effects include fatigue, insomnia, headaches, gastrointestinal

TABLE 27–2 Examples of Bullying Behavior by a Coworker

- Convincing liar; Jekyll and Hyde personality
- Verbally agile—nonspecific and evasive
- Sense of superiority
- Needs to control and attain power
- Compulsive need to criticize, intimidate, dominate, and humiliate
- Manipulative
- Acts out of self-interest and self-preservation
- Distorts or fabricates allegations for control
- Creates arbitrary rules and unreasonable demands
- Makes a fuss over trivia while ignoring important things
- Uses gossip, rumor, and innuendo to discredit and isolate target
- Excludes and "ices out"
- Tries to erode the confidence of the target
- Has a short, selective memory regarding what they said or did
- Does not value others or their achievements
- Cannot distinguish between aggression and assertive behavior
- Poor listening skills
- Tends to rely on written communication such as e-mail rather than face-to-face contact
- May take credit for others' work
- Threatens job loss

Adapted from materials available at http://bullyonline.org/ and "Battling the Workplace Bully," by R. Mezger, July 25, 2004, *Cleveland Plain Dealer.*

disorders, dermatological disorders, susceptibility to infection, hypertension, and heart disease (Farmer, Monahan, & Hekeler, 1984). Psychologically, a person may feel some degree of anxiety or depression. How the person perceives and eventually copes with chronic stress may in itself cause further problems. For example, skipping meals may lead to unnecessary weight loss, and self-medicating through the use of drugs, alcohol, or overeating may lead to dependency or health issues. Social withdrawal may lead to feelings of even greater despair. Stress can be brought on by a single catastrophic life event (e.g., death, moving to a new location, divorce) or by a series of events that, in combination, overwhelm the individual's capacity to cope.

Losing a job is particularly stressful. In addition to loss of income, there is also loss of professional identity, self-esteem, daily routine, purposeful activity, a social network, and sense of security (Helpguide, 2009a). Job loss is often associated with signs of grief. At some point you may cry and feel angry, rejected, and scared. How to deal with job loss is discussed later in the chapter. Table 27–1 lists a variety of sources of stress.

Burnout

A special effect of chronic stress is burnout. Maslach (1982) defines burnout as a "syndrome of emotional exhaustion, depersonalization, and reduced personal accomplishment that can occur among individuals who do 'people work' of some type" (p. 3). Burnout is a cumulative process rather than an event (Farber, 1983) and can emanate from the sustained burden in a caregiving relationship or in unresolved and prolonged workplace stress.

The issue of competing demands from job and family deserves special attention because the profession of speech-language pathology, in particular, is dominated by women. It should be remembered, however, that many professional men share in caregiving and homemaking duties and thus also experience difficulties in balancing competing demands of professional and family life. In a study of caregiving needs of our

TABLE 27–3 Signs of a Bad Boss

- Lacks organizational and leadership skills
- Inconsistent in mood and instructions
- Micromanages employees' work—often rigid
- Does not listen to employees' issues or ideas
- Criticizes employees in public
- Does not follow up on assignments
- Does not support employees' efforts
- Jumps to conclusions
- Unethical
- Jealous of employees' accomplishments
- Teases or tells sarcastic jokes
- Manipulative and mistrustful
- Self-pitying
- Rejects contradiction
- Can be mean or vicious

professions, Shewan and Blake (1991) found that while the median number of dependents for affiliates of ASHA was only one, caregiving duties consumed 20 hours per week. Full-time speech-language pathologists spent more time on caregiving duties than did audiologists; women spent more time on caregiving duties than did men.

Stages of Burnout

Burnout is similar to grief in that it evolves through several stages. Cherniss (1980) postulates that there are three major stages to the process of burnout in the helping professions. Stage 1 is an imbalance between the demands and resources to deal with job stress. There are too few personal or institutional resources to equalize increasing demands. This leads to Stage 2, when the individual reacts to this strain with feelings of anxiety, tension, fatigue, helplessness, and exhaustion. Finally, in Stage 3, defensive coping emerges, characterized by emotional detachment, withdrawal, cynicism, and rigidity. A vicious and insidious cycle emerges: The greater the demands placed on the professional, the greater the demand for and depletion of the individual's energy and resources for coping. By the final stage of complete burnout, professionals may lack affect, perform responsibilities without involvement, and consider leaving the profession (Alexander, 2009).

Effects of Burnout

The effects of burnout are as numerous and complex as the causes. Table 27–4 divides the effects of burnout into four major categories: professional effects, psychological effects, physiological effects, and effects on significant others. According to Maslach (1982), one of the most obvious signs of burnout is a sense of *emotional exhaustion* in which the professional feels frustrated, physically exhausted, and emotionally depleted. The individual feels hopeless and as though there is "no more to give." The natural strategy to cope with such emotional exhaustion is to try to distance oneself from work. The professional perceives that with self-withdrawal from the source(s) of the problem, particularly the people involved, stability will be recovered.

Unfortunately, this response leads to *depersonalization* in which the professional resents and denigrates clients, coworkers, or others who are perceived to be the root of the problem. Maslach adds that such a negative perception eventually leads to a sense of *personal inadequacy*. In this state, one feels a deep sense of failure and inability to accomplish one's goals. All of these feelings blend and lead to poor quality and quantity of work performance as well as depression. Consequently, some individuals may change careers or job positions, reduce workload, and/or seek counseling.

The psychological effects are also apparent and range from feelings of sadness, anger, and frustration to depression, suspicion, and paranoia. Conflicting feelings abound. Feelings such as being annoyed and frustrated lead to detachment; irritation and overload lead to depersonalization; reduced self-esteem leads to depression.

One of the most common physiological effects is a sense of chronic exhaustion. The persistent negative responses of emotional depletion, depersonalization, and sense of inadequacy combined with pervasive deleterious psychological effects may lead to serious health problems. These health problems can take any

TABLE 27–4 Signs and Effects of Burnout

Professional Effects

- Detachment/depersonalization
- Sense of inadequacy
- Irritation with clients
- Diminished listening skills
- Decreased work output
- Deteriorating work performance
- Leave work earlier than usual/increased absenteeism
- Negative impact on finances of individual or agency

Psychological Effects

- Sadness
- Anger
- Frustration
- Loss of satisfaction or accomplishment
- Overly self-critical
- Cynical and negative
- Tension
- Anxiety
- Depression
- Forgetfulness
- Feeling of helplessness
- Suspiciousness
- More risk taking
- Paranoia
- Suicide

Physiological Effects

- Feeling of exhaustion and chronic fatigue
- Reduced autoimmune response
- Increased susceptibility to illness and infection
- Rapid heart rate
- Hormonal abnormalities
- Shortness of breath
- Poor eating habits
- Addiction to controlled substances or alcohol
- Frequent headaches
- Teeth grinding
- Insomnia
- Gastrointestinal disorders
- Dermatological disorders (e.g., hives, eczema, acne)
- Back and neck disorders
- Hypertension
- Heart attack
- Stroke

Effects on Significant Others

- Marital conflict
- Family discord
- Domestic violence
- Loss of intimacy
- Estrangement from others

individual or combination of forms, such as headaches, susceptibility to infections, insomnia, gastrointestinal disorders, and hypertension. At the most serious end of the continuum, some individuals may suffer a heart attack or stroke. Numerous other obvious health problems may also occur such as poor eating habits, alcohol abuse, smoking, and overuse of or dependency on tranquilizers or other drugs. Some individuals may even resort to suicide.

The effects of stress and burnout are also evident in work productivity and efficiency. According to a 2003 study of the effects of depression on work productivity, Stewart (2003) found that the annual total cost of depression was $44 billion. Workers with depression lost more than eight hours of work per week whereas those who were not depressed lost only about one and a half hours of productive time.

The effects of burnout may reach to coworkers and family. For example, a professional who is experiencing burnout may withdraw from coworkers, view them in a suspicious manner, or become dependent on them for completing a job. When burnout is rampant within an agency, a negative climate may pervade the institution, and job satisfaction and morale are likely to be low (Cherniss, 1980). Frequent job turnover is also a result and has economic and quality improvement implications.

Family members are likely to bear some of the brunt of professional burnout. Marital conflict and family discord are well documented by many professionals who feel burned out (e.g., *social work*: Siefert, Jayaratne, & Chess, 1991; *teaching*: Sakharov & Farber, 1983; *medicine*: Mawardi, 1983; *nursing*: McLaughlin & Erdman, 1992; *day care workers*: Maslach & Pines, 1977). Spouses and children may make such comments as "Dad's grumpy all the time," "I can't seem to do anything right for Mom anymore," and "Since you got that job, you've not been the person I married." The professional may be unaware that the angry outbursts at home are a reflection of professional burnout. A professional who is emotionally and physically exhausted from stresses in the workplace cannot magically leave them at the door when family time begins. In addition, the effects of stresses associated with marriage, family life, finances, and other outside issues complicate and magnify professional stresses and their effects. A vicious and insidious cycle of stress and maladaptive coping is likely to occur. See Alexander (2009) for a comprehensive discussion of sources and effects of stress and burnout.

STRESS IN HUMAN SERVICE PROFESSIONS

A logical question you might ask is, "Why is burnout so common among human service professionals?" Peters (1985) calls it the "modern malady of helping." A helping relationship involves an investment of knowledge and skill blended with facilitating interpersonal qualities to effect change in another individual. Individuals drawn into helping professions such as speech-language pathology and audiology tend to be oriented to people rather than things and to helping those in trouble (Pines, 1983). Other helping professions include, but are not limited to, those related to teaching, psychology, counseling and social work, medicine, and nursing. The fact that so many human service professions work in impersonal institutions further complicates the situation. Farmer and colleagues (1984) identify at least four stressful factors inherent in helping professions: (1) the complexity of our clients and their needs, (2) the difficulty in evaluating "success" in the helping professions, (3) poor perception of helping relationships by others, and (4) the decision-making process inherent in many helping relationship agencies. Maslach (1982) calls burnout the "cost of caring."

The fact that human services are frequently offered through governmental and institutional settings further complicates the situation. Caplan and Jones (1975) list stresses particular to institutional settings, including role ambiguity, role conflict, and role overload. For example, in some institutional settings, job definitions, discipline boundaries, and criteria for success are unclear. Role conflict emerges from inappropriate or unclear demands on the professional or when faced with disparity between individual and institutional ethics and values. Role overload develops from caseloads that are too large or too demanding. The setting by its very nature may be insensitive to the demands on or needs of individual professionals. Farber (1983) cautions that this attitude may increase as economic resources to support human service programs decrease. Changes in Medicare and other insurance funding have caused instability in some health care settings and worry concerning employment. Such concern can exacerbate feelings of burnout.

BURNOUT IN SPEECH-LANGUAGE PATHOLOGY AND AUDIOLOGY

Several studies have addressed the topic of burnout among speech-language pathologists (Miller & Potter, 1982; Potter, Hellesto, Shute, & Dengerink, 1988; Potter & Rudensey, 1984). In Miller and Potter's 1982 study of speech-language pathologists, 43 percent of the respondents considered themselves to have experienced moderately severe burnout. Burnout appeared related to job dissatisfaction, job effectiveness, and lack of management and support services for coping.

Interestingly, burnout was not related to setting, years of employment, caseload, client severity level, paperwork demands, or collegial relationships.

In a second study that investigated how speech-language pathologists coped with burnout, Potter and Rudensey (1984) found that 16 percent of their respondents were leaving the profession because of burnout. Effective coping strategies included adapting personal career goals to be more realistic, understanding motivations for being within a helping profession, increasing communication with administrators, and developing a self-change attitude. They also found that agencies generated some effective strategies to reduce burnout among speech-language pathologists. These strategies included systematic solicitation and implementation of employee suggestions, group discussions, flexible scheduling, released time for continuing education, and clear communication about job expectations. Potter and Rudensey concluded that a team approach involving a speech-language pathologist and an administrator could be effective in improving the mental health of clinical staff.

Poche et al. (2003) studied stress among school speech-language pathologists in Louisiana. They found that time and workload management cause the most stress. Other major stressors included lack of preparation time, inflexible scheduling, too much work, and poorly motivated students. Hale, Kellum, and Burger (2006) in a similar survey found that the most highly identified stressors were paperwork and caseload issues followed by lack of budgetary support, imposed extra duties, and employer demands.

Two studies have specifically addressed burnout among audiologists (Potter et al., 1988). In the first study of 184 clinically certified audiologists, 40 percent of the respondents considered themselves mildly burned out, 30 percent as moderately or severely burned out, and 29 percent as not experiencing burnout. Factors contributing to burnout included feelings of job ineffectiveness and dissatisfaction. In a follow-up survey of audiologists that explored causes and coping strategies related to burnout, the same authors found 15 percent of their respondents were leaving the profession, with another 67 percent having considered this option. The authors concluded that strategies that might reduce burnout among audiologists include (1) having employees participate more in organizational policy setting, (2) reducing caseloads and paperwork, (3) including more uninterrupted flexible break time, (4) matching supervisors' and employees' role expectations, and (5) providing accurate job descriptions. Nemes (2004) cautioned audiologists to walk a fine line between deriving too much satisfaction from working with patients and burnout. Burnout is a real possibility for those professionals who work with hearing impaired clients for many years and make their professional work the total focus of their personal satisfaction.

Several themes emerge from this discussion of sources of burnout. The sources of burnout are idiosyncratic, diverse, and multiple. The stressors can range from mild to catastrophic. Given the combination of circumstances, anyone in a helping profession such as speech-language pathology or audiology is a candidate for burnout. Critical to prevention of burnout is awareness and self-perception of stressors and knowing how to access your internal and external resources for coping successfully with them.

REMEDIATION OF STRESS AND BURNOUT

Both professionals and their employment settings have a vital interest in remediating or preventing stress and burnout. Thus, changes that will reduce stress and foster productive coping strategies can emanate from you and/or your setting. You can take three basic approaches to this problem: (1) recognize the warning signs of stress and burnout, (2) reverse their effects by managing stress and seeking support, and (3) build resilience to stress by taking care of your physical and emotional health (Helpguide, 2009b, 2010a). Numerous studies on the effects of stress-reducing programs tend to show positive outcomes for the professional and the setting (e.g., Lees & Ellis, 1989). Keep in mind that if you want to cure your job stress, you must be proactive and make your choices carefully (McKay, 2011).

Recognizing the Warning Signs

Remediation begins with identifying the signs and symptoms of stress and burnout. Basically, if you feel every day is a "bad day," you may be at risk. If, when you review the list of characteristics in Table 27–4, you perceive that you are experiencing a number of these, you may be a candidate for stress and burnout. Simply identifying your body's response, such as tight muscles and shallow breathing, may help you recognize stressful situations and your response to them. Ask yourself about how you react to stress. For example, do you become over- or underexcited or do you freeze and exhibit both over- and underexcitement (Helpguide, 2010b)? Consultation with a mental health professional may be necessary to identify the problems and distinguish them from depression or other mental disorders. Administration of the Maslach Burnout Inventory (Maslach et al., 1996), the Burnout Risk Appraisal (Pfifferling, 2009), or other tools for depression or stress may provide more data. Professionals who feel burned out need to self-analyze goals, expectations, and value systems governing their professional and personal lives.

Reversing the Effects of Stress

The next step is to manage stress and avoid burnout. Begin by identifying your strengths. Professionals who feel stressed may ignore personal strengths. Farmer and colleagues (1984) suggest you begin by listing what you consider to be your physical, emotional, social, intellectual, spiritual, and other strengths. Such analysis may lead you to affirm your positive qualities, cultivate a more positive self-image, and call up these resources when stressed. You must regain control and sell yourself to yourself. In the case of bullies and bad bosses, remember that they have the problem, not you.

If you are feeling burned out professionally, you may need to analyze your own motivations influencing the practice of your job. Tschudin (1990) suggests that many professionals bring "personal luggage" to work such as carryover of childhood expectations to adulthood, guilt, vague resentments, perfectionism, inability to say no, overcaring for others, and lack of confidence. Examine your personal values and live by them. Tschudin states that when you look at the stress produced from within yourself, you begin to see that the responsibility lies with you, and within you. But it takes a lot of personal strength to accept this, cope with it, and use it *positively* (p. 41).

Working Smarter

Another strategy for reversing effects of stress and burnout is to work smarter. Professionals who feel burned out do not need to work harder but do need to make a more productive investment in their work life. Working smarter, according to Maslach (1982), involves changing your job to be less stressed and more efficient. You need to know and abide by your limits (Peters, 1985). This can be achieved by setting realistic goals, doing the same thing differently, improving time management, taking breaks, and taking things less personally. Some of you might want to talk to your employer about flexible work schedules, if this is possible in your setting.

Setting realistic goals stems from an analysis of what *really* needs to be done, resources for completion, and available time. "Setting realistic goals involves a recognition of your limitations as well as your abilities" (Maslach, 1982, p. 91). The value of changing how things are done is that you will feel more in control of the situation. This strategy begins with analysis of the steps involved in tasks and their eventual elimination or modification. For example, one clinician may want to begin the day at 7 a.m. with completion of paperwork from the previous day, whereas another would rather come in later and do this at the end of the day. Taking a planned break from work is also essential in remediation of burnout. Some professionals need quiet times dispersed between clients; others need to "go out for lunch," and still others divert some of their professional time to less intense or stressful tasks. You may also want to speak with your supervisor about changing duties or being reassigned to a different job role within your program. Finally, and perhaps most difficult, professionals need to perceive difficult situations as objectively as possible.

Working smarter may also involve taking action. It is critical that you learn how to communicate effectively with colleagues and clients and learn how to express your own needs (Maxon, 1999). Learn to say *no* to unreasonable demands or when you really do not want to participate. Documentation of difficult situations is also important. For example, you may keep a log of bullying behavior to identify patterns of such actions. Keep a copy of memos, e-mails, or other written or recorded harassment for future reference in a safe place. If harassment is the source of your stress and burnout, check your employer's harassment policy and work with your occupational health office ("How to Deal with Workplace Bullying," 2005). For example, if you choose to approach the bully, discuss your grievance with your grievance officer first and focus on the undesirable behaviors, not the person. At times, a formal written complaint may be necessary.

Nutrition

Proper nutrition is key to relieving stress. Alcohol and food abuse may only add to the problems and reduce your physiological reserve. Check with your physician and/or a nutritionist for dietary guidance regarding diet and vitamin regimens appropriate for you.

Decompression Activities

Taking care of yourself outside the work situation helps relieve burnout. Maslach (1982) states, "The demands of a caring profession necessitate that professionals take good care of their body and spirit" (p. 95). Examples of physical and psychological decompression activities include exercise, noncompetitive physical activities, a healthy diet, plenty of rest, yoga, meditation, massage, and relaxation techniques. You may also want to use sensory imagery to decompress. For example, if you are a visual person, surround yourself with favorite pictures or close your eyes and visualize a peaceful scene. Similarly, listening to soothing music may relieve stress. Other sensory avenues may be used including smell, touch, and taste to reduce stress (Helpguide, 2010b).

For some professionals, taking a "real vacation" is critical to coping. You may use vacation time, sick time, or ask for a leave of absence if need be. A surprise long weekend is rejuvenating for some, while for others a week or two away from work is necessary. A vacation will give you a chance to recharge and rethink your situation and strategies for working more productively and stress free.

Exercise, one of the most popular stress reduction techniques, helps to condition the cardiovascular system to withstand stress (e.g., Tatelbaum, 1989). Exercise activities such as walking, jogging, swimming, and other aerobics all result in direct medical, endurance, flexibility, and emotional benefits (Farmer et al., 1984). Relaxation activities include deep breathing, progressive muscle relaxation, autogenic training, biofeedback, yoga, imagery, and meditation (Peddicord, 1991). Many people find listening to music or reading "nonwork" books to be a natural "tranquilizer" (Parachin, 1991). Many of these relaxation activities can be done throughout the workday.

Psychological decompression activities include participation in meaningful and enjoyable outside activities. As the song goes, "accentuate the positive." Participation in recreation activities, such as hobbies, can help counterbalance a day of stress. Unfortunately, because of demanding caseloads, financial needs, and competing demands from work and home, some professionals have or make little time available just for themselves. Maslach (1982) states that "frustrations and failures can be put into perspective when balanced by satisfactions and successes" (p. 95). To help others effectively, you consistently need to fortify yourself physically and psychologically.

Other possible decompressions strategies include taking a break from technology (Helpguide, 2010a). Turn off your computer and phone and stop checking email for a specific time each day. This may be a good time to finish tasks that have been started but not completed or to participate in creative activities or other decompression programs.

Continuing Education

Participation in continuing education programs offered through the workplace or professional organizations is an excellent strategy for dealing with burnout. Continuing education helps you gain new skills to work more effectively and efficiently, stimulates creativity and problem solving, and opens networks with other professionals. In-services offered through your employment setting might focus not only on assessment and intervention issues related to communication disorders but also on time management, conflict resolution, and stress management.

Attendance at regional, state, or national meetings provides an opportunity for many professionals to combine educational enhancement with the opportunity to "get away" from the stresses of both work and family. Generally, there are social activities at these events where you can initiate or renew professional and personal friendships. So that you are not disappointed with the continuing education program offered, you should be sure to review announcements carefully and determine whether the stated objectives match your background and needs at the time. Finally, you may find yourself "recharged" when you are the presenter at a continuing education program. The challenge and intellectual stimulation inherent in the preparation and the positive feedback afterward may help relieve burnout.

Support and Counseling

Social support is defined as "information that leads individuals to believe that they are cared for and loved, esteemed, and valued and that they participate in a network of communication and mutual obligation" (Pines, 1983, p. 156). Support is an "immunization" against stress (Cobb, 1976). A supportive individual is an active listener who provides nonjudgmental emotional backup, assistance, insight, and feedback. The primary vehicles for offering support are open communication, active listening, and accessibility.

In many institutional settings, individual mentors are available to discuss technical and psychological aspects of the job. The Clinical Fellowship or fourth-year clinical experience supervisor may assume this role with the first-year professional. Pines, Aronson, and Kafry (1981) suggest that even staff meetings can help reduce burnout if they focus on articulation of shared problems and staff development. Similarly, in some settings, particularly large institutional settings such as school districts or hospitals, work-setting support groups may be available. These groups focus on developing staff effectiveness and problem solving through free expression of feelings, offering of suggestions and feedback, and realistic goal setting (Scully, 1983). Discussion may focus on techniques for stress management, methods of conflict management, development of self-esteem, and assertiveness (Tschudin, 1990).

Support offered by family and friends is also valuable, although "bringing home" stressful topics may exacerbate burnout rather than relieve it. Maslach (1982) states that family and friends tend to offer comfort, appreciation, and positive experiences. Her research has also identified the critical importance of a good marriage or intimate relationship in "counterbalancing" the stresses of a job. Some authors suggest that spirituality may sustain individuals through stressful times. Spirituality goes beyond participation in formal religious organizations and focuses on a person's perception of his or her place in the universe and the creation of a personal value system (Farmer et al., 1984). Prayer and meditation may provide relief and serve as decompression activities.

McKay (2011) states there are times when it is necessary to seek professional counseling to cope with job-related stress. This may be from a psychologist, psychiatrist, or social worker. Do not be afraid to seek such help or of any perceived stigma. If medications are prescribed, be sure to follow directions carefully and keep your therapist and physician informed of progress and possible side effects. You should also check your health insurance for possible coverage of services.

Finally, should you belong to a union in your workplace, you may want to discuss your situation with your union representative about any resources that may be available from the union. A union representative may also help with mediation if necessary (United Electrical Workers, 2010).

Humor

In his autobiography, Norman Cousins (1981) called humor a form of internal jogging. It moves your internal organs around, increases your heart rate, and reduces your blood pressure. It also enhances respiration. Laughter is an "igniter of great expectations" (p. 217). Maslach (1982) also states that humor is an important supportive coping technique. "Being able to joke and laugh about a stressful event reduces the tension and anxiety—it also serves to make the situation less serious and less overwhelming" (p. 60). These two quotes serve to remind us that humor is one of the most powerful techniques to reduce stress and to cope with burden. Murphy and Murphy (2000, p. 24) offer seven strategies on how to incorporate humor in our lives:

1. Select humor that complements your life and work.
2. Quantify humor by using it as part of your therapy goals and measure the results.
3. Keep in mind that the very best humor is when you can laugh at yourself.
4. Know where to find good, funny stuff fast.
5. Know and believe what humor can do for you and your patients.
6. Remember: You can't always be in control, but you always have choices.
7. Reward yourself.

Humor can be shared with clients, families, and coworkers through jokes, funny stories, quotes, and anecdotes, through nonverbal communication, through cartoons, posters, and bulletin boards, and via the Internet. Professionals should only use humor that is culturally and linguistically appropriate.

Coping with Bad Bosses

Vanzant-Stern (2011) states that the worst thing you could do when you have a bad boss is "nothing" while hoping that the problems will disappear. She suggests having an action plan that includes communicating with a trusted confidant or mentor within your workplace, reading about supervisory skills and how to acquire them, and finding other sources of positive reinforcement for doing a good job. You should also do an honest appraisal of your own actions and behaviors. Other strategies include making a list of supervisory behaviors that are frustrating and discussing these in an open but positive manner with your boss. You should also keep a written record of bad behaviors and, as a last resort, report your boss to his or her supervisor or human resources (Hansen, 2012).

Conflict Resolution on the Job

Remember that all of us experience some conflict in the course of our professional lives, but it must be handled carefully so that work can be meaningful and productive. Sometimes the strategies featured here do not help relieve stress and burden, particularly when the stress involves a conflict with a colleague. You will need to identify who is involved in the conflict, what critical issues are involved, what each person's position is regarding the conflict, and what strategies might be used to settle the conflict. Conflict resolution will involve your ability to create a dialogue with the other person. This conversation should stem from your basic sense of respect for this individual. It is best to have your dialogue in a neutral place that is physically and psychologically comfortable for you both. Be prepared to define the issue as something you need to solve together. Fittro (2005) suggests that you describe the behaviors, feelings, consequences, and desired changes you envision by starting sentences with "I" rather than "you." Empathic listening is critical to the process so that you understand the other person as a precursor to being understood. The next step is for each person to brainstorm possible solutions followed by a positive evaluation of each one. The goal is to identify solutions or compromises that are acceptable to each person and provide a "win-win" context. Solutions should be tried and evaluated after some period of time.

If personal conflict resolution does not solve the issue, a third party or mediator may be involved. Mediation provides both parties with a safe and neutral environment where they can offer their perspectives and solutions. Mediators create a context in which individuals feel they can speak openly. They also facilitate the meeting, clarify issues as needed, and provide possible suggestions. Mediation has been found to be a positive context for solving conflicts, particularly one in which individuals perceive they have had fair and equitable treatment (Roehl & Cook, 1989).

Unfortunately, the best strategies for resolving conflicts do not always work. Some individuals are so entrenched in their own perspectives and unwilling to work toward a solution that a positive resolution is impossible. Their own personalities and communication styles may be barriers to a productive dialogue. Still others may be unwilling to discuss issues and want to avoid any context in which the issues are openly discussed.

CHANGING JOBS

There may be times in your professional life when, despite your concerted efforts to adapt to and cope with stress, a change in employment may be the best alternative. Maslach (1982) cautions us to consider carefully what a change means and its expected outcome. "Change does not automatically guarantee success and happiness" (p. 107). Change may involve assuming another position within the same organization, such as becoming a supervisor or administrator. Pines et al. (1981) describe this as "quitting upward." It may also mean changing employment settings to work in a comparable position or a new one. Finally, change may mean leaving the profession of speech-language pathology or audiology.

In considering a change, you need to assess whether the new position really results in a removal of current stressors. It is possible a position in a new agency entails stressors similar to those of your present position. Further, a new position may have unique or additional stressors with which you are not prepared to cope. Before you change positions, remember there is a certain degree of stress inherent in changing positions. For example, the new position may involve unfamiliar duties and routines, philosophical differences in service delivery, and "great expectations" for performance. If you are changing geographical areas, there is the added stress of relocation, perhaps to an unfamiliar area that lacks a personal support system. Finally, consider the financial implications of changing jobs. You need to be ready to live without a paycheck for some time. In general, it is best not to leave your job until you have secured new employment.

Notwithstanding these cautions, change can be invigorating and challenging. A new position may be a true antidote for burnout. This may be the perfect opportunity to use coping skills learned in a previous position. It may also be a chance to demonstrate heretofore unrecognized abilities and to fulfill personal career goals.

ORGANIZATIONAL AND SUPERVISORY CONSIDERATIONS

Agencies and supervisors have a responsibility to create a workplace climate in which stress and burnout are prevented or minimized. Alexander (2009) advises that supervisors set realistic goals, create a supportive environment, share decision making, and encourage positive interpersonal relationships among staff. Supervisors have a responsibility to treat all employees in a fair and respectful manner, never tolerate bullying, design reasonable workloads and responsibilities, and recognize that some employees may be vulnerable to stress and burnout (Canadian Centre for Occupational Health and Safety, 2008). Some employers will offer wellness, lifestyle, or stress management programs; counseling; or continuing education that focuses on stress and burnout. Employers will find that psychologically healthy employees are better employees and offer better clinical services.

SUMMARY

Workplace stress may derive from a variety of personal and employment-related sources. Workplace stress and burnout are common among helping professionals, including speech-language pathologists and audiologists. One of the most important take-home messages of this chapter is that identification of stress and participation in stress relief activities take "practice, practice, and practice" (Helpguide, 2009b). Both audiologists and speech-language pathologists should actively make stress relief a natural part of their workday. The outcomes of these behaviors include better service delivery; physical and psychological health; and positive relationships with clients, colleagues, and family.

CRITICAL THINKING

1. Consider the following scenario. What are the sources of stress for Jim? What suggestions would you have for Jim? If you were his program director, what would you do?

   Jim is a 32-year-old audiologist who recently completed the requirements for an AuD at a university about 75 miles from his home. His position as an audiologist at a large medical center did not require this advanced degree, nor was it required for licensure in his state. Jim felt that the degree was to his advantage, although he knew it would consume his personal time and would involve financial expense. None of the other five audiologists in his program intended to do this and teased him about his motivation to "run the hospital" some day. Jim's wife was also skeptical but supportive about the added costs and the time it would take away from his job and family. Jim and his wife had adopted a preschooler with special needs two years previously. Jim worked full time while going to school for 18 months and traveled to classes two nights a week. During his second year, he was in a serious accident that totaled his car and resulted in minor injuries to his passenger. Jim then decided to take a three-month leave of absence so that he could finish his program, deal with his father's recent death, and provide support to his mother. When Jim returned to his job, he found that one of his colleagues had been promoted to program director and that his office had been moved. There was no public recognition of his having received the advanced degree and no salary increase. He overheard a colleague say, "Did he think we'd roll out the red carpet for him when he got a doctorate?" In the next several months following his return to work, Jim lost 15 pounds and resumed smoking. Feeling demoralized and depressed, Jim considered leaving audiology.

2. What societal factors do you believe contribute to burnout within human service professions?
3. You serve as a mentor to Chloe, a speech-language pathologist in her Clinical Fellowship in a public school setting. She has a 60-student caseload in two middle schools. Read the following description and consider what you would recommend to her.

   Chloe is a 25-year-old speech-language pathologist who graduated six months ago with a 4.0 GPA and excellent supervisor's evaluations in more than 600 hours of clinical practicum. Chloe graduated summa cum laude with a double major in biology and linguistics but decided against a medical career in favor of a graduate degree in speech-language pathology. Chloe was actively involved with her graduate student association, serving as its president, and she also served as a research assistant for her major professor. Chloe did a master's thesis and presented it and another paper at a state professional convention shortly before graduation. She continues to help her former professor with data analysis. She intends to start a weekend Executive MBA program in the near future. Chloe would like to start a private practice in the future. Her fiancé serves in the Army and recently incurred a traumatic brain injury in Afghanistan. He is in an Army hospital near Washington, DC. Chloe was also diagnosed with Graves' disease two months ago and has started a course of medication. Recently, Chloe abruptly broke down in tears, threw papers on the floor, and fled from a team meeting when asked to discuss a student's needs.
4. What are you doing as a graduate student or a professional to prevent stress and burnout in your personal and professional lives?
5. You have been asked by your employer to give a 15-minute presentation on Creating a More Positive Workplace Environment. What are the key points you would include in this presentation? What would be three or four key take-home messages you would want your audience to have?
6. One of your colleagues, Bob, always has something negative to say "under his breath" during staff meetings. Bob refers to his clients with severe communication problems as "dumbos" and has a ready joke for every type of client problem. He is a competent clinician but rarely does anything beyond what he has to do. What is going on here? Would you intervene? Why or why not?
7. What responsibility does a department supervisor have for monitoring the possible burnout of department clinicians? What is the difference between intruding and being proactive in preventing burnout among staff members?
8. Dana is an experienced clinician who works in a speech and hearing center of about 20 SLPs and audiologists. She is known as highly competent but bossy. When a new clinician, Marielle, was employed to develop a new preschool program, Dana was angry that she was passed over as she was also interested in creating the program. Dana's disappointment is obvious to the other staff, and many are dismayed that she avoids interacting with Marielle and at times "shrugs off" her ideas. Marielle has said nothing publicly about the difficulty but has intimated to friends that "It gets me that she feels threatened, but what would I say?" What is going on here? What should be done, if anything?

REFERENCES

Alexander, L. (2009). *Burnout: Impact on nursing.* Available from http://www.netcegroups.com/548/Course_3142.pdf

Canadian Centre for Occupational Health and Safety. (2008). *Workplace stress—General.* Retrieved from http://www.ccohs.ca/oshanswers/psychosocial/stress.html

Caplan, R., & Jones, K. (1975). Effects of workload, role ambiguity, and type A personality on anxiety, depression, and heart rate. *Journal of Applied Psychology, 60*, 713–719.

Cavaiola, A., & Lavender, N. (2000). *Toxic coworkers: How to deal with dysfunctional people on the job.* Oakland, CA: New Harbinger Publishers.

Cherniss, C. (1980). *Staff burnout: Job stress in the human services.* Beverly Hills, CA: Sage.

Cobb, S. (1976). Social support as a moderator of life stress. *Psychosomatic Medicine, 38*, 300–314.

Cousins, N. (1981). *Human options*. New York, NY: W.W. Norton.

Downs, M. (2005). *Putting a workplace bully back in line*. Available from http://my.webmd.com/

Farber, B. (1983). Dysfunctional aspects of the psychotherapeutic role. In B. Larker (Ed.), *Stress and burnout in the human service professions* (pp. 97–115). New York, NY: Pegasus.

Farmer, R., Monahan, L., & Hekeler, R. (1984). *Stress management for human services.* Beverly Hills, CA: Sage.

Fittro, J. (2005). *Resolving conflict constructively and respectfully*. Available from http://ohioline.osu.edu

Hale, S., Kellum, G., & Burger, C. (2006). *Burnout in speech-language pathologists employed in schools.* Paper presented at 2006 annual convention of American Speech-Language-Hearing Association. Retrieved from http://www.asha.org/Events/convention/handouts/2006/0446_Hale_Sue/

Hansen, R. (2012). *Dealing with a bad boss: Strategies for coping*. Retrieved from http://www.quintcareers.com/bad_bosses.html

Helpguide. (2009a). *Job loss and unemployment stress: Tips for staying positive during your job search*. Retrieved from http://www.helpguide.org/life/unemployment_job_loss_stress_coping_tips.htm

Helpguide. (2009b). *Understanding stress: Signs, symptoms, causes, and effects*. Retrieved from http://www.helpguide.org/mental/stress_signs.htm

Helpguide. (2010a). *Preventing burnout: Signs, symptoms, causes, and coping strategies*. Retrieved from http://www.helpguide.org/mental/burnout_signs_symptoms.htm

Helpguide. (2010b). *Quick stress relief: Surefire ways to rapidly reduce stress*. Retrieved from http://www.helpguide.org/mental/quick_stress_relief.htm

How to deal with workplace bullying: Advice, guidance and help with adult bullying. (2005). Available from http://www.bullyonline.org/

Lees, S., & Ellis, N. (1989). The design of a stress-management program for nursing personnel. *Journal of Advanced Nursing, 15*, 946–961.

Maslach, C. (1982). *Burnout: The cost of caring*. Englewood Cliffs, NJ: Prentice Hall.

Maslach C., Jackson S. E., & Leiter, M. P. (1996). *Maslach Burnout Inventory* (3rd ed.). Palo Alto, CA: Consulting Psychologists Press.

Maslach, C., & Pines, A. (1977). The 'burnout' syndrome in day care settings. *Child Care Quarterly, 6*, 100–113.

Mawardi, B. (1983). Aspects of the impaired physician. In B. Farber (Ed.), *Stress and burnout in the human service professions* (pp. 119–128). New York, NY: Pergamon Press.

Maxon, R. (1999). *Stress in the workplace: A costly epidemic*. Retrieved from http://www.fdu.edu/newspubs/magazine/99su/stress.html

McKay, D. R. (2011). *If you have job stress, here's what to do*. Retrieved from http://careerplanning.about.com/od/workrelated/a/stress.htm

McLaughlin, A., & Erdman, J. (1992). Rehabilitation staff stress as it relates to patient acuity and diagnosis. *Brain Injury, 6*, 59–64.

Mezger, R. (2004, July 25). Battling the workplace bully. *Cleveland Plan Dealer*.

Miller, M., & Potter, R. (1982). Professional burnout among speech-language pathologists. *ASHA, 24*, 177–180.

Monat, A., & Lazarus R. (Eds.). (1977). *Stress and coping*. New York, NY: Columbia University Press.

Murphy, J., & Murphy, A. (2000). Seven strategies for reducing stress. *Advance, 10*, 24.

Namie, G., & Namie, R. (2003). *The bully at work: What you can do to stop the hurt and reclaim your dignity on the job*. Naperville, IL: Sourcebooks.

Nemes, J. (2004). Professional burnout: How to stop it from happening to you. *The Hearing Journal. 57*, 21–22, 24, 26.

Parachin, V. (1991). Pressure-proof your life: Creative ways to reduce stress. *Today's Nurse, 13*, 9–11.

Peddicord, K. (1991). Strategies for promoting stress reduction and relaxation. *Nursing Clinics of North America, 26*, 867–874.

Peters, M. (1985). Burnout: The modern malady of helping. In D. Avila & A. Combs (Eds.), *Perspectives on helping relationships and the helping professions* (pp. 139–155). Boston, MA: Allyn & Bacon.

Pfifferling, J. (2009). *Burnout risk appraisal.* Available from http://www.cpwb.org/

Pines, A. (1983). On burnout and the buffering effects of social support. In B. Farber (Ed.), *Stress and burnout in the human service professions* (pp. 155–174). New York, NY: Pergamon Press.

Pines, A., Aronson, E., & Kafry, D. (1981). *Burnout.* New York, NY: The Free Press.

Poche, L., Tassin, J., Oliver, P., & Fellows, J. (2003). *Job stress in school-based speech-language pathologists.* 2003 Annual Convention of the American Speech-Language-Hearing Association, Chicago.

Potter, R., Hellesto, P., Shute, B., & Dengerink, J. (1988). Burnout among audiologists: Its incidence and causes. *The Hearing Journal, 41*, 18–25.

Potter, R., & Rudensey, K. (1984). Coping with burnout. *ASHA, 26*, 35–37.

Roehl, J., & Cook, R. (1989). Mediation in interpersonal disputes: Effectiveness and limitations. In K. Kressel, D. Pruitt, & Associates (Eds.), *Mediation research* (pp. 31–52). San Francisco, CA: Jossey-Bass.

Sakharov, M., & Farber, B. (1983). A critical study of burnout in teachers. In B. Farber (Ed.), *Stress and burnout in the human service professions.* New York, NY: Pergamon.

Scully, R. (1983). The work setting support group: A means of preventing burnout. In B. Farber (Ed.), *Stress and burnout in the human service professions.* New York, NY: Pergamon Press.

Shewan, C., & Blake, A. (1991). Caregiving: A common role for ASHA members. *ASHA, 35*, 35.

Siefert, K., Jayaratne, S., & Chess, W. (1991). Job satisfaction, burnout, and turnover in health care social workers. *Health and Social Work, 16*, 193–202.

Stewart, W. (2003). Cost of lost productive time among U.S. workers with depression. *Journal of the American Medical Association, 289*, 3135–3144.

Tatelbaum, J. (1989). *You don't have to suffer: A handbook for moving beyond life's crises.* New York, NY: Harper & Row.

The Serial Bully. (2005). Available from http://www.bullyonline.org/workbully/serial.htm

Tschudin, V. (1990). Support yourself. *Nursing Times, 86*, 40–42.

United Electrical Workers. (2010). *Stress in the workplace.* Retrieved from http://www.ueunion.org/stwd_stress.html

Vanzant-Stern, T. (2011). *Are you the victim of a bad boss?* Retrieved from http://humanresources.about.com/od/badmanagerboss/a/bad_boss2.htm

RESOURCES

Workplace Bullying Institute. (2010). *Being bullied? Start here.* Retrieved from http://www.workplacebullying.org/targets/starthere.html

Workplace Bullying Institute. (2010). *Definition of workplace bullying.* Retrieved from http://workplacebullying.org/targets/problem/definition.html

Workplace Bullying Institute. (2010). *Economic devastation.* Retrieved from http://workplacebullying.org/targets/impact/economic-harm.html

Workplace Bullying Institute. (2010). *Finding a lawyer: Tips and advice.* Retrieved from http://workplacebullying.org/targets/solution/selecting-a-lawyer.html

Workplace Bullying Institute. (2010). *How bullying happens.* Retrieved from http://workplacebullying.org/targets/problem/why-bullies-bully.html

Workplace Bullying Institute. (2010). *Physical health impairment: How bullying can affect your body.* Retrieved from http://workplacebullying.org/targets/impact/physical-harm.html

Workplace Bullying Institute. (2010). *Psychological-emotional-mental injuries*. Retrieved from http://workplacebullying.org/targets/impact/mental-harm.html

Workplace Bullying Institute. (2010). *Social harm: Ways bullying can impact other areas of your life*. Retrieved from http://workplacebullying.org/targets/impact/social-harm.html

Workplace Bullying Institute. (2010). *The WBI 3-step method: What bullied targets can do*. Retrieved from http://workplacebullying.org/targets/solution/three-step-method.html

Workplace Bullying Institute. (2010). *The WBI guide to selecting a therapist*. Retrieved from http://workplacebullying.org/targets/solution/selecting-a-therapist.html

Workplace Bullying Institute. (2010). *Who gets targeted.* Retrieved from http://workplacebullying.org/targets/problem/who-gets-targeted.html

Workplace Bullying Institute. (2010). *Why U.S. employers do so little*. Retrieved from http://workplacebullying.org/targets/problem/employer-resistance.html

SECTION V

Evidence-Based Practice

28

The Future of Science

Ray D. Kent, PhD

SCOPE OF CHAPTER

Research is intrinsically futuristic, always directed to the next experiment, the next theoretical advance, the next challenge to the standard or popular view. Research is a frontier phenomenon, and its practitioners work on a horizon of possibilities. To dare any specific forecast into what research may bring is uncertain at best, foolish or irrelevant at worst. Predictions about where science can take us are sometimes amusingly wrong, as described in *The Follies of Science* (Dregni & Dregni, 2006). And although it can be fun to look at predictions that went awry, there can be no argument that science has accomplished remarkable things. The advances can be spectacular. In 1924, Bertrand Russell wrote, "The effect of the biological sciences, so far, has been very small." This may have been an accurate assessment a few decades ago. But what would Russell say today about discoveries in genetics, biomolecular science, and nanomedicine? And what would he think about the ambitious project, the International Human Genome Sequencing Consortium, which has mapped the human genome ahead of schedule?

Science can be examined in many different ways, but three general aspects are critical in assessing the role of science in the world:

1. The intellectual and economic capital of science (the resources that support research, including scientific personnel)

2. The discoveries of science
3. The impact of science on society

The first of these is the infrastructure that leads to the second (discoveries), and the second is the foundation for the third (impact on society). Because research is a human enterprise that rests on intellectual and economic resources, it is possible to make some general projections about the future of science, taking into account the historic pattern and the present-day foundation for future development.

This chapter takes a general view of research in the discipline of communication sciences and disorders (CSD). The purpose is not to predict particular scientific accomplishments but rather to assay the socioeconomic trends and various influences that will govern funding for research and the parameters of its application. The expenditure for research on communication sciences and disorders is quite small compared to that for the major diseases such as cancer or heart disease, but all areas of research, whether large or small, are subject to the major forces of social policy. To put it in other words, "Science policy implements a social contract" (Pielke & Byerly, 1998, p. 42). The future of science will be defined by the social contract through which society provides the resources for science and, in turn, reaps the benefits of scientific achievements. The next section takes a closer look at the social contract.

SCIENCE AND THE SOCIAL CONTRACT

The social policy that provides economic support for science in the United States is in a period of fundamental change. Because this change has multiple ramifications, it is important to gain some understanding of it, beginning with a look at its history. For some time, the social policy that undergirded research support was the Bush contract, named after Vannevar Bush, who in 1945 published a document of extraordinary influence. As noted by Pielke and Byerly (1998), the Bush contract is based on three fundamental assumptions: (1) It assumes that scientific advances are essential to meet national needs. Few people would argue with this contention, and the expectation that science will benefit society is critical to the public support of science. (2) The way in which science meets national needs can be described through a simple linear/reservoir model. In this model, science creates a reservoir of knowledge that is tapped by society. (3) Science is practiced in relative autonomy, isolated from the direct influence of society. This isolation ensures a freedom of scientific inquiry. In this model, society provides the resources for, but does not govern, the scientific enterprise. Ideally, science would grow continuously, and as it does, the reservoir of knowledge would expand and society would benefit from this vast pool of information. At any one time, some of the information in the scientific reservoir may not be immediately applicable to the well-being of individuals in the society. It may take years, even decades, before some advances in basic science lead to successful application.

Science can become highly, even prohibitively, expensive, and some commentators believe that exponential growth is unlikely (Nalimov, 1981; Price, 1963). Inevitably, then, science must compete for resources with other social institutions, such as those addressing needs in defense, health, education, national disasters, and a range of social services. Even if there were general agreement that the reservoir of knowledge should be as large as possible, it may be economically prohibitive to support vigorous programs of research in all specialties at all times. Unharnessed growth of science is not sustainable. The conduct of science can also be affected by ethical issues, as in the case of reproduction science, the harvesting of fetal tissues for stem cell research, and genetic engineering.

Accordingly, the social contract may change in favor of a model in which economic and moral priorities are established for the support of science. These priorities would determine the allocation of funds for various areas of research. Some sense of the difficulties involved can be gained from an examination of the factors that determine funding for research by the National Institutes of Health. It has been proposed that the funding for different areas and disorders can be gauged by the burden of disease (Gross, Anderson, & Rowe, 1999) or by the amount and effectiveness of lobbying (Gottlieb, 1999). See Curran, Effinger, Pantel, & Curran, 1983, for further discussion of priorities and policy.

Some believe that science has come to a point that might be called "the end of growth," a period in which "the frontiers of knowledge still seem endless, but the financial and human resources needed to extend those frontiers now seem to be increasingly limited" (Sigma Xi, 1987, p. 32). The "end of growth" is not necessarily abrupt; indeed, warnings of a budgetary limitation for science have sounded for some time, even during periods when federal appropriations for science continued to increase. The expectation of change is evident in recent discussions that relate to definitions of what science should be in relation to society (Notturno, 2008), whether science is at a socioeconomic crossroads (Charlton & Andras, 2005), and whether a new model of leadership is needed for the research enterprise (Federoff & Rubin, 2010). It should not be assumed that science is immune to social, political, and economic forces; to the contrary, science is affected by each of these factors and the science of the future will be molded by exogenous influences. The dependency of science on its sociopolitical environment is captured in the following quotation: "Historians and economists have recognized that while scientific innovation has occurred in many settings, it has prospered most when talent, supportive institutions, mobility, free communications, and financing are available in significant measure" (Moses, Dorsey, Matheson, & Their, 2005, p. 1333).

Current and future scientists probably will have to consider very carefully how their work might be supported by the available resources. But this is not the only reason for a change in the social contract. It is also clear that many problems will not be solved solely by scientific methods. As Pielke and Byerly (1998) observed, "Infectious diseases develop resistance to antibiotics" and "Proliferation of wastes and weapons mars the nuclear option" (p. 44). Scientific accomplishments surely can produce benefits, but they also can incur side effects or long-term consequences that are not entirely desirable. Furthermore, some advances may bring about ethical dilemmas, as has been widely discussed with respect to modern genetics and various developments in molecular biology. The implication is that science today is not a completely autonomous enterprise but rather one that seeks solutions within a broader framework of personal and social benefits and risks. In certain circumstances, governments impose restrictions on the ways in which research can be done, especially when humans or human tissues are involved. One contemporary example is research with human embryonic stem cells. Pluripotent stem cells (cells that can develop into many different cell types) are isolated from human embryos that are a few days old. Pluripotent stem cell lines also can be developed from fetal tissue (i.e., tissue that is older than eight weeks of development).

A demand for immediate applicability of all research could greatly impair the health of the research enterprise. Frequently, research on fundamental scientific problems yields enormous benefits, not all of which were even imagined at the time of the initial discovery. Funding agencies must take care that research into fundamental questions is not harmed by a drastic reallocation of funds to research that addresses applied problems of high priority. The value of a given research project cannot always be determined from a narrow set of immediate priorities.

The Committee on Science of the U.S. House of Representatives took a major step in defining the new federal science policy with its report "Unlocking Our Future: Toward a New National Science Policy" (U.S. House of Representatives Committee on Science, 1998; excerpts of the report appear in *Science Communication, 20,* 328–336). Some basic issues are summarized here. An important point is that the report affirms the importance of federal funding for fundamental scientific, or basic, research. It also endorses a program of research grants to individual investigators that offset indirect costs and are evaluated by a peer-reviewed selection process. The report recommends that funding be provided for creative, groundbreaking research that might be considered too risky in a conservative review process. Mention also is made of the Governmental Results and Performance Act, which mandates a review of outcomes of federally supported programs, including research. The report recommends that funding agencies evaluate outcomes by using a research portfolio rather than evaluating outcomes for individual research grants.

An obligation that falls to scientists is to inform the public and policy makers about what kinds of scientific advances are likely and at what cost. For example, Feigin (2005) considers how research may affect the prospects for child health. The National Institutes of Health (NIH) accomplishes a similar goal with the preparation of strategic research plans that typically summarize major research accomplishments and identify particular opportunities for new discoveries and their clinical application. The NIDCD Strategic Plan for 2012-2016 is available (National Institute on Deafness and Other Communication Disorders, 2012).

In meeting its obligations to society, science must accomplish a broad agenda of discovery and application. To accomplish this goal, science has a diversified nature, as described next.

THE RESEARCH LANDSCAPE: TYPES OF RESEARCH

Research is not a monolithic entity but rather a combination of several types of investigative approaches that are complementary to one another. The following types are among the most widely recognized and are defined here in terms suitable for the CSD field. But a note of caution is in order: these terms have been defined in somewhat different ways by different authors and agencies.

Basic research (also known as fundamental or preclinical research) is aimed at the study of processes that are universal in their application to scientific knowledge. Although basic research in CSD is often understood as research on normal processes of speech, language, and hearing, that is not necessarily the case because this kind of research can be conducted with a combination of normal and abnormal behaviors. Basic research is conducted to discover fundamental principles of communication, often without an objective of immediate clinical application. Basic research not only illuminates mechanisms and processes in communication but also establishes normative data that are indispensible referents in the assessment of communicative disorders.

Basic biomedical research (a type of basic research) is directed to increase understanding of fundamental life processes, such as genetics, molecular biology, or functional patterns of neural activity. Much of this research focuses on normal or typical processes, such as the pattern of neural activation underlying processes of language comprehension or expression.

Applied research seeks specific knowledge needed to improve the treatment of a particular disorder. Frequently, then, this research is couched in terms of a given communication disorder (e.g., deafness, stuttering, speech sound disorder, specific language impairment, voice disorder).

Clinical research is conducted to learn about normal function and disorder in human subjects, with the aim of informing the understanding, assessment, and treatment of disorders.

Directed research is research undertaken by an investigator in response to an outside request for study of a particular problem or question. This kind of research opportunity is often announced in a program announcement (PA) or a request for applications (RFA), which is one mechanism that the NIH uses to solicit applications for research on a given topic or problem. The NIH and several private organizations use this method to solicit research proposals that are congruent with the major aims of the funding agency.

Interdisciplinary research is not defined consistently by those who use the term, but two common definitions are (1) the formation of research collaborations to focus on a common problem that is outside the boundaries of any one scientific discipline (e.g., the genetics of language impairment in children) and (2) the creation of hybrid disciplines such as biochemistry, psychoneuroimmunology, or neurolinguistics.

Investigator-initiated research is a research project defined by the individual investigator or a team of investigators. Typically, this kind of research falls within broad parameters defined by the funding agency, but applicants have considerable latitude in selecting a particular topic of research. Both private and governmental agencies may support this type of research. Later in this section, attention is given to a major source of financial support, the NIH.

Patient-oriented research is conducted with human subjects (or on material of human origin such as tissues, specimens, and behavioral phenomena) and addresses functional mechanisms in health and disease, developing and testing preventive and therapeutic principles or developing diagnostic tests.

Population health research pertains to the distribution and determinants of health status as influenced by social, economic, and physical environments; human biology; and health policy and services, with the general goal of prevention and health promotion at the population levels.

Outcome research is concerned with the end results of particular practices or interventions (see discussion in the next section).

Translational (or translative) research is of two types. The first, called T1, takes a discovery from basic science and studies its applicability to a clinical or human problem (sometimes called "bench to bedside"). The second type, T2, takes a result from clinical research, such as a prevention or treatment strategy, and explores its use in population-based studies to define best practices in the community. The relationships can be summarized with the notation, Bench > Bedside > Population. Ideally, the flow would be bidirectional so that observations at bedside (clinical application) can influence further work at the bench (basic research).

A "translation gap" results from disproportionate efforts in basic research and clinical applications. Several factors contribute to this gap, including industry's preference for late-stage clinical trials, a static distribution of NIH support for basic and applied research, and the inclination of venture investors to seek companies that have products that are close to market (Moses et al., 2005). The degree of concern that NIH has for this problem is reflected in the recent plans for the "NIH Roadmap," which features initiatives to encourage clinical and translational research (Zerhouni, 2005).

The proportion of research activity in these categories can change over time. For example, an analysis of research grants on autism by Singh, Illes, Lazzeroni, and Hallmayer (2009) showed the following: First, the number of funded grants increased 15 percent per year from 1997 to 2006. Second, over the total period of the analysis, basic science accounted for 65 percent of the projects; clinical research, 15 percent; and translational research, 20 percent. Third, the proportion of basic research grants decreased significantly per year while there was a significant increase in the proportion of translational grants per year.

A demand for immediate applicability of all research could greatly impair the health of the research enterprise. Frequently, research on fundamental scientific problems yields enormous benefits, not all of which were even imagined at the time of the initial discovery. The value of a given research project cannot always be determined from a narrow set of immediate priorities. Consider the instructions (see the appendix at the end of the chapter) that the National Institutes of Health provides to the reviewers of research grant applications. The fundamental dimensions by which an application is judged are the significance of the research, the approach to be used, the innovation of the proposed research, the capabilities of the investigator, and the appropriateness of the environment. These five yardsticks are the evaluation tools used by the world's largest funding agency for research on human health.

OUTCOME RESEARCH: CLINICAL TRIALS

There are many different research designs, as discussed in a number of books written on this subject. But it is important to mention here at least the different types of trials used in clinical research. These are known as four phases of research. Phase 0 is a designation for exploratory research that is first used in humans. Phase I trials are the initial stage of testing in humans and are designed to assess safety, tolerability, and basic mechanisms of an intervention. Phase II trials are performed on larger groups of participants (usually in the range of 20 to 300) and are designed to assess how well the treatment works, as well as to continue Phase I safety assessments in a larger group of individuals. Phase III studies are randomized, controlled, multicenter trials on large groups of participants (in the range of 300 to 3,000 or more depending on the condition under study) and are aimed at offering a definitive assessment of how effective the intervention is compared with a current "gold standard" treatment. Phase III studies are expensive, with costs typically running into millions of dollars, and they are logistically demanding. Phase III trials are considered to be the strongest evidence in support of a treatment. But it sometimes happens that different Phase III trials on the same treatment yield discrepant results, in which case a meta-analysis is in order to provide an overall assessment of the evidence. Meta-analyses are discussed by Robey and Dalebout (1998).

NIH GRANTS FOR RESEARCH AND RESEARCH TRAINING

The NIH supports more health research than any other agency in the world. Several types of research support are available through the NIH. The main types are identified by an activity code, and the different types have an availability and purpose that vary somewhat among the various member institutes. For example, the National Institute on Deafness and Other Communication Disorders (NIDCD) may have a different implementation than the National Institute on Child Health and Human Development (NICHD). The activity codes are listed in Table 28–1. Of primary interest to most career researchers is the vaunted R01 (Research Project Grant), the original and historically oldest grant mechanism used by NIH. The R01 provides support for health-related research and development consistent with the mission of the NIH. R01s can be investigator-initiated or can be in response to a program announcement or request for application. The NIH has both intramural (within NIH) and extramural

TABLE 28–1 Activity Codes for Types of Research Support Available from NICHD

R series	K series	T & F series	P series
R01: Research Project	K01: Mentored Research Scientist Development	T32: Institutional NRSA Training Grants	P20: Exploratory Grants
R03: Small Research Project	K07: Academic Career	F30: Individual MD/PhD Predoctoral Fellowship	P30: Core Center Grants
R13/U13: Conferences and Scientific Meetings	K08: Mentored Clinical Development Scientist	F31: PhD Individual Predoctoral Fellowship	P40: Animal and Biological Resource Grants
R15: Academic Research Enhancement Award (AREA)	K12: Institutional Clinical Scientist Development Program	F32: Postdoctoral Fellowship	P41: Biotechnology Resource Grants
R21: Exploratory/ Developmental Research	K23: Mentored Patient-oriented Research Career Development		P42: Hazardous Substances Basic Research
R41-R44: Small Business Grants (SBIR-STTR)	K25: Mentored Quantitative Research Career Development		P50: Specialized Center
Several others—see NIH website	K00/R00: NIH Pathway to Independence		P60: Comprehensive Center

Based on information from the National Institute on Child Health and Human Development (NICHD)

(outside NIH) programs. The former are located primarily in the facilities of the NIH, and the latter are based in universities and research institutions.

The topic of research training is taken up in a later section of this chapter, especially with regard to funding opportunities.

DISSEMINATION: THE FIRST FRUITS OF RESEARCH

The discovery of new information in any scientific domain is exciting and satisfying to the scientists involved, but unless the knowledge is disseminated, it could well be of little or no real value to the general public. Research is not only discovery but also the accurate and effective dissemination of the new knowledge to other researchers, clinical practitioners, and the public. Dissemination of research information is already changing quickly because of (1) new technologies such as the World Wide Web, (2) an increasingly active role of the media in presenting new results to the public, and (3) the urgent demands by insurers and others for certain kinds of data (e.g., data on the value of clinical interventions). Dissemination is not a simple pipeline between the scientific laboratory and the consumer of research. Rather, dissemination presents its own complex decisions about quality control, reliability, efficiency, and access. The ethical burden on authors of scientific articles is considerable, as considered in the excellent papers by Benos and colleagues (2005) and Claxton (2005a, 2005b).

The editor in chief of the *New England Journal of Medicine* commented that "The capacity to convert information of all kinds (print, audio, video) into a digitized form and to send digitized data out over an expanding number of networks has the potential of completely revolutionizing our definition of a journal" (Kassirer, 1993, p. 178). Today, we witness that continuing revolution as more and more journals move to online publication, sometimes with open access, meaning online access to scientific journal articles without charge to readers or libraries. Although some obstacles remain in the legal and economic domains, it is relatively simple to replace (or partner) print journals with electronic versions made available over the World Wide Web. Today, some journals give subscribers the choice of a traditional hard copy, a compact disc, or a website, and other journals have moved entirely to online publication. In 2009, the Publications Board of the American Speech-Language-Hearing Association (ASHA) announced that the online version of each of ASHA's four scholarly journals is now the official version, or "journal of record."

A positive result of the new technology is that recently acquired knowledge can be accessed quickly by anyone with the technological resources. This includes the lay public. Clinical specialists frequently discover that patients and clients (or their caregivers) have searched the World Wide Web for information on diseases or disabilities. Consequently, consumers may be considerably better informed today than was the case even a decade or so ago. Another advantage of online publication is that it relaxes the problem of journal pages. For budgetary reasons, print-only journals typically fix limits on the number of pages in a given issue of the journal. But online publication readily accommodates lengthy articles that can include elaborate graphs, large data sets, and audio or video recordings.

The media play an important role in announcing new scientific knowledge to the public. Many major discoveries attract the attention of the broadcast and print media almost as soon as they are released to the scientific community. Coverage by the media can be crucial to science because it demonstrates to the public the fast pace of discovery and the potential benefits to society. But at times, the advantages of such public dissemination are offset by inattention to limitations of the research or the need for corroboration of the findings. On occasion, clinical practitioners may feel caught between consumer demands for services (which may be fueled by powerful statements in the public media) and the need for scientific investigation into a type of intervention. The public may fail to understand that acceptance of a new intervention is not necessarily straightforward. Frequently, scientific studies may yield conflicting, or not entirely consistent, results. Some of the ways in which this problem is addressed are meta-analyses (mentioned earlier in connection with clinical trials) and consensus conferences, which convene a group of experts to consider the research on a particular topic (Ferguson, 1993).

Dissemination enables the next step in the research-to-practice sequence, the application of evidence to clinical practice. The ultimate goal of clinical research is to improve clinical assessment and intervention. The vitality of research in a clinical discipline can be gauged by the responsiveness of clinical practice to new discoveries. Obviously, research by itself will not accomplish this goal. It is imperative that the results of research be disseminated to clinicians who have the discernment to use these results to modify clinical practice as indicated. This is not a simple process. It demands a breed of practitioner who is committed to a vigorous kind of professional education. This education can be summarized as follows:

> Eventually, self-directed lifelong learning and the teaching of evidence-based medicine may take hold, so that practitioners learn during their training how to learn for the rest of their professional lives, becoming adept at keeping up with new evidence and applying it to the betterment of their patients' health. (Haynes, 1993, p. 220)

The new evidence can come in several forms, but it is well to recognize that certain types of evidence have a higher degree of acceptability than others.

TECHNOLOGY

Technology and science are not the same thing, although some in the lay public may confuse them. Science, as an enterprise that produces new ideas, typically uses technology, and often produces new technologies, but technologic proficiency alone does not define a science or a scientist. And yet technologic sophistication often is perceived to be an important credential of the scientist, and technologic apparatus may be taken to define the scientific workplace. Technology extends the faculties and senses of the scientist, making possible a degree of accuracy and sensitivity that can be quite remarkable. Unquestionably, technology will have profound effects on research in all disciplines. Technology also may facilitate the transfer of knowledge from the laboratory to the clinic. For example, computer-generated analyses perfected in the laboratory may be transported to the clinic to increase the power and accuracy of clinical observations. Of course, technological transfer demands resources. Clinical personnel must be trained in the use of the technology, and the necessary instruments must be acquired and maintained.

As Nalimov (1981, p. 153) observed, "science creates the ecological situation favorable for itself." That is, science promotes education in the sciences, communication of scientific information, technological and engineering resources, and even the demand for more science. It is difficult to separate science from its resources, especially as the resources, including technology, enable the growth of science and the social impact of its discoveries. Science is not an encapsulated human activity but rather an activity that tends to affect the way we conceptualize the world and the way we work in the world. Sweeping technological advances undoubtedly will affect science. As one example, consider the opportunities that lie in cloud computing.

INTERDISCIPLINARY RESEARCH AND TEAM SCIENCE

Both the complexity of many research problems and the powerful benefits of hybrid expertise favor the continued development of interdisciplinary research. Teams of investigators and technicians are often required in areas such as neuroimaging, prosthetics (mechanical and electrical), genetic studies, surgical monitoring, nanotechnology, tissue engineering, and many others. Collaborations and consortia will be the rule rather than the exception in certain kinds of research, and disciplinary specialists need to learn the skills of interdisciplinary and multidisciplinary communication and project management.

It is almost bromidic to say that the field of communication sciences and disorders draws from many different disciplines. But mere proclamation does not guarantee the desired result. The most sophisticated kind of interdisciplinary or multidisciplinary research requires an aggressive crossing of borders and an enlightened understanding of what each discipline has to offer. The future of science will require scientific personnel to seek interdisciplinary and multidisciplinary projects. Multidisciplinary centers are being formed in several areas and are particularly suited to fields of study in which there are ample data but difficult problems. Ideally, the multidisciplinary center integrates scientists with different specialties to work on a complex problem.

One of the most important divides to be bridged in interdisciplinary or multidisciplinary initiatives is that between behavioral and natural sciences. Poor behavioral choices by individuals can induce, maintain, or exacerbate health problems. Just one behavioral issue—compliance with a clinical specialist's recommendations—is critical to the success of intervention. Behavioral and natural science can be mutually informative, but bringing them together in the desired symbiotic relationship is not as easy as one might hope. Glass and McAtee (2006) recommended three innovations to promote the integration of behavior and natural sciences. The first is an elaboration of the "stream of causation" metaphor along the two axes of time and levels of nested systems of social and biological organization. The second is an inquiry into the proposition that "upstream" features of social context are themselves causes of disease. The third is the concept of a risk regulator to advance the investigation of behavior and health in populations.

In their analysis of team science, Wuchty, Jones, and Uzzi (2007) reviewed 19.9 million research articles over five decades and also examined 2.1 million patents. The data were grouped in three main areas: science and engineering (171 subfields), social sciences (54 subfields), and arts and humanities (27 subfields). The results indicated that teams increasingly dominate in knowledge production, and a strong shift toward collective research was evident in science and engineering, social sciences, and patents. A smaller shift was seen in the arts and humanities. In each area, work by teams dominated the top of the citation distribution. This transition to team science affects the way in which research is conceived and performed, while also redefining the roles of individual scientists.

INTERNATIONAL PERSPECTIVES

Many scientific advances have a value that is not limited by cultural or national boundaries, and a major scientific advance can have the potential for worldwide benefit.

Discovery of a new vaccine, a potent antibiotic, a new source of fuel, or an efficient means of waste management can affect people in every continent and every nation for generations to come. Research in communication sciences and disorders also can bring benefits to the international community, but these benefits are not always as straightforward as in other sciences.

Particularly when a discovery is in some way specific to a given dialect or language, the application to other speech communities or languages cannot be immediately assumed. Nonetheless, it is clear from cross-language studies that important commonalities can exist. But aside from the question of the immediate application of scientific discoveries, there is a fundamental issue concerning international cooperation. The issue is the education of scientists and the development of research facilities on the international stage. The United States is one of the world's leaders in research on communicative disorders, and it is not surprising that students from many other nations have come to the United States to study in the disciplines of speech-language pathology and audiology. Academic programs therefore have the potential for international influence. Thinking about communication and its disorders should become increasingly international in its character, even as the new communication technologies (e.g., machine translation) begin to erase linguistic barriers in their careers.

TRAINING THE NEXT GENERATION OF SCIENTISTS IN CSD

The lifeblood of science in any discipline is the preparation and retention of investigators. The future of science in CSD hinges on the generation of the next generations of scientists. Unlike many, if not most, specialties, CSD has faced, and apparently continues to face, a shortage of trained research personnel. This problem has been recognized for many years and has been addressed by initiatives within ASHA and the Council of Academic Programs in Communication Sciences and Disorders (CAPCSD). In 1997, ASHA and CAPCSD formed a joint committee, the Working Group on Recruitment, Retention, and Academic Preparation of Researchers and Teacher-Scholars. This working group made a number of recommendations, some of which were realized in the development of an ASHA-focused initiative in 2004 and 2005. This initiative, called the *Doctoral (Ph.D.) Shortage,* identified three issues:

Issue 1: There is a critical shortage and continuing attrition of PhD-level faculty in higher education that will affect preparation of professionals as well as the conduct of research in communication sciences and disorders.

Issue 2: Tradition has limited the role of research instruction in all levels of the curriculum, resulting in a lack of coordinated academic culture and scientific/research personnel-preparation experiences in the discipline that promote careers as teachers/researchers in higher education.

Issue 3: There is no coordinated data collection and dissemination system related to doctoral programs that allows for the exchange of information on research training experiences, funding levels, scholarship activities, and those who enter academia upon completing the PhD degree.

A subsequent committee, jointly composed of representatives from ASHA and CAPCSD, prepared a report titled "Crisis in the Discipline: A Plan for Reshaping our Future" (Council of Academic Programs in Communication Sciences and Disorders, 2002).

The challenge of preparing future generations of researchers is formidable, but the attention given to this problem is the first step toward a solution. At least two points are clear: (1) newly graduated PhD students should find excellent professional opportunities in the field, and (2) educational programs must increase their generation of PhD students. With respect to the second point, the need is not only for more PhD graduates but for PhD graduates who are prepared to work in a research and scholarly environment that is increasingly multidisciplinary and international. Revamping graduate programs in the current economic climate is challenging, but realignment and pooling of resources may be one way of enhancing doctoral research education even though resources are basically static. An example of a new approach that specifically targets interdisciplinary collaboration was described by Humphrey, Cote, Walton, Meininger, and Laine (2005). The approach incorporates three major ways for students to learn about the value of interdisciplinary partnerships: (1) study of successful case studies of cooperation, (2) increased mutual interactions, and

(3) experience in interdisciplinary approaches through team-based problem solving (collaborative problem-based learning). As applied to research education in CSD, these ideas would encourage interdisciplinary efforts with other academic units such as psychology, engineering, neuroscience, physics, and biology.

Financial support for research training is available from several sources, with two major sources of support being the NIH (funding opportunities listed in Table 28–1) and the American Speech-Language-Hearing Foundation (ASHF), which offers a variety of educational and mentoring programs (see the ASHF website: http://www.ashfoundation.org/). A listing of various kinds of support also is available at http://www.scangrants.com, which is a public service listing of grants and other funding types to support health research, programs, and scholarship. General advice on research careers is available in Ludlow and Kent (2011).

SUMMARY

The field of communicative disorders and sciences is but one small slice of a gigantic research enterprise. To some degree, the progress of research in any one discipline is affected by the overall vigor of science in its broadest scope. For example, the budgets for major federal funding agencies determine the number of research grants that will be funded in a given fiscal period. Directly or indirectly, budgets can also determine the amount and kind of preparation of new scientists. Different priorities for funding can enrich one area while impoverishing others. It is likely that there will be intense competition among scientific disciplines for financial support of research. Especially because there appears to be a major change in the social contract that underlies science policy, those who are concerned about the state of the science in the discipline should be prepared to take an active role in encouraging scientists and in providing the resources needed for a healthy research environment.

CRITICAL THINKING

1. What is the Bush contract? Why is this contract important to understanding the public policy behind scientific research?
2. For what reasons might the proportion of grant funding for basic versus clinical or translational research on a given topic change over time?
3. Discuss the relationship between science and technology. How do they differ? How do they benefit one another? Think of some examples of the interaction between science and technology from communication sciences and disorders. In these examples, delineate science from technology.
4. What experiences in your undergraduate or graduate education encouraged you to participate in research? Discouraged you? How and why should a practicing clinician participate in research?
5. What can graduate programs do to encourage students to participate in research opportunities during their graduate studies and prepare them for doing research once they become practicing professionals?
6. How does "qualitative research" contribute to the need for evidence-based research? What types of qualitative research can practicing clinicians do in their everyday work?

REFERENCES

Benos, D. J., Fabres, J., Farmer, J., Gutierrez, J. P., Hennessy, K., Kosek, D., et al. (2005). Ethics and scientific publication. *Advances in Physiology Education, 29,* 59–74.

Bush, V. (1945; reprinted 1960). *Science: The endless frontier.* Report to the president on a program for postwar scientific research. Washington, DC: U.S. Government Printing Office.

Charlton, B. G., & Andras, P. (2005). Medical research funding may have over-expanded and may be due for collapse. *QJM, 98,* 53–55.

Claxton, L. D. (2005a). Scientific authorship. Part 1. A window into scientific fraud? *Mutation Research, 589,* 17–30.

Claxton, L. D. (2005b). Scientific authorship. Part 2. History, recurring issues, practices, and guidelines. *Mutation Research, 589,* 31–45.

Council of Academic Programs in Communication Sciences and Disorders. (2002). *Crisis in the discipline: A plan for reshaping our future*. Joint Ad Hoc Committee on the Shortage of PhD Students and Faculty in Communication Sciences and Disorders. Retrieved from http://www.capcsd.org/reports/JointAdHocCmteFinalReport.pdf

Curran, A. S., Effinger, A. W., Pantel, E. S., & Curran, J. P. (1983). Public health: Priorities and policy-setting in the real world. In F. S. Sterret (Ed.), Science and public policy III. *Annals of the New York Academy of Sciences* (Vol. 403). New York, NY: New York Academy of Sciences.

Dregni, E., & Dregni, J. (2006). *Follies of science: 20th century visions of our fantastic future*. Denver, CO: Speck Press.

Federoff, H. J., & Rubin, E. R. (2010). A new research and development policy framework for the biomedical research enterprise. *Journal of the American Medical Association, 304*, 1003–1004.

Feigin, R. A. (2005). Prospects for the future of child health through research. *Journal of the American Medical Association, 294,* 1373–1379.

Ferguson, J. H. (1993). NIH consensus conferences: Dissemination and impact. In K. S. Warren & F. Mosteller (Eds.), Doing more good than harm: The evaluation of health care interventions. *Annals of the New York Academy of Sciences* (Vol. 703, pp. 180–198). New York, NY: New York Academy of Sciences.

Glass, T. A., & McAtee, M. J. (2006). Behavioral science at the crossroads in public health: Extending horizons, envisioning the future. *Social Sciences and Medicine, 62,* 1650–1671.

Gottlieb, S. (1999). U.S. research funding depends on lobbying, not need. *British Medical Journal, 318,* 1715.

Gross, C. P., Anderson, G. F., & Rowe, N. R. (1999). The relation between funding by the National Institutes of Health and the burden of disease. *New England Journal of Medicine, 340,* 1881–1887.

Haynes, R. B. (1993). Some problems in applying evidence in clinical practice. In K. S. Warren & F. Mosteller (Eds.), Doing more good than harm: The evaluation of health care interventions. *Annals of the New York Academy of Sciences* (Vol. 703, pp. 210–225). New York, NY: New York Academy of Sciences.

Humphrey, J. D., Cote, G. L., Walton, J. R., Meininger, G. A., & Laine, G. A. (2005). A new paradigm for graduate research and training in the biomedical sciences and engineering. *Advances in Physiological Education, 29,* 98–102.

Kassirer, J. P. (1993). Dissemination of medical information: A journal's role. In K. S. Warren & F. Mosteller (Eds.), Doing more good than harm: The evaluation of health care interventions. *Annals of the New York Academy of Sciences* (Vol. 703, pp. 173–179). New York, NY: New York Academy of Sciences.

Ludlow, C. L., & Kent, R. D. (2011). *Building a research career*. San Diego, CA: Plural Publishing.

Moses, H., Dorsey, E. R., Matheson, D. H. M., & Their, S. O. (2005). Financial anatomy of biomedical research. *Journal of the American Medical Association, 294,* 1333–1342.

Nalimov, V. V. (1981). *Faces of science.* Philadelphia, PA: ISI Press.

National Institute on Child Health and Human Development (NICHD). Retrieved from http://www.nichd.nih.gov/funding/mechanism/index.cfm

National Institute on Deafness and Other Communication Disorders. (2012). *Strategic Plan: FY 2012–2016.* Retrieved from http://www.nidcd.nih.gov/about/plans/2012-2016/Pages/2012-2016-Strategic-Plan.aspx

Notturno, M. (2008). Nine governance choices pertaining to science. *Medical Hypotheses, 71,* 168–177.

Pielke, R. A., Jr., & Byerly, R., Jr. (1998, February). Beyond basic and applied. *Physics Today,* 42–46.

Price, D. J. D. (1963). *Little science, big science.* New York, NY: Columbia University Press.

Robey, R. R., & Dalebout, S. D. (1998). A tutorial on conducting meta-analyses of clinical outcomes research. *Journal of Speech, Language, and Hearing Research, 40,* 1227–1241.

Russell, B. (1924). *Icarus: Or, the future of science.* Available from http://onlinebooks.library.upenn.edu/webbin/book/lookupid?key=olbp27562

Sigma Xi. (1987). *A new agenda for science.* New Haven, CT: Author.

Singh, J., Illes, J., Lazzeroni, L., & Hallmayer, J. (2009). Trends in U.S. autism research funding. *Journal of Autism and Developmental Disorders, 39*, 788–795.

U.S. House of Representatives Committee on Science. (1998). Unlocking our future: Toward a new national science policy (Document No. Y 4.SCI 2:105B, Item 1025-A-01). Available from http://www.gpo.gov/fdsys/pkg/GPO-CPRT-105hprt105-b/pdf/GPO-CPRT-105hprt105-b.pdf

Wuchty, S., Jones, B. F., & Uzzi, B. (2007). The increasing dominance of teams in production of knowledge. *Science, 316*, 1036–1039.

Zerhouni, E. A. (2005). U.S. biomedical research: Basic, translational, and clinical sciences. *Journal of the American Medical Association, 294*, 1352–1358.

Appendix 28-A

Criteria for Review of Extramural Research Grants Submitted to NIH (updated in 2008)

The goals of NIH-supported research are to advance our understanding of biological systems, to improve the control of disease, and to enhance health. In their written critiques, reviewers will be asked to comment on each of the following criteria in order to judge the likelihood that the proposed research will have a substantial impact on the pursuit of these goals. Each of these criteria will be addressed and considered in assigning the overall score, weighting them as appropriate for each application. Note that an application does not need to be strong in all categories to be judged likely to have major scientific impact and thus deserve a high priority score. For example, an investigator may propose to carry out important work that by its nature is not innovative but is essential to move a field forward.

1. **Significance.** Does this study address an important problem? If the aims of the application are achieved, how will scientific knowledge or clinical practice be advanced? What will be the effect of these studies on the concepts, methods, technologies, treatments, services, or preventative interventions that drive this field?
2. **Approach.** Are the conceptual or clinical framework, design, methods, and analyses adequately developed, well integrated, well reasoned, and appropriate to the aims of the project? Does the applicant acknowledge potential problem areas and consider alternative tactics?
3. **Innovation.** Is the project original and innovative? For example: Does the project challenge existing paradigms or clinical practice; address an innovative hypothesis or critical barrier to progress in the field? Does the project develop or employ novel concepts, approaches, methodologies, tools, or technologies for this area?
4. **Investigators.** Are the investigators appropriately trained and well suited to carry out this work? Is the work proposed appropriate to the experience level of the principal investigator and other researchers? Does the investigative team bring complementary and integrated expertise to the project (if applicable)?
5. **Environment.** Does the scientific environment in which the work will be done contribute to the probability of success? Do the proposed studies benefit from unique features of the scientific environment, or subject populations, or employ useful collaborative arrangements? Is there evidence of institutional support?

SOURCE: National Institute of Health. (2008). NIH announces updated criteria for evaluating research grant applications. Available from http://grants.nih.gov/grants/guide/notice-files/NOT-OD-05-002.html

29

Applying Evidence to Clinical Practice

Karen E. Brown, PhD
Lee Ann C. Golper, PhD

SCOPE OF CHAPTER

Audiologists and speech-language pathologists are increasingly being asked to justify their procedures and methods by evidence-based practices (EBPs). Looking to research evidence and using decision tools that are a part of evidence-based practices can help answer basic clinical questions: Is my diagnosis correct? Is this test needed? What is the expected outcome, or prognosis, with and without treatment? Is this particular intervention likely to improve my client's condition? Could this intervention cause harm? What is the cost-benefit of an assessment or treatment protocol?

Evidence-based practice is based on the premise that the answers to these questions lie with "the integration of the best research evidence with clinical expertise and patient values" (Sackett, Straus, Richardson, & Haynes, 2000, p. 1). These authors define *best research evidence* as coming from clinically relevant research examining the precision and accuracy of diagnostic tests and the efficacy of treatment and its application to everyday practices. That evidence is to be considered in the context of the clinician's own expertise and the client's expressed wishes and values.

In this chapter, we consider some of the terminology, concepts, practices, and methodologies that are a part of evidence-based practices. We look at how we can examine research and draw recommendations from systematic reviews (SRs); how research is ranked, or classified; how the predictive validity of assessment methods and diagnostic tests might be evaluated; and what these analyses mean to clinical practice. The goal of this chapter is to convince you that all clinicians have the tools at hand to evaluate the strength of the evidence available to guide their clinical decisions.

RANKING RESEARCH AND RECOMMENDATIONS

When we talk about the "best" evidence, we are referring to applying specific criteria to determine the credibility of a research study or a group of studies under review. It is important that our diagnostic and treatment decisions be guided by the least biased sources. Systematic reviews and rankings of the evidence are key features of evidence-based practices. There are several different general approaches to ranking evidence. Some provide fine-tuned distinctions and criteria within levels (e.g., the Oxford Centre for Evidence-Based Medicine Levels of Evidence), while others might group different types of studies into a single category if they appear to have equivalent risks for bias. Rating systems for the strength of the recommendations are typically graded in some manner. For example, Grade A recommendations are supported by one or more randomized controlled trials; Grade B recommendations are supported by at least one well-designed retrospective, prospective, or outcome study; Grade C recommendations are supported by case series reports of outcome studies without a control or comparison group; and Grade D recommendations are supported by expert opinion without explicit appraisal (Centre for Evidence-Based Medicine, 1999). Other reviewers apply descriptive systems with recommendations designated as based on experimental (highest ranked), observational, or authoritative (lowest ranked) evidence (Beukelman, 2001).

Evidence-ranking systems are applied in systematic reviews; examples include the approach used by the Quality Standards Subcommittee of the American Academy of Neurology (Miller et al., 1999):

- Class I: Evidence provided by one or more well-designed, randomized controlled trial(s) (RCTs)
- Class II: Evidence provided by one or more well-designed, observational clinical study(ies) with concurrent controls (such as single case-controlled or cohort-controlled studies)
- Class III: Evidence provided by expert opinion, case series, case reports, and studies with historical controls

The Research and Scientific Affairs Committee (RSAC) of the American Speech-Language-Hearing Association (2004) presented an adaptation of a rating scale used in the Scottish Intercollegiate Guideline Network (SIGN), provided in Table 29–1.

Such rankings of evidence and classifications of recommendations allow for a systematic assessment of the strength of the evidence in support of a given approach to treatment or a specific procedure—the higher the ranking, the more credible the evidence. Within these ratings, *meta-analyses* (discussed in detail later in this chapter) that include at least one RCT and/or a systematic review (SR) that includes at least one RCT are viewed as highly credible, while committee recommendations, expert opinions, or other sources not explicitly supported by research (such as in textbooks) are the least credible. That does not imply that less credible sources are bogus, only that the evidence available has not been tested with the level of scrutiny of higher-ranked evidence. When considering the evidence, one goes to the "best available," most highly ranked evidence. When Level I or II evidence is not available to answer a clinical question, we move to the next level of evidence for guidance, appreciating that uncertainty increases as a function of an increased potential for bias (Figure 29–1).

The various methods for rating research quality can create confusion when several rating systems are applied to the same body of evidence. In the future, we may see fewer, more highly standardized evaluation systems. One attempt to develop a common international evaluation guide was undertaken by the Grading of Recommendations, Assessment, Development and Evaluation (GRADE) Working Group (Atkins et al., 2004). The GRADE system is a guide for rating

TABLE 29–1 Levels of Evidence for Studies of Efficacy

Level	Description
	Evidence is ranked according to quality and credibility from highest/most credible to lowest/least credible.
Ia	Well-designed meta-analysis of more than one RCT
Ib	Well-designed randomized control study
IIa	Well-designed controlled study without randomization
IIb	Well-designed quasi-experimental study
III	Well-designed nonexperimental studies (i.e., correlational and case studies)
IV	Expert committee report, consensus conference, clinical experience, or respected authorities

ASHA, 2004, Research and Scientific Affairs Committee. Adapted from the Scottish Intercollegiate Guideline Network, http://www.sign.ac.uk.

"the quality of evidence in systematic reviews and guidelines and grading strength of recommendations in guidelines" (Guyatt et al., 2011, p. 384). This system rates the quality of evidence as high, moderate, low, or very low. RCTs start with the highest rating, and observational studies start with the lowest rating. Points are added or subtracted based on a comprehensive set of quality markers to obtain the final rating. Although this system is relatively new, 57 organizations have endorsed the GRADE system, including the Agency for Healthcare Research and Quality (AHRQ), the Cochrane Collaboration, SIGN, and the World Health Organization (WHO) (GRADE Working Group, 2010; Oxman, 2009). Detailed instructions for using GRADE are available on the GRADE Working Group website, and software—GRADEpro—is available on the Cochrane Collaboration website (Cochrane IMS, n.d.).

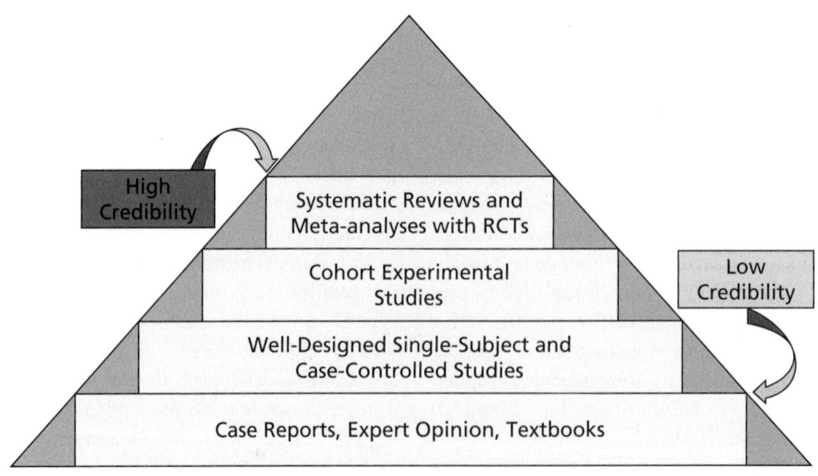

FIGURE 29–1 Ranking Sources of Evidence

Research and Scientific Affairs Committee (RSAC) Report

The ASHA RSAC report (ASHA, 2004) identified five themes to consider when you are looking at evidence rankings and evidence reviews:

1. **Independent confirmation and converging evidence:** Systematic reviews of evidence are encouraged and supported by a number of organizations. The purpose behind these reviews is to look for converging evidence from multiple, credible studies. At times, these systematic reviews reveal conflicting findings in the literature; thus, the reviewers may be more persuaded by the higher-ranked evidence or may advise caution in interpreting the evidence.
2. **Experimental control:** Systematic reviews include a close examination of the controls imposed and design of the study. The RSAC report points out that evidence from quasi-experimental studies ranks lower than that of controlled studies, only because controls and random assignment ought to reduce experimenter bias.
3. **Avoidance of subjectivity and bias:** Any steps taken to reduce subjectivity and bias will increase a study's credibility. For example, the extent to which both the participant and the experimenter are "blinded" to the therapy would enhance the credibility of the results. The extent to which the outcome measurements are taken by someone other than the investigator would also presumably reduce bias. The investigators should explain what happened to any participants who did not complete the study as there should be an "intention to treat" all participants.
4. **Effect size and confidence intervals:** Another prominent theme in EBP is the expectation that studies specify the magnitude of differences and provide data to indicate that there was sufficient statistical power to detect a clinically important effect in the sample (e.g., the *effect size* should be reported). Several standardized metrics are now routinely applied to calculate effect size (Robey, 2004; Wilkinson & APA Task Force on Statistical Inference, 1999). Investigators should also report the *confidence interval* (CI) that is associated with a given effect. Statistical significance does not provide evidence of the strength of an observed association (Riegelman, 2005). The underlying assumption in any statistical sampling is that there is potential for a sampling error—that is, that the findings occurred by chance rather than by design. The CI is the range within which the investigator predicts "with confidence" that a given value is the true value for the trait being studied. The CI is the estimated difference range or variation around the "true" value. A narrow CI provides stronger evidence than a wide CI. For this reason, studies with more subjects are likely to be ranked higher than studies with smaller samples. In EBP, it is common for reviewers to look for a CI of 95 percent (Riegelman, 2005).
5. **Relevance and feasibility:** Finally, the RSAC report suggests EBP looks for the applicability, relevance, and feasibility of the research. Can this treatment or test be applied to the real world?

Meta-analysis

Meta-analysis is a statistical method for combining data from two or more published studies in a manner somewhat similar to conducting multisite studies (Riegelman, 2005). Meta-analysis is usually intended to examine the effect of a given procedure or area of treatment by applying statistical methods to combine the results from a group of studies examining the same or similar questions and hypotheses. Meta-analyses can be performed only when the data in the reference studies have been presented in sufficient detail. Meta-analysis presents a number of limitations and confounding variables. For example, the reference studies may contain bias or methodological flaws; also, since positive findings are more likely to be published than negative findings, the problem of a selection bias is always a consideration with meta-analyses. The analysis itself is not unlike the type of analysis required in any clinical investigation: estimating effect size, testing the statistical significance, adjusting for confounding variables, and looking for homogeneities (Riegelman, 2005; Sackett et al., 2000). Robey's (1998) meta-analysis of the efficacy of aphasia treatment provides an excellent step-by-step illustration of its application to clinical questions.

Although the inclusion of single-subject research (SSR) in meta-analyses for systematic reviews (Robey & Schultz, 1998) has elicited debate among statisticians,

Schlosser (2009) and Schlosser and Sigafoos (2008) provide persuasive arguments in support of including single-subject research in meta-analysis. Methods for conducting meta-analysis of SSR studies and the use of parametric approaches for analysis and nonparametric effect-size estimation have been proposed as having utility with this type of N=1 research (see Shadish, Rindskopf, & Hedges, 2008, for example).

Conducting Systematic Reviews

Several organizations and groups support and conduct ongoing systematic reviews of research evidence across many professional enterprises, including law, medicine, rehabilitation, and education, and information in this area is expanding rapidly. There has been a high degree of interest in evidence reviews in audiology and speech-language pathology to support clinical decisions. For example, in 1997 the Academy of Neurologic Communication Disorders and Sciences (ANCDS) identified the need for a systematic analysis of the research evidence related to neurogenic communication disorders and has an ongoing project aimed at a systematic review across neurogenic communication disorders and treatment procedures (Academy of Neurologic Communication Disorders and Sciences, 2010; Golper et al., 2001).

Reviews such as these require considerable time and effort to complete. The introduction to the ANCDS project provides a model for conducting systematic searches and reviews, which includes forming the review committee, defining the questions, identifying the references, establishing criteria for classifying and ranking the evidence, conducting the searches, preparing the evidence table(s), identifying the strength of the recommendations for procedures or therapies based on the best evidence, and publishing evidence-based practice guidelines in clinical articles (Yorkston et al., 2001).

ASHA's 2004 Focused Initiative aimed to educate its members about EBP and emphasized EBP in research to improve the availability of systematic reviews and research-guided clinical practices (ASHA, 2004). A 2005 survey in *The ASHA Leader* asked members to identify barriers to using EBP principles (Mullen, 2005). The most frequent responses were (1) not enough time to search and analyze research articles and (2) insufficient clear evidence. ASHA's National Center for Evidence-Based Practice in Communication Disorders (N-CEP) was established in 2005 to address these and other member concerns. N-CEP coordinates ASHA's EBP initiative and communicates the findings, information, and positions to its members. Also in 2005, N-CEP launched a series of evidence-based systematic reviews (EBSRs) of relevant, clinical research (Frymark et al., 2009). The first N-CEP EBSR was completed in 2007, and to date, more than 15 EBSRs have been completed on a wide range of research topics such as drug-induced hearing loss, nonspeech oral motor exercises, and behavioral treatment for dysphagia. Nine EBSRs are in progress, and ASHA members are encouraged to nominate additional topics for review (ASHA, 2011).

CONDUCTING PHASED RESEARCH

As Kent states in Chapter 28 of this text, one of the problems with conducting systematic reviews of research evidence is that the pool of published research literature in any given area does not necessarily accumulate in a logical, systematic way, and widespread application of a given therapy can proceed before the efficacy has been examined. An exciting finding may be reported on the evening news immediately after the preliminary results are presented at a professional meeting or released by the public relations service in the investigator's university. Often these are premature findings that have not undergone controlled investigation. These headline-making claims will be followed by a caveat from the principal investigator who, if interviewed, might say something like, "Although the findings are encouraging, further research is required to verify and understand the clinical significance."

Robey and Schultz (1998) help us to frame and conceptualize a logical plan for experimentation, one that progresses from discovery to real-world application. These concepts and terminology were proposed nearly 35 years ago by the Office of Technology Assessment (1978). We include this model in our discussion of EBP for two purposes: (1) when conducting systematic reviews of research evidence, it may be useful to consider where a given investigation fits within the ideal schema for systematic investigation, from discovery to application, and (2) readers will encounter the terms *outcomes, efficacy,* and *effectiveness* used interchangeably in the research literature, when in fact these terms refer to different types and phases of investigation.

Outcomes, Efficacy, and Effectiveness

An *outcome* merely designates an observed consequence, usually an observation made at one point in time compared to an observation made later. An outcome does not index efficacy or effectiveness (Wertz & Irwin, 2001). Clinicians are constantly engaged in collecting "outcomes." If an individual clinician conducts outcome ratings and submits the data in the prescribed manner, outcome data can be pooled, as with the National Outcomes Measurement System (NOMS), an ASHA-sponsored program. This project requires systematic collection of pre- and post-treatment data, including the use of functional rating scale measures, to evaluate treatment outcomes across communication disorders by a number of variables (e.g., service delivery setting, diagnosis type, number of visits).

In individual cases, the clinician's own clinical data and the clients' preferences are key factors in treatment decisions. As empirical evidence, however, the clinician expert opinion based on clinical experience and clinician-gathered treatment data could be viewed as potentially biased. Clinicians sometimes refer to their clinical experience and outcomes data as "practice-based evidence." Case study reports are cited as a form of practice-based evidence, but in a research-ranking schema, such evidence would be ranked lower than outcomes gathered under some amount of experimental control. That is where single-subject research designs can help the clinician. Most SSR designs require measuring and establishing a stable baseline prior to treatment implementation, and the conditions (sequence, timing, methods, and procedures) are controlled and applied systematically in an individual subject.

Another form of practice-based evidence comes from aggregated outcome data increasingly used for a variety of purposes. Outcome data are sometimes gathered to make comparisons between facilities, such as infection rates or morbidity and mortality data comparisons among hospitals. Or outcome data may be examined within a payer type (e.g., Medicare) for benchmarking cost versus benefits of particular procedures, for fiscal adjustment purposes, or to determine whether particular provider groups or facilities have better or worse outcomes than their peers. Since most billing data must be submitted electronically to third-party payers, transparent comparisons of national outcomes can be made from large data pools across various service settings (schools, hospitals, inpatient rehabilitation, nursing homes) and providers.

Collecting and comparing outcome data are problematic. Cornett (1998) points out that outcome measures in health service delivery often are not statistically meaningful, not comparable across institutions, and not adjusted for severity or risk and other key variables. Outcome measures may have no direct link to a provider action, the data may be difficult to collect due to technological constraints and expense, and they are easily manipulated. Nonetheless, treatment outcome information is increasingly important in service delivery, and the clinician's own data may be the best available and only evidence upon which to justify treatment recommendations. Individual outcome data can also be used to examine whether assessment methods, particularly screening assessments, are under- or overselecting individuals with certain conditions, by applying EBP methods for making calculations of sensitivity, specificity, and likelihood ratios, which we discuss later.

To better appreciate the universe of outcome measurement as applied to our discipline, the reader is directed to Frattali (1998); however, the important caution to note here is that an outcome, whether it is derived from observing an individual client or a pool of thousands of clients, does not tell us much about either the efficacy or effectiveness of a given procedure. Let us consider why the Office of Technology Assessment (1978) and Robey and Schultz (1998) advise care in the use of the terms *efficacy* and *effectiveness*:

> *Efficacy*: The probability of benefit to individuals in a defined population from a procedure applied for a given disorder in *ideal* conditions (Office of Technology Assessment, 1978)

> *Effectiveness*: The probability of benefit of a given procedure in the general population of individuals with a given disorder under *average* conditions (Robey & Schultz, 1998)

Ideally, effectiveness studies would be conducted after efficacy has been demonstrated. Unfortunately, the distinctions among outcomes, efficacy, and effectiveness are not always appreciated nor consistently applied in the literature; consequently, claims regarding efficacy are made from studies that lack the required controls, particularly in early literature looking at the efficacy of various treatments in single-subject experiments or small group studies. As Robey and Schultz (1998) observe,

> ... efficacy is a property of a treatment delivered to a population and inference to a population requires a group experiment ... and, as single-subject experiments do not provide inference to a population ... they do not and cannot index efficacy. (p. 805)

In regard to working within a phased research framework, Rogers (2011) captured the challenges facing researchers who investigate the wide variety of topics in the discipline:

> In the discipline of Communication Sciences and Disorders (CSD), intervention research aimed at informing clinical practice has proceeded for nearly a century now without a clear set of expectations about what the necessary, or at least desirable, steps ought to be to develop foundational knowledge that can later support inferences of causality as well as conclusions that can be generalized to the larger population being sampled. (p. 1)

Robey and Schultz (1998) developed a model of five progressive phases of research applicable to treatments for aphasia and other communication disorders. Their model was adapted from a standard medical model for clinical research. A clear understanding of this model provides a solid foundation for evaluating subsequent developments and adaptations of phased clinical research.

Phase I: Discovery In this phase of research, hypotheses are initially developed and refined. A new treatment is introduced and tested with a small number of cases, typically patients who have not been adequately treated by other methods. A hypothesis based on a theory, or perhaps an incidental observation, is tested on a small sample without a control group, to see if the treatment might be fruitful. In this phase of research, the experimenter is asking, "Is this therapy *active*? Does this help?"

Let's look at Botox therapy for an illustrative example: Dolly, Black, Williams, and Melling (1984) published a report in *Nature* on the effect that botulinum neurotoxin has on motor nerve terminals, producing paralysis without loss of sensation. Shortly afterward, clinical applications of this therapy with various dystonias were explored by researchers, and botulinum toxin (Botox) was found to have therapeutic effects for segmental dystonias of the face and neck. It seemed reasonable, therefore, to predict that Botox might have a therapeutic benefit in treating a focal dystonia of the laryngeal musculature in patients with spasmodic dysphonia (SD). Once the drug was approved for clinical investigations in the late 1980s, patients were recruited to determine if a small injection of Botox into the vocal folds could effectively reduce SD without inordinate risk to the patient. Pre- and post-treatment outcome measures were taken and case reports were published (Miller, Woodson, & Jankovic, 1987; Friedman, Grybauskas, Toriumi, & Applebaum, 1987). At that point, randomized controlled trials had not been conducted (efficacy studies), nor had there been any subsequent or large-scale examination of the application in real clinical practice (effectiveness studies).

Clinicians did not know yet what the efficacy or effectiveness of Botox was for SD. We knew only that Botox therapy was "active." That is, it could be demonstrated to be a treatment that resulted in a desired outcome surpassing what might be expected from other therapies, such as behavioral voice therapy and surgery, and the risks and complications were minimal. Studies examining variables to determine ideal candidacy for Botox (e.g., age, gender, duration of the disorder, associated medical problems, smokers versus nonsmokers, abductor versus adductor types of SD, severe versus mild disorders) had not been conducted. Studies of the best injection sites, injection methods, dosages, or the optimal assessment and follow-up protocols did not appear until the mid-1990s (Inagi, Ford, Bless, & Heisey, 1996; Langeveld, Drost, & Baatenburg de Jong, 1998; Meleca, Hogikyan, & Bastian, 1997). A systematic review of research in the use of Botox for SD completed by Duffy and colleagues (2003) showed strong, converging evidence to support the effectiveness of Botox with certain SD candidates, but the development of much of this body of evidence lagged behind the routine use of Botox in clinical practice. This is a common pattern in many medical, surgical, and behavioral therapies.

Since its introduction, Botox has undergone testing in a number of Phase I and Phase II type studies, in addition to clinical trials for several conditions. A variety of therapeutic uses are being studied in National Institutes of Health-sponsored randomized controlled clinical trials with studies ranging from treatment of drooling in amyotrophic lateral sclerosis (ALS) to idiopathic toe walking in children. Information on these types of studies is available online at PubMed, a service sponsored by the National Library of Medicine and the National Institutes of Health (see Resources at the end of this chapter).

Phase II: Refinement of the Methods The investigator continues the experimentation begun in Phase I by refining the methods, establishing the participant selection criteria, determining the variables that need to be controlled, establishing the assessment protocol, and laying out a plan for the conditions required to test the efficacy of the treatment. Phases I and II are preliminary steps needed prior to initiating large group clinical trials.

Phase III: Efficacy Research In this clinical trial phase of research, studies are conducted with rigid experimental controls applied according to the ideal conditions defined in Phase II. In Phase III, the experimenter applies criteria to the subject selection and recruits robust numbers of subjects who are randomly assigned to groups. Ideally, both participants and investigators are blinded to the treatment (i.e., neither the participants nor investigators are aware of who did or did not receive the treatment under investigation). Treatment versus no treatment designs or a comparison of two treatment designs may be also applied, if more appropriate. Note that well-designed randomized controlled studies are rated level Ib in Table 29–1. RCTs are the hallmark of Phase III efficacy studies and thus are often referred to as the "gold standard" index of evidence-based practice.

Robey and Schultz (1998) point out that during this phase, new discoveries may be made and refinement of methods may take place; however, all research activities today must be highly scrutinized and governed by institutional review boards (IRBs). IRB review and approval is required with any change in a research protocol, however tantalizing, to ensure the Health Insurance and Portability and Accountability Act (HIPAA) protections are maintained. All clinical investigators are required to follow strict guidelines enforced by their IRBs regarding the protection of human subjects and information about them, that is, protected health information (PHI) or protected research information (PRI). These guidelines were delineated in the *Belmont Report* from the National Commission for the Protection of Human Subjects of Biomedical and Behavioral Research (1976). This statement addresses basic ethical principles and guidelines to assist researchers in resolving ethical problems that may arise in the conduct of research with human subjects.

Phase IV: Effectiveness Research In this phase, treatment procedures found to be efficacious in Phase III are tested in subpopulations in real-life clinical practice to determine their effectiveness. Effectiveness research tests the therapeutic applications in less-than-ideal, average, and noncontrolled conditions. In this phase, variations in participant compliance, clinician training, and amount (dosage), duration, frequency, and timing of the treatment can be evaluated.

Phase V: Application Research The final step in the analysis involves exploration of the efficiency and relevance of treatment by considering client satisfaction, cost-effectiveness of the treatment, cost utility (quality of life outcome), and the cost-benefit ratio.

Levels of Evidence for Communication Sciences and Disorders

In her discussion of the myths and realities of evidence-based practices, Dollaghan (2004) reminds us:

> The EBP orientation disavows the longstanding belief that all basic science findings are relevant to clinical practice. The goals, designs, and methods of studies aimed at providing strong answers to questions about clinical practice are in some respects quite different from those of studies aimed at understanding basic mechanisms of disease. In the EBP framework, evidence from studies of basic mechanisms plays a similar role to evidence derived from personal experience or the opinions of authorities; all of those sources can provide fruitful "leads," but these must be followed up in subsequent studies explicitly designed to address questions about clinical practice. (p. 4)

ASHA and other organizations, most notably the National Institutes of Health (NIH), recognize the need for translational research, that is, research aimed at "translating" discoveries at the basic science level into clinical techniques (Justice, 2010; "Translational Research," 2011). Due to the typical one-on-one therapeutic approach for the remediation of communication disorders, a significant portion of the treatment research in our field is conducted in single-subject design case studies and case series studies. Few of the medical-based systems for grading levels of evidence recognize the contributions of well-designed and well-conducted single-subject studies. While such studies will not be given the same weight as RCTs, neither should they be summarily excluded from the evaluation of research evidence for communication disorders (Mullen, 2007).

With the five-phase model of clinical research as the starting point, ASHA's N-CEP and the Advisory Committee on Evidence-Based Practice (ACEBP) developed a levels of evidence (LOE) evaluation system specific to communication sciences and disorders.

ASHA's LOE system is a four-step process that involves assessing the extent to which a study meets quality indicators, deciding the stage of research to which a study applies, "scoring" the quality of the study in the context of the stage of research, and finally, synthesizing this information for all studies to give an overall picture of the level of evidence available on a particular clinical issue (Mullen, 2007).

The system includes a decision tree (see Figure 29–2) to determine which stage (or phase) of research is represented by individual studies. Exploratory studies encompass the *discovery* and *refinement* phases of the five-phase model discussed above. Efficacy studies, consistent with Phase III, are carefully designed RCTs conducted under ideal conditions. Effectiveness studies test the intervention in average or typical clinical settings. Cost-benefit or public policy research investigates the value of the intervention relative to economic or environmental factors (Mullen, 2007). Currently, the ASHA LOE system is being used to produce evidence-based systematic reviews of treatments for communication disorders.

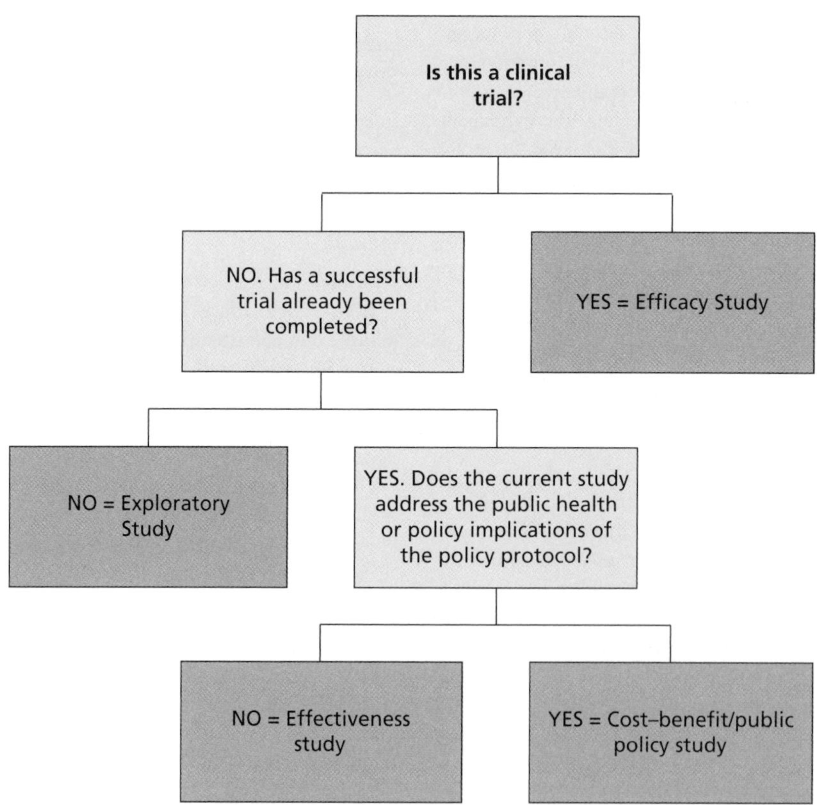

FIGURE 29–2 ASHA LOE System: Stages of Research

From "The State of Evidence: ASHA Develops Levels of Evidence for Communication Sciences and Disorders," by B. Mullen, 2007, *The ASHA Leader*. Adapted with permission.

ASHA's Compendium of Clinical Practice Guidelines and Systematic Reviews

Does the prospect of finding, reading, and systematically evaluating all the relevant research literature for any given treatment seem like an overwhelming task? Fortunately, the N-CEP evidence-based systematic reviews are available on the ASHA website. N-CEP actively promotes EBP by making EBSRs and other EBP materials readily available and easy to access. A wealth of information is available on the N-*CEP* Compendium of Evidence-Based Systematic Reviews and Clinical Guidelines. In addition to N-CEP EBSRs, the compendium provides links to EBSRs and clinical guidelines from around the world. The compendium is updated monthly as new systematic reviews and clinical guidelines become available. Each clinical guideline is evaluated using the Appraisal of Guidelines for Research and Evaluation (AGREE) framework, and only those that are rated "highly recommended" or "recommended with provisos" are included in the compendium (Mullen, n.d.).

As noted at the beginning of this chapter, EBP is not based on research evidence alone but on "the integration of the best research evidence with clinical expertise and patient values" (Sackett et al., 2000, p. 1). In 2010, N-CEP launched ASHA's evidence maps to "provide clinicians, researchers, clients, and caregivers with tools and guidance to engage in evidence-based decision making" (ASHA, 2010). Evidence maps are organized by topic (disorder). They provide links to information about research evidence in the compendium as well as links to resources for incorporating client values in clinical practice and links to resources for developing clinical expertise. ASHA currently has evidence maps available for the following:

- Amyotrophic Lateral Sclerosis
- Aphasia
- Autism Spectrum Disorders
- Cerebral Palsy
- Cleft Lip & Palate
- Dementia
- Head & Neck Cancer
- Parkinson's Disease
- Pediatric Dysphagia
- Traumatic Brain Injury (Adults)
- Traumatic Brain Injury (Children)

ASHA's evidence maps give clinicians a clear picture of the resources they need to be evidence-based practitioners.

EVALUATING DIAGNOSTIC AND SCREENING PROCEDURES

Clinicians use a variety of tests to help make assessment and management decisions for their clients. Testing can be time consuming and expensive, and it is important to conduct the appropriate amount of testing necessary to arrive at an accurate diagnosis. Most diagnostic tests that are quick and easy to administer (checklists, screening tests) may or may not be completely accurate. They are typically used to determine whether further evaluation with a more sophisticated instrument is needed. Since additional testing can be costly and difficult to access, clinicians should know how much confidence to place in the results of a preliminary or screening test. In some cases, it may not be possible to conduct further testing or to refer the client for more comprehensive assessment, which makes it all the more important for clinicians to understand the strengths and weaknesses of the tests they administer.

Sensitivity and Specificity

The practice of using the results of one test to determine the need for further evaluation with another test, or a battery of tests, is common in the field of medicine, where there is great concern about the costs of ordering multiple expensive procedures and tests of dubious or redundant diagnostic value. For example, a person with a family history of diabetes and positive test results on a blood glucose screening is likely to be referred for a glucose tolerance test and careful evaluation of clinical symptoms to rule in or rule out diabetes (Pagana & Pagana, 2002). In the practice of speech-language pathology and audiology, many times the results of a screening test prompt the clinician to pursue further testing. A school-age child's poor performance on a hearing screening may result in a referral to an audiologist for a comprehensive hearing evaluation. A bedside screening for dysphagia that suggests the presence of aspiration may be followed by a modified barium swallow study to confirm or rule out aspiration. A child who performs poorly on an articulation screening test may be scheduled for comprehensive speech and language testing to determine whether the child will qualify for school-based speech-language pathology services. In such cases, clinicians must interpret the results of the screening test and decide whether the evidence supports the need for further testing to ensure an accurate diagnosis.

Decisions based on test results should take into account the statistical probability that the results are wrong. Clinicians need to know how likely it is that a test will fail to identify an individual with a specific disorder or, conversely, that the test will incorrectly indicate that an individual has the disorder when, in fact, it is not present. Determining the *sensitivity* and *specificity* of a diagnostic finding is one of the tools available in EBP to evaluate the diagnostic accuracy of a test, what Riegelman (2005) referred to as "testing a test" (p. 137). Using fairly simple 2 × 2 table calculations, sensitivity measures how well a test identifies individuals who have the target disorder, and specificity measures how well a test identifies individuals who do not have the target disorder. Both provide uniquely important information, and both are reported as the percentage of correct results.

To evaluate the specificity and sensitivity of a particular measure, we usually need to index an established measure or "gold standard" test for comparison. A gold standard is a test, or some other measurement, that is consistently close to 100 percent accurate for diagnosing the target condition. This standard is the reference for determining the accuracy of screening test results. To calculate sensitivity and specificity, a screening test is given to a group of individuals, and the same individuals are given the gold standard, or reference, test. The results of the screening test are then compared to the results of the gold standard test. Sensitivity is the percentage of positive screening test results that correctly identify individuals who have the target condition, as verified by the reference test. Specificity is the percentage of negative screening test results that correctly identify individuals who do not have the target condition, as verified by the reference test. Figure 29–3 shows the calculations for sensitivity and specificity.

The results of the screening test and the reference test are entered into a 2 × 2 contingency table (see Figure 29–4). Test results that are positive for both the screening test and the reference test are referred to as *true positive* results. The number of true positive results is entered into quadrant *a* on the table. When the screening test result is negative for a disorder that was positively identified by the gold standard test, the screening test result is known as a *false negative* result. The number of false negative results is entered into quadrant *c* on the table. Test results that are negative for both the screening test and the reference test are known as *true negative* results, and that number is entered into quadrant *d*. Finally, if the target condition is absent, as confirmed by the gold standard test, but the screening test results are positive, the results are referred to as *false positives*. The number of false positives is entered into quadrant *b*.

Sensitivity = The percentage of true positives: (number of True Positives)/(number of True Positives + number of False Negatives), or the proportion of affected individuals caught by screening

Specificity = The percentage of true negatives: (number of True Negatives)/(number of True Negatives + number of False Positives), or the proportion of unaffected individuals who pass screening

FIGURE 29–3 Calculating Specificity and Sensitivity

The formula for sensitivity is $a \div (a + c)$. A screening test with high sensitivity produces a large percentage of true positives. The formula for specificity is $d \div (b + d)$. A screening test with high specificity produces a large percentage of true negatives.

For example, consider a group of 183 children who are given a screening test to detect developmental language delay. If 95 of the children actually have developmental language delays, and 80 of those children are correctly identified with positive screening test results (true positives), the sensitivity of the test would be $80 \div (80 + 15)$, or 84 percent. If the remaining 88 children have typically developing language skills, and 81 of those children are correctly identified with negative test results (true negatives), the specificity of the test would be $81 \div (7 + 81)$, or 92 percent. The 2 × 2 table and calculations for this example are shown in Figure 29–4.

Describing how well a test performs in terms of its sensitivity alone or specificity alone is problematic. Sensitivity alone does not provide information for distinguishing between true positive results and false positive results. Sensitivity would be 100 percent for

		Gold standard test for language delay	
		Language delay: Present	Language delay: Absent
Screening test for language delay	Positive screening test results	80 True Positives *a*	*b* 7 False Positives
	Negative screening test results	15 False Negatives *c*	*d* 81 True Negatives
	Totals	*a* + *c* 95	*b* + *d* 88

Sensitivity = $a/(a+c)$ = 80/95 = .84 (84%)
Specificity = $d/(b+d)$ = 81/88 = .92 (92%)

FIGURE 29–4 2 × 2 Contingency Table for Calculating Sensitivity and Specificity of a Hypothetical Screening Test for Developmental Language Delay

a test that simply identified every person who took it as having the target condition. Obviously, such a test would produce many false positive results. A clinician reviewing test results could not state with confidence that positive results were true positives.

Likewise, specificity alone does not provide information for distinguishing between true negative results and false negatives results. A test would achieve 100 percent specificity by identifying every person who took it as being free of the target condition. Such a test would misidentify (with false negative results) all individuals who had the disorder. Such a test would be useless for helping a clinician distinguish between individuals who did and did not have the target condition.

Reports of sensitivity and specificity, when considered in isolation, can be misleading. Both must be known for a clinician to determine how much confidence to place in the results of a screening test. Sensitivity, in particular, can overrepresent the value of a test. For example, consider a hearing screening test for which the sensitivity is 95 percent. This means the test correctly identified 95 percent of the test takers who actually had significant hearing loss. Without knowing the specificity of the test, 95 percent sensitivity sounds pretty good. Now consider what happens if the specificity for that test is only 25 percent. Look at quadrants *a* and *b* in Figure 29–5. Imagine that 200 individuals (100 with significant hearing loss and 100 with normal hearing) were given the test, and the test produced 75 false positive results. A total of 170 individuals had positive screening test results, and 44 percent of those positive results were wrong. A clinician would have very little confidence that a positive result on that test was a true positive rather than a false positive.

The same type of example can be used to demonstrate the problems that would arise from a similar screening test that had excellent specificity and poor sensitivity. Figure 29–6 shows the results of a screening procedure that had 98 percent specificity and 30 percent sensitivity. The test correctly ruled out hearing loss in all but two of the individuals who had normal hearing; however, the 70 false negative results show that this test failed to identify hearing loss in most of the individuals who actually had significant hearing loss.

The closer sensitivity and specificity are to 100 percent, the more predictive information they provide about the presence or absence of the target disorder. Sackett and colleagues (2000) state that high sensitivity is most useful for ruling out the disorder in individuals with negative test results, and they suggest applying the mnemonic *SnNout* (**Sen**sitivity high, **N**egative result - rule **out**) to such findings. They also propose that high specificity is

		Gold standard test results	
		Disorder Present	Disorder Absent
Screening test results	Positive	95 True Positives *a*	*b* 75 False Positives
	Negative	*c* 5 False Negatives	*d* 25 True Negatives
	Totals	$a + c = 100$	$b + d = 100$

Sensitivity = $a/(a+c)$ = 95/100 = .95 (95%)
Specificity = $d/(b+d)$ = 25/100 = .25 (25%)

FIGURE 29-5 Example of a Hearing Screening Procedure with Excellent Sensitivity and Poor Specificity

most useful for ruling in the disorder in individuals with positive test results. They suggest that *SpPin* (**Sp**ecificity high, **P**ositive result - rule **in**) is an appropriate mnemonic for these findings. This is the opposite of how many clinicians tend to think about sensitivity and specificity.

To understand how to use SnNout and SpPin, look again at Figure 29–5. The high sensitivity of this test, 95 percent, is of limited use because it would not help a clinician distinguish between true positive and false positive test results. But notice that the negative screening test results are primarily true negatives. Since most of the individuals who had the disorder (as verified by the gold standard test) produced true positive screening test results, there were very few false negative results. Although positive screening test results would not be diagnostically meaningful, a clinician could feel confident that an individual with a negative screening test result probably did not have the disorder. When sensitivity is high and the test result is negative, the condition may be ruled out (SnNout).

Figure 29–6 illustrates how SpPin is applied. The high specificity of this test (98 percent) indicates that

		Gold standard test results	
		Disorder Present	Disorder Absent
Screening test results	Positive	30 True Positives *a*	*b* 2 False Positives
	Negative	*c* 70 False Negatives	*d* 98 True Negatives
	Totals	$a + c = 100$	$b + d = 100$

Sensitivity = $a/(a+c)$ = 30/100 = .30 (30%)
Specificity = $d/(b+d)$ = 98/100 = .98 (98%)

FIGURE 29-6 Example of a Hearing Screening Test with Excellent Specificity and Poor Sensitivity

most individuals who did not have the disorder had negative screening test results. Of the 100 individuals who were free of the disorder, only two had positive screening results. Therefore, a clinician whose client had a positive result on this screening test could feel confident that additional testing or management strategies were appropriate for that individual. When specificity is high and the test result is positive, the condition may be ruled in (SpPin).

When test makers create a screening test for a specific disorder, they must consider the consequences of erroneous results. Tests with high sensitivity and low specificity err on the side of overidentifying the disorder. This may result in referrals for unneeded additional testing or unneeded treatment. On the other hand, tests with low sensitivity and high specificity err on the side of missing the condition, but correctly rule out most individuals who are disorder free. This could mean that some individuals who would benefit from further evaluation and treatment are missed. A decision to use a test that tends to overidentify or underidentify a disorder must balance the risks of failing to detect the condition relative to the risks of subjecting individuals to unneeded testing and treatment.

In choosing a test, the clinician must consider the consequences of failing to identify the condition as well as the consequences of misdiagnosing a condition that is not present. Where possible outcomes are serious, the clinician may choose to be overly cautious. A clinician working in an acute care setting may choose a bedside screening test for dysphagia that has high sensitivity, but low specificity, for the presence of aspiration. Referrals for instrumental swallowing evaluations, such as the modified barium swallow study (MBS) or fiberoptic endoscopic evaluation of swallowing (FEES), can be expensive and require specialized equipment. Nevertheless, the risks and cost-benefit ratio associated with misidentifying an aspirator as a nonaspirator usually outweigh the risks associated with performing an instrumental evaluation on a person who does not aspirate. On the other hand, a school-based clinician who wants an articulation screener for preschool children may choose a test with greater specificity than sensitivity. Missing the chance to provide early intervention for a child with speech deficits is not desirable, but neither is it life threatening. In addition, overidentifying articulation problems at the preschool level can produce problems related to caseload levels and availability of resources.

Likelihood Ratios

Sensitivity and specificity are the most basic and the most frequently reported test evaluation statistics, but they have some inherent limitations that can be addressed with other statistics. The 2 × 2 contingency table is used to calculate a number of other statistics that are useful for test evaluations, including *likelihood ratios* and *predictive values*. These metrics take into consideration the demonstrated accuracy of the screening instrument and the prevalence of the target condition within a particular population. Sackett and colleagues (2000) refer to the "old-fashioned concepts of sensitivity and specificity and the new-fangled and more powerful ideas around likelihood ratios" (p. 72). They suggest that clinicians become familiar with the more advanced assessment tools. An excellent discussion of the expanded roles of sensitivity and specificity to aid in clinical decision making is presented in Riegelman's *Studying a Study and Testing a Test* (2005).

Calculating Likelihood Ratios

Likelihood ratios (LRs) are easy to calculate if the test manual reports sensitivity and specificity (see Figure 29–7). Likelihood ratios for positive tests (LR+) compare the proportion of true positive screening test results to the proportion of false positive screening test results. As discussed previously, one problem with sensitivity is that it does not provide any information about the relationship between true positive results and false positive results. For the example shown in Figure 29–4, the proportion of true positive results (sensitivity) is 84 percent. The proportion of false positive results is 8 percent. The calculation is 100% − specificity = 100% − 92% = 8%. (Alternatively, you could simply calculate the

Likelihood Ratio (LR) for a Positive Test =

$$\frac{\text{Probability of a true positive (sensitivity)}}{\text{Probability of a false positive (100\% − specificity)}}$$

Likelihood Ratio (LR) for a False Test =

$$\frac{\text{Probability of a false negative (100\% − sensitivity)}}{\text{Probability of a true negative (specificity)}}$$

FIGURE 29-7 Calculating Likelihood Ratios

percentage in quadrant *b*.) The formula for the likelihood ratio for positive tests is *sensitivity / (100% − specificity)*. A simpler way to express that equation is the percentage of true positive results divided by the percentage of false positive results: 84% / 8% = 10.5. This means that a positive test result is 10.5 times more likely to have been produced by a person with the target condition than a person who is free of the target condition. The greater the LR+, the higher the likelihood that a positive test result is a true positive.

Likelihood ratios for negative tests (LR−) compare the proportion of false negative screening test results to the proportion of true negative results. This statistic shows how likely it is that a negative test result is a *false* negative. In other words, how likely is it that a negative test result is wrong and that the individual being examined actually has the target condition? The lower the LR−, the better. A low LR− means there is little chance that a negative test result was produced by a person who has the target condition. For the example in Figure 29–4, the proportion of false negative results is 16 percent. The calculation is: 100% − sensitivity = 100% − 84% = 16%. (As noted previously, you could simply calculate the percentage in quadrant *c*.) The proportion of true negative results (specificity) is 92 percent. The formula for the likelihood ratio for negative tests is (*100% − sensitivity) / specificity*, or the proportion of false negative results divided by the proportion of true negative results: 16% / 92% = 0.174. Therefore, a negative test result is much less likely to have been produced by a person with the target condition than to have been produced by a person without the condition. Since equal likelihood is represented by a LR of 1.0, a LR− of 0.174 indicates that there is little likelihood that a negative screening test result would be wrong.

How can an understanding of sensitivity, specificity, and likelihood ratios help clinicians make the best use of a screening test? Here is an example. Suppose a new screening test has been developed for the early detection of children with specific language disability. A clinician administers the screening test to a child, and the result is positive. Based on the positive result, should the clinician rule in the diagnosis of specific language disability and conclude that the child is a candidate for a diagnostic evaluation and/or intervention? The test manual reports that during the development phase, it was administered to 1,120 children. The resulting sensitivity was moderate, 60 percent, and specificity was high, 93 percent. The results are shown in Figure 29–8. The clinician sees that the test

		Gold standard test for autism	
		Autism Present	Autism Absent
Screening test for early detection of autism	Positive	263 (60%) True Positives *a*	*b* 51 (7%) False Positives
	Negative	173 (40%) *c* False Negatives	*d* 633 (93%) True Negatives
	Totals	*a* + *c* = 436	*b* + *d* = 684

N = 436 + 684 = 1120

Sensitivity 263/436 = 60% false positives = 51/684 = 7%
Specificity 633/684 = 93% false negatives =173/436 = 40%

LR + = 60/7 = 8.6
LR − = 40/93 = .43

FIGURE 29-8 Hypothetical Screening Test for Early Detection of Autism

failed to identify 40 percent of children with specific language disability, but it correctly ruled out specific language disability in almost all children who did not have the condition. The SpPin mnemonic can be applied here to rule in specific language disability because specificity is high. The test produced relatively few false positive results. Therefore, it would be reasonable to think that the positive result for the child who was just tested is probably a true positive.

When discussing the result of the test with the parents, or making a referral for further evaluation, the clinician would like to have a more precise way of describing the child's performance. This is where the likelihood ratio can help. How *likely* is it that the positive result is correct? The likelihood ratio for a positive test result is 8.6 (60% / 7% = 8.6). The clinician can say that the positive result indicates the child is about eight and a half times more likely to have specific language disability than he or she would be if the test result was negative.

What if the same test was administered to a child and the result was negative? The clinician would know that during test development, 40 percent of the children with specific language disability had false negative test results. The clinician would wonder if the negative test result for the child just tested was a false negative. Comparing the proportion of false negatives to the proportion of true negatives shows that the likelihood ratio for a negative test is an unimpressive 0.43 (40% / 93% = 0.43). Remember that equal likelihood is a likelihood ratio of 1.0. It appears unlikely that the screening test result is wrong, but is that enough information to rule out specific language disability? This is where clinical judgment plays a critical role. The screening test alone is not strong enough to engender confidence that a negative test result is accurate. This is a situation in which the long-term effects of failure to identify the condition are usually worse than subjecting a child who is free of the condition to more extensive testing. Clinical expertise, based on the clinician's experience and critical evaluation of the child's performance, medical history, and other pertinent factors, must be employed to determine whether further assessment is needed.

Predictive Values Predictive value (PV) is another statistic that can be calculated from the 2 × 2 contingency table. PVs reflect the ability of a screening test to predict the presence or absence of a disorder. The predictive value for a positive finding, or positive predictive value (PPV), refers to the proportion of individuals who actually have a disorder after producing positive screening test results for the disorder. The formula for PPV is *True Positive* / (*True Positive* + *False Positive*), or, as applied to our 2 × 2 table, $a / (a + b)$. Conversely, the predictive value for a negative finding, or negative predictive value (NPV), refers to the proportion of individuals who do not have the disorder after testing negative for that disorder on the screening test. The formula for NPV is *True Negative* / (*True Negative* + *False Negative*), or, as applied to our 2 × 2 table, $d / (c + d)$.

To be meaningful, PVs require an additional element. Accurate pretest probability must be reflected in the 2 × 2 table. Riegelman (2005) explains that pretest probability for a condition has a tremendous impact on predictive value—that is, the predictive value of a screening test will be dramatically different for groups that have different probabilities for the target condition. Some tests may have high PV when used to screen populations with high probability for a given disorder, but the same screening instrument may not be nearly as accurate in the general, healthy population where the incidence of the disorder is low. An example is screening for hearing loss. Positive results on hearing screenings are more reliable (more likely to identify individuals with significant hearing loss) when they occur in the population of individuals over the age of 65 than when they occur in the population of younger people. In other words, positive results for hearing loss are more likely to be true positive within the older population, and the younger population will produce proportionately more false positives.

Predictive values for communication disorders screening tests are sometimes reported in the literature. In general, they tend to be less useful tools for the clinician than other metrics because they "should only be calculated from cohort studies or studies that legitimately reflect the number of people in the population who have the condition of interest at that time" (Family Practice Notebook, n.d.). To calculate accurate PVs, the 2 × 2 contingency table must accurately reflect the prevalence of the condition for the population of interest. Care must be exercised when applying PVs to screening tests for communication disorders if the prevalence of the target condition is not known or not reliable. The interested reader is directed to Riegelman (2005) for an excellent discussion of positive and negative predictive values.

SUMMARY

Clinicians are expected to demonstrate the efficacy and effectiveness of their treatment methods. Access to systematic reviews across several topics is as easy as visiting the ASHA website. Dollaghan (2004) described these searches as good "high yield" sources for busy clinicians. Unfortunately, these reviews make it apparent that, as in other areas of health service delivery, audiologists and speech-language pathologists do not yet have a deep pool of Level I or Level II research evidence to guide them in every clinical decision. Thus, clinicians must look to the best available evidence, which frequently will be Phase I or Phase II types of studies, or Level III studies, such as case reports and/or consensus or expert opinions. Those sorts of evidence are not as highly ranked as investigations using random assignment to group or other controls (RCTs), so recommendations to guide clinical decisions are made with caution. Randomized controlled trials are referenced as the "gold standard" for evidence; however, such studies are not explicitly designed to answer real-world clinical questions in audiology and speech-language pathology, and it is difficult to construct RCTs with a complete "blinding" of patients and clinicians (Dollaghan, 2004). The ongoing project of ASHA's N-CEP to systematically review and rate current research evidence and practice guidelines puts vital research information within reach of all clinicians. The reports in the Compendium of EBP Guidelines and Systematic Reviews allow clinicians to quickly identify consensus opinion about the state of the research for many clinical conditions. The compendium does not make the need to read and evaluate research articles obsolete, but it is a valuable, time-saving resource for busy clinicians. It is the responsibility of clinicians to make informed decisions that take into account the best evidence available coupled with their own clinical expertise and the unique treatment conditions and attributes of an individual client.

CRITICAL THINKING

1. Under the current Medicare regulations for skilled nursing facilities and rehabilitation facilities, the costs of off-site diagnostic studies (hearing tests, modified barium swallow studies, and so on) for clients receiving care in the facilities are borne by the facility. Consequently, the medical director in an inpatient rehabilitation facility has decided to reduce orders for outpatient evaluations, including modified barium swallow studies that require transportation and costly evaluation in another facility. The medical director has recommended implementing an in-house bedside dysphagia screening program as first-line assessment to guide feeding and swallowing management with residents who have trouble swallowing. The medical director has announced a goal of reducing the number of orders for outside radiologic studies by 50 percent and has asked you, the SLP member of the care team, to design a "best practices" protocol for the new bedside dysphagia screening program. How might you use EBP tools and methodologies to help determine the best practices for appropriately diagnosing and evaluating dysphagia? Are there any studies or evidence-based guidelines currently available related to evaluation or management of dysphagia that might be brought into the discussion? Apply what you know about determining specificity and sensitivity of a screening test to determine best practices. How can the research evidence and your own clinical records guide you in assessing the cost-benefit factor of misdiagnosing the type and severity of dysphagia?
2. What does the current evidence tell us about the usefulness of newborn hearing screening? How can we evaluate the reliability of that evidence?
3. What are some of the issues or difficulties faced when designing a randomized, double-blind controlled study in audiology and speech-language pathology? Can you think of ways to circumvent those difficulties?
4. Based on the evidence at hand, do we know if *not treating* a person with aphasia is harmful?

5. What are the implications of identifying a child as having a mild hearing loss? Conversely, what are the implications of *not* identifying a child as having a mild hearing loss?
6. Locate a current journal in communication sciences and disorders, and select and review a research article. Describe the following: type of study (single-subject research design, case report, treatment/no treatment design, comparison of treatments design, other); number of participants; variables controlled (e.g., age, gender, handedness, health status, medications); and random or nonrandom assignment to groups. Where might this study fit in the Robey and Schultz (1998) phases of research? Is this an efficacy or effectiveness study? Was the effect size reported? Can you rank the evidence in the article using the rankings provided in Table 29–1?
7. Your department is committed to using evidence-based practice in providing clinical services. You are chair of a small committee to gather this information for several clinical areas including aphasia, traumatic brain injury, child language disorders, and fluency. Where can you find information about evidence-based practice in these areas? What type of resource do you think would be useful for the practicing clinicians?

REFERENCES

Academy of Neurologic Communication Disorders and Sciences. (2010). *ANCDS strategic plan: Goals, objectives, plans, and outcome metrics 2009–2014.* Retrieved from http://www.ancds.org/pdf/ANCDS_Strategic_Plan_Final.pdf

American Speech-Language-Hearing Association. (2004). *Evidence-based practice in communication disorders: An introduction.* Retrieved from http://www.asha.org/docs/html/TR2004-00001.html

American Speech-Language-Hearing Association. (2010). *Welcome to ASHA's evidence maps.* Retrieved from http://www.ncepmaps.org/

American Speech-Language-Hearing Association. (2011). *ASHA/N-CEP evidence-based systematic reviews.* Retrieved from http://www.asha.org/members/ebp/EBSRs.htm

Atkins, D., Eccles, M., Flottorp, S., Guyatt, G. H., Henry, D., Hill, S. L., et al. (2004). Systems for grading the quality of evidence and the strength of recommendations I: Critical appraisal of existing approaches. The GRADE Working Group. *BMC Health Services Research, 4,* 38–45.

Beukelman, D. (2001). *State of the science report, 2001.* Rehabilitation Research Center in Communication Enhancement. Durham, NC: Duke University.

Centre for Evidence-Based Medicine. (1999). *Levels of evidence and grades of recommendation.* Retrieved from http://www.cebm.net/index.aspx?o=1025

Cochrane IMS. (n.d.). *GRADEpro.* Retrieved from http://ims.cochrane.org/gradepro

Cornett, B. S. (1998). Outcomes measure in health care settings. In C. Frattali (Ed.), *Measuring outcomes in speech-language pathology* (pp. 453–476). New York, NY: Thieme.

Dollaghan, C. (2004, April 13). Evidence-based practice: Myths and realities. *The ASHA Leader, 12,* 4–5.

Dolly, J. O., Black, J., Williams, R. S., & Melling, J. (1984). Acceptors for botulinum neurotoxin reside on motor nerve terminals and mediate its internalization. *Nature, 307,* 457–460.

Duffy, J. R., Yorkston, K. M., Beukelman, D., Golper, L. A., Miller, R., Spencer, K., et al. (2003). *Medical interventions for spasmodic dysphonia and some related conditions: A systematic review* (ANCDS Technical Report No. 2). Available from http://ancds.org/

Family Practice Notebook. (n.d.). *Positive predictive value of diagnostic tests.* Retrieved from http://www.fpnotebook.com/prevent/epi/PstvPrdctvVl.htm

Frattali, C. M. (Ed.). (1998). *Measuring outcomes in speech-language pathology.* New York, NY: Thieme.

Friedman, M., Grybauskas, V., Toriumi, D. M., & Applebaum, E. L. (1987). Treatment of spastic dysphonia without nerve section. *Annals of Otology, Rhinology & Laryngology, 96,* 590–596.

Golper, L. A., Wertz, R. T., Frattali, C. M., Yorkston, K., Myers, P., Katz, R., Beeson, P., et al. (2001). *Evidence-based practice guidelines for the management of communication disorders in neurologically impaired individuals: An introduction*. Available from http://www.ancds.org

GRADE Working Group. (2010). *Grading the quality of evidence and the strength of recommendations*. Available from http://www.gradeworkinggroup.org

Guyatt, G., Oxman, A. D., Akl, E. A., Kunz, R., Vist, G., Brozek, J., Norris, S., et al. (2011). GRADE guidelines: 1. Introduction—GRADE evidence profiles and summary of findings tables. *Journal of Clinical Epidemiology, 64*(4), 383–394.

Inagi, K., Ford, C. N., Bless, D. M., & Heisey, D. (1996). Analysis of features affecting botulinum toxin results in spasmodic dysphonia. *Journal of Voice, 10,* 306–313.

Justice, L. (2010). Truly translational research. *American Journal of Speech-Language Pathology, 19,* 95–96.

Langeveld, T. P. M., Drost, H. A., & Baatenburg de Jong, R. J. (1998). Unilateral versus bilateral botulinum toxin injections in adductor spasmodic dysphonia. *Annals of Otology, Rhinology & Laryngology, 107,* 280.

Meleca, R. J., Hogikyan, N. D., & Bastian, R. W. (1997). A comparison of methods of botulinum toxin injection for abductor spasmodic dysphonia. *Otolaryngology–Head and Neck Surgery, 117,* 487–492.

Miller, R. G., Rosenberg, J. A., Gelinas, D. F., Mitsumoto, H., Newman, D., Sufit, R., et al. (1999). Practice parameter: The care of the patient with amyotrophic lateral sclerosis (an evidence-based review). *Neurology, 52,* 1311–1325.

Miller, R. H., Woodson, G. E., & Jankovic, J. (1987). Treatment options for spasmodic dysphonia. *Otolaryngology Clinics of North America, 24,* 1227–1237.

Mullen, R. (2005, August 16). Evidence-based practice planning addresses member needs, skills. *The ASHA Leader*. Retrieved from http://www.asha.org/Publications/leader/2005/050816/050816b.htm

Mullen, R. (2007, March 6). The state of the evidence. *The ASHA Leader*. Retrieved from http://www.asha.org/Publications/leader/2007/070306/f070306b/

Mullen, R. (n.d.). The N-CEP compendium of clinical practice guidelines and systematic reviews. Retrieved from http://www.asha.org/members/ebp/compendium/N-CEP-background.htm

National Commission for the Protection of Human Subjects of Biomedical and Behavioral Research. (1979). *The Belmont report*. Retrieved from http://www.hhs.gov/ohrp/humansubjects/guidance/belmont.html

Office of Technology Assessment. (1978). *Assessing the efficacy and safety of medical technologies* (OTA-H-75). Washington, DC: U.S. Government Printing Office.

Oxman, A. (2009). *Making judgments about the quality of evidence.* GRADE and SIGN: A discussion of grading systems. Retrieved from http://www.sign.ac.uk/pdf/gradeao.pdf

Pagana, K. D., & Pagana, T. J. (Eds.). (2002). *Mosby's manual of diagnostic and laboratory tests* (2nd ed.). St. Louis, MO: Mosby.

Riegelman, R. K. (2005). *Studying a study and testing a test* (5th ed.). Philadelphia, PA: Lippincott, Williams & Wilkins.

Robey, R. R. (1998). A meta-analysis of clinical outcomes in the treatment of aphasia. *Journal of Speech, Language, and Hearing Research, 41,* 172–187.

Robey, R. R. (2004). Reporting point and interval estimates of effect-size for planned contrasts: Fixed within effect analyses of variance. *Journal of Fluency Disorders, 29,* 307–341.

Robey, R. R., & Schultz, M. C. (1998). A model of conducting clinical-outcome research: An adaptation of the standard protocol for use in aphasiology (review). *Aphasiology, 12,* 787–810.

Rogers, M. A. (2011). *What are the phases of intervention research?* Retrieved from http://www.asha.org/academic/questions/PhasesClinicalResearch/

Sackett, D. L., Straus, S. E., Richardson, W. S., & Haynes, R. B. (2000). *Evidence-based medicine: How to practice and teach EBM* (2nd ed.). New York, NY: Churchill Livingstone.

Schlosser, R. W. (2009). The role of single-subject experimental designs in evidence-based practice time. *Focus: Technical Brief No. 22,* unnumbered.

Schlosser, R. W., & Sigafoos, J. (2008). Meta-analysis of single-subject experimental designs: Why now? *Evidence-Based Communication Assessment and Intervention, 2*(3), 117–119.

Shadish, W. R., Rindskopf, D. M., & Hedges, L. V. (2008). The state of the science in the meta-analysis of single-case experimental designs. *Evidence-Based Communication Assessment and Intervention, 2*(3), 188–196.

Translational research. (2011). NIH Common Fund, Division of Program Coordination, Planning, and Strategic Initiatives. Retrieved from http://commonfund.nih.gov/clinicalresearch/overview-translational.aspx

Wertz, R. T., & Irwin, W. (2001). Darley and the efficacy of language rehabilitation in aphasia. *Aphasiology, 15,* 231–247.

Wheeler-Hegland, K., Frymark, T., Schooling, T., McCabe, D., Ashford, J., Mullen, R., Smith Hammond, C., et al. (2009). Evidence-based systematic review: Oropharyngeal dysphagia behavioral treatments. Part I—Background and methodology. *Journal of Rehabilitation, Research and Development 46*(2), 175–184.

Wilkinson, L., & American Psychological Association Task Force on Statistical Inference. (1999). Statistical methods in psychology journals: Guidelines and explanations. *American Psychologist, 54,* 594–604.

Yorkston, K. M., Spencer, K., Duffy, J., Beukelman, D., Golper, L. A., Miller, R., Strand, E., et al. (2001). Evidence-based practice guidelines: An application to the field of speech-language pathology. *Journal of Medical Speech-Language Pathology, 4,* 243–256.

RESOURCES

Edlund, W., Gronseth, G., So, Y., Franklin, G., & American Academy of Neurology. (2004). *Clinical practice guideline process manual.* Retrieved from http://www.aan.com/professionals/practice/pdfs/2004_Guideline_Process.pdf

Guyatt, G., Rennie, D., Meade, M., & Cook, D. (2008). *Users' guides to the medical literature: Essentials of evidence-based clinical practice.* New York, NY: McGraw Hill Professional.

Liberati, A., Altman, D. G., Tetzlaff, J., Mulrow, C., Gotzsche, P. C., Ioannidis, J. P., Clarke, M., et al. (2009). The PRISMA statement for reporting systematic reviews and meta-analyses of studies that evaluate health care interventions: Explanation and elaboration. *Journal of Clinical Epidemiology, 62*(10), e1–34.

Internet Sources

Academy of Neurologic Communication Disorders and Sciences
http://www.ancds.org

Agency for Healthcare Research and Quality (AHRQ)
http://www.ahrq.gov

American Speech-Language-Hearing Association (ASHA)
http://www.asha.org/research/

Center for Reviews and Dissemination
http://www.york.ac.uk/inst/crd/report4.htm

ClinicalTrials.gov, National Institutes of Health
http://clinicaltrials.gov

Cochrane Collaboration
http://www.cochrane.org

National Center for the Dissemination of Disability Research
http://www.ncddr.org/

National Guideline Clearinghouse
http://www.guideline.gov

Oxford Centre for Evidence-Based Medicine Levels of Evidence
http://www.cebm.net/toolbox.asp

PubMed, U.S. National Library of Medicine, National Institutes of Health
http://www.pubmed.gov

Scottish Intercollegiate Guideline Network
http://www.sign.ac.uk

Index

A

B

C

D

E

F

I

M

N

O

R

S

U

V

W